Worldmark Global Health and Medicine Issues

Worldmark Global Health and Medicine Issues

VOLUME 1

A–M

Brenda Wilmoth Lerner & K. Lee Lerner, Editors

GALE
CENGAGE Learning·

Farmington Hills, Mich • San Francisco • New York • Waterville, Maine
Meriden, Conn • Mason, Ohio • Chicago

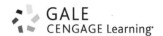

Worldmark Global Health and Medicine Issues

K. Lee Lerner and Brenda Wilmoth Lerner, Editors

Project Editor: Elizabeth P. Manar

Acquisition Editor: Michele P. LaMeau

Editorial: Kathleen J. Edgar, Jacqueline Longe, Rebecca Parks

Rights Acquisition and Management: Moriam Aigoro, Ashley M. Maynard

Imaging: John L. Watkins

Product Design: Kristine A. Julien

Composition: Evi Abou-El-Seoud

Manufacturing: Wendy Blurton

New Products Manager: Douglas A. Dentino

Cover photographs: Image of pollution © Kairos69/Shutterstock.com; Image of world map © PHOTOCREO Michal Bednarek/Shutterstock.com; Image of hand washing © africa924/Shutterstock.com; and Image of scientist in laboratory © A and N photography/Shutterstock.com.

Inside art: Image of DNA strands © vitstudio/Shutterstock.com

While every effort has been made to ensure the reliability of the information presented in this publication, Gale, a part of Cengage Learning, does not guarantee the accuracy of the data contained herein. Gale accepts no payment for listing; and inclusion in the publication of any organization, agency, institution, publication, service, or individual does not imply endorsement of the editors or publisher. Errors brought to the attention of the publisher and verified to the satisfaction of the publisher will be corrected in future editions.

LIBRARY OF CONGRESS CATALOGING-IN-PUBLICATION DATA

Worldmark global health and medicine issues / K. Lee Lerner & Brenda Wilmoth Lerner, editors.
　　p. ; cm.
　　Includes bibliographical references and index.
　　ISBN 978-1-4103-1752-0 (set : alk. paper) — ISBN 978-1-4103-1753-7 (v. 1 : alk. paper) — ISBN 978-1-4103-1754-4 (v. 2 : alk. paper) — ISBN 978-1-4103-1755-1 (e-book)
I. Lerner, K. Lee, editor.　II. Lerner, Brenda Wilmoth, editor.
　　[DNLM: 1. Global Health—Encyclopedias—English.　2. Disease—Encyclopedias—English.　3. International Agencies—Encyclopedias—English.　WB 13]
　　RC81.A2
　　616.003—dc23
　　　　　　　　　　　　　　　　　　　　　　　　　　　　2015010922

Gale
27500 Drake Rd.
Farmington Hills, MI 48331-3535

978-1-4103-1752-0 (set)
978-1-4103-1753-7 (vol. 1)
978-1-4103-1754-4 (vol. 2)

This title is also available as an e-book.
ISBN-13: 978-1-4103-1755-1
Contact your Gale sales representative for ordering information.

Printed in China
1 2 3 4 5 6 7 19 18 17 16 15

Table of Contents

VOLUME 2: N-Z

Introduction

Many of the great successes in public health and medicine also serve as important social milestones for humanity, especially with regard to the prevention and treatment of disease. While civic sanitation, water purification, immunization, and antibiotics have dramatically reduced the overall morbidity and the mortality of disease in advanced nations, much of the world is still ravaged by disease and epidemics, and new threats—including lifestyle diseases—constantly appear to challenge the most advanced medical and public health systems.

A collection of 90 entries on topics covering current global health issues, *Worldmark Global Health and Medicine Issues* is devoted to helping students and general readers quickly grasp the essence and complexities of often quickly-evolving global health issues.

At its core, *Worldmark Global Health and Medicine Issues* contains accessible explanations of many recent scientific advances in public health, as well as advances in medicine, molecular biology, genetics, epidemiology, and related fields.

Another key and distinguishing feature of *Worldmark Global Health and Medicine Issues* is an attempt to articulate links between science and social facets of global health issues. Health and medicine issues cannot be distantly cast from their intimate influence over daily life, economic impacts, and social context. Accordingly, a focus of *Worldmark Global Health and Medicine Issues* is the identification of the social determinants of health.

Global health issues can also arouse passionate debate as to effective and appropriate solutions. By illuminating global health issues as a nexus of science, ethics, economics, and policy, *Worldmark Global Health and Medicine Issues* serves both scientists and nonscientists searching to formulate rational opinions on an array of issues. In turn, issues that were once purely social or ethical issues (such as sexuality or alcoholism) are explained as aspects of human behavior and personality determined or influenced by genetics.

Worldmark Global Health and Medicine Issues also attempts to capture the increasing influence of wellness and preventative health measures in responding to public health issues.

The pace of change in facets of global health issues dealing with emerging diseases is daunting, and it is inevitable that as soon as this book went to press, some new threat emerged or some exiting threat reasserted its peril. For this reason, *Worldmark Global Health and Medicine Issues* attempts to lay a broader foundation supporting an understanding of how scientists detect novel diseases and how policy makers have responded to such challenges in the past.

Social and political issues can still arise out of even the most effective and seemingly well-intended of medical advances. For example, although childhood diseases such as measles, mumps, whooping cough, and diphtheria have been effectively controlled by childhood vaccinations, some parents resist or reject vaccinating their own children because they feel that the small personal risk is not mitigated by the larger social benefit of disease control. By opting out of the system (by relying on the immunizations of others to reduce the risk of disease), they simultaneously leave their own children vulnerable while lowering protection for some of most immunologically vulnerable members of their community (infants and immunocompromised individuals).

The interplay of complex ethical and social considerations is also evident when considering the general rise of infectious diseases that sometimes occurs as an unintended side effect of the otherwise beneficial use of medications. Nearly half the world's population, for example, is infected with the bacterium that causes tuberculosis, or TB (although for most people the infection is inactive), yet the organism causing some new cases of TB is evolving toward a greater resistance to the antibiotics that were once effective in treating TB. Such statistics take on added social dimension when considering that TB disproportionately impacts certain social groups, such as the elderly, minority groups, and people infected with HIV.

In an age of globalization, our common biology and biochemistry unite us across culture and geography, but also make us susceptible to contracting and transmitting infectious disease. Increased contact between societies raises new biomedical concerns about the potential spread of disease and sparks social debate regarding the nature and extent of medical cooperation across a varied political landscape. A shrinking global village, beneficial in many cultural and economic aspects, also increases the possibility that the terrible loss of life associated with the plagues of the Middle Ages or with the pandemic influenza outbreak of 1918–1919 might once again threaten humanity on a worldwide scale. Often ominous social and political implications of global health issues cannot be ignored when death continues to cast a disproportionately longer shadow over the poorest nations.

Although specific diseases may be statistically associated with particular regions or other demographics, disease does not recognize social class or political boundary. In our intimately connected world, an outbreak of disease in a remote area may quickly transform into a global threat. Given the opportunity, the agents of disease may spread at the speed of modern travel, and also leap from animals to humans.

Contributors to *Worldmark Global Health and Medicine Issues* include an array of experienced scientists and journalists with expertise in global health issues and a real-world appreciation for the proper context in which issues must be framed.

Brenda Wilmoth Lerner & K. Lee Lerner, Editors
Cambridge, Massachusetts
2015

Organization

All entries in *Worldmark Global Health and Medicine Issues* share a common structure, providing consistent coverage of topics and a simple way of comparing basic elements of one topic with another. Each entry has six parts: introduction, historical background, impacts and issues, future implications, bibliography, and a sidebar, which discusses a related topic, such as an important organization or concept. Some entries also contain an excerpt from a relevant historical text or contemporary article illustrating the topic. The entries are organized A to Z.

Worldmark Global Health and Medicine Issues contains other elements to help guide students studying these topics. It includes a chronology of important historical events; a general bibliography on health and medicine resources; a glossary of important terms in the field; a list of organizations and advocacy groups; about 80 line art images, such as tables and charts, that illustrate various aspects of health and medicine issues; and more than 200 full-color photographs related to the entry topics. Coverage of specific health and medicine subjects can be located in the general index.

Suggestions Welcome

Comments on *Worldmark Global Health and Medicine Issues* are cordially invited. Please write:

The Editors

Worldmark Global Health and Medicine Issues

Gale

27500 Drake Rd.

Farmington Hills, Michigan 48331-3535

Gale, a part of Cengage Learning, does not endorse any of the organizations, products, or methods mentioned in this title.

The websites appearing in *Worldmark Global Health and Medicine Issues* have been reviewed by Gale to provide additional information. Gale is not responsible for the content or operations policies of these websites. Further, Gale is not responsible for the conduct of website providers who offer electronic texts that may infringe on the legal right of copyright holders.

Using Primary Sources

Many of the entries in *Worldmark Global Health and Medicine Issues* contain documents written by or transcribed from (in the case of interviews and speeches) key players in the field covered in the entry. These documents, formally known as *primary sources*, provide insight into the historical setting during which they were produced and offer direct, firsthand witness to the events of their day or thoughts of important people in a particular activity or field. Primary sources come from a wide spectrum of resources, and the definition of what constitutes a primary source depends a great deal on the course of study or the institution of higher learning offering the definition. For the purposes of *Worldmark Global Health and Medicine Issues*, categories of primary sources include:

- Documents containing firsthand accounts of historic events by witnesses and participants. This category includes diaries, journal entries, and blogs; letters and e-mails; newspaper articles; interviews and oral histories; memoirs and autobiographies; and testimony in legal proceedings.

- Documents or works representing the official views of both government leaders and leaders of other organizations. These include policy statements, speeches, interviews, press releases, government reports, and legislation.

- Works of art, including (but not limited to) photographs, poems, and songs, as well as advertisements and reviews of those works that help establish an understanding of the cultural environment with regard to attitudes and perceptions of events.

- Secondary and tertiary sources. In some cases, secondary or tertiary sources may be considered primary sources. For example, a work written many years after an event or to summarize the event that includes quotes, recollections, or retrospectives by participants in the earlier event.

Analysis of Primary Sources

The primary material in *Worldmark Global Health and Medicine Issues* is intended to generate interest and lay a foundation for further inquiry and study.

In order to analyze a primary source properly, readers should remain skeptical and develop probing questions about the source. Using historical documents requires that readers analyze them carefully and extract specific information. However, readers must also read "beyond the text" to garner larger clues about the social impact of the primary source.

In addition to providing information about the topics, primary sources may also supply a wealth of insight into their creator's viewpoint. For example, when reading a news article about an event, consider whether the reporter's words also indicate something about his or her origin, bias, prejudices, or intended audience.

It is important to view the primary source within the historical and social context existing at its creation. Readers should remember that primary sources may contain information later proven to be false or viewpoints and terms unacceptable to future generations. If, for example, a newspaper article is written within hours or days of an event, later developments may reveal some assertions in the original article as false or misleading.

Test Conclusions and Ideas

It is critical to test whatever opinion or working hypothesis you, the reader, form from reading the primary source(s) against other facts and sources related to the incident. For example, it might be wrong to conclude that factual mistakes are deliberate unless evidence can be produced of a pattern and practice of such mistakes with an intent to promote a false idea.

Despite the fact that some primary sources can contain false information or lead readers to false conclusions based on the facts presented, they remain an invaluable resource regarding past events. Primary sources allow readers and researchers to come as close as possible to understanding the perceptions and context of events and thus to more fully appreciate how and why misconceptions occur.

Glossary of Terms

A

ACQUIRED (ADAPTIVE) IMMUNITY: Immunity is the ability to resist infection and is subdivided into innate immunity, with which an individual is born, and acquired, or adaptive, immunity, which develops according to circumstances and is targeted to a specific pathogen. There are two types of acquired immunity, known as active and passive. Active immunity is either humoral, involving production of antibody molecules against a bacterium or virus, or cell-mediated, in which T-cells are mobilized against infected cells. Infection and immunization can both induce acquired immunity. Passive immunity is induced by injection of the serum of a person who is already immune to a particular infection.

ACQUIRED IMMUNE DEFICIENCY SYNDROME (AIDS): A disease of the immune system caused by the human immunodeficiency virus (HIV). It is characterized by the destruction of a particular type of white blood cell and increased susceptibility to infection and other diseases.

ACTIVE INFECTION: An active infection is one that is currently producing symptoms or in which the infective agent is multiplying rapidly. In contrast, a latent infection is one in which the infective agent is present but not causing symptoms or damage to the body nor reproducing at a significant rate.

ADAPTIVE IMMUNITY: Adaptive immunity is another term for acquired immunity, referring to the resistance to infection that develops through life and is targeted to a specific pathogen. There are two types of adaptive immunity, known as active and passive. Active immunity is either humoral, involving production of antibody molecules against a bacterium or virus, or cell-mediated, in which T-cells are mobilized against infected cells. Infection and immunization can

both induce acquired immunity. Passive immunity is induced by the transfer of antibodies from one person to another, and occurs when antibodies in blood products from a person who is immune to a particular disease are injected into a susceptible person.

AIDS (ACQUIRED IMMUNE DEFICIENCY SYNDROME): A disease of the immune system caused by the human immunodeficiency virus (HIV). It is characterized by the destruction of a particular type of white blood cell and increased susceptibility to infection and other diseases.

AIRBORNE PRECAUTIONS: Airborne precautions are procedures that are designed to reduce the chance that certain disease-causing (pathogenic) microorganisms will be transmitted through the air.

AIRBORNE TRANSMISSION: Airborne transmission refers to the ability of a disease-causing (pathogenic) microorganism to be spread through the air by droplets expelled during sneezing or coughing.

ALLELE: Any of two or more alternative forms of a gene that occupy the same location on a chromosome.

ALLERGIES: An allergy is an excessive or hypersensitive response of the immune system to substances (allergens) in the environment. Instead of fighting off a disease-causing foreign substance, the immune system launches a complex series of actions against the particular irritating allergen. The immune response may be accompanied by a number of stressful symptoms, ranging from mild to life threatening. In rare cases, an allergic reaction leads to anaphylactic shock—a condition characterized by a sudden drop in blood pressure, difficulty in breathing, skin irritation, collapse, and possible death.

AMEBIC DYSENTERY: Amebic (or amoebic) dysentery, which is also referred to as amebiasis or amoebiasis, is an inflammation of the intestine caused by the parasite *Entamoeba histolytica*. The severe form of the malady is characterized by the formation of localized lesions (ulcers) in the intestine, especially in the colon; abscesses in the liver and the brain; vomiting; severe diarrhea with fluid loss leading to dehydration; and abdominal pain.

ANAEROBIC BACTERIA: Bacteria that grow without oxygen, also called anaerobic bacteria or anaerobes. Anaerobic bacteria can infect deep wounds, deep tissues, and internal organs where there is little oxygen. These infections are characterized by abscess formation, foul-smelling pus, and tissue destruction.

ANTHRAX: Anthrax refers to a disease that is caused by the bacterium *Bacillus anthracis*. The bacterium can enter the body via a wound in the skin (cutaneous anthrax), via contaminated food or liquid (gastrointestinal anthrax), or can be inhaled (inhalation anthrax).

ANTIBACTERIAL: A substance that reduces the number of or kills germs (bacteria and other microorganisms but not viruses). Also often a term used to describe a drug used to treat bacterial infections.

ANTIBIOTIC: A drug, such as penicillin, used to fight infections caused by bacteria. Antibiotics act only on bacteria and are not effective against viruses.

ANTIBIOTIC RESISTANCE: The ability of bacteria to resist the actions of antibiotic drugs.

ANTIBIOTIC SENSITIVITY: Antibiotic sensitivity refers to the susceptibility of a bacterium to an antibiotic. Each type of bacteria can be killed by some types of antibiotics and not be affected by other types. Different types of bacteria exhibit different patterns of antibiotic sensitivity.

ANTIBODIES: Antibodies, or Y-shaped immunoglobulins, are proteins found in the blood that help to fight against foreign substances called antigens. Antigens, which are usually proteins or polysaccharides, stimulate the immune system to produce antibodies. The antibodies inactivate the antigen and help to remove it from the body. While antigens can be the source of infections from pathogenic bacteria and viruses, organic molecules detrimental to the body from internal or environmental sources also act as antigens. Genetic engineering and the use of various mutational mechanisms allow the construction of a vast array of antibodies (each with a unique genetic sequence).

ANTIGEN: Antigens, which are usually proteins or polysaccharides, stimulate the immune system to produce antibodies. The antibodies inactivate the antigen and help to remove it from the body. While antigens can be the source of infections from pathogenic bacteria and viruses, organic molecules detrimental to the body from internal or environmental sources also act as antigens. Genetic engineering and the use of various mutational mechanisms allow the construction of a vast array of antibodies (each with a unique genetic sequence).

ANTIHELMINTHIC: Antihelminthic drugs are medicines that rid the body of helminths (parasitic worms).

ANTIMICROBIAL: An antimicrobial material slows the growth of bacteria or is able to kill bacteria. Antimicrobial materials include antibiotics (which can be used inside the body) and disinfectants (which can only be used outside the body).

ANTIRETROVIRAL THERAPY (ART): Antiretroviral treatment (ART) with antiretroviral (ARV) drugs prevents the reproduction of a type of virus called a retrovirus. The human immunodeficiency virus (HIV), which causes acquired immune deficiency syndrome (AIDS, also known as acquired immunodeficiency syndrome), is a retrovirus. ARV drugs are therefore used to treat HIV infections. These medicines cannot prevent or cure HIV infection, but they help to keep the virus in check.

ANTISEPTIC: A substance that prevents or stops the growth and multiplication of microorganisms in or on living tissue.

ANTITOXIN: An antidote to a toxin that neutralizes its poisonous effects.

ANTIVIRAL DRUGS: Antiviral drugs are compounds that are used to prevent or treat viral infections, via the disruption of an infectious mechanism used by the virus, or to treat the symptoms of an infection.

ARBOVIRUS: An arbovirus is a virus that is typically spread by blood-sucking insects, most commonly mosquitoes. Over 100 types of arboviruses cause disease in humans. Yellow fever and dengue fever are two examples.

ARENAVIRUS: An arenavirus is a virus that belongs in a viral family known as *Arenaviridae*. The name arenavirus derives from the appearance of the spherical virus particles when cut into thin sections and viewed using a transmission electron microscope. The interior of the particles is grainy or sandy in appearance, due to the presence of ribosomes that have been acquired from the host cell. The Latin designation *arena* means "sandy."

ARTHROPOD-BORNE VIRUS: A virus caused by one of a phylum of organisms characterized by exoskeletons and segmented bodies, such as insects.

ASEPSIS: Asepsis means without germs, more specifically without microorganisms.

ASYMPTOMATIC: A state in which an individual does not exhibit or experience symptoms of a disease.

ATROPHY: Decreasing in size or wasting away of a body part or tissue.

ATTENUATED: An attenuated bacterium or virus has been weakened and is often used as the basis of a vaccine against the specific disease caused by the bacterium or virus.

ATTENUATED STRAIN: A specific strain of bacteria that has been killed or weakened, often used as the basis of a vaccine against the specific disease caused by the bacterium.

AUTOIMMUNE DISEASE: A disease in which the body's defense system attacks its own tissues and organs.

AUTOINFECTION: Autoinfection is the reinfection of the body by a disease organism already in the body, such as eggs left by a parasitic worm.

B

BACTERIA: Single-celled microorganisms that live in soil, water, plants, and animals. Their activities range from the development of disease to fermentation. They play a key role in the decay of organic matter and the cycling of nutrients. Bacteria exist in various shapes, including spherical, rod-shaped, and spiral. Some bacteria are agents of disease. Different types of bacteria cause many sexually transmitted diseases, including syphilis, gonorrhea, and chlamydia. Bacteria also cause diseases such as typhoid, dysentery, and tetanus. Bacterium is the singular form of bacteria.

BACTERIOCIDAL: Bacteriocidal is a term that refers to the treatment of a bacterium such that the organism is killed. A bacteriocidal treatment is always lethal and is also referred to as sterilization.

BACTERIOLOGICAL STRAIN: A bacterial subclass of a particular tribe and genus.

BED NETS: A type of netting that provides protection from diseases caused by insects such as flies and mosquitoes. It is often used when sleeping to allow air to flow through its mesh structure while preventing insects from biting.

BIOINFORMATICS: Bioinformatics, or computational biology, refers to the development of new database methods to store genomic information (information related to genes and the genetic sequence), computational software programs, and methods to extract, process, and evaluate this information. Bioinformatics also refers to the refinement of existing techniques to acquire the genomic data. Finding genes and determining their function, predicting the structure of proteins and sequence of ribonucleic acid (RNA) from the available sequence of deoxyribonucleic acid (DNA), and determining the evolutionary relationship of proteins and DNA sequences are aspects of bioinformatics.

BIOLOGICAL WEAPON: A weapon that contains or disperses a biological toxin, disease-causing microorganism, or other biological agent intended to harm or kill plants, animals, or humans.

BIOSAFETY LEVEL 4 FACILITY: A specialized biosafety laboratory that deals with dangerous or exotic infectious agents or biohazards that are considered high risks for spreading life-threatening diseases, either because the disease is spread through aerosols or because there is no therapy or vaccine to counter the disease.

BIOTECHNOLOGY: Use of biological organisms, systems, or processes to make or modify products.

BLOOD-BORNE PATHOGENS: Disease-causing agents carried or transported in the blood. Blood-borne infections are those in which the infectious agent is transmitted from one person to another via contaminated blood.

BLOOD-BORNE ROUTE: Via the blood. For example, blood-borne pathogens are pathogens (disease-causing agents) carried or transported in the blood. Bloodborne infections are those in which the infectious agent is transmitted from one person to another via contaminated blood. Infections of the blood can occur as a result of the spread of an ongoing infection caused by bacteria such as *Yersinia pestis*, *Haemophilus influenzae*, or *Staphylococcus aureus*.

BOTULINUM TOXIN: Botulinum toxin is among the most poisonous substances known. The toxin, which can be ingested or inhaled, and which disrupts transmission of nerve impulses to muscles, is naturally produced by the bacterium *Clostridium botulinum*. Certain strains of *C. baratii* and *C. butyricum* can also be capable of producing the toxin.

BOTULISM: Botulism is an illness generally produced by a toxin that is released by the soil bacterium *Clostridium botulinum*. Some strains of *C. baratii* and *C. butyricum* produce the toxin, as well. The toxins affect nerves and can produce paralysis. The paralysis can affect the functioning of organs and tissues that are vital to life.

BROAD-SPECTRUM ANTIBIOTICS: Broad-spectrum antibiotics are drugs that kill a wide range of bacteria rather than just those from a specific family. For example, amoxicillin is a broad-spectrum antibiotic that is used against many common illnesses such as ear infections, pneumonia, and urinary tract infections.

C

CAMPYLOBACTERIOSIS: Campylobacteriosis is a bacterial infection of the intestinal tract of humans. The infection, which typically results in diarrhea, is caused by members of the genus *Campylobacter*. Worldwide, approximately 5 to 14 percent of all diarrhea may be the result of campylobacteriosis.

CARBOLIC ACID: An acidic compound that, when diluted with water, is used as an antiseptic and disinfectant.

CARCINOGEN: A carcinogen is any biological, chemical, or physical substance or agent that can cause cancer. There are over 100 different types of cancer, which can be distinguished by the type of cell or organ that is affected, the treatment plan employed, and the cause of the cancer. Most of the carcinogens that are commonly discussed come from chemical sources artificially produced by humans. Some of the better-known carcinogens are the pesticide DDT (dichlorodiphenyltrichloroethane), asbestos, and the carcinogens produced when tobacco is smoked.

CASE FATALITY RATE: The rate of patients suffering disease or injury that die as a result of that disease or injury during a specific period of time.

CASE FATALITY RATIO: A ratio indicating the amount of persons who die as a result of a particular disease, usually expressed as a percentage or as the number of deaths per 1,000 cases.

CATALYST: Substance that speeds up a chemical process without actually changing the products of reaction.

CD4 T CELLS: CD4 cells are a type of T cell found in the immune system that are characterized by the presence of a CD4 antigen protein on their surface. These are the cells most often destroyed as a result of HIV infection.

CENTERS FOR DISEASE CONTROL AND PREVENTION (CDC): The Centers for Disease Control and Prevention (CDC) is one of the primary public health institutions in the world. The CDC is headquartered in Atlanta, Georgia, with facilities at nine other sites in the United States. The centers are the focus of U.S. government efforts to develop and implement prevention and control strategies for diseases, including those of microbiological origin.

CESTODE: A class of worms characterized by flat, segmented bodies, commonly known as tapeworms.

CHAGAS DISEASE: Chagas disease is a human infection that is caused by a microorganism that establishes a parasitic relationship with a human host as part of its life cycle. The disease is named for the Brazilian physician Carlos Chagas, who in 1909 described the involvement of the flagellated protozoan known as *Trypanosoma cruzi* in a prevalent disease in South America.

CHAIN OF TRANSMISSION: Chain of transmission refers to the route by which an infection is spread from its source to a susceptible host. An example of a chain of transmission is the spread of malaria from an infected animal to humans via mosquitoes.

CHILDBED FEVER: Childbed fever, also known as puerperal infection or postpartum infection, is a bacterial infection occurring in women following childbirth, causing fever and in some cases blood poisoning and possible death.

CHRONIC INFECTION: A chronic infection persists for a prolonged period of time—months or even years—in the host. This lengthy persistence is due to a number of factors, which can include masking of the disease-causing agent (e.g., bacteria) from the immune system, invasion of host cells, and the establishment of an infection that is resistant to antibacterial agents.

CIRRHOSIS: Cirrhosis is a chronic, degenerative, irreversible liver disease in which normal liver cells are damaged and are then replaced by scar tissue. Cirrhosis changes the structure of the liver and the blood vessels that nourish it. The disease reduces the liver's ability to manufacture proteins and process hormones, nutrients, medications, and poisons.

CLINICAL TRIALS: According to the U.S. National Institutes of Health, a clinical trial is "a research study to answer specific questions about vaccines or new therapies or new ways of using known treatments." These studies allow researchers to determine whether new drugs or treatments are safe and effective. When conducted carefully, clinical trials can provide fast and safe answers to these questions.

CLUSTER: In epidemiology, cluster refers to a grouping of individuals contracting an infectious disease or food-borne illness very close in time or place.

COHORT: A cohort is a group of people (or any species) sharing a common characteristic. Cohorts are identified and grouped in cohort studies to determine the frequency of diseases or the kinds of disease outcomes over time.

COHORTING: Cohorting is the practice of grouping persons with similar infections or symptoms together, sometimes in order to reduce transmission of infection to others.

COMMUNITY-ACQUIRED INFECTION: Community-acquired infection is an infection that develops outside of a hospital, in the general community. It differs from hospital-acquired infections in that those who are infected are typically in better health than hospitalized people.

CONTACT PRECAUTIONS: Contact precautions are actions developed to minimize the transfer of microorganisms directly by physical contact and indirectly by touching a contaminated surface.

CONTAGIOUS: A disease that is easily spread among a population, usually by casual person-to-person contact.

CONTAMINATED: The unwanted presence of a microorganism or compound in a particular environment. That environment can be in the laboratory setting, for example, in a medium being used for the growth of a species of bacteria during an experiment. Another environment can be the human body, where contamination by bacteria can produce an infection. Contamination by bacteria and viruses can occur on several levels, and their presence can adversely influence the results of experiments. Outside the laboratory, bacteria and viruses can contaminate drinking water supplies, foodstuffs, and other products, thus causing illness.

CREUTZFELDT-JAKOB DISEASE (CJD): Creutzfeldt-Jakob disease (CJD) is a transmissible, rapidly progressing, fatal neurodegenerative disorder related to bovine spongiform encephalopathy (BSE), commonly called mad cow disease.

CULL: A cull is the selection, often for destruction, of a part of an animal population. Often done just to reduce numbers, a widespread cull was carried out during the epidemic of bovine spongiform encephalopathy (BSE or mad cow disease) in the United Kingdom during the 1980s and has also been carried out in bird populations during outbreaks of avian influenza.

CULTURE: A culture is a single species of microorganism that is isolated and grown under controlled conditions. The German bacteriologist Robert Koch first developed culturing techniques in the late 1870s. Following Koch's initial use of cultures, medical scientists quickly sought to identify other pathogens using such techniques. Today bacterial cultures are used as basic tools in microbiology and medicine.

CULTURE AND SENSITIVITY: Culture and sensitivity refer to laboratory tests that are used to identify the type of microorganism causing an infection and the compounds to which the identified organism is sensitive and resistant. In the case of bacteria, this approach permits the selection of antibiotics that will be most effective in dealing with the infection.

CUTANEOUS: Pertaining to the skin.

CYST: Refers to either a closed cavity or sac or the stage of life during which some parasites live inside an enclosed area. In a protozoan's life, it is a stage when it is covered by a tough outer shell and has become dormant.

CYTOKINE: Cytokines are a family of small proteins that mediate an organism's response to injury or infection. Cytokines operate by transmitting signals between cells in an organism. Minute quantities of cytokines are secreted, each by a single cell type, and regulate functions in other cells by binding with specific receptors. Their interactions with the receptors produce secondary signals that inhibit or enhance the action of certain genes within the cell. Unlike endocrine hormones, which can act throughout the body, most cytokines act locally near the cells that produced them.

D

DEFINITIVE HOST: The organism in which a parasite reaches reproductive maturity.

DEHYDRATION: Dehydration is the loss of water and salts essential for normal bodily function. It occurs when the body loses more fluid than it takes in. Water is very important to the human body because it makes up about 70 percent of the muscles, around 75 percent of the brain, and approximately 92 percent of the blood. A person who weighs about 150 pounds (68 kilograms) will contain about 80 quarts (just over 75 liters) of water. About two cups of water are lost each day just from regular breathing. If the body sweats more and breathes more heavily than normal, the human body loses even more water. Dehydration occurs when that lost water is not replenished.

DEMENTIA: Dementia, which is from the Latin word *dement* meaning "away mind," is a progressive deterioration and eventual loss of mental ability that is severe enough to interfere with normal activities of daily living; lasts more than six months; has not been present since birth; and is not associated with a loss or alteration of consciousness. Dementia is a group of symptoms caused by gradual death of brain cells.

Dementia is usually caused by degeneration in the cerebral cortex, the part of the brain responsible for thoughts, memories, actions, and personality. Death of brain cells in this region leads to the cognitive impairment that characterizes dementia.

DEMOGRAPHICS: The characteristics of human populations or specific parts of human populations, most often reported through statistics.

DEOXYRIBONUCLEIC ACID (DNA): Deoxyribonucleic acid (DNA) is a double-stranded, helical molecule that forms the molecular basis for heredity in most organisms.

DIAGNOSIS: Identification of a disease or disorder.

DIARRHEA: To most individuals, diarrhea means an increased frequency or decreased consistency of bowel movements; however, the medical definition is more exact than this explanation. In many developed countries, the average number of bowel movements is three per day. However, researchers have found that diarrhea, which is not a specific disease, best correlates with an increase in stool weight; a stool weight above 10.5 ounces (300 grams) per day generally indicates diarrhea. This is mainly due to excess water, which normally makes up 60 to 85 percent of fecal matter. In this way, true diarrhea is distinguished from diseases that cause only an increase in the number of bowel movements (hyperdefecation) or incontinence (involuntary loss of bowel contents). Diarrhea is also classified by physicians into acute, which lasts one to two weeks, and chronic, which continues for longer than four weeks. Viral and bacterial infections are the most common causes of acute diarrhea.

DIPHTHERIA: Diphtheria is a potentially fatal, contagious bacterial disease that usually involves the nose, throat, and air passages, but may also infect the skin. Its most striking feature is the formation of a grayish membrane covering the tonsils and upper part of the throat.

DISINFECTANT: Disinfection and the use of chemical disinfectants is one key strategy of infection control. Disinfectants reduce the number of living microorganisms, usually to a level that is considered to be safe for the particular environment. Typically, this entails the destruction of those microbes that are capable of causing disease.

DISSEMINATION: The spreading of a disease in a population, or of disease organisms in the body, is dissemination. A disease that occurs over a large geographic area.

DNA: Deoxyribonucleic acid, a double-stranded, helical molecule that is found in almost all living cells and that determines the characteristics of each organism.

DNA FINGERPRINTING: DNA fingerprinting is the term applied to a range of techniques that are used to show similarities and dissimilarities between the DNA present in different individuals (or organisms).

DROPLET: A droplet is a small airborne drop or particle—less than 5 microns (a millionth of a meter) in diameter—of fluid, such as may be expelled by sneezing or coughing.

DROPLET TRANSMISSION: Droplet transmission is the spread of microorganisms from one space to another (including from person to person) via droplets that are less than 5 microns in diameter. Droplets are typically expelled into the air by coughing and sneezing.

DRUG RESISTANCE: Drug resistance develops when an infective agent, such as a bacterium, fungus, or virus, develops a lack of sensitivity to a drug that would normally be able to control or even kill it. This tends to occur with overuse of anti-infective agents, which selects out populations of microbes most able to resist them, while killing off those organisms that are most sensitive. The next time the anti-infective agent is used, it will be less effective, leading to the eventual development of resistance.

DYSENTERY: Dysentery is the inflammation of the intestines and resulting bloody diarrhea due to infection with the bacteria *Shigella* or the amoeba *Entamoeba histolytica*. Both bacterial and amoebic dysentery are infectious and are still a major problem in developing countries with primitive sanitary facilities.

E

ELECTROLYTES: Compounds that ionize in a solution; electrolytes dissolved in the blood play an important role in maintaining the proper functioning of the body.

EMERGING DISEASE: New infectious diseases such as SARS and West Nile virus, as well as previously known diseases such as malaria, tuberculosis, and bacterial pneumonias that are appearing in forms resistant to drug treatments, are termed emerging infectious diseases.

ENDEMIC: Present in a particular area or among a particular group of people.

ENTERIC: Involving the intestinal tract or relating to the intestines.

ENTEROBACTERIAL INFECTIONS: Enterobacterial infections are caused by a group of bacteria that dwell in the intestinal tract of humans and other warm-blooded animals. The bacteria are all gram-negative and rod-shaped. As a group they are termed Enterobacteriaceae. A prominent member of this group is *Escherichia coli*.

ENTEROVIRUS: Enteroviruses are a group of viruses that contain ribonucleic acid (RNA) as their genetic material. They are members of the picornavirus family. The various types of enteroviruses that infect humans are referred to as serotypes, in recognition of their different antigenic patterns. The different immune response is important, as infection with one type of enterovirus does not necessarily confer protection to infection by a different type of enterovirus. The serotypes include polio viruses, coxsackie A and B viruses, echoviruses, and a large number of what are referred to as non-polio enteroviruses.

ENZYME: Enzymes are molecules that act as critical catalysts in biological systems. Catalysts are substances that increase the rate of chemical reactions without being consumed in the reaction. Without enzymes, many reactions would require higher levels of energy and higher temperatures than exist in biological systems. Enzymes are proteins that possess specific binding sites for other molecules (substrates). A series of weak binding interactions allows enzymes to accelerate reaction rates. Enzyme kinetics is the study of enzymatic reactions and mechanisms. Enzyme inhibitor studies have allowed researchers to develop therapies for the treatment of diseases, including AIDS.

EPIDEMIC: The word *epidemic* comes from the Greek word meaning prevalent among the people and is most commonly used to describe an outbreak of an illness or disease in which the number of individual cases significantly exceeds the usual or expected number of cases in any given population.

EPIDEMIOLOGY: Epidemiology is the study of the various factors that influence the occurrence, distribution, prevention, and control of disease, injury, and other health-related events in a defined human population. By the application of various analytical techniques, including mathematical analysis of the data, the probable cause of an infectious outbreak can be pinpointed.

EPSTEIN-BARR VIRUS (EBV): Epstein-Barr virus (EBV) is part of the family of human herpes viruses. Infectious mononucleosis (IM) is the most common disease manifestation of this virus, which, once established in the host, can never be completely eradicated. Very little can be done to treat EBV; most methods can only alleviate resultant symptoms.

ERADICATE: To get rid of; the permanent reduction to zero of global incidence of a particular infection.

ETIOLOGY: The study of the cause or origin of a disease or disorder.

EXECUTIVE ORDER: Presidential orders that implement or interpret a federal statute, administrative policy, or treaty.

EXOTOXIN: A toxic protein produced during bacterial growth and metabolism and released into the environment.

F

FECAL-ORAL TRANSMISSION: The spread of disease through the transmission of minute particles of fecal material from one organism to the mouth of another organism. This can occur by drinking contaminated water, eating food that was exposed to animal or human feces (perhaps by watering plants with unclean water), or by the poor hygiene practices of those preparing food.

FILOVIRUS: A filovirus is any RNA virus that belongs to the family *Filoviridae*. Filoviruses infect primates. Marburg virus and Ebola virus are filoviruses.

FLEA: A flea is any parasitic insect of the order *Siphonaptera*. Fleas can infest many mammals, including humans, and can act as carriers (vectors) of disease.

FLORA: In microbiology, flora refers to the collective microorganisms that normally inhabit an organism or system. Human intestines, for example, contain bacteria that aid in digestion and are considered normal flora.

FOCUS: In medicine, a focus is a primary center of some disease process (for example, a cluster of abnormal cells). Foci is plural for focus (more than one focus).

FOMITE: A fomite is an object or a surface to which infectious microorganisms such as bacteria or viruses can adhere and be transmitted. Papers, clothing, dishes, and other objects can all act as fomites. Transmission is often by touch.

FOOD PRESERVATION: The term food preservation refers to any one of a number of techniques used to prevent food from spoiling. It includes methods such as canning, pickling, drying and freeze-drying, irradiation, pasteurization, smoking, and the addition of chemical additives. Food preservation has become an increasingly important component of the food industry as fewer people eat foods produced on their own lands, and as consumers expect to be able to purchase and consume foods that are out of season.

FULMINANT: A fulminant infection is an infection that appears suddenly and the symptoms of which are immediately severe.

G

GAMETOCYTE: A germ cell with the ability to divide for the purpose of producing gametes, either male gametes called spermatocytes or female gametes called oocytes.

GAMMA GLOBULIN: Gamma globulin is a term referring to a group of soluble proteins in the blood, most of which are antibodies that can mount a direct attack upon pathogens and can be used to treat various infections.

GANGRENE: Gangrene is the destruction of body tissue by a bacteria called *Clostridium perfringens* or a combination of streptococci and staphylococci bacteria. *C. perfringens* is widespread; it is found in soil and the intestinal tracts of humans and animals. It becomes dangerous only when its spores germinate, producing toxins and destructive enzymes, and germination occurs only in an anaerobic environment (one almost totally devoid of oxygen). While gangrene can develop in any part of the body, it is most common in fingers, toes, hands, feet, arms, and legs, the parts of the body most susceptible to restricted blood flow. Even a slight injury in such an area is at high risk of causing gangrene. Early treatment with antibiotics, such as penicillin, and surgery to remove the dead tissue will often reduce the need for amputation. If left untreated, gangrene results in amputation or death.

GASTROENTERITIS: Gastroenteritis is an inflammation of the stomach and the intestines. More commonly, gastroenteritis is called the stomach flu.

GENE: A gene is the fundamental physical and functional unit of heredity. Whether in a microorganism or in a human cell, a gene is an individual element of an organism's genome and determines a trait or characteristic by regulating biochemical structure or metabolic process.

GENE THERAPY: Gene therapy is the name applied to the treatment of inherited diseases by corrective genetic engineering of the dysfunctional genes. It is part of a broader field called genetic medicine, which involves the screening, diagnosis, prevention, and treatment of hereditary conditions in humans. The results of genetic screening can pinpoint a potential problem to which gene therapy can sometimes offer a solution. Genetic defects are significant in the total field of medicine, with up to 15 out of every 100 newborn infants having a hereditary disorder of greater or lesser severity. More than 2,000 genetically distinct inherited defects have been classified so far, including diabetes, cystic fibrosis, hemophilia, sickle-cell anemia, phenylketonuria, and cancer.

GENETIC ENGINEERING: Genetic engineering is the altering of the genetic material of living cells in order to make them capable of producing new substances or performing new functions. When the genetic material within the living cells (i.e., genes) is working properly, the body can develop and function smoothly. However, should a single gene—even a tiny segment of a gene go awry—the effect can be dramatic: deformities, disease, and even death are possible.

GENOME: All of the genetic information for a cell or organism. The complete sequence of genes within a cell or virus.

GENOTYPE: The genetic information that a living thing inherits from its parents that affects its makeup, appearance, and function.

GEOGRAPHIC FOCALITY: The physical location of a disease pattern, epidemic, or outbreak; the characteristics of a location created by interconnections with other places.

GEOGRAPHIC INFORMATION SYSTEM (GIS): A system for archiving, retrieving, and manipulating data that has been stored and indexed according to the geographic coordinates of its elements. The system generally can utilize a variety of data types, such as imagery, maps, tables, etc.

GEOGRAPHIC MEDICINE: Geographic medicine, also called geomedicine, is the study of how human health is affected by climate and environment.

GERM THEORY OF DISEASE: The germ theory is a fundamental tenet of medicine that states that microorganisms, which are too small to be seen without the aid of a microscope, can invade the body and cause disease.

GLOBAL OUTBREAK ALERT AND RESPONSE NETWORK (GOARN): A collaboration of resources for the rapid identification, confirmation, and response to outbreaks of international importance.

GLOBALIZATION: The integration of national and local systems into a global economy through increased trade, manufacturing, communications, and migration.

H

HARM-REDUCTION STRATEGY: In public health, a harm-reduction strategy is a public-policy scheme for reducing the amount of harm caused by a substance such as alcohol or tobacco. The phrase may refer to any medical strategy directed at reducing the harm caused by a disease, substance, or toxic medication.

HELMINTHIC DISEASE: Helminths are parasitic worms such as hookworms or flatworms. Helminthic disease by such worms is infectious. A synonym for helminthic is verminous.

HELSINKI DECLARATION: A set of ethical principles governing medical and scientific experimentation on human subjects; it was drafted by the World Medical Association and originally adopted in 1964.

HEMOLYSIS: The destruction of blood cells, an abnormal rate of which may lead to lowered levels of these cells. For example, hemolytic anemia is caused by destruction of red blood cells at a rate faster than they can be produced.

HEMORRHAGE: Very severe, massive bleeding that is difficult to control.

HEMORRHAGIC FEVER: A hemorrhagic fever is caused by viral infection and features a high fever and copious (high volume of) bleeding. The bleeding is caused by the formation of tiny blood clots throughout the bloodstream. These blood clots—also called microthrombi—deplete platelets and fibrinogen in the bloodstream. When bleeding begins, the factors needed for the clotting of the blood are scarce. Thus, uncontrolled bleeding (hemorrhage) ensues.

HEPA FILTER: A HEPA (high efficiency particulate air) filter is a filter that is designed to nearly totally remove airborne particles that are 0.3 microns (millionth of a meter) in diameter or larger. Such small particles can penetrate deeply into the lungs if inhaled.

HEPADNAVIRUSES: *Hepadnaviridae* is a family of hepadnaviruses comprised by two genera, *Avihepadnavirus* and *Orthohepadnavirus*. Hepadnaviruses have partially double-stranded DNA, and they replicate their genome in the host cells using an enzyme called reverse transcriptase. Because of this, they are also termed retroviruses. The viruses invade liver cells (hepatocytes) of vertebrates. When hepadna retroviruses invade a cell, a complete viral double-stranded (ds) DNA is made before it randomly inserts into one of the hosta's chromosomes. Once part of the chromosomal DNA, the viral DNA is then transcribed into an intermediate messenger RNA (mRNA) in the host's nucleus. The viral mRNA then leaves the nucleus and undergoes reverse transcription, which is mediated by the viral reverse transcriptase.

HEPATITIS: Hepatitis is an inflammation of the liver, a potentially life-threatening disease most frequently caused by viral infections but which may also result from liver damage caused by toxic substances such as alcohol and certain drugs. There are five major types of viruses that cause hepatitis: hepatitis A (HAV), hepatitis B (HBV), hepatitis C (HCV), hepatitis D (HDV), and hepatitis E (HEV). Hepatitis G (HGV, also known as GB virus C) is also a potential cause.

HERD IMMUNITY: Herd immunity is a resistance to disease that occurs in a population when a large proportion of the population has been immunized against it. The theory is that it is less likely that an infectious disease will spread in a group in which many individuals are unlikely to contract it.

HERPESVIRUS: Herpesvirus is a family of viruses, many of which cause disease in humans. The herpes simplex type 1 and herpes simplex type 2 viruses cause infection in the mouth or on the genitals. Other common types of herpesvirus include chicken pox, Epstein-Barr virus, and cytomegalovirus. Herpesvirus is notable for its ability to remain latent, or inactive, in nerve cells near the area of infection, and to reactivate long after the initial infection. Herpes simplex types 1 and 2, along with chicken pox, cause skin sores. Epstein-Barr virus causes mononucleosis. Cytomegalovirus is also a herpesvirus infection. It usually does not cause symptoms, however it can be dangerous to the developing fetuses of pregnant women, the elderly, infants, and those with weakened immune systems.

HIGHLY ACTIVE ANTIRETROVIRAL THERAPY (HAART): Highly active antiretroviral therapy (HAART) is the name given to the combination of drugs used to treat people with human immunodeficiency virus (HIV) infection to slow or stop the progression of their condition to AIDS (acquired human immune deficiency syndrome). HIV is a retrovirus, and the various components of HAART block its replication by different mechanisms.

HISTOCOMPATIBILITY: The histocompatibility molecules (proteins) on the cell surfaces of one individual of a species are unique. Thus, if a cell from one person is transplanted into another person, the cell will be recognized by the immune system as being foreign. The histocompatibility molecules act as antigens in the recipient and so can also be called histocompatibility antigens or transplantation antigens. This is the basis of the rejection of transplanted material.

HISTOPATHOLOGY: Histopathology is the study of diseased tissues. A synonym for histopathology is pathologic histology.

HIV (HUMAN IMMUNODEFICIENCY VIRUS): The virus that causes AIDS (acquired immune deficiency syndrome).

HOMOZYGOUS: A condition in which two alleles for a given gene are the same.

HORIZONTAL GENE TRANSFER: Horizontal gene transfer is a major mechanism by which antibiotic resistance genes get passed between bacteria. It accounts for many hospital-acquired infections.

HORIZONTAL TRANSMISSION: Horizontal transmission refers to the transmission of a disease-causing microorganism from one person to another, unrelated person by direct or indirect contact.

HOST: An organism that serves as the habitat for a parasite or possibly for a symbiont. A host may provide nutrition to the parasite or symbiont, or it may simply provide a place in which to live.

HUMAN IMMUNODEFICIENCY VIRUS (HIV): The human immunodeficiency virus (HIV) belongs to a class of viruses known as the retroviruses. These viruses are known as RNA viruses because they have RNA (ribonucleic acid) as their basic genetic material instead of DNA (deoxyribonucleic acid).

HUMAN T-CELL LEUKEMIA VIRUS: Two types of human T-cell leukemia virus (HTLV) are known. They are also known as human T-cell lymphotrophic viruses. HTLV-I often is carried by a person with no obvious symptoms. However, HTLV-I is capable of causing a number of maladies. These include abnormalities of the T cells and B cells, a chronic infection of the myelin covering of nerves that causes a degeneration of the nervous system, sores on the skin, and an inflammation of the inside of the eye. HTLV-II infection usually does not produce any symptoms. However, in some people a cancer of the blood known as hairy cell leukemia can develop.

HYGIENE: Hygiene refers to the health practices that minimize the spread of infectious microorganisms between people or between other living things and people. Inanimate objects and surfaces such as contaminated cutlery or a cutting board may be a secondary part of this process.

HYPERENDEMIC: A disease that is endemic (commonly present) in all age groups of a population is hyperendemic. A related term is holoendemic, meaning a disease that is present more in children than in adults.

I

IMMIGRATION: The relocation of people to a different region or country from their native lands; also refers to the movement of organisms into an area in which they were previously absent.

IMMUNE RESPONSE: The body's production of antibodies or some types of white blood cells in response to foreign substances.

IMMUNE SYSTEM: The body's natural defense system that guards against foreign invaders and that includes lymphocytes and antibodies.

IMMUNOCOMPROMISED: A reduction of the ability of the immune system to recognize and respond to the presence of foreign material.

IMMUNODEFICIENCY: In immunodeficiency disorders, part of the body's immune system is missing or defective, thus impairing the body's ability to fight infections. As a result, the person with an immunodeficiency disorder will have frequent infections that are generally more severe and last longer than usual.

IMMUNOLOGY: Immunology is the study of how the body responds to foreign substances and fights off infection and other disease. Immunologists study the molecules, cells, and organs of the human body that participate in this response.

IMMUNOSUPPRESSION: A reduction of the ability of the immune system to recognize and respond to the presence of foreign material.

IMPORTED CASES OF DISEASE: Imported cases of disease happen when an infected person who is not yet showing symptoms travels from his home country to another country and develops symptoms of his disease there.

IN SITU: A Latin term meaning "in place" or in the body or natural system.

INACTIVATED VACCINE: An inactivated vaccine is a vaccine that is made from disease-causing microorganisms that have been killed or made incapable of causing the infection. The immune system can still respond to the presence of the microorganisms.

INACTIVATED VIRUS: An inactivated virus is incapable of causing disease but still stimulates the immune system to respond by forming antibodies.

INCIDENCE: The number of new cases of a disease or injury that occur in a population during a specified period of time.

INCUBATION PERIOD: Incubation period refers to the time between exposure to a disease-causing virus or bacteria and the appearance of symptoms of the infection. Depending on the microorganism, the incubation time can range from a few hours (for example, food poisoning due to *Salmonella*) to a decade or more (for example, acquired immune deficiency syndrome, or AIDS).

INFECTION CONTROL: Infection control refers to policies and procedures used to minimize the risk of spreading infections, especially in hospitals and health care facilities.

INFORMED CONSENT: An ethical and informational process in which a person learns about a procedure or clinical trial, including potential risks or benefits, before deciding to voluntarily participate in a study or undergo a particular procedure.

INNATE IMMUNITY: Innate immunity is the resistance against disease that an individual is born with, as distinct from acquired immunity, which develops with exposure to infectious agents.

INPATIENT: A patient who is admitted to a hospital or clinic for treatment, typically requiring the patient to stay overnight.

INSECT-BORNE VIRUS: A virus carried and transmitted by an insect, such as a mosquito.

INSECTICIDE: A chemical substance used to kill insects.

INTERMEDIATE HOST: An organism infected by a parasite while the parasite is in a developmental form, not sexually mature.

INTERNATIONAL HEALTH REGULATIONS (IHR): International regulations introduced by the World Health Organization (WHO) that aim to control, monitor, prevent, protect against, and respond to the spread of disease across national borders while avoiding unnecessary interference with international movement and trade.

INTRAVENOUS: In the vein. For example, the insertion of a hypodermic needle into a vein to instill a fluid, withdraw or transfuse blood, or start an intravenous feeding.

IONIZING RADIATION: Any electromagnetic or particulate radiation capable of direct or indirect ion production in its passage through matter. In general use: Radiation that can cause tissue damage or death.

IRRADIATION: A method of preservation that treats food with low doses of radiation to deactivate enzymes and to kill microorganisms and insects.

ISOLATION: Within the health community, isolation refers to the precautions that are taken in a hospital to prevent the spread of an infectious agent from an infected or colonized patient to susceptible persons. Isolation practices are designed to minimize the transmission of infection.

ISOLATION AND QUARANTINE: Public health authorities rely on isolation and quarantine as two important tools among the many they use to fight disease outbreaks. Isolation is the practice of keeping a disease victim away from other people, sometimes by treating them in their homes or by the use of elaborate isolation systems in hospitals. Quarantine separates people who have been exposed to a disease but have not yet developed symptoms from the general population. Both isolation and quarantine can be entered voluntarily by patients when public health authorities request it, or it can be compelled by state or national governments or government agencies, such as the U.S. Centers for Disease Control and Prevention.

J

JAUNDICE: Jaundice is a condition in which a person's skin and the whites of the eyes are discolored a shade of yellow due to an increased level of bile pigments in the blood as a result of liver disease. Jaundice is sometimes called icterus, from a Greek word for the condition.

K

KOCH'S POSTULATES: Koch's postulates are a series of conditions that must be met for a microorganism to be considered the cause of a disease. German microbiologist Robert Koch (1843–1910) proposed the postulates in 1890.

L

LATENT: A condition that is potential or dormant, not yet manifest or active, is latent.

LESION: The tissue disruption or the loss of function caused by a particular disease process.

LIVE VACCINE: A live vaccine uses a virus or bacteria that has been weakened (attenuated) to cause an immune response in the body without causing disease. Live vaccines are preferred to killed vaccines, which use a dead virus or bacteria, because they cause a stronger and longer-lasting immune response.

LYMPHATIC SYSTEM: The lymphatic system is the body's network of organs, ducts, and tissues that filters harmful substances out of the fluid that surrounds body tissues. Lymphatic organs include the bone marrow, thymus, spleen, appendix, tonsils, adenoids, lymph nodes, and Peyer's patches (in the small intestine). The thymus and bone marrow are called primary lymphatic organs, because lymphocytes are produced in them. The other lymphatic organs are called secondary lymphatic organs. The lymphatic system also includes thin vessels, capillaries, valves, ducts, nodes, and organs that run throughout the body, helping protect and maintain the internal fluids system of the entire body by both producing and filtering lymph and by producing various blood cells. The three main purposes of the lymphatic system are to drain fluid back into the bloodstream from the tissues, to filter lymph, and to fight infections.

LYMPHOCYTE: A type of white blood cell; includes B and T lymphocytes. These white blood cells function as part of the lymphatic and immune systems by stimulating antibody formation to attack specific invading substances.

M

MAJOR HISTOCOMPATIBILITY COMPLEX (MHC): The proteins that protrude from the surface of a cell that identify the cell as "self." In humans, the proteins coded by the genes of the major histocompatibility complex (MHC) include human leukocyte antigens (HLA), as well as other proteins. HLA proteins are present on the surface of most of the body's cells and are important in helping the immune system distinguish "self" from "non-self" molecules, cells, and other objects.

MALAISE: Malaise is a general or nonspecific feeling of unease or discomfort, often the first sign of disease infection.

MALIGNANT: A general term for cancer cells that can dislodge from the original tumor, then invade and destroy other tissues and organs.

MEASLES: Measles is an infectious disease caused by a virus of the paramyxovirus group. It infects only humans, and the infection results in life-long immunity to the disease. It is one of several exanthematous (rash-producing) diseases of childhood, the others being rubella (German measles), chicken pox, and the now rare scarlet fever. The disease is particularly common in both preschool and young school children.

MENINGITIS: Meningitis is an inflammation of the meninges—the three layers of protective membranes that line the spinal cord and the brain. Meningitis can occur when there is an infection near the brain or spinal cord, such as a respiratory infection in the sinuses, the mastoids, or the cavities around the ear. Disease organisms can also travel to the meninges through the bloodstream. The first signs may be a severe headache and neck stiffness followed by fever, vomiting, a rash, and then convulsions leading to loss of consciousness and potentially death. Meningitis generally involves two types: non-bacterial meningitis, which is often called aseptic meningitis, and bacterial meningitis, which is referred to as purulent meningitis.

MESSENGER RIBONUCLEIC ACID (MRNA): A molecule of RNA that carries the genetic information for producing one or more proteins; mRNA is produced by copying one strand of DNA, but in eukaryotes it is able to move from the nucleus to the cytoplasm (where protein synthesis takes place).

METHICILLIN-RESISTANT *STAPHYLOCOCCUS AUREUS* (MRSA): Methicillin-resistant *Staphylococcus aureus* (MRSA) are bacteria resistant to most penicillin-type antibiotics, including methicillin.

MICROBICIDE: A microbicide is a compound that kills microorganisms such as bacteria, fungi, and protozoa.

MICROFILIAE: Live offspring produced by adult nematodes within the host's body.

MICROORGANISM: Microorganisms are minute organisms. With only a single currently known exception (i.e., *Epulopiscium fishelsonia*, a bacterium that is billions of times larger than the bacteria in the human intestine and is large enough to view without a microscope), microorganisms are minute organisms that require microscopic magnification to view. To be seen, they must be magnified by an optical or electron microscope. The most common types of microorganisms are viruses, bacteria, blue-green bacteria, some algae, some fungi, yeasts, and protozoans.

MIGRATION: In medicine, migration is the movement of a disease symptom from one part of the body to another, apparently without cause.

MMR VACCINE: The MMR (measles, mumps, and rubella) vaccine is a vaccine that is given to protect someone from measles, mumps, and rubella. The vaccine is made up of viruses that cause the three diseases. The viruses are incapable of causing the diseases but can still stimulate the immune system.

MONO SPOT TEST: The mononucleosis (mono) spot test is a blood test used to check for infection with the Epstein-Barr virus, which causes mononucleosis.

MONOCLONAL ANTIBODIES: Antibodies produced from a single cell line that are used in medical testing and, increasingly, in the treatment of some cancers.

MONOVALENT VACCINE: A monovalent vaccine is one that is active against just one strain of a virus, such as the one that is in common use against the poliovirus.

MORBIDITY: The term "morbidity" comes from the Latin word *morbus*, which means sick. In medicine it refers not just to the state of being ill, but also to the severity of the illness. A serious disease is said to have a high morbidity.

MORPHOLOGY: The study of form and structure of animals and plants. The outward physical form possessed by an organism.

MORTALITY: Mortality is the condition of being susceptible to death. The term mortality comes from the Latin word *mors*, which means death. Mortality can also refer to the rate of deaths caused by an illness or injury, i.e., rabies has a high mortality rate.

MOSQUITO COILS: Mosquito coils are spirals of flammable paste that, when burned, steadily release insect repellent into the air. They are often used in Asia, where many coils release octachlorodipropyl ether, which can cause lung cancer.

MOSQUITO NETTING: Fine meshes or nets hung around occupied spaces, especially beds, to keep out disease-carrying mosquitoes. Mosquito netting is a cost-effective way of preventing malaria.

MRSA: MRSA is an abbreviation for methicillin-resistant *Staphylococcus aureus*, which are bacteria resistant to most penicillin-type antibiotics, including methicillin.

MULTI-DRUG RESISTANCE: Multi-drug resistance is a phenomenon that occurs when an infective agent loses its sensitivity against two or more of the drugs that are used against it.

MULTI-DRUG THERAPY: Multi-drug therapy is the use of a combination of drugs against infection, each of which attacks the infective agent in a different way. This strategy can help overcome resistance to anti-infective drugs.

MUTABLE VIRUS: A mutable virus is one whose DNA changes rapidly so that drugs and vaccines against it may not be effective.

MUTATION: A mutation is a change in an organism's DNA that occurs over time and may render it less sensitive to the drugs that are used against it.

MYCOBACTERIA: *Mycobacteria* is a genus of bacteria that includes the bacteria causing leprosy and tuberculosis. The bacteria have unusual cell walls that are harder to dissolve than the cell walls of other bacteria.

MYCOTIC: Mycotic means having to do with or caused by a fungus. Any medical condition caused by a fungus is a mycotic condition, also called a mycosis.

N

NECROPSY: A necropsy is a medical examination of a dead body; also called an autopsy.

NECROTIC: Necrotic tissue is dead tissue in an otherwise living body. Tissue death is called necrosis.

NEEDLESTICK INJURY: Any accidental breakage or puncture of the skin by an unsterilized medical needle (syringe) is a needlestick injury. Health-care providers are at particular risk for needlestick injuries (which may transmit disease) because of the large number of needles they handle.

NEGLECTED TROPICAL DISEASE: Many tropical diseases are considered to be neglected because, despite their prevalence in less-developed areas, new vaccines and treatments are not being developed for them. Malaria was once considered to be a neglected tropical disease, but a great deal of research and money have been devoted to its prevention, treatment, and cure in the twenty-first century.

NEMATODES: Also known as roundworms; a type of helminth characterized by long, cylindrical bodies.

NODULE: A nodule is a small, roundish lump on the surface of the skin or of an internal organ.

NONGOVERNMENTAL ORGANIZATION (NGO): A voluntary organization that is not part of any government; often organized to address a specific issue or perform a humanitarian function.

NORMAL FLORA: The bacteria that normally inhabit some part of the body, such as the mouth or intestines, are normal flora. Normal flora are essential to health.

NOROVIRUS: Norovirus is a type of virus that contains ribonucleic acid as the genetic material and causes an intestinal infection known as gastroenteritis. A well-known example is Norwalk virus.

NOSOCOMIAL INFECTION: A nosocomial infection is an infection that is acquired in a hospital. More precisely, the U.S. Centers for Disease Control in Atlanta, Georgia, defines a nosocomial infection as a localized infection or an infection that is widely spread throughout the body that results from an adverse reaction to an infectious microorganism or toxin that was not present at the time of admission to the hospital.

NOTIFIABLE DISEASES: Diseases that the law requires must be reported to health officials when diagnosed, including active tuberculosis and several sexually transmitted diseases; also called reportable diseases.

NUCLEOTIDE: The basic unit of a nucleic acid. It consists of a simple sugar, a phosphate group, and a nitrogen–containing base.

NUCLEUS, CELL: Membrane-enclosed structure within a cell that contains the cell's genetic material and controls its growth and reproduction. The plural of nucleus is nuclei.

NUTRITIONAL SUPPLEMENTS: Nutritional supplements are substances necessary to health, such as calcium or protein, that are taken in concentrated form to compensate for dietary insufficiency, poor absorption, unusually high demand for a specific nutrient, or other reasons.

O

ONCOGENIC VIRUS: An oncogenic virus is a virus that is capable of changing the cells it infects so that the cells begin to grow and divide uncontrollably.

OPPORTUNISTIC INFECTION: An opportunistic infection is so named because it occurs in people whose immune systems are diminished or are not functioning normally; such infections are opportunistic insofar as the infectious agents take advantage of their hosts' compromised immune systems and invade to cause disease.

ORAL REHYDRATION THERAPY: Patients who have lost excessive water from their tissues are said to be dehydrated. Restoring body water levels by giving the patient fluids through the mouth (orally) is oral rehydration therapy. Often, a special mixture of water, glucose, and electrolytes called oral rehydration solution is given.

OUTBREAK: The appearance of new cases of a disease in numbers greater than the established incidence rate or the appearance of even one case of an emergent or rare disease in an area.

OUTPATIENT: A person who receives health care services without being admitted to a hospital or clinic for an overnight stay.

P

PANDEMIC: Pandemic, which means all the people, describes an epidemic that occurs in more than one country or population simultaneously.

PARAMYXOVIRUS: Paramyxovirus is a type of virus that contains ribonucleic acid as the genetic material and has proteins on its surface that clump red blood cells and assist in the release of newly made viruses from the infected cells. Measles virus and mumps virus are two types of paramyxoviruses.

PARASITE: An organism that lives in or on a host organism and that gets its nourishment from that host. The parasite usually gains all the benefits of this relationship, while the host may suffer from various diseases and discomforts, or show no signs of the infection. The life cycle of a typical parasite usually includes several developmental stages and morphological changes as the parasite lives and moves through the environment and one or more hosts. Parasites that remain on a host's body surface to feed are called ectoparasites, while those that live inside a host's body are called endoparasites. Parasitism is a highly successful biological adaptation. There are more known parasitic species than nonparasitic ones, and parasites affect just about every form of life, including most all animals, plants, and even bacteria.

PASTEURIZATION: Pasteurization is a process in which fluids such as wine and milk are heated for a predetermined time at a temperature that is below the boiling point of the liquid. The treatment kills any microorganisms that are in the fluid but does not alter the taste, appearance, or nutritive value of the fluid.

PATHOGEN: A disease-causing agent or microorganism, such as a bacteria, virus, fungus, etc., that can cause or is capable of causing disease.

PATHOGENIC: Something causing or capable of causing disease.

PAUCIBACILLARY: Paucibacillary refers to an infectious condition, such as a certain form of leprosy, characterized by few, rather than many, bacilli, which are a rod-shaped type of bacterium.

PCR (POLYMERASE CHAIN REACTION): The polymerase chain reaction, or PCR, refers to a widely used technique in molecular biology involving the amplification of specific sequences of genomic DNA.

PERSISTENCE: Persistence is the length of time a disease remains in a patient. Disease persistence can vary from a few days to life-long.

PESTICIDE: Substances used to reduce the abundance of pests, any living thing that causes injury or disease to people, animals, or crops.

PHENOTYPE: The visible characteristics or physical shape produced by an organism's genotype.

PNEUMONIA: Pneumonia is inflammation of the lung accompanied by filling of some air sacs with fluid (consolidation). It can be caused by a number of infectious agents, including bacteria, viruses, and fungi.

POTABLE: Water that is clean enough to drink safely is potable water.

PREVALENCE: The actual number of cases of disease (or injury) that exist in a population.

PRIMARY HOST: The primary host is an organism that provides food and shelter for a parasite while allowing it to become sexually mature, while a secondary host is one occupied by a parasite during the larval or asexual stages of its life cycle.

PRIONS: Prions are proteins that are infectious. The name prion is derived from "proteinaceous infectious particles." The discovery of prions and confirmation of their infectious nature overturned a central dogma that infections were caused only by intact organisms, particularly microorganisms such as bacteria, fungi, parasites, or viruses. Because prions lack genetic material, the prevailing attitude was that a protein could not cause disease.

PROPHYLAXIS: Pre-exposure treatment (e.g., immunization) that prevents or reduces severity of disease or symptoms upon exposure to the causative agent.

PROSTRATION: A condition marked by nausea, disorientation, dizziness, and weakness caused by dehydration and prolonged exposure to high temperatures; also called heat exhaustion or hyperthermia.

PROTOZOA: Single-celled animal-like microscopic organisms that live by taking in food rather than making it by photosynthesis and must live in the presence of water. (Singular: protozoan.) Protozoa are a diverse group of single-celled organisms, with more than 50,000 different types represented. The vast majority are microscopic, many measuring less than 0.0002 inches (0.005 millimeters), but some, such as the freshwater *Spirostomun*, may reach 0.17 inches (3 millimeters) in length, large enough to enable them to be seen with the naked eye.

PUERPERAL: An interval of time around childbirth, from the onset of labor through the immediate recovery period after delivery.

PUERPERAL FEVER: Puerperal fever is a bacterial infection present in the blood (septicemia) that follows childbirth. The Latin word *puer* meaning boy or child, is the root of this term. Puerperal fever was much more common before the advent of modern aseptic practices, but infections still occur. Louis Pasteur showed that puerperal fever is most often caused by *Streptococcus* bacteria, which is now treated with antibiotics.

PULMONARY: Having to do with the lungs or respiratory system. The pulmonary circulatory system delivers deoxygenated blood from the right ventricle of the heart to the lungs and returns oxygenated blood from the lungs to the left atrium of the heart. At its most minute level, the alveolar capillary bed, the pulmonary circulatory system is the principle point of gas exchange between blood and air that moves in and out of the lungs during respiration.

Q

QUANTITATED: An act of determining the quantity of something, such as the number or concentration of bacteria in an infectious disease.

QUARANTINE: Quarantine is the practice of separating people who have been exposed to an infectious agent but have not yet developed symptoms from the general population. This can be done voluntarily or involuntarily. In the United States, it can be enacted by the authority of states and the U.S. Centers for Disease Control and Prevention (CDC).

R

RECEPTOR: Protein molecules on a cell's surface that acts as a "signal receiver" and allow communication between cells.

RECOMBINANT DNA: DNA that is cut using specific enzymes so that a gene or DNA sequence can be inserted.

RECOMBINATION: Recombination is a process during which genetic material is shuffled during reproduction to form new combinations. This mixing is important from an evolutionary standpoint because it allows the expression of different traits between generations. The process involves a physical exchange of nucleotides between duplicate strands of deoxyribonucleic acid (DNA).

RED TIDE: Red tides are a marine phenomenon in which water is stained a red, brown, or yellowish color because of the temporary abundance of a particular species of pigmented dinoflagellate (these events are known as "blooms"). Also called phytoplankton, or planktonic algae, these single-celled organisms of the class Dinophyceae move using a tail-like structure called a flagellum. They also photosynthesize, and it is their photosynthetic pigments that can tint the water during blooms. Dinoflagellates are common and widespread. Under appropriate environmental conditions, various species can grow very rapidly, causing red tides. Red tides occur in all marine regions within temperate or warmer climates.

RE-EMERGING INFECTIOUS DISEASE: Re-emerging infectious diseases are illnesses such as malaria, diphtheria, and tuberculosis that were once nearly absent from the world but are starting to cause greater numbers of infections once again. These illnesses are reappearing for many reasons. Malaria and other mosquito-borne illnesses increase when mosquito-control measures decrease or they spread to new areas. Other diseases are spreading because people have stopped being vaccinated, as happened with diphtheria after the collapse of the Soviet Union. A few diseases are re-emerging because drugs to treat them have become less available or drug-resistant strains have developed.

REHYDRATION: Dehydration is excessive loss of water from the body; rehydration is the restoration of water after dehydration.

REPLICATE: To replicate is to duplicate something or make a copy of it. All reproduction of living things depends on the replication of DNA molecules or, in a few cases, RNA molecules. Replication may be used to refer to the reproduction of entire viruses and other microorganisms.

REPLICATION: A process of reproducing, duplicating, copying, or repeating something, such as the duplication of DNA or the recreation of characteristics of an infectious disease in a laboratory setting.

REPORTABLE DISEASE: By law, occurrences of some diseases must be reported to government authorities when observed by health-care professionals. Such diseases are called reportable diseases or notifiable diseases. Cholera and yellow fever are examples of reportable diseases.

RESERVOIR: The animal or organism in which a specific virus or parasite normally resides.

RESISTANCE: Immunity developed within a species (especially bacteria) to an antibiotic or other drug via evolution. For example, in bacteria, the acquisition of genetic mutations that render the bacteria invulnerable to the action of antibiotics.

RESISTANT BACTERIA: Resistant bacteria are microbes that have lost their sensitivity to one or more antibiotic drugs through mutation.

RESISTANT ORGANISM: An organism that has developed the ability to counter something trying to harm it. With infectious diseases, the causative organism, such as a bacterium, has developed a resistance to drugs, such as antibiotics, normally used to fight the disease.

RESPIRATOR: A respirator is any device that assists a patient in breathing or takes over breathing entirely for them.

RESTRICTION ENZYME: A special type of protein that can recognize and cut DNA at certain sequences of bases to help scientists separate out a specific gene. Restriction enzymes recognize certain sequences of DNA and cleave the DNA at those sites. The enzymes are used to generate fragments of DNA that can be subsequently joined together to create new stretches of DNA.

RETROVIRUS: Retroviruses are viruses in which the genetic material consists of ribonucleic acid (RNA) instead of the usual deoxyribonucleic acid (DNA). Retroviruses produce an enzyme known as reverse transcriptase that can transform RNA into DNA, which can then be permanently integrated into the DNA of the infected host cells.

REVERSE TRANSCRIPTASE: An enzyme that makes it possible for a retrovirus to produce DNA (deoxyribonucleic acid) from RNA (ribonucleic acid).

RHINITIS: An inflammation of the mucous lining of the nose. A nonspecific term that covers infections, allergies, and other disorders whose common feature is the location of their symptoms. These symptoms include infected or irritated mucous membranes, production of a discharge, nasal congestion, and swelling of the tissues of the nasal passages. The most widespread form of infectious rhinitis is the common cold.

RIBONUCLEIC ACID (RNA): Any of a group of nucleic acids that carry out several important tasks in the synthesis of proteins. Unlike DNA (deoxyribonucleic acid), RNA has only a single strand. Nucleic acids are complex molecules that contain a cell's genetic information and the instructions for carrying out cellular processes. In eukaryotic cells, the two nucleic acids, ribonucleic acid (RNA) and deoxyribonucleic acid (DNA), work together to direct protein synthesis. Although it is DNA that contains the instructions for directing the synthesis of specific structural and enzymatic proteins, several types of RNA actually carry out the processes required to produce these proteins. These include messenger RNA (mRNA), ribosomal RNA (rRNA), and transfer RNA (tRNA). Further processing of the various RNAs is carried out by another type of RNA called small nuclear RNA (snRNA). The structure of RNA is very similar to that of DNA, however, instead of the base thymine, RNA contains the base uracil in its place.

RING VACCINATION: Ring vaccination is the vaccination of all susceptible people in an area surrounding a case of an infectious disease. Since vaccination makes people immune to the disease, the hope is that the disease will not spread from the known case to other people. Ring vaccination was used in eliminating the smallpox virus.

RNA VIRUS: An RNA virus is one whose genetic material consists of either single- or double-stranded ribonucleic acid (RNA) rather than deoxyribonucleic acid (DNA).

ROUNDWORM: Also known as nematodes; a type of helminth characterized by long, cylindrical bodies. Roundworm infections are diseases of the digestive tract and other organ systems that are caused by roundworms. Roundworm infections are widespread throughout the world, and humans acquire most types of roundworm infection from contaminated food or by touching the mouth with unwashed hands that have come into contact with the parasite larva. The severity of infection varies considerably from person to person. Children are more likely to have heavy infestations and are also more likely to suffer from malabsorption and malnutrition than adults.

ROUS SARCOMA VIRUS: Rous sarcoma virus, named after American doctor Francis Peyton Rous (1879–1970), is a virus that can cause cancer in some birds, including chickens. It was the first virus known to be able to cause cancer.

RUMINANTS: Cud-chewing animals with four-chambered stomachs and even-toed hooves, including cows.

S

SANITATION: Sanitation is the use of hygienic recycling and disposal measures that prevent disease and promote health through sewage disposal, solid waste disposal, waste material recycling, and food processing and preparation.

SCHISTOSOMES: Blood flukes that infect an estimated 200 million people.

SEIZURE: A seizure is a sudden disruption of the brain's normal electrical activity accompanied by altered consciousness and/or other neurological and behavioral abnormalities. Epilepsy is a condition characterized by recurrent seizures that may include repetitive muscle jerking called convulsions. Seizures are traditionally divided into two major categories: generalized seizures and focal seizures. Within each major category, however, there are many different types of seizures. Generalized seizures come about due to abnormal neuronal activity on both sides of the brain,

while focal seizures, also named partial seizures, occur in only one part of the brain.

SELECTION: Process that favors one feature of organisms in a population over another feature found in the population. This occurs through differential reproduction—those with the favored feature produce more offspring than those with the other feature, such that they become a greater percentage of the population in the next generation.

SELECTION PRESSURE: Selection pressure (or selective pressure) refers to factors that influence the evolution of an organism and the tendency of an organism that has a certain characteristic to be eliminated from an environment or to increase in numbers. An example is the overuse of antibiotics, which provides a selection pressure for the development of antibiotic resistance in bacteria and an increased prevalence of bacteria that are resistant to multiple kinds of antibiotics.

SENTINEL: A sentinel is a guard or watcher; in medicine, a sentinel node is a lymph node near the breast in which cancer cells from a breast tumor are likely to be found at an early stage of the cancer's spreading (metastasization).

SENTINEL SURVEILLANCE: Sentinel surveillance is a method in epidemiology where a subset of the population is surveyed for the presence of communicable diseases. Also, a sentinel is an animal used to indicate the presence of disease within an area.

SEPSIS: Sepsis refers to a bacterial infection in the bloodstream or body tissues. This is a very broad term covering the presence of many types of microscopic disease-causing organisms. Sepsis is also called bacteremia. Closely related terms include septicemia and septic syndrome.

SEPTIC: The term "septic" refers to the state of being infected with bacteria, particularly in the bloodstream.

SEPTICEMIA: Prolonged fever, chills, anorexia, and anemia in conjunction with tissue lesions.

SEQUENCING: Finding the order of chemical bases in a section of DNA.

SEROTYPES: Serotypes or serovars are classes of microorganisms based on the types of molecules (antigens) that they present on their surfaces. Even a single species may have thousands of serotypes, which may have medically quite distinct behaviors.

SEXUALLY TRANSMITTED DISEASE (STD): Sexually transmitted diseases (STDs) vary in their susceptibility to treatment, their signs and symptoms, and the consequences if they are left untreated. Some are caused by bacteria. These usually can be treated and cured. Others are caused by viruses and can typically be treated but not cured.

SHED: To shed is to cast off or release. In medicine, the release of eggs or live organisms from an individual infected with parasites is often referred to as shedding.

SHOCK: Shock is a medical emergency in which the organs and tissues of the body are not receiving an adequate flow of blood. This condition deprives the organs and tissues of oxygen (carried in the blood) and allows the buildup of waste products. Shock can result in serious damage or even death.

SOCIOECONOMIC: Concerning both social and economic factors.

SPECIAL PATHOGENS BRANCH: A group within the U.S. Centers for Disease Control and Prevention (CDC) whose goal is to study highly infectious viruses that produce diseases within humans.

SPIROCHETE: A bacterium shaped like a spiral. Spiral-shaped bacteria live in contaminated water, sewage, soil, and decaying organic matter, as well as inside humans and animals.

STANDARD PRECAUTIONS: Standard precautions are the safety measures taken to prevent the transmission of disease-causing bacteria. These include proper hand washing; wearing gloves, goggles, and other protective clothing; proper handling of needles; and sterilization of equipment.

STRAIN: A subclass or a specific genetic variation of an organism.

STREPTOCOCCUS: A genus of bacteria that includes species such as *Streptococci pyogenes*, a species of bacteria that causes strep throat.

SUPERINFECTION: When a new infection occurs in a patient who already has some other infection, it is called a superinfection. For example, a bacterial infection appearing in a person who already had viral pneumonia would be a superinfection.

SURVEILLANCE: The systematic analysis, collection, evaluation, interpretation, and dissemination of data. In public health, it assists in the identification of health threats and the planning, implementation, and evaluation of responses to those threats.

SYSTEMIC: Any medical condition that affects the whole body (i.e., the whole system) is systemic.

T

T CELL: Immune-system white blood cells that enable antibody production, suppress antibody production, or kill other cells. When a vertebrate encounters substances that are capable of causing it harm, a protective system known as the immune system comes into play. This system is a network of many different organs that work together to recognize foreign substances and destroy them. The immune system can respond to the presence of a disease-causing agent (pathogen) in two ways. In cell-mediated immunity, T cells produce special chemicals that can specifically isolate the pathogen and destroy it. The other branch of immunity is called humoral immunity, in which immune cells called B cells can produce soluble proteins (antibodies) that can accurately target and kill the pathogen.

T-CELL VACCINE: A T-cell vaccine is one that relies on eliciting cellular immunity, rather than humoral antibody-based immunity, against infection. T cell vaccines are being developed against the human immunodeficiency virus (HIV) and hepatitis C.

TAPEWORM: Tapeworms are parasitic flatworms of class *Cestoidea*, phylum *Platyhelminthes*, that live inside the intestine. Tapeworms have no digestive system, but absorb predigested nutrients directly from their surroundings.

TICK: A tick is any blood-sucking parasitic insect of suborder *Ixodides*, superfamily *Ixodoidea*. Ticks can transmit a number of diseases, including Lyme disease and Rocky Mountain spotted fever.

TOPICAL: Any medication that is applied directly to a particular part of the body's surface is termed topical; for example, a topical ointment.

TOXIC: Something that is poisonous and that can cause illness or death.

TRANSFUSION-TRANSMISSIBLE INFECTIONS: Any infection that can be transmitted to a person by a blood transfusion (addition of stored whole blood or blood fractions to a person's own blood) is a transfusion-transmissible infection. Some diseases that can be transmitted in this way are AIDS, hepatitis B, hepatitis C, syphilis, malaria, and Chagas disease.

TRANSMISSION: Microorganisms that cause disease in humans and other species are known as pathogens. The transmission of pathogens to a human or other host can occur in a number of ways, depending upon the microorganism.

TREMATODES: Trematodes, also called flukes, are a type of parasitic flatworm. In humans, flukes can infest the liver, lung, and other tissues.

TYPHUS: A disease caused by various species of *Rickettsia*, characterized by fever, rash, and delirium. Insects such as lice and chiggers transmit typhus. Two forms of typhus, epidemic typhus and scrub typhus, are fatal if untreated.

U

UNIVERSAL PRECAUTION: Universal precaution refers to an infection control strategy in which all human blood and other material is assumed to be potentially infectious, specifically with organisms such as human immunodeficiency virus (HIV) and hepatitis B virus. The precautions are aimed at preventing contact with blood or the other materials.

V

VACCINATION: Vaccination is the inoculation, or use of vaccines, to prevent specific diseases within humans and animals by producing immunity to such diseases. It is the introduction of weakened or dead viruses or microorganisms into the body to create immunity by the production of specific antibodies.

VACCINE: A substance that is introduced to stimulate antibody production and thus provide immunity to a particular disease.

VACCINIA VIRUS: The vaccinia virus is a usually harmless virus that is closely related to the virus that causes smallpox, a dangerous disease. Infection with the vaccinia virus confers immunity against smallpox, so vaccinia virus has been used as a vaccine against smallpox.

VARICELLA ZOSTER IMMUNE GLOBULIN (VZIG): Varicella zoster immune globulin is a preparation that can give people temporary protection against chicken pox after exposure to the Varicella virus. It is used for children and adults who are at risk of complications of the disease or who are susceptible to infection because they have weakened immunity.

VARICELLA ZOSTER VIRUS (VZV): Varicella zoster virus is a member of the alpha herpes virus group and is the cause of both chicken pox (also known as varicella) and shingles (herpes zoster).

VARIOLA VIRUS: Variola virus (or variola major virus) is the virus that causes smallpox. The virus is one of the members of the poxvirus group (Family Poxviridae). The virus particle is brick shaped and contains a double strand of deoxyribonucleic acid. The variola virus is among the most dangerous of all the potential biological weapons.

VARIOLATION: Variolation was the pre-modern practice of deliberately infecting a person with smallpox in order to make them immune to a more serious form of the disease. It was dangerous, but did confer immunity on survivors.

VECTOR: Any agent that carries and transmits parasites and diseases. Also, an organism or chemical used to transport a gene into a new host cell.

VECTOR-BORNE DISEASE: A vector-borne disease is one in which the pathogenic microorganism is transmitted from an infected individual to another individual by an arthropod or other agent, sometimes with other animals serving as intermediary hosts. The transmission depends upon the attributes and requirements of at least three different living organisms: the pathologic agent, either a virus, protozoa, bacteria, or helminth (worm); the vector, commonly arthropods such as ticks or mosquitoes; and the human host.

VENEREAL DISEASE: Venereal diseases are diseases that are transmitted by sexual contact. They are named after Venus, the Roman goddess of female sexuality. They are now more commonly called sexually transmitted diseases.

VESICLE: A membrane-bound sphere that contains a variety of substances in cells.

VIRAL SHEDDING: Viral shedding refers the period of time in which a person with a virus is contagious, allowing the movement of a virus from one person to another. For example, when the herpes virus moves from the nerves to the surface of the skin. During shedding, the herpes virus can be passed on through skin-to-skin contact.

VIRION: A virion is a mature virus particle, consisting of a core of ribonucleic acid (RNA) or deoxyribonucleic acid (DNA) surrounded by a protein coat. This is the form in which a virus exists outside of its host cell.

VIRULENCE: Virulence is the ability of a disease organism to cause disease: a more virulent organism is more infective and liable to produce more serious disease.

VIRUS: A virus is a small, infectious agent that consists of a core of genetic material—either deoxyribonucleic acid (DNA) or ribonucleic acid (RNA)—surrounded by a shell of protein. Viruses are essentially nonliving repositories of nucleic acid that require the presence of a living prokaryotic or eukaryotic cell for the replication of the nucleic acid. Very simple microorganisms, viruses are much smaller than bacteria that enter and multiply within cells. There are a number of different viruses that challenge the human immune system and that may produce disease in humans. Viruses often exchange or transfer their genetic material (DNA or RNA) to cells and can cause diseases such as chicken pox, hepatitis, measles, and mumps.

VISCERAL: Visceral means pertaining to the viscera. The viscera are the large organs contained in the main cavities of the body, especially the thorax and abdomen, for example, the lungs, stomach, intestines, kidneys, and liver.

W

WATERBORNE DISEASE: Waterborne disease refers to diseases that are caused by exposure to contaminated water. The exposure can occur by drinking the water or having the water come in contact with the body. Examples of waterborne diseases are cholera and typhoid fever.

WEAPONIZATION: The use of any bacterium, virus, or other disease-causing organism as a weapon of war. Among other terms, it is also called germ warfare, biological weaponry, and biological warfare.

WILD VIRUS: Wild- or wild-type virus is a genetic description referring to the original form of a virus, first observed in nature. It may remain the most common form in existence but mutated forms develop over time and sometimes become the new wild type virus.

Z

ZOONOTIC: A zoonotic disease is a disease that can be transmitted between animals and humans. Examples of zoonotic diseases are anthrax, plague, and Q-fever.

Chronology of Events

Nineteenth Century

1854 English physician John Snow traces the source of a cholera epidemic to a public water pump in Soho, London. This discovery is generally considered to be the foundation of modern epidemiology.

1857 Louis Pasteur demonstrates that lactic acid fermentation is caused by a living organism. Between 1857 and 1880, he performs a series of experiments that refute the doctrine of spontaneous generation. He also introduces vaccines for fowl cholera, anthrax, and rabies, based on attenuated strains of viruses and bacteria.

1858 Rudolf Virchow publishes his landmark paper "Cellular Pathology" and establishes the field of cellular pathology. Virchow asserts that all cells arise from preexisting cells (*Omnis cellula e cellula*). He argues that the cell is the ultimate locus of all disease.

1859 Charles Darwin publishes his landmark book *On the Origin of Species by Means of Natural Selection*.

1860 Ernst Heinrich Haeckel describes the essential elements of modern zoological classification.

1860 Max Johann Sigismund Schultze describes the nature of protoplasm and shows that it is fundamentally the same for all life forms.

1865 An epidemic of rinderpest kills 500,000 cattle in Great Britain. Government inquiries into the outbreak pave the way for the development of contemporary theories of epidemiology and the germ theory of disease.

1865 French physiologist Claude Bernard publishes *Introduction to the Study of Human Experimentation* that advocates "Never perform an experiment which might be harmful to the patient even if advantageous to science."

1866 The Austrian botanist and monk Johann Gregor Mendel discovers the laws of heredity and writes the first of a series of papers on heredity (1866–1869). The papers formulate the laws of hybridization. Mendel's work is disregarded until 1900, when Hugo de Vries rediscovers it. Unbeknownst to both Darwin and Mendel, Mendelian laws provide the scientific framework for the concepts of gradual evolution and continuous variation.

1870 Lambert Adolphe Jacques Quetelet shows the importance of statistical analysis for biologists and provides the foundations of biometry.

1871 Ferdinand Cohn coins the term bacterium.

1875 Ferdinand Cohn publishes a classification of bacteria in which the genus name Bacillus is used for the first time.

1867 Robert Koch publishes a paper on anthrax that establishes the role of bacteria in causing anthrax, providing the final piece of evidence in support of the germ theory of disease. Koch later formulates postulates that established steps for determining the cause, such as a specific bacteria or virus, of a particular infectious disease.

1877 Paul Erlich recognizes the existence of the mast cells of the immune system.

1877   Robert Koch describes new techniques for fixing, staining, and photographing bacteria.

1878   Joseph Lister publishes a paper describing the role of a bacterium he names *Bacterium lactis* in the souring of milk.

1878   Thomas Burrill demonstrates for the first time that a plant disease (pear blight) is caused by a bacterium (*Micrococcus amylophorous*).

1879   Albert Nisser identifies *Neiserria gonorrhoeoe* as the cause of gonorrhea.

1880   C. L. Alphonse Laveran isolates malarial parasites in erythrocytes of infected people and demonstrates that the organism can replicate in the cells. He is awarded the 1907 Nobel Prize in Medicine or Physiology for this work.

1880   The passage of a nationwide food and drug law is first attempted in the U.S. Congress. Although defeated in Congress, the U.S. Department of Agriculture's findings of widespread food adulteration spur continued interest in food and drug legislation.

1882   The German bacteriologist Robert Koch discovers the tubercle bacillus, the cause of tuberculosis.

1883   Edward Theodore Klebs and Frederich Loeffler independently discover *Corynebacterium* diphtheriae, the bacterium that causes diphtheria.

1884   Elie Metchnikoff discovers the antibacterial activity of white blood cells, which he calls "phagocytes," and formulates the theory of phagocytosis. He also develops the cellular theory of vaccination.

1884   Hans Christian J. Gram develops the Gram stain.

1884   Robert Koch enunciates "Koch's postulates," four steps for determining the source of an infection or disease.

1884   Louis Pasteur and coworkers publish *A New Communication on Rabies*. Pasteur proves that the causal agent of rabies can be attenuated, and the weakened virus can be used as a vaccine to prevent the disease. This work serves as the basis of future work on virus attenuation, vaccine development, and the concept that variation is an inherent characteristic of viruses.

1885   Francis Galton devises a new statistical tool, the correlation table.

1885   French chemist Louis Pasteur inoculates a boy, Joseph Meister, against rabies. Meister had been bitten by an infected dog. The treatment saves his life. This is the first time Pasteur uses an attenuated germ on a human being.

1885   Theodor Escherich identifies a bacterium inhabiting the human intestinal tract that he names *Bacterium coli* and shows that the bacterium causes infant diarrhea and gastroenteritis. The bacterium is subsequently named *Escherichia coli*.

1886   Adolf Mayer publishes the landmark article "Concerning the Mosaic Disease of Tobacco." This paper is considered the beginning of modern experimental work on plant viruses. Mayer assumes that the causal agent was a bacterium, although he was unable to isolate it.

1888   Martinus Beijerinck uses a growth medium enriched with certain nutrients to isolate the bacterium *Rhizobium*, demonstrating that nutritionally-tailored growth media are useful in bacterial isolation.

1888   The Institut Pasteur is formed in France as an international research institute to advance science, medicine, and public health.

1891   Charles-Edouard Brown-Sequard suggests the concept of internal secretions (hormones).

1891   Paul Ehrlich proposes that antibodies are responsible for immunity.

1891   The Prussian State dictates that even jailed prisoners must give consent prior to treatment (even for tuberculosis).

1892   Dmitri Ivanowski demonstrates that filterable material causes tobacco mosaic disease. The infectious agent is subsequently showed to be the tobacco mosaic virus. Ivanowski's discovery creates the field of virology.

1892   George M. Sternberg publishes *Practical Results of Bacteriological Researches*. Sternberg's realization that a specific antibody was produced after infection with vaccinia virus and that immune serum could neutralize the virus becomes the basis of virus serology. The neutralization test provides a technique for diagnosing viral infections, measuring the immune response, distinguishing antigenic similarities and differences among viruses, and conducting retrospective epidemiological surveys.

1892   In an experiment to try to prevent syphilis, Albert Neisser injects human subjects with serum from syphilis patients without their consent. Instead of conferring immunity, the subjects subsequently acquire the disease.

1894   Alexandre Yersin isolates *Yersinia (Pasteurella) pestis,* the bacterium responsible for bubonic plague.

1894   Wilhelm Konrad Roentgen discovers x rays.

1895   Heinrich Dreser, working for the Bayer Company in Germany, produces a drug he believes to be as effective an analgesic as morphine, but without its harmful side effects. Bayer begins mass production of diacetylmorphine, and in 1898 markets the new drug as a cough sedative under the brand name heroin.

1898   Friedrich Loeffler and Paul Frosch publish their *Report on Foot-and-Mouth Disease.* They prove that this animal disease is caused by a filterable virus and suggests that similar agents might cause other diseases.

1898   The First International Congress of Genetics is held in London.

1898   Frederick Manson cites British colonization in the tropics as justification for the new discipline of tropical medicine.

1899   A meeting to organize the Society of American Bacteriologists is held at Yale University. The society will later become the American Society for Microbiology.

Twentieth Century

1900   Carl Correns, Hugo de Vries, and Erich von Tschermak independently rediscover Mendel's laws of inheritance. Their publications mark the beginning of modern genetics. Using several plant species, de Vries and Correns perform breeding experiments that parallel Mendel's earlier studies and independently arrive at similar interpretations of their results. Therefore,

upon reading Mendel's publication, they immediately recognize its significance. William Bateson describes the importance of Mendel's contribution in an address to the Royal Society of London.

1900   Karl Landsteiner discovers the blood-agglutination phenomenon and the four major blood types in humans.

1900   Paul Erlich proposes the theory concerning the formation of antibodies by the immune system.

1900   Walter Reed demonstrates that yellow fever is caused by a virus transmitted by mosquitoes. This is the first demonstration of a viral cause of a human disease. Reed injects paid Spanish immigrant workers in Cuba with the agent, paying them if they survive and paying them still more should they contract the disease.

1901   Jokichi Takamine, Japanese-American chemist, and T. B. Aldrich first isolate epinephrine from the adrenal gland. Later known by the trade name Adrenalin, it is eventually identified as a neurotransmitter. This is also the first time a pure hormone is isolated.

1902   The Pan American Health Organization (PAHO), one of the earliest international public health agencies, is founded. PAHO works to improve health and quality of life in the Americas, eventually becoming the Regional Office for the Americas of the World Health Organization and a member of the United Nations system.

1902   Carl Neuberg introduces the term biochemistry.

1903   Willem Einthoven invents the electrocardiograph (EKG).

1906   The U.S. Congress passes, and President Theodore Roosevelt signs, the Pure Food and Drug Act.

1906   Viennese physician and immunological researcher Clemens von Pirquet coins the term allergy to describe the immune reaction to certain compounds.

1906   Doctor of tropical medicine (and later Harvard professor) Richard Strong experiments with cholera on prisoners in the Philippines. Some of the prisoners die because the injections they are given are contaminated by plague.

1909	Sigurd Orla-Jensen proposes that the physiological reactions of bacteria are primarily important in their classification.
1911	(Francis) Peyton Rous publishes the landmark paper "Transmission of a Malignant New Growth by Means of a Cell-Free Filtrate." His work provides the first rigorous proof of the experimental transmission of a solid tumor and suggests that a filterable virus is the causal agent.
1912	Casimir Funk, Polish-American biochemist, coins the term vitamine. Since the dietary substances he discovers are in the amine group, he calls all of them vita-amines (using the Latin word for life, *vita*).
1912	Paul Ehrlich discovers a chemical cure for syphilis. This is the first chemotherapeutic agent for a bacterial disease.
1912	The U.S. Public Health Service is established.
1914	Frederick William Twort, English bacteriologist, and Felix Hubert D'Herelle, Canadian-Russian physician, independently discover bacteriophages, viruses that destroy bacteria.
1916	Felix Hubert D'Herelle carries out further studies of the agent that destroys bacterial colonies and gives it the name "bacteriophage" (bacteria eating agent). D'Herelle and others unsuccessfully attempt to use bacteriophages as bactericidal therapeutic agents.
1918	A global influenza pandemic caused by a virulent strain of Spanish influenza kills more people than the number of soldiers who died fighting during World War I (1914–1918). By the end of 1918, approximately 25 million people have died from influenza.
1918	Thomas Hunt Morgan and coworkers publish *The Physical Basis of Heredity,* a survey of the development of the new science of genetics.
1919	James Brown uses blood agar to study the destruction of blood cells by the bacterium *Streptococcus.* He observes three reactions that he designates alpha, beta, and gamma.
1919	The Health Organization of the League of Nations is established for the prevention and control of disease around the world.

1920	Frederick Grant Banting, Canadian physician, Charles Best, Scottish-American physiologist, and James B. Collip, Canadian biochemist, discover insulin. They develop a method of extracting insulin from the human pancreas. The insulin is then injected into the blood of diabetics to lower their blood sugar.
1922	Elmer Verner McCollum, American biochemist, discovers vitamin D.
1922	Herbert McLean Evans, American physician, and colleagues discover vitamin E.
1924	Albert Jan Kluyver publishes *Unity and Diversity in the Metabolism of Microorganisms.* He demonstrates that different microorganisms have common metabolic pathways of oxidation, fermentation, and synthesis of certain compounds. Kluyver also states that life on Earth depends on microbial activity.
1927	Thomas Rivers publishes a paper that differentiates bacteria from viruses, establishing virology as a field of study that is distinct from bacteriology.
1928	Fred Griffith discovers that certain strains of pneumococci could undergo some kind of transmutation of type. After injecting mice with living R type pneumococci and heat-killed S type, Griffith is able to isolate living virulent bacteria from the infected mice. Griffith suggests that some unknown "principle" had transformed the harmless R strain of the pneumococcus to the virulent S strain.
1929	Francis O. Holmes introduces the technique of local lesion as a means of measuring the concentration of tobacco mosaic virus. The method becomes extremely important in virus purification.
1929	Frank M. Burnet and Margot McKie report critical insights into the phenomenon known as lysogeny (the inherited ability of bacteria to produce bacteriophage in the absence of infection). Burnet and McKie postulate that the presence of a lytic unit is a normal hereditary component of lysogenic bacteria. The lytic unit is proposed to be capable of liberating bacteriophage when it is activated by certain conditions. This concept is confirmed in the 1950s.

1929   Scottish biochemist Alexander Fleming discovers penicillin. He observes that the mold *Penicillium notatum* inhibits the growth of some bacteria. This is the first antibacterial agent, and it opens a new era of "wonder drugs" to combat infection and disease.

1930   Max Theiler demonstrates the advantages of using mice as experimental animals for research on animal viruses. Theiler uses mice in his studies of the yellow fever virus.

1930   The U.S. Food, Drug, and Insecticide Administration is renamed the Food and Drug Administration (FDA).

1931   Alice Miles Woodruff and Ernest W. Goodpasture demonstrate the advantages of using the membranes of the chick embryo to study the mechanism of viral infections.

1931   Joseph Needham publishes his landmark work *Chemical Embryology,* which emphasizes the relationship between biochemistry and embryology.

1931   Rules outlined in Germany's "Regulation on New Therapy and Experimentation" call for consent of patients in medical experimentation and for experiments to be tried on animal subjects prior to testing in humans, as well as other ethical standards for medical experimentation.

1931   Ernst Ruska and Max Knoll develop the first electron microscope. Ruska is awarded the Nobel Prize in 1986 for his work on electron microscopy.

1932   Hans Adolf Krebs, German biochemist, describes and names the citric acid cycle.

1932   William J. Elford and Christopher H. Andrewes develop methods of estimating the sizes of viruses by using a series of membranes as filters. Later studies prove that the viral sizes obtained by this method were comparable to those obtained by electron microscopy.

1932   In an experiment based in Tuskegee, Alabama, African-American sharecroppers become unknowing and unwilling subjects of experimentation on the untreated natural course of syphilis. Even after penicillin came into use in the 1940s, the men remained untreated.

1933   The Twenty-first Amendment to the Constitution repeals the Eighteenth Amendment, reversing the prohibition laws that ban the sale and consumption of alcohol in United States.

1934   John Marrack begins a series of studies that lead to the formation of the hypothesis governing the association between an antigen and the corresponding antibody.

1935   Wendall Meredith Stanley, American biochemist, discovers that viruses are partly protein-based. By purifying and crystallizing viruses, he enables scientists to identify the precise molecular structure and propagation modes of several viruses.

1936   George P. Berry and Helen M. Dedrick report that the Shope virus could be "transformed" into myxomatosis/Sanarelli virus. This virological curiosity was variously referred to as "transformation," "recombination," and "multiplicity of reactivation." Subsequent research suggests that it is the first example of genetic interaction between animal viruses, but some scientists warn that the phenomenon might indicate the danger of reactivation of virus particles in vaccines and in cancer research.

1937   The Marijuana Tax Act effectively criminalizes the use and possession of marijuana, even for medical reasons.

1938   Emory L. Ellis and Max Delbrück perform studies on phage replication that mark the beginning of modern phage work. They introduce the one-step growth experiment, which demonstrates that after bacteriophages attack bacteria, replication of the virus occurs within the bacterial host during a latent period, after which viral progeny are released in a burst.

1938   The Federal Food, Drug, and Cosmetics Act gives regulatory powers over such products to the Food and Drug Administration.

1938   Japanese scientists conduct experiments on Chinese prisoners.

1939   Ernest Chain and H. W. Florey refine the purification of penicillin, allowing the mass production of the antibiotic.

1939   Richard E. Shope reports that the swine influenza virus survived between epidemics in an intermediate host. This discovery is an important step in revealing the role of intermediate hosts in perpetuating specific diseases.

1940 Helmuth Ruska, brother of Ernst Ruska, the inventor of the electron microscope, obtains the first electron microscopic image of a virus.

1941 Nazi scientists perform experiments exposing Buchenwald and Natzweiler concentration camp prisoners to typhus and, in separate experiments, phosphorus burns.

1942 Jules Freund and Katherine McDermott identify adjuvants (e.g., paraffin oil) that act to boost antibody production.

1942 Salvador Luria and Max Delbrück demonstrate statistically that inheritance of genetic characteristics in bacteria follows the principles of genetic inheritance proposed by Charles Darwin. For their work, the two (along with Alfred Day Hershey) are awarded the 1969 Nobel Prize in Medicine or Physiology.

1942 Selman Waksman suggests the word antibiotics be used to identify antimicrobial compounds that are made by bacteria.

1942 Nazi scientists perform experiments subjecting Dachau concentration camp prisoners to high altitude conditions (freezing and low pressure) and, in other experiments, diseases such as malaria.

1944 Salvador E. Luria and Alfred Day Hershey prove that mutations occur in bacterial viruses, and develop methods to distinguish the mutations from other alterations.

1944 A Manhattan Project subprogram experiments with the effects of radioactive implants on U.S. soldiers at Oak Ridge, Tennessee.

1944 U.S. Public Health Service Act passed.

1944 University of Chicago Medical School professor Dr. Alf Alving conducts malaria experiments on more than 400 Illinois prisoners.

1945 Joshua Lederberg and Edward L. Tatum demonstrate genetic recombination in bacteria.

1946 The Communicable Disease Center is organized in Atlanta, Georgia, as part of the U.S. Public Health Service. Its first mission is to prevent the spread of malaria. The agency eventually becomes the Centers for Disease Control and Prevention, a division of the U.S. Department of Health and Human Services.

1946 Felix Bloch and Edward Mills Purcell develop nuclear magnetic resonance (NMR) as a viable tool for observation and analysis.

1946 Max Delbrück and W. T. Bailey, Jr. publish a paper titled *Induced Mutations in Bacterial Viruses*. Despite some confusion about the nature of the phenomenon in question, this paper establishes the fact that genetic recombinations occur during mixed infections with bacterial viruses. Alfred Hershey and R. Rotman make the discovery of genetic recombination in bacteriophage simultaneously and independently. Hershey and his colleagues prove that this phenomenon can be used for genetic analyses. They construct a genetic map of phage particles and show that phage genes can be arranged in a linear fashion.

1948 James V. Neel reports evidence that sickle-cell disease is caused by a Mendelian autosomal recessive trait.

1948 The World Health Organization's Constitution comes into force, as proposed by diplomats at the formation of the United Nations in 1945.

1948 Alfred Kinsey publishes *Sexual Behavior in the Human Male*.

1949 Atomic Energy Commission's "Green Run" study takes place, using intentional release of radioactive iodine and xenon 133 over Hanford, Washington.

1949 John F. Ender, Thomas H. Weller, and Frederick C. Robbins publish "Cultivation of Polio Viruses in Cultures of Human Embryonic Tissues." The report by Enders and coworkers is a landmark in establishing techniques for the cultivation of poliovirus in cultures on non-neural tissue and for further virus research. The technique leads to the polio vaccine and other advances in virology.

1949 Macfarlane Burnet and his colleagues begin studies that lead to the immunological tolerance hypothesis and the clonal selection theory. Burnet receives the 1960 Nobel

Prize in Physiology or Medicine for this research.

1949   The role of mitochondria is revealed. These slender filaments within the cell, which participate in protein synthesis and lipid metabolism, are the cell's source of energy.

1950   British physician Douglas Bevis demonstrates that amniocentesis can be used to test fetuses for Rh-factor incompatibility.

1950   Robert Hungate develops the roll-tube culture technique, which is the first technique that allows anaerobic bacteria to be grown in culture.

1950   Dr. Joseph Stokes of the University of Pennsylvania infects 200 women prisoners with viral hepatitis.

1951   Esther M. Lederberg discovers a lysogenic strain of *Escherichia coli*, K12, and isolates a new bacteriophage, called lambda.

1952   Alfred Hershey and Martha Chase publish their landmark paper "Independent Functions of Viral Protein and Nucleic Acid in Growth of Bacteriophage." The famous "blender experiment" suggests that DNA is the genetic material. When bacteria are infected by a virus, at least 80 percent of the viral DNA enter the cell and at least 80 percent of the viral protein remain outside.

1952   James T. Park and Jack L. Strominger demonstrate that penicillin blocks the synthesis of the peptidoglycan of bacteria. This represents the first demonstration of the action of a natural antibiotic.

1952   Karl Maramorosch demonstrates that some viruses could multiply in both plants and insects. This work leads to new questions about the origins of viruses.

1952   Esther and Joshua Lederberg develop the replica plating method that allows for the rapid screening of large numbers of genetic markers. They use the technique to demonstrate that resistance to antibacterial agents such as antibiotics and viruses is not induced by the presence of the antibacterial agent.

1952   Renato Dulbecco develops a practical method for studying animal viruses in cell cultures. His so-called plaque method is comparable to that used in studies of bacterial viruses, and the method proves to be important in genetic studies of viruses. These methods are described in his paper *Production of Plaques in Monolayer Tissue Cultures by Single Particles of an Animal Virus.*

1952   William Hayes isolates a strain of *Escherichia coli* that produces recombinants thousands of times more frequently than previously observed. The new strain of K12 is named Hfr (high-frequency recombination) Hayes.

1953   Jonas Salk begins testing a polio vaccine comprised of a mixture of killed viruses.

1954   Seymour Benzer deduces the fine structure of the rII region of the bacteriophage T4 of *Escherichia coli*, and coins the terms cistron, recon, and muton.

1955   Fred L. Schaffer and Carlton E. Schwerdt report on their successful crystallization of the polio virus. Their achievement is the first successful crystallization of an animal virus.

1955   Heinz Fraenkel-Conrat and Robley C. Williams prove that tobacco mosaic virus can be reconstituted from its nucleic acid and protein subunits. The reconstituted particles exhibit normal morphology and infectivity.

1956   Alfred Gierer and Gerhard Schramm demonstrate that naked RNA from tobacco mosaic virus is infectious. Subsequently, infectious RNA preparations are obtained for certain animal viruses.

1956   The American Medical Association defines alcoholism as a disease.

1957   Alick Isaacs and Jean Lindemann discover interferon, a protein made by the immune system that responds to pathogens such as viruses.

1957   The World Health Organization advances the oral polio vaccine developed by Albert Sabin as a safer alternative to the Salk vaccine.

1959   English biochemist Rodney Porter begins studies that lead to the discovery of the structure of antibodies. Porter receives the 1972 Nobel Prize in Physiology or Medicine for this research.

1959   Sydney Brenner and Robert W. Horne publish a paper titled "A Negative Staining

Method for High Resolution Electron Microscopy of Viruses." The two researchers develop a method for studying the architecture of viruses at the molecular level using the electron microscope.

1961   French pathologist Jacques Miller discovers the role of the thymus in cellular immunity.

1961   Noel Warner establishes the physiological distinction between the cellular and humoral immune responses.

1961   Rachel Carson publishes *Silent Spring,* exposing harmful effects of pollutants, including DDT, a commonly used insecticide.

1962   After thousands of birth deformities are blamed on the drug, Thalidomide is withdrawn from the market.

1962   The U.S. Food and Drug Administration requires multiphase human clinical trials before drugs can be released to market.

1964   The first Surgeon General's Report on Smoking and Health is released, and the U.S. government first acknowledges and publicizes that cigarette smoking is a leading cause of cancer, bronchitis, and emphysema.

1964   The World Medical Association adopts the Helsinki Declaration, a set of ethical principles governing the use of human subjects in medical experimentation.

1965   At the height of tobacco use in America, surveys show 52 percent of adult men and 32 percent of adult women use tobacco products.

1966   Bruce Ames develops a test to screen for compounds that cause mutations, including those that are cancer causing. The so-called Ames test utilizes the bacterium *Salmonella typhimurium.*

1966   The U.S. Food and Drug Administration and National Academy of Sciences begin investigation of the effectiveness of 4,000 drugs previously approved because they were safe, though they had not been proven effective.

1966   The United States passes the Fair Packaging and Labeling Act.

1966   The U.S. National Institutes of Health Office for Protection of Research Subjects (OPRR) is created.

1967   Dr. Christiaan Barnard performs the first successful transplant of a human heart. The recipient, Louis Washkansky, survives for 18 days.

1967   British physician M. H. Pappworth publishes "Human Guinea Pigs," advising "No doctor has the right to choose martyrs for science or for the general good."

1968   The U.S. Food and Drug Administration administratively moves to the U.S. Public Health Service.

1968   Werner Arber discovers that bacteria defend themselves against viruses by producing DNA-cutting enzymes. These enzymes quickly become important tools for molecular biologists.

1969   Julius Adler discovers protein receptors in bacteria that function in the detection of chemical attractants and repellents. The so-called chemoreceptors are critical for the directed movement of bacteria that comes to be known as chemotaxis.

1969   Max Delbrück, Alfred D. Hershey, and Salvador E. Luria are awarded the Nobel Prize in Medicine or Physiology for their discoveries concerning the replication mechanism and the genetic structure of viruses.

1970   The Controlled Substance Act (CSA) puts strict controls on the production, import, and prescription of amphetamines. Many amphetamine forms, particularly diet pills, are removed from the over-the-counter market.

1970   The U.S. Food and Drug Administration requires a patient information package insert in oral contraceptives. The insert must contain information regarding specific risks and benefits.

1970   The U.S. Congress passes the Controlled Substance Act (CSA).

1971   Médecins Sans Frontières (MSF) is founded by a group of young French doctors to aid victims of conflict and disaster. Known in English as Doctors Without Borders, MSF is awarded the Nobel Peace Prize in 1999 "in recognition of the organization's pioneering humanitarian work on several continents."

1972   Recombinant technology emerges as one of the most powerful techniques of molecular biology. Scientists are able to splice together pieces of DNA to form recombinant genes. As the potential uses, therapeutic and industrial, became increasingly clear, scientists and venture capitalists establish biotechnology companies.

1973   Herbert Wayne Boyer and Stanley H. Cohen create recombinant genes by cutting DNA molecules with restriction enzymes. These experiments mark the beginning of genetic engineering.

1974   Peter Doherty and Rolf Zinkernagl discover the basis of immune determination of self and non-self.

1975   César Milstein and George Kohler create monoclonal antibodies.

1975   David Baltimore, Renato Dulbecco, and Howard Temin share the Nobel Prize in Medicine or Physiology for their discoveries concerning the interaction between tumor viruses and the genetic material of the cell and the discovery of reverse transcriptase.

1975   John R. Hughes, Scottish physiologist, and others discover enkephalin. This first known opioid peptide, popularly called brain morphine, occurs naturally in the brain, indicating that the brain's chemicals block the transmission of pain signals.

1975   Scientists at an international meeting in Asilomar, California, call for the adoption of guidelines regulating recombinant DNA experimentation.

1975   E. O. Wilson publishes *Sociobiology*, proposing the interrelation of biology, human behavior, and culture.

1976   The U.S. Federal Bureau of Investigation (FBI) warns "crack" cocaine use and cocaine addiction are on the rise in the United States.

1976   The first outbreak of Ebola virus is observed in Zaire, Africa. There are more than 300 cases with a 90 percent death rate.

1976   Michael J. Bishop, Harold Elliot Varmus, and coworkers establish definitive evidence of the oncogene hypothesis. They discover that normal genes can malfunction and cause cells to become cancerous.

1976   Swine flu is identified in soldiers stationed in New Jersey. The virus, identified as H1N1, causes concern due to its similarities to H1N1 responsible for Spanish flu pandemic of 1918. President Gerald Ford

calls for an emergency vaccination program. More than 20 deaths result from Guillain-Barre syndrome related to the vaccine.

1977   Philip Allen Sharp and Richard John Roberts independently discover that the DNA making up a particular gene could be present in the genome as several separate segments. Although both Roberts and Sharp use a common cold-causing virus, called adenovirus, as their model system, researchers later find split genes in higher organisms, including humans. Sharp and Roberts are subsequently awarded the Nobel Prize in Medicine or Physiology in 1993 for the discovery of split genes.

1977   The first known human fatality from H5N1 avian flu occurs in Hong Kong.

1977   The World Health Organization develops the first list of essential medicines, describing them as "those drugs that satisfy the health care needs of the majority of the population; they should therefore be available at all times in adequate amounts and in appropriate dosage forms, at a price the community can afford."

1977   The last reported smallpox case is recorded. Ultimately, the World Health Organization declares the disease eradicated in 1980.

1978   The Alma Ata Declaration, one of the first declarations to promote health as a basic human right, is adopted at the International Conference on Primary Health Care in Almaty (present day Kazakhstan). The resolution calls for building health care capacity in rural as well as urban areas and encourages partnership with community health workers and traditional healers for extending the reach of health care providers.

1978   Louise Brown, the world's first "test-tube baby," is born.

1981   The U.S. Centers for Disease Control and Prevention recognizes acquired immune deficiency syndrome (AIDS) as an emergent infectious disease.

1981   Karl Illmensee clones baby mice.

1982   The U.S. Food and Drug Administration approves the first genetically engineered drug, a form of human insulin produced by bacteria.

1983   *Escherichia coli* O157:H7 is identified as a human pathogen.

1983   Luc Montainer and Robert Gallo discover the human immunodeficiency virus (HIV) that is believed to cause acquired immune deficiency syndrome (AIDS).

1984   Steen A. Willadsen successfully clones a sheep.

1985   Alec Jeffreys develops genetic fingerprinting, a method of using DNA polymorphisms (unique sequences of DNA) to identify individuals. The method, which has been used in paternity, immigration, and murder cases, is generally referred to as DNA fingerprinting.

1985   American molecular biologist and physician Leroy Hood leads a team that discovers the genes that code for the T cell receptor.

1985   Japanese molecular biologist Susuma Tonegawa discovers the genes that code for immunoglobulins. He receives the 1986 Nobel Prize in Physiology or Medicine for this discovery.

1986   Congress passes the National Childhood Vaccine Injury Act, requiring patient information on vaccines and reporting of adverse events after vaccination.

1986   Robert A. Weinberg and coworkers isolate a gene that inhibits growth and appears to suppress retinoblastoma (a cancer of the retina).

1986   The U.S. Food and Drug Administration approves the first genetically engineered human vaccine for hepatitis B.

1986   A U.S. Surgeon General's report focuses on the hazards of environmental tobacco smoke (secondhand smoke) to nonsmokers.

1987   The U.S. Congress charters a Department of Energy (DOE) advisory committee, the Health and Environmental Research Advisory Committee (HERAC), that recommends a 15-year, multidisciplinary, scientific, and technological undertaking to map and sequence the human genome. DOE designates multidisciplinary human genome centers. National Institute of General Medical Sciences at the National Institutes of Health begins funding genome projects.

1988   Harvard and Dow Chemical patent a genetically engineered mouse with plans to use it in cancer studies.

1988   The Human Genome Organization (HUGO) is established by scientists in order to coordinate international efforts to sequence the human genome.

1989   Cells from one cow embryo are used to produce seven cloned calves.

1990   Michael R. Blaese and French W. Anderson conduct the first gene replacement therapy experiment on a four-year-old girl with adenosine deaminase (ADA) deficiency, an immune-system disorder. T cells from the patient are isolated and exposed to retroviruses containing an RNA copy of a normal ADA gene. The treated cells are returned to her body where they help restore some degree of function to her immune system.

1990   The U.S. National Council on Alcoholism and Drug Dependence, along with the American Society of Addictive Medicine, defines alcoholism as a chronic disease influenced by genetic, psychological, and environmental factors. Alcoholism is described as a loss of control over drinking and a preoccupation with drinking despite negative consequences to one's physical, mental, and emotional makeup as well as one's work and family life.

1990   The U.S. Supreme Court decides in *Employment Division v. Smith* that the religious use of peyote by Native Americans is not protected by the First Amendment.

1990   The U.S. Congress passes the Nutrition Labeling and Education Act, permitting manufacturers to make some health claims for foods, including dietary supplements.

1991   Mary-Claire King concludes, based on her studies of the chromosomes of women in cancer-prone families, that a gene on chromosome 17 causes the inherited form of breast cancer and also increases the risk of ovarian cancer.

1991   The gender of a mouse is changed at the embryo stage.

1991   The Genome Database, a human chromosome mapping data repository, is established.

1992   The United Nations' Earth Summit is held in Rio de Janeiro, Brazil. The United Nations Framework Convention on Climate Change (UNFCCC) is adopted, with the goal of stabilizing "greenhouse gas concentrations in the atmosphere at a level that would prevent dangerous anthropogenic interference with the climate system."

1992   American and British scientists develop a technique for testing embryos *in vitro* for genetic abnormalities such as cystic fibrosis and hemophilia.

1992   U.S. Congress passes the Prescription Drug User Fee Act requiring the U.S. Food and Drug Administration to use product application fees collected from drug manufacturers to hire more reviewers to assess applications.

1992   Craig Venter establishes The Institute for Genomic Research (TIGR) in Rockville, Maryland. TIGR later sequences the genome of *Haemophilus influenzae* and many other bacterial genomes.

1992   The U.S. Army begins collecting blood and tissue samples from all new recruits as part of a "genetic dog tag" program aimed at better identification of soldiers killed in combat.

1993   An international research team led by Daniel Cohen of the Center for the Study of Human Polymorphisms in Paris produces a rough map of all 23 pairs of human chromosomes.

1993   George Washington University researchers clone human embryos and nurture them in a Petri dish for several days. The project provokes protests from ethicists, politicians, and critics of genetic engineering.

1993   Hantavirus emerges in the United States in a 1993 outbreak on a Four Corners area (the juncture of Utah, Colorado, New Mexico, and Arizona) Native American Reservation. The resulting hantavirus pulmonary syndrome (HPS) has a 43 percent mortality rate.

1993   Scientists identify p53, a tumor suppressor gene, as the crucial factor preventing uncontrolled cell growth. In addition, scientists find that p53 performs a variety of functions ensuring cell health.

1994   Geneticists determine that DNA repair enzymes perform several vital functions, including preserving genetic information and protecting the cell from cancer.

1994   The Human Genome Project website is made available to researchers and the public.

1994   The U.S. Congress passes the Dietary Supplement Health and Education Act expressly defining a dietary supplement as a vitamin, a mineral, an herb or other botanical, an amino acid, or any other "dietary substance." This law prohibits claims that herbs can treat diseases or disorders, but it allows more general health claims about the effect of herbs on the "structure or function" of the body or about the "well-being" they induce. Under this law, the Food and Drug Administration bears the burden of having to prove an herbal supplement is unsafe before restricting its use. This law also establishes the Office of Dietary Supplements within the National Institutes of Health to promote and compile research on dietary supplements.

1995   Public awareness of the potential use of chemical or biological weapons by terrorist groups increases following the release of sarin gas in a Tokyo subway by the Japanese cult Aum Shinrikyo. The gas kills a dozen people and sends thousands to hospitals.

1995   Researchers at Duke University Medical Center report that they have transplanted hearts from genetically altered pigs into baboons. All three transgenic pig hearts survive at least a few hours, suggesting that xenotransplants (cross-species organ transplantation) might be possible.

1995   The sequence of *Mycoplasma genitalium* is completed. *Mycoplasma genitalium*, regarded as the smallest known bacterium, is considered a model of the minimum number of genes needed for independent existence.

1996   Chris Paszty and co-workers successfully employ genetic engineering techniques to create mice with sickle-cell anemia, a serious human blood disorder.

1996   H5N1 avian flu virus is identified in Guangdong, China.

1996   Researchers C. Cheng and L. Olson demonstrate that the spinal cord can be regenerated in adult rats. Experimenting on rats with severed spinal cords, Cheng and Olson use peripheral nerves to connect white matter and gray matter.

1996   Researchers find that abuse and violence can alter a child's brain chemistry, placing him or her at risk for various problems including drug abuse, cognitive disabilities, and mental illness later in life.

1996   Scientists discover a link between apoptosis (cellular suicide, a natural process whereby the body eliminates useless cells) gone awry and several neurodegenerative conditions, including Alzheimer's disease.

1996   Dolly, the world's first cloned sheep, is born. Several European Union nations ban human cloning. The U.S. Congress debates a bill to ban human cloning.

1996   Scientists report further evidence that individuals with two mutant copies of the CC-CLR-5 gene are generally resistant to HIV infection.

1996   The South Carolina Supreme Court decides in favor of the Medical University of South Carolina (MUSC) policy to secretly test pregnant patients for cocaine use. The court upholds MUSC's drug testing in an effort to protect the unborn. Cocaine greatly increases the chances of a miscarriage. Low birth weight "crack babies" have 20 times as great a risk of dying in their first month of life as normal weight babies. Those who survive are at increased risk for birth defects. Subsequently, in 2001 the U.S. Supreme Court rules that based on the Fourth Amendment, hospitals cannot test pregnant women for drugs without their consent and then inform the police.

1996   William R. Bishai and coworkers report that SigF, a gene in the tuberculosis bacterium, enables the bacterium to enter a dormant stage.

1997   The Kyoto Protocol, an international treaty on climate change, is adopted by the United Nations. Signatories are legally bound to emission reduction targets.

1997   Donald Wolf and coworkers announce that they have cloned rhesus monkeys from early stage embryos, using nuclear transfer methods.

1997   Researchers identify a gene that plays a crucial role in establishing normal left-right configuration during organ development.

1997   The DNA sequence of *Escherichia coli* is completed.

1997   The United States passes the Food and Drug Administration Modernization Act and reauthorizes the Prescription Drug User Fee Act of 1992. The changes in policy allow for a more rapid review of drugs and delivery devices. The Act also expands U.S. Food and Drug Administration regulatory powers over advertising, especially with regard to health claims.

1997   William Jacobs and Barry Bloom create a biological entity that combines the characteristics of a bacterial virus and a plasmid (a DNA structure that functions and replicates independently of the chromosomes). This entity is capable of triggering mutations in *Mycobacterium tuberculosis*.

1998   Craig Venter forms a company (later named Celera), and predicts that the company will decode the entire human genome within three years. Celera plans to use a "whole genome shotgun" method, which would assemble the genome without using maps.

1998   The U.S. Department of Energy funds bacterial artificial chromosome and sequencing projects.

1998   Dolly, the first cloned sheep, gives birth to a lamb that had been conceived by a natural mating with a Welsh Mountain ram. Researchers say the birth of Bonnie proves that Dolly is a fully normal and healthy animal.

1998   Immunologist Ellen Heber-Katz, researcher at the Wistar Institute in Philadelphia, reports that a strain of laboratory mice can regenerate tissue in their ears, closing holes which scientists had created for identification purposes. This discovery reopens the discussion on possible regeneration in humans.

1998   Scientists find that an adult human's brain can replace cells. This discovery heralds potential breakthroughs in neurology.

1998   Two research teams succeed in growing embryonic stem cells.

1999   Scientists announce the complete sequencing of the DNA making up human chromosome 22. The first complete human chromosome sequence is published in December 1999.

Twenty-First Century

2000   The United Nations, at its Millennium Summit, establishes eight international Millennium Development Goals. They are: (1) eradicate extreme poverty and hunger; (2) achieve universal primary education; (3) promote gender equality and empower women; (4) reduce child mortality; (5) improve maternal health; (6) combat HIV/AIDS, malaria, and other diseases; (7) ensure environmental stability; and (8) create a global partnership for development. These goals are agreed to by all countries of the world.

2000   The first volume of *Annual Review of Genomics and Human Genetics* is published. Genomics is defined as the new science dealing with the identification and characterization of genes and their arrangement in chromosomes and human genetics as the science devoted to understanding the origin and expression of human individual uniqueness.

2000   The National Cancer Institute (NCI) estimates that 3,000 lung cancer deaths, and as many as 40,000 cardiac deaths per year among adult nonsmokers in the United States can be attributed to passive smoke or environmental tobacco smoke (ETS).

2000   The U.S. Congress considers but does not pass the Pain Relief Promotion Act, which would have amended the Controlled Substances Act to say that relieving pain or discomfort—within the context of professional medicine—is a legitimate use of controlled substances. The bill does not pass in the Senate.

2000   The U.S. Congress passes a transportation spending bill that includes the establishment of a national standard for drunk driving for adults at a 0.08 percent blood alcohol level. States are required to adopt this stricter standard by 2004 or face penalties. By 2001, more than half the states adopt this stricter standard. All states adopt it by 2005.

2000   The U.S. Drug Addiction Treatment Act allows opioids to be distributed to physicians for the treatment of opioid dependence.

2001   In February 2001, the complete draft sequence of the human genome is published. The public sequence data is published in the British journal *Nature* and the Celera sequence is published in the American journal *Science*. Increased knowledge of the human genome allows greater specificity in pharmacological research and drug interaction studies.

2001   Scientists from the Whitehead Institute announce test results that show patterns of errors in cloned animals that might explain why such animals die early and exhibit a number of developmental problems. The report stimulates new debate on ethical issues related to cloning. In the journal *New Scientist*, Ian Wilmut, the scientist who headed the research team that cloned the sheep Dolly, argues that the findings demand "a universal moratorium against copying people."

2001   The company Advanced Cell Technology announces that its researchers have created cloned human embryos that grew to the six cell stage.

2001   The United States announces that the National Institutes of Health will fund research on only 64 embryonic stem cell lines created from human embryos.

2001   Research conducted by the U.S. National Institute of Drug Abuse asserts that children exposed to cocaine prior to birth sustain long-lasting brain changes. Eight years after birth, children exposed to cocaine prior to birth had detectable brain chemistry differences from children not exposed to the drug prior to birth.

2001   The U.S. Office of National Drug Control Policy's annual report asserts that about 80 percent of Americans abusing illegal drugs used marijuana.

2001   Study titled "Global Illicit Drug Trends," conducted by the United Nations Office for Drug Control and Crime Prevention, estimates that 14 million people use cocaine worldwide.

2001   The annual Monitoring the Future study, conducted by the University of Michigan and funded by the National Institute on Drug Abuse, finds that 17.1 percent of eighth-graders had abused inhalants at some point in their lives.

2001 The U.S. military endorses the situational temporary usefulness of caffeine, recommending it as a safe and effective stimulant for its soldiers in good health.

2001 The U.S. Supreme Court rules 8 to 0 in *United States vs. Oakland Cannabis Buyers' Cooperative* that the cooperatives permitted under California law to sell marijuana to medical patients who had a physician's approval to use the drug were unconstitutional under federal law.

2001 In August 2001, U.S. President George W. Bush announces the United States will allow and support limited forms of stem cell growth and research.

2001 Terrorists attack the United States on September 11, 2001, and kill thousands by crashing airplanes into the World Trade Center buildings in New York City. Several weeks later, an unknown terrorist sends four mailings, including letters to U.S. government leaders, that contain anthrax. The anthrax ultimately kills five people.

2002 Following the September 11, 2001, terrorist attacks on the United States, the Public Health Security and Bioterrorism Preparedness and Response Act of 2002 is passed in an effort to improve ability to prevent and respond to public health emergencies.

2002 Health Canada, the Canadian health regulatory agency, requests a voluntary recall of products containing both natural and chemical ephedra.

2002 In June 2002 traces of biological and chemical weapon agents are found in Uzbekistan on a military base used by U.S. troops fighting in Afghanistan. Early analysis dates and attributes the source of the contamination to former Soviet Union biological and chemical weapons programs that formerly utilized the base.

2002 The Best Pharmaceuticals for Children Act passes in an effort to improve safety and efficacy of patented and off-patent medicines for children.

2002 The planned destruction of stocks of smallpox causing Variola virus at the two remaining depositories in the United States and Russia is delayed over fears that large scale production of vaccine might be needed in the event of a bioterrorist action.

2003 An unusual pneumonia is reported in Hanoi, Vietnam. It is later identified as SARS.

2003 World Health Organization (WHO) officer Dr. Carlo Urbani identifies sudden acute respiratory syndrome or SARS. Urbani later dies of the disease.

2003 The U.S. Commissioner of Food and Drugs establishes an obesity working group to deal with the U.S. obesity epidemic. In March 2004 the group releases "Calories Count: Report of the Obesity Working Group."

2003 Differences in influenza outbreaks in Hong Kong between 1997 and 2003 cause investigators to conclude that the H5N1 virus has mutated.

2003 The United States invades Iraq and finds chemical, biological, and nuclear weapons programs but no actual weapons.

2003 The U.S. Food and Drug Adminsitration requires food labels to include trans fat content. This is the first major change to the nutrition facts panel on foods since 1993.

2003 SARS is added to the list of quarantinable diseases in the United States.

2003 The World Health Organization Global Influenza Surveillance Network intensifies work on development of a H5N1 vaccine for humans.

2004 Based on results from controlled clinical studies indicating that Cox-2 selective agents may be connected to an elevated risk of serious cardiovascular events, including heart attack and stroke, the U.S. Food and Drug Administration issues a public health advisory urging health professionals to limit the use of these drugs.

2004 The U.S. Food and Drug Administration bans dietary supplements containing ephedrine.

2004 The U.S. Food Allergy Labeling and Consumer Protection Act requires the labeling of foods that contain proteins derived from peanuts, soybeans, cow's milk, eggs, fish, crustacean shellfish, tree nuts, and wheat, which account for a majority of food allergies.

2004   In the United States, the Project BioShield Act of 2004 authorizes U.S. government agencies to expedite procedures related to rapid distribution of treatments as countermeasures to chemical, biological, and nuclear attack.

2004   The most powerful earthquake in more than 40 years occurs underwater off the Indonesian island of Sumatra. The resulting tsunami produces a disaster of unprecedented proportion in the modern era, affecting 14 countries and killing over 230,000 by some estimates. Some experts stated it was one of the costliest, longest, and most difficult recovery periods ever endured as a result of a natural disaster.

2005   H5N1 virus, responsible for avian flu, moves from Asia to Europe. The World Health Organization attempts to coordinate multinational disaster and containment plans. Some nations begin to stockpile antiviral drugs.

2005   Hurricane Katrina slams into the U.S. Gulf Coast, causing levee breaks and massive flooding in New Orleans. Damage is extensive across the coasts of Louisiana, Mississippi, and Alabama. The Federal Emergency Management Agency is widely criticized for lack of coordination in relief efforts. Three other major hurricanes make landfall in the United States within a two-year period, straining relief and medical supply efforts. Long-term health studies begin of populations in devastated areas.

2005   The World Health Assembly adopts International Health Regulations (IHR) 2005, the purpose of which is "to prevent, protect against, control and provide a public health response to the international spread of disease in ways that are commensurate with and restricted to public health risks, and which avoid unnecessary interference with international traffic and trade." The IHR, which would enter into force in 2007, are binding on 194 countries.

2005   The U.S. Food and Drug Administration Drug Safety Board is founded.

2005   A massive 7.6-magnitude earthquake leaves more than three million homeless and without food or basic medical supplies in the Kashmir mountains between India and Pakistan. Approximately 80,000 die.

2006   More than a dozen people are diagnosed with avian flu in Turkey, but United Nations health experts assure the public that human-to-human transmission is still rare and only suspected in a few cases in Asia.

2006   The European Union bans the importation of avian feathers (non-treated feathers) from countries neighboring or close to Turkey.

2006   In an effort to aid vaccine development, the WHO influenza pandemic task force officials ask that all countries share H5N1 (avian flu) virus samples and genetic sequencing results.

2006   Mad cow disease (bovine spongiform encephalopathy) is confirmed in an Alabama cow as the third reported case in the United States.

2007   The Intergovernmental Panel on Climate Change scientists, composed of scientists from 113 countries, issues a consensus report stating that global warming is caused by humans and predicting that warmer temperatures and rises in sea level will continue for centuries, unless humans begin to control their pollution.

2007   Studies announced in 2007 show the ability to create stem cells from cloned monkey embryos and normal adult skin cells rather than from destroyed human embryos. Stem cells are undifferentiated cells that can give rise to diverse types of differentiated (specialized) cells. The results of the studies offer a potential solution to ethical concerns about the origins of stem cells.

2007   Henrik Clausen at the University of Copenhagen in Denmark announces in the journal *Nature Biotechnology* the discovery of enzymes (proteins that help control the rates of reaction) and a method to convert any blood type into the universal Type O, a discovery that could lead to reduction in blood shortages.

2007 The U.S. Food and Drug Administration concludes that food products containing meat or products from cloned animals and their offspring are safe for human consumption.

2007 The environmental group Greenpeace launches an attack on genetically modified corn developed by U.S. biotech company Monsanto, saying that rats fed on one variety developed liver and kidney problems.

2008 Agricultural testing demonstrates that a genetically modified, drought-tolerant wheat developed to boost harvests in water-challenged areas yields up to 20 percent more harvestable wheat than similar non-modified crops used as research controls.

2008 The 1000 Genome Project embarks on its mission to sequence the profiles of a large group of people in order to catalog and better understand variation in humans.

2008 Trials of an HIV vaccine on nonhuman primates show that the vaccine, based on cell-mediated immunity, fails to prevent HIV-1 infection. The vaccine also fails to produce significant reductions in levels of the virus in newly infected specimen. Researchers continue to test whether cell-mediated immune responses might reduce replication of the HIV virus.

2008 Oil and food prices rise sharply on a global scale, increasing dangers of famine and poverty. Critics contend increased prices for petroleum lead to the diversion of food crops to biofuel production.

2009 Pandemic influenza H1N1 is confirmed in over 208 countries and territories, leading to at least 12,220 deaths, according to the World Health Organization.

2009 Yellow fever outbreaks in several African nations lead to large scale emergency vaccination programs.

2009 The U.S. Food and Drug Administration (FDA) approves clinical trials for human embryonic stem cell therapies.

2010 The Patient Protection and Affordable Care Act is signed into law by U.S. President Barack Obama, making quality health care affordable and accessible to all U.S. citizens. The law brings the United States into line with the rest of the developed world of middle- and high-income countries in the provision of universal health coverage.

2010 The *Deepwater Horizon* oil spill in the Gulf of Mexico is effectively stopped when a well cap is successfully placed. Cleanup efforts include use of microorganisms selected, modified, and tested using an array of biotechnology.

2011 The U.S. Department of Agriculture introduces MyPlate, a nutrition guide using a graphic of a plate to illustrate recommended serving proportions from the five food groups. MyPlate is widely praised as simpler and easier to understand than food pyramid diagrams, which it replaces.

2011 An international team of researchers construct the first carbon-nanotube yarns to build artificial muscles.

2012 The first reported cases of Middle East respiratory syndrome (MERS), a new coronavirus, are noted in Saudi Arabia. MERS is linked to countries in or near the Arabian Peninsula.

2014 The World Health Organization (WHO) reports the largest outbreak of Ebola virus disease to date, beginning in Guinea, West Africa. The WHO statement says, "The Ebola epidemic ravaging parts of West Africa is the most severe acute public health emergency seen in modern times. Never before in recorded history has a biosafety level four pathogen infected so many people so quickly, over such a broad geographical area, for so long."

2014 The World Health Organization announces that the spread of polio—a serious vaccine-preventable disease—presents a renewed global public health risk, and requires a coordinated international response.

2015 Measles cases in the United States reach a 20-year high, fueled by an 18-state outbreak traced to unvaccinated children exposing others at California's Disneyland amusement park.

2015 On May 9, Liberia is declared Ebola free following the West African Ebola outbreak that began the previous year. The World Health Organization estimates that by that date, almost 27,000 people had been infected by Ebola and more than 11,000 had died in the outbreak.

Air Pollution: Urban, Industrial, and Transborder

⊕ Introduction

Air pollution is the contamination of air with substances known as pollutants that are harmful to the health of humans, animals, or plants, or which damage property. Air pollutants are either gases, liquids, or solids, and they come from a variety of sources, including industrial processes, transport, and domestic stoves.

According to the World Health Organization (WHO), air pollution was linked to around 7 million deaths around the world in 2012, mainly in low- and middle-income countries. Of these, around 4.3 million died as a result of exposure to indoor air pollution and 3.7 from outdoor air pollution. (Some deaths were linked to exposure to both indoor and outdoor pollution.) This means that air pollution is now considered to be the leading environmental health risk. In developed countries, air pollution levels have fallen in recent years because of strong environmental legislation and the adoption of cleaner energy technologies. The main problems arise in emerging economies, like China and India, where growth in industry and traffic have been allowed to emit unprecedented levels of air pollution. The other major issue is exposure to indoor air pollution from solid fuel stoves used for cooking and heating, which causes half of all deaths from pneumonia among children under the age of five.

The nature of air pollution varies with time and place, and it does not recognize national boundaries. The main gaseous pollutants are sulfur dioxide, nitrogen oxides, carbon monoxide, and hydrocarbons. Sulfur dioxide comes from burning fossil fuels, which have up to 7 percent sulfur content. Most sulfur dioxide comes from coal-fueled energy generation. If inhaled, sulfur dioxide causes, or exacerbates, respiratory disease. It also combines with moisture in the air to form sulfuric acid, or acid rain, which then deposits on surfaces. Such acid deposition damages buildings and works of art. Acid rain also affects water and soil, which damages fish and plants.

Nitrogen oxides is an umbrella term for a mixture of pollutants formed by the combustion of fossil fuels and emitted by vehicles, power stations, and industrial processes. They are formed when the combustion process oxidizes both atmospheric nitrogen and nitrogen present in the fuel itself. Initially, nitric oxide, which is harmless, is emitted, but that is soon oxidized in air to a number of secondary pollutants, including nitrogen dioxide and ground level ozone. Both have a negative impact on lung health.

Motor vehicles are also the main source of the two other major gaseous air pollutants. Carbon monoxide is a colorless, odorless gas formed through the incomplete combustion of fossil fuels. Exposure is dangerous to health because carbon monoxide binds to hemoglobin, which normally transports oxygen throughout the body. Reduced oxygenation exacerbates heart disease, and a reduced oxygen supply to the brain may be fatal. Meanwhile, hydrocarbons are also formed by incomplete fossil fuel combustion. Several hydrocarbons, such as benzene and formaldehyde, are classed as carcinogens. Hydrocarbons also contribute to the formation of ground level ozone by combining with nitrogen oxides in the presence of sunlight. Ozone is a major component of photochemical smog, a toxic combination of pollutants that contributes to poor air quality in cities like Los Angeles, California, where climatic condition and geographic location favor its formation. The smog causes coughing, chest pain, eye irritation, asthma, and bronchitis.

Particulate matter (PM) is the other significant type of air pollution and refers to a mixture of solid particles and liquid droplets present in the atmosphere. Such mixtures are known as aerosols and are composed of materials from many different sources. Major components of PM are sulfate, nitrates, ammonia, sodium chloride, black carbon, and water. Particles that come from combustion of fossil fuels are called smoke or soot and may have a particularly complex composition.

PM pollution is generally classified, and regulated, according to particle size. PM10s, also known as coarse particles, are those whose sizes range from 10 to 2.5 microns, while PM2.5s, also known as fine particles,

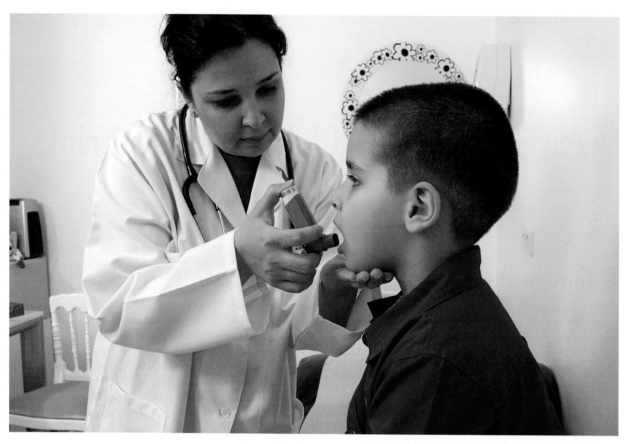

A doctor helps a little boy with an inhaler for his asthma. According to the U.S. Environmental Protection Agency, asthma can be caused or triggered by some types of air pollution. *© Levent Konuk/Shutterstock.com.*

range in size from 2.5 to 0.1 microns. The third category, ultrafine particles, are below 0.1 microns in size.

PM comes from industrial processes, vehicle exhausts, friction between tires and roads, and many other kinds of human activity. Particles larger than 10 microns tend to settle rapidly, but smaller ones remain airborne and may be inhaled. The distance they can penetrate into the respiratory system depends upon their size. Ultrafine particles can get into the bloodstream from the alveoli of the lungs. PM pollution has been shown to cause a number of health problems, including respiratory disease, heart disease, and lung cancer. Exposure to high levels of PM is linked to overall increases in rates of hospital admission and mortality, both daily and over time. More people are affected by PM than by any other form of pollution, according to the WHO.

Air pollution can be reduced and its impact on human health minimized by a combination of new technologies, environmental legislation and behavioral change. In the United States, the Clean Air Act was introduced in 1970 in response to concern about visible smog in many cities. It sets standards of levels of the main pollutants described above, plus lead. To achieve these standards, technologies such as catalytic converters are mandatory. Since pollution is not confined within national boundaries,

legislation on a multinational and global basis is also essential. Thus the European Commission has many policies designed to combat the ill effects of air pollution. Its clean air policy package, adopted in 2013, contains measures to ensure that existing targets are met in the short term and that new air quality objectives are met by 2030. This will be done by encouraging research and innovation and promoting international cooperation on transborder air pollution.

Air quality standards vary greatly around the world. While developed countries are now seeing the fruits of environmental legislation put into place many years ago, rapid urbanization is taking its toll on developing nations, particularly India and China. In recognition of the fact that air pollution is a global health issue, the United Nations Environmental Programme and WHO have put in place many partnerships and programs aimed at improving both outdoor and indoor air quality.

⊕ Historical Background

The idea that "bad" air causes disease is an old one, found in early Indian, Chinese, and Roman writings. The miasmatic theory of disease held that cholera, the Black

Death, and other infectious diseases arose from breathing in noxious particles in polluted air. Indeed, the word miasma comes from the Greek word for pollution. The miasmatic theory was used to explain the spread of cholera through London and Paris in the mid-19th century, even though work on the germ theory of disease was quite advanced by this stage.

Miasma was said to be a mixture of vapor from rotting vegetation, polluted waterways, and human waste, all exacerbated by overcrowding. The diseases attributed to miasma were not the ones known today to result from air pollution. They were infectious diseases, and the miasmatic theory was eventually overtaken by the germ theory of disease. The legacy of the miasmatic theory was that it laid the basis for better sanitation from the 19th century onward, because it was recognized that there was a genuine link between foul smells and disease. However, the idea that "bad air" itself can be harmful to health, as the result of particulates from air pollution, has proven to be true.

The Industrial Revolution

With the exception of the smog that often appears over some Asian cities, most pollution today is invisible. In the past, coal smoke was the first notable form of air pollution. As early as 1273, when coal was first introduced into London, its residents were banned from burning "dirty coal." The use of coal, both as a domestic fuel and power both factories and the railways, then rose dramatically during the Industrial Revolution.

Chimneys emitting black smoke were a common sight, and people breathing it in suffered from many health problems. Therefore, governments started to make moves to bring the emissions under control. For instance, the U.S. city governments of Chicago, Illinois, and Cincinnati, Ohio, brought in regulation to regulate emissions from factories and locomotives in the late 1800s. However, these measures could not, seemingly, keep pace with the rate of industrial development, with coal as its engine. Exposure to coal smoke continued to be a major cause of respiratory problems until the 1960s.

The Great Smog of 1952

Also known as the Big Smoke, the Great Smog descended on London on December 5, 1952, and lasted for five days, claiming the lives of about 4,000 people. There was nothing unusual about this smoke-laden fog, for similar incidents had occurred in London in 1813, 1873, 1882, 1891, 1892, and 1948. It was brought about by exceptionally cold weather, which meant that more coal was being burned than usual and also the pollution near ground level was trapped.

Analysis of the Great Smog showed that it contained tons of smoke particles, hydrochloric acid, and—probably most dangerous to health—sulfur dioxide, which was converted in the moist air into sulfuric acid. This was a toxic cocktail for all who were forced to breathe it in as they hurried home. So high was the death toll that the government took action through the Clean Air Acts of 1956 and 1968 to ban black smoke emission and require conversion to smokeless fuel. Although there was another smog in London in 1962, which killed 750 people, nothing like the Great Smog ever happened again, thanks to legislation and the spread of central heating, which has now largely replaced the coal fire in developed nations.

⊕ Impacts and Issues

In 2012, the WHO estimated that air pollution accounted for 12.5 percent (7 million) of all deaths globally, making air pollution the greatest single environmental health risk in the world. More deaths were attributed to indoor pollution (4.3 million) than outdoor (3.7 million), however there is overlap, as many people are exposed to both sources of pollution. Data collected by the WHO show a strong link between air pollution exposure and cardiovascular disease (e.g., heart disease and stroke) and cancer. It also has been linked to lung disease.

Estimates of exposure gathered by the WHO show that it is the low- and middle-income countries in the WHO regions of South-East Asia and the Western Pacific with the highest air pollution-linked mortality rates, with 3.3 million deaths linked to indoor air pollution and 2.6 million linked to outdoor air pollution, representing around 80 percent of all air pollution-related deaths.

Outdoor Air Pollution

Outdoor air pollution, also known as ambient or urban air pollution, arises from many different sources. Industrial processes may emit mixtures of toxic gases and particles whose nature depends upon the type of operation involved. Transport still largely relies upon gasoline and diesel, both of which emit polluting gases and particles when they are burned in an engine. As cities and countries develop, the volume of both industrial production and traffic tend to increase. Thus, development tends to go hand in hand with increased pollution, as has been the case in some countries in Southeast Asia and China.

Not all outdoor air pollution occurs in cities. It may be assumed that the air in the countryside must be cleaner than that in the city, but this is not always so. There have also been problems, particularly in developing countries, with burning agricultural wastes, deliberate setting of forest fires to clear land, and agro forestry activities such as charcoal production. The issue is compounded because there is less monitoring of pollution in rural areas.

An analysis of the 2012 WHO data shows that 40 percent of outdoor air pollution-related deaths arise from heart disease and 40 percent from stroke. The rest are from chronic obstructive pulmonary disease (11 percent), lung cancer (6 percent), and acute lower respiratory infection in children (3 percent). In 2013, WHO's

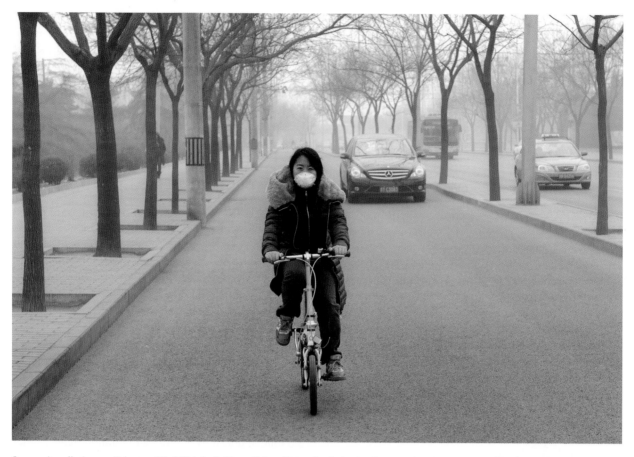

Severe air pollution on February 25, 2014, in Beijing, China. Air quality index levels were classed as "Beyond Index" (PM2.5 of over 500 micrograms per cubic meter). © *Hung Chung Chih/Shutterstock.com.*

International Agency for Research on Cancer stated that outdoor air pollution is carcinogenic to humans, with PM exposure being particularly linked to increased cancer incidence, particularly cancer of the lung.

Action on Outdoor Air Pollution

Controlling outdoor air pollution is a complex challenge requiring action on the part of governments at city, national, and international levels. Responsible management of industrial waste and the adoption of processes based upon "green" chemistry and clean/ alternative energy are essential to control industrial emissions. Agricultural processes should also be regulated to minimize emissions.

Regulation of transport in order to minimize air pollution is perhaps even more difficult than the regulation of industry. In many parts of the world, gasoline is cheap, and people feel they have a right to a car as their personal means of transport. It is important to shift as soon as possible to cleaner forms of energy for transport, such as hydrogen, electricity, and biodiesel. People need to be encouraged to walk, cycle, and take public transport. To support this, investment should be made in the public transport infrastructure. Urban planning also has

an important role to play, ensuring that towns and cities become more pedestrian-friendly.

Indoor Air Pollution

Indoor air pollution has received less attention than outdoor air pollution as a health issue. However, people can spend up to 90 percent of their time indoors, whether in an office or other workplace, in school, or at home. Furthermore, levels of air pollution indoors can be many times higher than they are outdoors, especially where ventilation is poor.

One particular indoor air pollution issue is exposure to fumes from solid fuel stoves. Three billion people, mostly in low- to middle-income countries, use either simple stoves or open fires that burn biomass and coal. This leads to exposures to high levels of soot particles, which can penetrate deep into the lungs. Women and young children are most at risk from these exposures, as they spend the most time around the domestic hearth.

Exposure to this so-called household air pollution leads to 4.3 million premature deaths a year, according to 2012 WHO data. These deaths come from stroke, heart disease, chronic obstructive pulmonary disease, and lung cancer. Exposure also doubles the risk for childhood pneumonia.

AIR POLLUTION IN CHINA

At present, and for the foreseeable future, the population of China is set to pay a heavy price for its rapid economic development. The WHO Global Burden of Disease report states that 1.2 million people died in China and North Korea in 2010 as a result of air pollution. Research published in the *Proceedings of the National Academy of Sciences* in 2013 sounded a further alarm by noting that air pollution in recent years has led to the loss of more than 2.5 billion years of life expectancy in China. In other words, prosperity is being accompanied by a reduction of 5.5 years in life expectancy for the average Chinese citizen.

China's air pollution problems are well known. First of all, the smog that often envelops Beijing and other Chinese cities is highly visible, even from space. Late in 2013, the moderate resolution imaging spectroradiometer aboard the National Aeronautics and Space Administration satellite Terra captured a 750 mile swath of smog stretching between Beijing and Shanghai. Second, the U.S. embassy in Beijing monitors PM2.5 levels every hour and posts these online and on Twitter, so anyone in the world can become aware of air quality in the city in real time. From this information, it is evident that PM2.5 levels in the city are often far beyond the 25 micrograms per cubic meter ($\mu g/m^3$) 24-hour mean set by the WHO. On occasion, they have reached 500 $\mu g/m^3$ or even as high as 1,000 $\mu g/m^3$.

China's growing economy relies very heavily on coal. Beginning early in the first decade of the 21st century, the country has undergone mass industrialization, with an accompanying dramatic growth in road transport, serving to compound the air pollution problem. The smog that often hangs over Chinese cities and towns resembles that which plagued London in earlier years. However, the Chinese smog likely also contains sulfur dioxide, nitrogen oxides, carbon monoxide, ground level ozone, and PM2.5s (the exact composition is not known because sources are said to be various and complicated).

The problems caused by China's smog are both immediate and long term. On several occasions, reduced visibility has caused the closure of airports in several cities. Children have also been kept away from school when PM2.5 levels have soared, out of concern for the health of those with asthma. These air pollution emergencies hit both tourism and business, with people fearing they will become ill if they visit China during an air pollution episode.

Air pollution is also exacting a severe toll on the health of the Chinese population. According to Greenpeace China, PM2.5 exposure caused nearly 10,000 premature deaths and 70,000 hospital visits or admissions in the Beijing-Tianjin-Hebei region in 2011. Meanwhile, Chinese scientists are noting a change in the pattern of lung cancer seen in Beijing in recent years. There are more cases of adenocarcinoma, which is linked to air pollution, and fewer cases of squamous cell lung cancer, which is more likely to be caused by smoking. They expect to see many more cases of adenocarcinoma in the next few years because even if there is a dramatic improvement in air quality in Beijing, lung cancer takes many years to develop; in most cases, damage to cells that will develop into a tumor has already been done. The researchers are also linking exposure to PM2.5 pollution to reduced birth weight and premature birth.

To improve the quality of air in its towns and cities, China needs to reduce its dependence on coal. If possible, the government needs to find ways of doing this without compromising the continued economic growth that its population expects. In 2013, the government released its national Airborne Pollution Action Plan. This calls for a 10 percent reduction of PM10 levels by 2017 in 338 of China's cities. In Beijing, Tianjin, and Hebei, where pollution problems are generally worse than elsewhere, PM2.5 levels must be reduced by 25 percent by 2017.

Other measures include banning heavily polluting vehicles from city streets by 2017 and extending air monitoring to all Chinese cities. Natural gas and nuclear power capacity will be increased in order to decrease dependence on coal. The proportion of coal in China's energy mix should therefore fall 3 percent by 2017. There are also local plans to improve air quality. For instance, Beijing aims to reduce it PM2.5 levels to 60 $\mu g/m^3$, which may be a realistic target, but that is still higher than the WHO 24-hour mean level of 25 $\mu g/m^3$.

Action on Household Air Pollution

The WHO has issued new air quality guidelines that contain recommendations on performance of solid fuel heaters and stoves. It is also working to integrate guidance and resources for clean household energy into global child health initiatives. There are a number of specific measures that could reduce household pollution. The most important is a switch from solid fuels to cleaner and more efficient fuels and technologies, including liquefied petroleum gas, biogas, producer gas, electricity, and solar power.

Where access to these clean fuels is still limited, the focus should be upon using improved stoves, which emit less smoke if they are properly designed, installed, and maintained. Improved ventilation of the cooking and living area should also be encouraged to reduce exposures to smoke. Installation of chimneys, smoke hoods, enlarged windows, and eave spaces can help get away from the dangerously confined cooking or heating space. Finally, advising users to dry their fuel before burning it and keeping young children away from smoke supports the other smoke reduction measures.

Air Quality Guidelines

The WHO first issued guidelines on selected air pollutants in 1987, updated these in 1997, and again in 2005. In the guidelines, upper limits are set for PM, ozone, nitrogen oxides, and sulfur dioxide, according to the latest scientific evidence on the effects of air pollution on health. The guidelines provide targets for various policy options aimed at improving air quality around the world. There are also, in many countries, national air quality standards that may vary according to local conditions and capacity to make improvements.

Particulate matter pollution is measured as μg/m³ and levels for PM10 are 20 (annual mean) and 50 (24-hour mean) and for PM2.5 10 (annual mean) and 25 (24-hour mean). The upper limit for PM2.5 reflects the greater health hazard associated with the smaller particles. For ground level ozone, the upper limit is 100 μg/m³ (8-hour mean), for nitrogen oxides 40 μg/m³ (annual mean) and 700 μg/m³ (1-hour mean), and for sulfur dioxide 20 μg/m³ (24-hour mean) and 500 μg/m³ (10-minute mean). Air quality monitoring stations can be found at many locations in cities around the world, and they regularly post data on the Internet, so it is clear how well the location is performing with respect to WHO guidelines.

⊕ Future Implications

Air pollution is an inevitable consequence of human activity. It cannot be eliminated and will only grow as countries continue to develop. To mitigate the effect of both indoor and outdoor pollution on human health, it will be necessary to apply new and cleaner technologies for industry, transport, and household activities, within a strong framework on environmental legislation.

Reports in 2014 that the European Commission (EC) would consider relaxing air pollution legislation in the interest of reducing debt and creating jobs highlighted that bringing air pollution to the top of the political agenda will continue to be a challenge. The EC has proposed delegating air pollution legislation to national level, which would make it harder to deal with transborder pollution. Opponents of tough legislation argue that businesses will locate to countries where environmental law is weak or nonexistent. There is clearly still some way to go in convincing both the public and industry of the short- and long-term benefits of cleaner air.

PRIMARY SOURCE

Ambient (Outdoor) Air Quality and Health

SOURCE *"Ambient (Outdoor) Air Quality and Health," Fact Sheet No. 313, Updated March 2014, World Health Organization (WHO). http://www.who.int/mediacentre/factsheets/fs313/en/ (accessed January 25, 2015).*

INTRODUCTION *The primary source that follows is taken from a fact sheet compiled by the World Health Organization. It presents the background and key points of the air pollution issue from a global perspective.*

Key facts

- Air pollution is a major environmental risk to health. By reducing air pollution levels, countries can reduce the burden of disease from stroke, heart disease, lung cancer, and both chronic and acute respiratory diseases, including asthma.

- The lower the levels of air pollution, the better the cardiovascular and respiratory health of the population will be, both long- and short-term.

- The "WHO Air quality guidelines" provide an assessment of health effects of air pollution and thresholds for health-harmful pollution levels.

- Ambient (outdoor air pollution) in both cities and rural areas was estimated to cause 3.7 million premature deaths worldwide in 2012.

- Some 88% of those premature deaths occurred in low- and middle-income countries, and the greatest number in the WHO Western Pacific and South-East Asia regions.

- Policies and investments supporting cleaner transport, energy-efficient housing, power generation, industry and better municipal waste management would reduce key sources of urban outdoor air pollution.

- Reducing outdoor emissions from household coal and biomass energy systems, agricultural waste incineration, forest fires and certain agro-forestry activities (e.g. charcoal production) would reduce key rural and peri-urban air pollution sources in developing regions.

- Reducing outdoor air pollution also reduces emissions of CO_2 and short-lived climate pollutants such as black carbon particles and methane, thus contributing to the near- and long-term mitigation of climate change.

- In addition to outdoor air pollution, indoor smoke is a serious health risk for some 3 billion people who cook and heat their homes with biomass fuels and coal.

Background

Outdoor air pollution is a major environmental health problem affecting everyone in developed and developing countries alike.

WHO estimates that some 80% of outdoor air pollution-related premature deaths were due to ischaemic heart disease and strokes, while 14% of deaths were due to chronic obstructive pulmonary disease or acute lower respiratory infections; and 6% of deaths were due to lung cancer.

Some deaths may be attributed to more than one risk factor at the same time. For example, both smoking and ambient air pollution affect lung cancer. Some lung cancer deaths could have been averted by improving ambient air quality, or by reducing tobacco smoking.

A 2013 assessment by WHO's International Agency for Research on Cancer (IARC) concluded that outdoor air pollution is carcinogenic to humans, with the particulate matter component of air pollution most closely associated with increased cancer incidence, especially cancer of the lung. An association also has been observed between outdoor air pollution and increase in cancer of the urinary tract/bladder.

Ambient (outdoor air pollution) in both cities and rural areas was estimated to cause 3.7 million premature deaths worldwide per year in 2012; this mortality is due to exposure to small particulate matter of 10 microns or less in diameter (PM_{10}), which cause cardiovascular and respiratory disease, and cancers....

The latest burden estimates reflect the very significant role air pollution plays in cardiovascular illness and premature deaths—much more so than was previously understood by scientists.

SEE ALSO *Global Health Initiatives; Noncommunicable Diseases (Lifestyle Diseases); World Health Organization: Organization, Funding, and Enforcement Powers*

BIBLIOGRAPHY

Books

Godish, Thad, Wayne Davis, and Joshua Fu. *Air Quality*, 5th ed. Boca Raton, FL: CRC Press, 2014.

Gurjar, Bhola, and Luisa Molina. *Air Pollution: Health and Environmental Impact*. Boca Raton, FL: CRC Press, 2010.

Jackson, Lee. *Dirty Old London: The Victorian Fight against Filth*. New York: Yale University Press, 2014.

Khare, Mukesh. *Air Pollution—Monitoring, Modelling and Health*. Rijeka, Croatia: InTech, 2012.

Websites

"Ambient (Outdoor) Air Quality and Health," Fact Sheet No. 313. *World Health Organization (WHO)*, March 2014. http://www.who.int/mediacentre/factsheets/fs313/en/ (accessed February 10, 2015).

"Burden of Disease from Air Pollution for 2012." *World Health Organization (WHO)*. http://www.who.int/phe/health_topics/outdoorair/databases/FINAL_HAP_AAP_BoD_24March2014.pdf? (accessed February 10, 2015).

"The Great London Smog of 1952." *Met Office Education*. http://www.metoffice.gov.uk/education/teens/case-studies/great-smog (accessed February 10, 2015).

Kaiman, Jonathan. "China's Toxic Air Pollution Resembles Nuclear Winter, Say Scientists." *Guardian*, February 25, 2014. http://www.theguardian.com/world/2014/feb/25/china-toxic-air-pollution-nuclear-winter-scientists (accessed February 10, 2015).

Susan Aldridge

Alcohol Use and Abuse

⊕ Introduction

Alcohol is the most widely used addictive substance in the world. Addiction, primarily a brain disorder caused by compulsive substance-seeking without regard for consequences, is accompanied by chemical changes in the brain. While the majority of people can use alcohol without difficulties, many either use it to excess or become addicted. The condition of being addicted to alcohol is called alcoholism. Excess drinking is defined as either binge drinking (more than five drinks on a single occasion for men or four drinks for women), any drinking under the age of 21, or drinking by pregnant women. It is important to note that not everyone who drinks excessively is an alcoholic.

Alcohol is a substance that effects changes, not only on the brain, but in almost every cell in the body. It can affect the neurons (nerve cells) and the neurotransmitters (chemical messengers); it can also affect blood flow in areas of the brain. These changes affect behavior and alter mood and motor function. The exact mechanism is unknown. Long-term effects include permanent damage to organs including the brain and nervous system, liver, heart, and pancreas. Cholesterol levels increase and bones and the immune system weaken. Pregnant women who drink during pregnancy risk spontaneous abortions or damage to the fetus.

⊕ Historical Background

Beer jugs dating to the Stone Age (10,000 BCE) have been found. Tests on Chinese jars dating from 7000 to 6600 BCE revealed residue of fermented drinks. Beer and wine were important to the everyday life of the ancient Egyptians, who believed beer was created by the god Osiris. Home brewed beer and wine were used for religious rites, medical purposes, pleasure, and even for nutrition. The code of Hammurabi (circa 1750 BCE) mentions alcohol as part of fair trade.

Other early civilizations also left records of wine and beer use. The ancient Greeks originally drank mead, but by 2000 BCE wine making was introduced. In Athens, drinking wine was considered a civic duty. According to scholars, the concept of *demokratia* (democracy) arose from the practice of ensuring everyone had an equal share of wine during festivals. Originally used for religious purposes, it was soon incorporated into everyday life. In Greece, those not using alcohol were considered lethargic and odoriferous (morally offensive), but drunkenness was frowned upon. The cult of Dionysus was an exception, as followers believed drunkenness brought them closer to the god of wine.

Around 475 CE, as the Roman Empire fell, brewing and wine making were taken over by monasteries. Bartholomaeus of Salerno, a physician in the early 12th century, is thought to have written about distillation. Albertus Magnus (c. 1200–1280) of Cologne is the author of the first comprehensive description of distilling, as part of his work in alchemy. These distilled liquids were called spirits. As knowledge of alcohol brewing increased, different areas became known for different alcohols produced there. Germany excelled in beer making, Ireland and Scotland were praised for their whiskey, and the French became known for wine. Laws were passed related to alcohol, such as the German Beer Purity Law of 1516, which made it illegal to brew beer with anything other than barley, hops, and pure water. The incidence of excessive drinking rose throughout the 16th century so that in 1606, the English Parliament passed "The Act to Repress the Odious and Loathesome Sin of Drunkenness."

As distillation increased, governments began to tax spirits. The practice of taxation on alcohol traveled to the New World with the Puritans, who initially held the view that alcohol, a natural food, was good in moderation. In 1791, U.S. Secretary of State Alexander Hamilton (1755–1804) proposed an excise tax on spirits distilled in the new nation. The distillers of Pennsylvania refused to pay this tax, and by 1794,

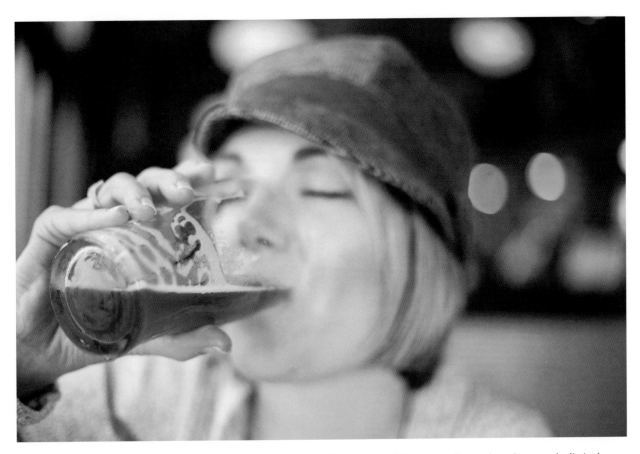

Most adults can enjoy a glass of beer or wine without any negative health impacts, and there are studies to show there may be limited benefits to moderate consumption. However, excessive use of alcohol has been proven to be linked to multiple negative health impacts and is a costly global burden.   © *Robert Brown Stock/Shutterstock.com.*

protests became violent. President George Washington (1732–1799) was forced to send militia into Pennsylvania. The rebels dispersed before the militia arrived, ending what would be called the Whiskey Rebellion. As time passed, other taxes on spirits would help to pay for wars, including the War of 1812 and the American Civil War (1861–1865).

Increased industrialization across the globe, especially in the 19th century, changed attitudes about inebriation. Factories needed a workforce that was competent, dependable, and sober. Drunkenness began to be associated with inefficiency. Advocates of moderation soon turned to temperance.

In the United States, the temperance movement led to the 18th Amendment to the Constitution, which took effect in January 1920. The amendment prohibited the making, selling, or drinking of alcohol outside the home. An exception was made for medical use, and doctors began writing prescriptions for alcohol, including beer. These could be filled at any pharmacy across the country. An illicit alcohol trade also developed to foil the prohibition on alcoholic beverages. The 18th Amendment was repealed in December 1933; the 13-year period that the law was in effect is known as Prohibition.

⊕ Impacts and Issues

With the advent of trade and taxation of alcohol, the production and sale of alcohol became essential to national economies. However, with increasing drinking, those economies are burdened with the costs of excess drinking and alcoholism.

According to the U.S. Centers for Disease Control and Prevention (CDC), alcohol use caused approximately 88,000 deaths in the United States each year from 2006 to 2010. In 2012, the World Health Organization (WHO) estimated there were as many as 3.3 million deaths worldwide due to alcohol consumption. Excess alcohol use leads to debilitating and often fatal diseases. It is linked to cirrhosis of the liver, seizures, pancreatitis, poisonings, birth defects, and brain damage, and it is associated with injuries including motor vehicle accidents.

Alcohol also has an impact on social issues such as poverty and crime. Its excessive use costs the United States more than US$484 billion each year, according to both the CDC and the National Institute on Drug Abuse (NIDA). This includes health-care issues, lost earnings, and crime-related costs such as damages, court costs, and

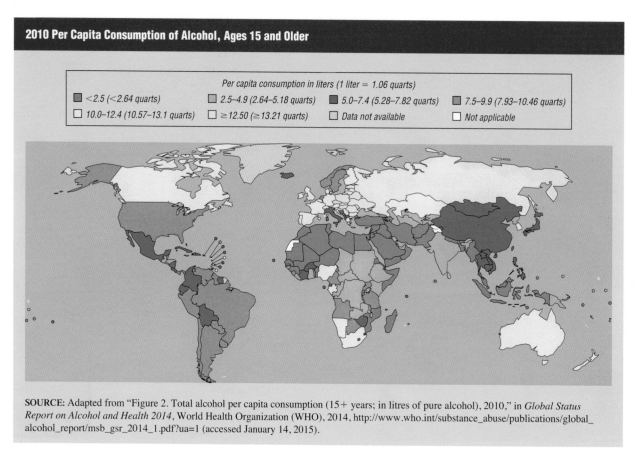

2010 Per Capita Consumption of Alcohol, Ages 15 and Older

Per capita consumption in liters (1 liter = 1.06 quarts)

- <2.5 (<2.64 quarts)
- 2.5–4.9 (2.64–5.18 quarts)
- 5.0–7.4 (5.28–7.82 quarts)
- 7.5–9.9 (7.93–10.46 quarts)
- 10.0–12.4 (10.57–13.1 quarts)
- ≥12.50 (≥13.21 quarts)
- Data not available
- Not applicable

SOURCE: Adapted from "Figure 2. Total alcohol per capita consumption (15+ years; in litres of pure alcohol), 2010," in *Global Status Report on Alcohol and Health 2014*, World Health Organization (WHO), 2014, http://www.who.int/substance_abuse/publications/global_alcohol_report/msb_gsr_2014_1.pdf?ua=1 (accessed January 14, 2015).

In 2012, the World Health Organization (WHO) estimated there were as many as 3.3 million deaths worldwide due to alcohol consumption. Excess alcohol use leads to debilitating and often fatal diseases.

prison expenses. According to a 2015 WHO data sheet, Europe has the world's largest consumption rate of alcohol. This varies by area, with Eastern and Central-Eastern Europe reporting higher levels than Southern Europe and the Nordic countries. In the European Union, 12 percent of all deaths of people aged 15–64 were due to alcohol-related problems. Additionally, statistics from the Crime Survey for England and Wales show that 40–47 percent of violent crimes in England and Wales involve alcohol, while crimes in Scotland involve alcohol 63 percent of the time. In Russia, a study reported by *The Lancet* reveals that 25 percent of deaths in men before the age of 55 are attributed directly to vodka consumption.

Asia has not been spared the effects and costs of alcohol abuse. According to the *Japan Times*, an estimated 6.45 million people in Japan suffer from alcohol-related problems. Of those cases, 800,000 are severe enough to require medical treatment. Yearly costs are more than 4.15 trillion yen (about US$34 billion), with 35,000 deaths.

Drinking habits in China are somewhat unique, according to *Science Daily*. While most countries are dealing with younger users, in China drinking amounts, frequency, and binge drinking increase with age.

Chinese culture expects their youth to concentrate on education and avoid alcohol, while older people are encouraged to drink to build friendships and business contacts. Most alcohol consumed in China is spirits instead of wine or beer. Other parts of Asia have varying degrees of consumption; in Indonesia, according to an Institute of Alcohol Studies report, only 2.7 percent of the population reports use compared to 40 percent in Bali. Poor areas of Sri Lanka report that up to 93 percent of villagers use locally produced alcohol, which is not reported in national consumption data.

Both the WHO and *The Lancet* report that alcohol use in India is on the rise. Production, distribution, and sales are increasing; 30 percent of the population reports consumption, and 11 percent indulges in heavy or binge drinking. As in China, most of the alcohol used is spirits. Despite the increase, India as a country remains one of the lowest consumers of alcohol.

Another public health issue is the consumption of alcohol by pregnant women. The exact amount of alcohol that will damage the fetus is unknown, but a range of problems can ensue. Discussing drinking with a pregnant woman can be difficult because of the implications for both the health-care worker and mother. According to the

FETAL ALCOHOL SYNDROME

Fetal alcohol syndrome (FAS) was first described in 1968 in France and officially named in the United States in 1973. Recently, the term fetal alcohol spectrum syndrome has been used to describe a wide range of effects, with FAS being the worst form of damage.

When a pregnant woman drinks alcohol, it readily crosses the placenta and enters the fetal bloodstream. Although the exact mechanism is unknown, it is speculated that several events take place. Because the fetus has only 10 percent of the amount of alcohol dehydrogenase found in adults, it cannot break down and detoxify the alcohol. Alcohol can disrupt DNA, modify the metabolism of nutrients, and cause fetal hypoxia (lack of oxygen).

Worse effects are seen when drinking occurs during the first 12 weeks after conception, a time when many women do not know they are pregnant. Damage continues throughout the rest of the pregnancy. Children born with FAS have a distinctive facial structure. They have a short bridge of the nose, smaller eyes, and a thin upper lip with the area above the lip very smooth and thin. Their skulls and brains are smaller, and they are small for their age. Those affected may have behavioral, neurologic, and learning disabilities.

It is now believed that incidence of FAS in the United States may be double what was originally thought, with 2 to 5 percent of children affected. South Africa has the highest number of FAS children in the world.

While some countries are officially addressing the problem, most programs are nongovernmental. The expense to society is immense, costing US$321 million annually in the United States alone. The worst affected children need specialized health and educational programs for life. The effects are not reversible. Although lower socioeconomic populations are disproportionally affected due to cultural or educational issues, this syndrome knows no economic or racial boundaries. There is still much work to do in eliminating this preventable problem.

American Congress of Obstetricians and Gynecologists, trust is an important issue between patient and doctor. Pregnant women who drink may fear being reported to child services and may not be honest in reporting, or may not seek care at all. Doctors must consider the well-being of both mother and fetus.

⊕ Future Implications

With both incidence and costs of alcohol abuse rising, it is clear that understanding the illness and dealing with it efficiently are of paramount importance. Throughout history, alcohol has held an important role in society. It can serve as a relaxant that allows for better social interaction, provides pharmaceutical pleasure, and enhances flavors of food. The majority of users can drink without health concerns; however, those who abuse alcohol need medical and social interventions.

For those already abusing or addicted, recognizing the problem and getting treatment is essential. If drinking interferes with work; if a person drives while drinking, gets into legal trouble because of drinking, harms themselves or others while drinking; or if there are arguments with loved ones about the drinking, then that person is probably abusing alcohol. Dependence is a physiologic response that involves needing more amounts of alcohol to be satisfied (tolerance), drinking to avoid withdrawal, inability to reduce use, and spending time trying to obtain alcohol. Recognizing alcoholism can be thwarted by belief systems. Although alcohol abuse was once deemed a moral issue, many countries now consider it an illness. The *Japan Times* reports that nationally, one of the major problems in treating alcoholism is that it is still viewed as a personal weakness.

Treatment must address causes and treat symptoms. No one knows exactly why some people can drink without becoming addicted and others begin abusing after their first exposure. Genetics plays a part in the development of alcohol addiction. The exact mechanism is unknown but the U.S. National Council on Alcoholism and Drug Dependence reports that twin studies show a higher rate of similarity in addiction between identical twins than fraternal twins. Adoption studies show that sons who were adopted at birth and did not know their biologic fathers had a higher rate of alcoholism if the biologic father was an alcoholic. There was no difference if the adoptive father was an alcoholic. These data support the theory that alcoholism runs in families. The single most reliable indicator of risk is family history. This does not mean that everyone who has an alcoholic parent is doomed to become an alcoholic, but the genetic potential exists.

Treatment must also address other causes of the disease, especially factors that can cause relapse. Mental and emotional stress, social pressures, internal temptations, and personal relationships are all factors. Alcoholism is a chronic disease; relapses are not uncommon and should not be thought of as failure.

A *New York Times* health article summarizes treatment for alcoholics as follows: goals must be individualized; inpatient treatment may be required if there is eminent danger of harm; the best goal is full abstinence but drinking less may be the goal for some. Both medical and behavioral techniques are used, and treatment may address concurrent psychiatric problems. Relapse is common and statistics vary.

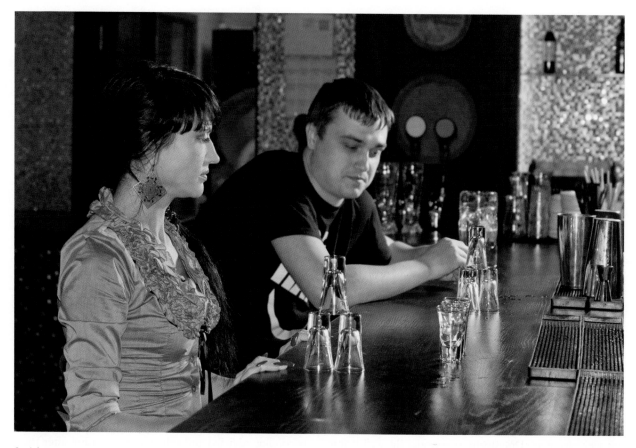

Social pressure can be a factor in how much people drink and can have either a positive or negative effect. © *Viacheslav Nikolaenko/ Shutterstock.com.*

Prevention remains the focus of worldwide organizations. It has been shown that the earlier people start drinking, the more likely they are to abuse alcohol. Legal drinking age differs worldwide: the average age is 15.9, with the majority of countries setting the legal age to drink at 18. Some have no minimum age. Enforcement of these laws varies widely. In some Muslim countries, non-Muslims over the age of 17 can purchase alcohol but must consume it in their homes. Although it is widely believed that those under 21 cannot drink in the United States, many states have laws that allow drinking within the home or private clubs under the supervision of a guardian. Programs by schools and agencies, both governmental and nongovernmental, are needed to start alcohol education, prevention, and treatment at early ages. A study in the *Journal of Adolescent Health* suggests that school curricula based on a social influence model may reduce the occurrence of alcohol-related behavioral problems. According to *The Lancet*, some countries, including India, concentrate on acute care instead of prevention, pouring precious resources into preventable problems.

The WHO is backing policies that regulate pricing, target drinking and driving, and restrict marketing of alcohol. The BBC reports that in 1985, Soviet leader Mikhail Gorbachev (1931–) cut vodka production and prohibited its sale prior to lunchtime. The death rate dropped, correlating with the restrictions. Governments should set minimum age limits and enforce the laws. The U.S. surgeon general's report recommends mandatory installation of ignition interlocks in vehicles belonging to those convicted of impaired driving. Norway has one of the lowest burdens of harmful use in Europe. They have been effective in creating very high alcohol taxes, regulating accessibility through operation hours of bars, and enacting a complete ban on advertising. However, despite their success, consumption is still rising in Norway.

The countries with the fastest-growing consumption of alcohol are in Asia and Africa, areas that can ill afford to spend limited resources on preventable problems. Other areas of concern, such as starvation, infectious diseases, clean water, and adequate housing suffer when money is spent on alcohol-related illnesses, crimes, and injuries. Future issues will include dealing with cultural bias in recognizing alcohol excess as a problem, enacting tax regulations, limiting availability to young people, and prevention of abuse. This is a global problem that will require global solutions.

PRIMARY SOURCE

Global Status Report on Alcohol and Health 2014

SOURCE *"Executive Summary," in* Global Status Report on Alcohol and Health 2014, *World Health Organization (WHO), 2014, xiii–xiv. http://www.who.int/substance_abuse/publications/global_alcohol_report/msb_gsr_2014_1.pdf (accessed January 25, 2015).*

INTRODUCTION *This primary source is from the Executive Summary section of the World Health Organization's* Global Status Report on Alcohol and Health 2014, *published in 2014. It outlines the topics covered in the full report and summarizes the main findings outlined in each of the four chapters in the report, which include alcohol consumption from a global perspective; the consumption of alcohol in select populations; negative health consequences; and what countries are doing to combat alcohol abuse.*

Chapter 1: Alcohol and Public Health

Alcohol is a psychoactive substance with dependence-producing properties that has been widely used in many cultures for centuries. The harmful use of alcohol causes a large disease, social and economic burden in societies.

- Environmental factors such as economic development, culture, availability of alcohol and the level and effectiveness of alcohol policies are relevant factors in explaining differences and historical trends in alcohol consumption and related harm.

- Alcohol-related harm is determined by the volume of alcohol consumed, the pattern of drinking, and, on rare occasions, the quality of alcohol consumed.

- The harmful use of alcohol is a component cause of more than 200 disease and injury conditions in individuals....

- The latest causal relationships suggested by research are those between harmful use of alcohol and infectious diseases such as tuberculosis and HIV/AIDS.

- A wide range of global, regional and national policies and actions are in place to reduce the harmful use of alcohol.

Chapter 2: Alcohol Consumption

- Worldwide consumption in 2010 was equal to 6.2 litres of pure alcohol consumed per person aged 15 years or older, which translates into 13.5 grams of pure alcohol per day.

- A quarter of this consumption (24.8 percent) was unrecorded, i.e., homemade alcohol, illegally produced or sold.... Of total recorded alcohol consumed worldwide, 50.1 percent was consumed in the form of spirits.

- Worldwide 61.7 percent of the population aged 15 years or older (15+) had not drunk alcohol in the past 12 months. In all WHO regions, females are more often lifetime abstainers than males. There is a considerable variation in prevalence of abstention across WHO regions.

- Worldwide about 16.0 percent of drinkers aged 15 years or older engage in heavy episodic drinking.

- In general, the greater the economic wealth of a country, the more alcohol is consumed and the smaller the number of abstainers....

Chapter 3: Health Consequences

- In 2012, about 3.3 million deaths, or 5.9 percent of all global deaths, were attributable to alcohol consumption.

- There are significant sex differences in the proportion of global deaths attributable to alcohol, for example, in 2012 7.6 percent of deaths among males and 4.0 percent of deaths among females were attributable to alcohol.

- In 2012 139 million DALYs (disability-adjusted life years), or 5.1 percent of the global burden of disease and injury, were attributable to alcohol consumption.

- There is also wide geographical variation in the proportion of alcohol-attributable deaths and DALYs, with the highest alcohol-attributable fractions reported in the WHO European Region.

Chapter 4: Alcohol Policy and Interventions

- Alcohol policies are developed with the aim of reducing harmful use of alcohol and the alcohol-attributable health and social burden in a population and in society. Such policies can be formulated at the global, regional, multinational, national and subnational level.

- Many WHO Member States have demonstrated increased leadership and commitment to reducing harmful use of alcohol in recent years. A higher percentage of the reporting countries indicated having written national alcohol policies and imposing stricter blood alcohol concentration limits in 2012 than in 2008.

SEE ALSO *Drug/Substance Abuse; Health-Related Education and Information Access; Maternal and Infant Health; Noncommunicable Diseases (Lifestyle Diseases)*

BIBLIOGRAPHY

Books

Boyle, Peter, et al., eds. *Alcohol: Science, Policy and Public Health.* Oxford: Oxford University Press, 2013.

Dasgupta, Amitava. *The Science of Drinking: How Alcohol Affects Your Body and Mind.* Lanham, MD: Rowman & Littlefield, 2011.

Myers, Peter L., and Richard Isralowitz. *Alcohol.* Santa Barbara, CA: Greenwood, 2011.

National Institute on Alcohol Abuse and Alcoholism (U.S.). *Rethinking Drinking: Alcohol and Your Health.* Bethesda, MD: National Institute on Alcohol Abuse and Alcoholism, 2010.

National Institute on Alcohol Abuse and Alcoholism (U.S.) and American Academy of Pediatrics. *Alcohol Screening and Brief Intervention for Youth: A Practitioner's Guide.* Rockville, MD: National Institute on Alcohol Abuse and Alcoholism, U.S. Dept. of Health and Human Services, National Institutes of Health, 2011.

Periodicals

Caria, M. P., et al. "Effects of a School-Based Prevention Program on European Adolescents' Patterns of Alcohol Use." *Journal of Adolescent Health* 48, no. 2 (2011): 182–188.

"Fetal Alcohol Syndrome: Dashed Hopes, Damaged Lives." *Bulletin of the World Health Organization* 89 (2011): 398–399. Available online at http://www.who.int/bulletin/volumes/89/6/11-020611/en/ (accessed February 17, 2015).

Laramée, P. "The Economic Burden of Alcohol Dependence in Europe." *Alcohol* 48, no. 3 (2013): 259–269.

Prasad, Raekha. "Alcohol Use Is on the Rise in India." *The Lancet* 373, no. 9657 (2009): 17–18. Available online at http://www.thelancet.com/journals/lancet/article/PIIS0140-6736(08)61939-X/fulltext?ictd%5Bmaster%5D=vid~a8ad52e7-ecc7-4a05-93bd-4b9d7382afe4&ictd%5Bil726%5D=rlt~14223 48221~land~2_4757_direct_ (accessed February 17, 2015).

Websites

"Alcohol Dependency in Japan." *Japan Times,* January 27, 2014. http//www.japantimes.co.jp/opinion/2014/01/17/editorials/alcohol-dependency-in-Japan (accessed February 17, 2015).

"Alcohol Use Disorder." *New York Times.* http://www.nytimes.com/health/guides/disease/alcoholism/causes.html (accessed February 17, 2015).

"At-Risk Drinking and Illicit Drug Use: Ethical Issues in Obstetrics and Gynecologic Practice." ACOG Committee Opinion Number 422. *American Congress of Obstetricians and Gynecologists,* December 2008. http://www.acog.org/Resources-And-Publications/Committee-Opinions/Committee-on-Ethics/At-Risk-Drinking-and-Illicit-Drug-Use-Ethical-Issues-in-Obstetric-and-Gynecologic-Practice (accessed February 17, 2015).

"Drug Abuse and Addiction: One of America's Most Challenging Public Health Problems." *National Institute on Drug Abuse (U.S.).* http://archives.drugabuse.gov/about/welcome/aboutdrugabuse/magnitude/ (accessed February 17, 2015).

"Fact Sheets—Alcohol Use and Your Health." *Centers for Disease Control and Prevention.* http://www.cdc.gov/alcohol/fact-sheets/alcohol-use.htm (accessed February 17, 2015).

"Family History and Genetics." *National Council on Alcoholism and Drug Dependence (U.S.).* http://ncadd.org/for-parents-overview/family-history-and-genetics/226-family-history-and-genetics (accessed February 17, 2015).

Mazumdar, Tulip. "Vodka Blamed for High Death Rates in Russia." *BBC News Health,* January 31, 2014. http://www.bbc.com/news/health-25961063 (accessed February 17, 2015).

"Preventing Drug Abuse and Excessive Alcohol Use." *U.S. Department of Health and Human Services.* http://www.surgeongeneral.gov/initiatives/prevention/strategy/preventing-drug-abuse-excessive-alcohol-use.html (accessed February 17, 2015).

"UK Alcohol-Related Crime Statistics." *Institute of Alcohol Studies (UK).* http://www.ias.org.uk/Alcohol-knowledge-centre/Crime-and-social-impacts/Factsheets/UK-alcohol-related-crime-statistics.aspx (accessed February 17, 2015).

"Worldwide Alcohol Trends." *World Health Organization (WHO).* http://www.who.int/mediacentre/multimedia/podcasts/2011/alcohol_20110315/en/ (accessed February 17, 2015).

Virginia Herbert McDougall

Antibiotic/Antimicrobial Resistance

⊕ Introduction

Antimicrobials are compounds that harm or kill microorganisms, and the term is an umbrella for agents that include antibiotics, antifungals, antiprotozoals, and antivirals. Antibiotics kill or inhibit the growth of bacteria; antifungals are active against fungi; antiprotozoals destroy protozoa (single-celled organisms) or inhibit their growth and ability to reproduce; and antivirals kill viruses or suppress their ability to replicate. The ways in which antimicrobials damage or destroy pathogens (disease causing microorganisms) vary, and they may be active against a variety of different microbes (broad-spectrum activity) or specific to a few or just one species of bacteria, virus, fungi, or protozoa (narrow spectrum activity).

Most bacteria are classified as either gram-positive or gram-negative depending on whether they retain a specific stain color. Gram-positive bacteria stain purple, and gram-negative bacteria appear pink or red. Narrow-spectrum antibiotics are useful against particular species of bacteria. For example, bacitracin is only effective against gram-positive bacteria, while polymixins are usually only effective against gram-negative bacteria. In contrast, broad-spectrum antibiotics are active against both gram-positive and gram-negative organisms. Examples include tetracyclines, phenicols, and fluoroquinolones. Bacteria also may be classified an aerobic, which means they are able to use oxygen, or anaerobic, which means they can live without oxygen. Some antibiotics are only effective against aerobic bacteria while others work against anaerobic bacteria.

Narrow-spectrum antibiotics are often prescribed when the specific bacterium causing illness is known. Broad-spectrum antibiotics may be prescribed when there is uncertainty about which bacterium is responsible for the infection.

Antibacterial resistance in particular, and antimicrobial resistance more generally, essentially involves a change in the targeted microorganism. The change can be general, such as a change in the cell membrane that makes it more difficult for the antibacterial/antimicrobial agent to bind to the cell surface or pass across the membrane to get to the cell interior. Changes also may be specific, involving the actual site of activity of the antibacterial/antimicrobial agent. A common example is the development of a mutation that changes the three-dimensional structure of the target enzyme; the binding site of the differently-shaped enzyme becomes inaccessible, and the antimicrobial agent is no longer effective against the microorganism.

Genes encoding resistance to antibiotics are usually not located on the chromosome; instead they are located on mobile genetic material termed a plasmid. All or part of a plasmid can be transferred from one bacterium to another, which provides a means of spreading resistance. If the resistance is advantageous to the bacterium, such as occurs when the cell is in an environment containing the antibiotic, the genetic trait is more likely to be maintained. This is the genetic basis of antibiotic and antimicrobial resistance.

⊕ Historical Background

While some antibiotics have likely existed naturally for millennia, it was only in the 20th century that they were discovered and put into use. The first antibiotic, penicillin, was accidentally discovered in the 1930s by Sir Alexander Fleming (1881–1955). Prior to that time, bacterial illnesses like pneumonia, tuberculosis, and typhoid fever were untreatable and frequently serious or lethal to those who became infected. The discovery of penicillin opened the floodgates, and in the next few decades, many antibiotics were discovered or synthesized.

In the natural world, antibiotics are produced by bacteria, fungi, and some plants. They help protect the producing organism against bacteria that could otherwise kill it. The serendipitous discovery of penicillin by Fleming came when a petri dish (a specialized plastic dish that can be filled with a growth medium such as agar) containing growing bacteria was accidentally left open. The vessel became contaminated with a mold (later found to be *Penicillium*, which was the basis of the name given to the antibiotic). Fleming noted that bacterial growth near the mold was curtailed. He was the first to publish about its ability to kill bacteria. In 1938, Oxford researchers developed techniques for extracting, cultivating, and purifying penicillin.

In the first decades following the discovery of penicillin, myriad different antibiotics proved to be phenomenally effective in controlling infectious bacteria. During this antibiotic era, infections plummeted in number. Antibiotics quickly became (and to a large extent remain) a vital tool in the physician's arsenal against many bacterial infections. Indeed, by the 1970s the success of antibiotics led to the widely held view that bacterial infectious diseases would soon be eliminated. The general consensus was that effective treatment for most, if not all, bacterial diseases had been found.

History has proven that the confidence that bacterial infections could all be easily vanquished was hasty and incorrect. Resistance to antibiotics and antimicrobials began to appear fairly soon after their introduction. This acquisition of resistance to many antibiotics by bacteria has proved to be very problematic. In the 21st century, as bacteria become resistant to the arsenal of antibiotics and multiple resistance spreads globally, the consensus is that the antibiotic era may be over.

⊕ Impacts and Issues

Antibiotic development has progressed considerably from accidental discovery to focused, intentional research. Sophisticated screening now can be carried out with a compound of interest that has been isolated from various materials, including plants and soil. The compound can be tested for activity against thousands of different bacteria in the same automated screening run. The structural tailoring of a compound to a selected target has been greatly advanced by molecular sequencing technologies and the ability to produce three-dimensional images based on sequence data. Knowing the shape of the target is crucial, since real-world applications involve a lock-and-key fit between the antibiotic and its target.

Unfortunately, even with a multitude of antibacterial drugs, bacteria may adapt to the antibiotics used to combat them. This adaptation, which can involve structural changes or the production of enzymes that partially destroy the antibiotic, can render a particular bacterial species resistant to a particular antibiotic. The graphic offers a simple depiction of how antibiotic resistance occurs. This resistance has spawned antibiotic and antimicrobial resistant microbes that are a problem in hospitals and in agriculture on a global scale. Furthermore, for a given bacterial species, some antibiotics may be very effective and others ineffective. For another bacterial species, the pattern of antibiotic sensitivity and resistance will be different. This is why it is so important to accurately

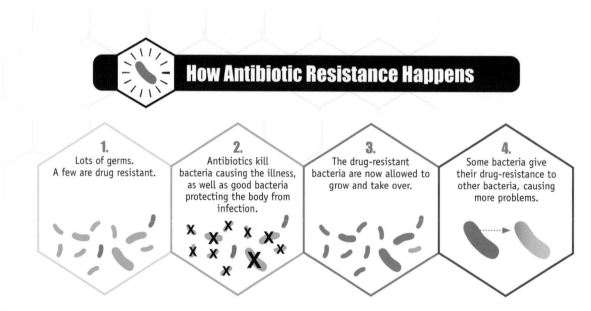

This infographic from the U.S. Centers for Disease Control and Prevention (CDC) illustrates in very simple terms how antibiotic resistance happens, in a four step process. (1) Lots of bacteria. (2) Antibiotics kill the bacteria causing the illness, as well as good bacteria protecting the body from infection. (3) The drug-resistant bacteria remain to grow and take over. (4) Some of the drug-resistant bacteria pass on their drug-resistance to other, nonresistant bacteria, increasing the numbers that are resistant. *Melissa Brower/U.S. Centers for Disease Control and Prevention.*

determine the bacteria responsible for infection. Without knowledge of the specific bacterial cause, treatment of the infection may be ineffective.

Sometimes resistance to an antibiotic can be overcome through modifying the antibiotic slightly by the addition of a different chemical group. This changes the three-dimensional structure of the antibiotic. Unfortunately, such a modification may confer susceptibility to the new antibiotic only for a relatively short time until resistance develops again.

A standard method of testing for antibiotic resistance involves growth of the bacteria in the presence of increasing concentrations of the particular antibiotic. Typically, this test is performed in a petri dish. The dish is sterile and is covered with a lid to avoid contamination, which would undermine the test results.

Some of the bacterial suspension is spread over the surface of the agar in the dish, and discs soaked in the different concentrations of the antibiotic are spaced apart on the surface. The hardened agar surface receives a suspension of the test bacteria, which is then spread out evenly over the surface of the agar. As growth of the bacteria occurs, antibiotic diffuses out from each disc into the agar. If the concentration of the antibiotic effectively inhibits bacterial growth, then there will be a clear zone around the disc. Some concentrations of antibiotic will not be sufficient to completely inhibit bacterial growth

and will recur. The concentration of antibiotic necessary can be determined, and comparisons with established data are made to establish whether the bacteria are resistant or susceptible to the antibiotic. The test was once performed manually, and still can be, but automated plate readers are now available.

Fluorescent indicators have become popular for evaluation of antibiotics. Many compounds will fluoresce when illuminated at certain wavelengths. For example, fluorescence can be used to determine if bacteria are killed by a specific antibiotic. The fluorescence test uses a specialized microscope called a confocal laser microscope. Another measurement technique uses a machine called a flow cytometer. This machine funnels a suspension of bacteria or other cells through an opening that is so small that only one bacterium at a time can pass. Each cell goes by a sensor that monitors for fluorescence (living) or nonfluorescence (dead). The entire process can be completed so quickly that it occurs almost in real-time assessment. If the number of bacteria that are scanned that are living reaches a predetermined threshold, the antibiotic is considered not effective (i.e., the bacterial population is resistant).

Antibiotic effectiveness testing must be done in a controlled way using standard types (strains) of bacteria that are resistant and susceptible to the particular antibiotic. The bacteria concentration is also important; too

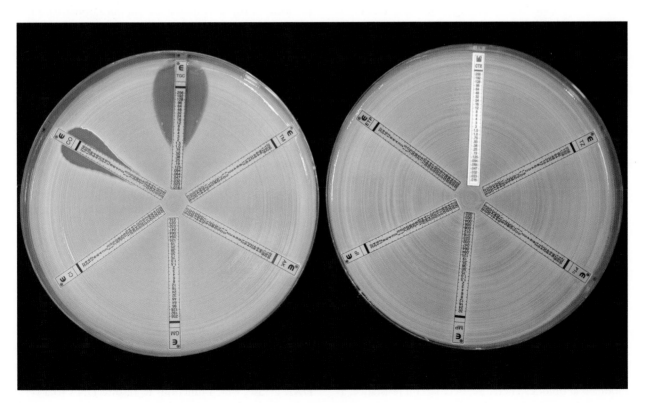

Two plates that were coated with an antibiotic-resistant bacteria called *Klebsiella* with a mutation called NDM 1 and then exposed to various antibiotics are seen at the Health Protection Agency in north London, England. The clear areas in the top left quarter of the plate on the left show that the *Klebsiella* with NDM 1 was sensitive to the respective antibiotics tigecycline and colistin. © *Suzanne Plunkett/Reuters.*

many cells can reduce the level of antibiotic that any one bacterium is exposed to, producing a false indication of resistance. Other controls rule out contamination. This is important, because if the contaminating microbe is resistant to the antibiotic, the positive result will be unreliable.

In cases of a sample from a patient, resistance would mean that the antibiotic being tested is not appropriate for use and another is necessary. Only a few generations ago, the second choice would not be difficult, as many antibiotics swiftly killed a variety of bacteria. The present day outlook is less optimistic because of the increase in antibiotic-resistant strains of bacteria and the emergence of extensively drug-resistant (XDR) organisms that resist nearly all existing antibiotics.

Penicillin is one of the members of a class of antibiotics termed beta-lactams. The name denotes the chemical ring that forms the core structure of beta-lactam. Other subclasses of beta-lactams include cephalosporins, monobactams, and carbapenems, which differ in the nature of the various side groups that are attached to the ring.

One action of antibiotics, including the nearly four dozen beta-lactam antibiotics, is to disrupt the peptidoglycan, which consists of long chains of sugar molecules that are chemically linked together by short stretches of protein (peptides) to form a complex, mesh like, and rigid polymer that completely encases a bacterium. The peptidoglycan is the stress-bearing network of a bacterium. Without an intact peptidoglycan, the bacterium is unable to withstand the pressure difference between the interior of the cell and the outside environment. Beta-lactams act by preventing the cross-linking of the sugar chains by the peptides.

There are several mechanisms of resistance to beta-lactam antibiotics. The first is the production of an enzyme termed beta-lactamase. The enzyme catalyzes the structural disruption of the beta-lactam ring, which destroys the activity of the antibiotic. Both gram-positive and gram-negative bacteria produce beta-lactamase. In the case of gram-positive bacteria, which have one membrane, the enzyme is released from the surface and diffuses outward. With gram-negative bacteria, the enzyme is trapped in the region between the inner and outer membranes, where it degrades beta-lactam antibiotics as they diffuse into the bacteria.

Strategies to cope with beta-lactamase production include the tweaking of antibiotics, typically by modification of the chemical side groups bound to the beta-lactam ring. The altered three-dimensional configuration of the modified antibiotic can be sufficient to diminish or restrict entirely the association of beta-lactamase. However, this strategy is not an absolute solution. Over time, bacteria will evolve other strategies to inactivate the modified antibiotic. Therefore, beta-lactam resistance, as with resistance to other antibiotics, is a never-ending race between the introduction of potent antibiotics and the development of resistance to them.

Vancomycin, a glycopeptide antibiotic, also blocks the cross-linking of peptidoglycan chains, but it does so in a different way than beta-lactam antibiotics. Vancomycin binds to the cross-linking peptides and blocks their ability to knit together the long sugar chains. The binding of vancomycin is to the last two amino acid residues of the peptide fragment; both are D-Alanine. If the very last D-Alanine is missing or replaced with another amino acid then vancomycin is blocked from its action.

Other antibiotics act by blocking the manufacture of different proteins by bacteria. Depending on the protein that is deficient, the bacterium can be weakened and rendered more susceptible to other compounds, or can be killed outright. Antibiotics that act by preventing protein synthesis include aminoglycosides (streptomycin, amikacin, tobramycin, and neomycin), tetracyclines (doxycycline, oxytetracycline, demeclocycline, and minocycline), macrolides (erythromycin and azithromycin), lincosamides (clindamycin), streptogramin (quinupristin and dalfopristin), oxazolidone (linezolid), and mupirocin.

Antibiotics that block protein synthesis do so by targeting a molecule called a ribosome, a complex molecule comprising 52 proteins and 3 types of ribonucleic acid (RNA). Different types of antibiotics bind to different regions on the ribosome. The binding disrupts the function of the ribosome, to match up the sequence of information in molecules called messenger RNA present in the form of triplet combinations of nucleotides with the amino acid specified by each nucleotide triplet. The amino acids are linked together to form the specified protein.

If the target site of the ribosome can be changed in a way that does not affect ribosome function and accuracy, then resistance can develop to the particular antibiotic. Fortunately, the many different sites on the ribosome means that a different antibiotic can be used. However, if a ribosome site is the target for more than one antibiotic, mutation of that site can confer resistance to all the antibiotics; this is termed cross-resistance. Cross-resistance to ribosome-targeted antibiotics can also occur if a bacterium undergoes a surface change that impedes the antibiotics from getting to the interior of the cell where ribosomes are located.

Macrolide antibiotics act at the ribosome, but do so in a different way, by blocking the growth of the protein chain instead of blocking protein formation. The truncated protein will likely be functionally defective. Quinolone antibiotics disrupt an enzyme that catalyzes the uncoiling of the double helix of deoxyribonucleic acid (DNA), which in turn can stop DNA replication.

Other antibiotics have targets other than bacterial membrane(s) or the ribosome. Fluoroquinolones (the best-known of which is ciprofloxacin) target the enzyme DNA gyrase, which functions to restore DNA to a very tightly wound (supercoiled) state after it has unwound so that replication can occur. Fluoroquinolones also target another enzyme called topoisomerase IV, which participates in compacting replicated DNA so that it will physically fit into the new bacterium. Mutations that change these enzymes, but still allow the bacterium to replicate DNA, can make the bacterium fluoroquinolone-resistant. While fluoroquinolone resistance has been relatively rare, the exploding popularity of fluoroquinolone antibiotics in 21st century, including as an additive to poultry feed, has encouraged the emergence of bacterial resistance.

The sulfonamide antibiotic sulfanilamide is often prescribed in combination with trimethoprim as an means of interfering with the production of tetrahydrofolic acid, a vitamin that is crucial for bacterial growth. The combination administered together can be effective, but resistance can develop to either compound administered alone.

Antimicrobial Resistance

Other antimicrobial compounds include antiviral, antifungal, and antiprotozoal compounds. While some antibiotics are active against a wide spectrum of bacteria, antiviral compounds tend to be specific in their action. Because viruses are not alive and because the nature of their replication depends of the use of the host cell's genetic replication machinery, the options for combatting viruses are limited, compared to bacteria.

Antivirals Efforts to eradicate viruses can harm the host cells, which can be bad for the host. Antiviral strategies focus on several aspects of the viral infection cycle: attachment of the virus to a recognized receptor on the surface of the host, the release of the viral genetic material inside the host cell (uncoating), integration of the viral genetic material into the host genome and replication of the viral genes along with the host genes, assembly of new virus, and release of the new virus. The steps preceding virus manufacture are the preferred targets, since they prevent new virus from being made.

After viruses enter the host cell, the release of viral DNA or RNA occurs as the virus particle dissolves. Stabilizing the molecules that make up the virus shell can prevent the dissolution and so the release of the genetic material. Examples of antiviral agents that act in this way include pleconaril, which is being tested for the treatment of rhinovirus (a cause of the common cold), and amantadine, which has been used to treat influenza (flu). Amantadine is not completely effective in preventing infection, but it does lessen the symptoms of flu. However, resistance can develop, which limits the practical use of amantadine to patients such as older adults or persons with chronic respiratory diseases who are at greater risk of developing pneumonia after contracting influenza.

Other antiviral drugs interfere with the active replication of the viral genetic material once the virus has released its payload of genetic material inside the host cell. Examples include zidovudine (INN) and azidothymidine (AZT), which disrupt the activity of a crucial enzyme needed for replication of human immunodeficiency virus (HIV). AZT combined with other compounds forms the basis of highly effective antiretroviral therapy (HAART), which has proven beneficial for millions of people infected with the two types of HIV. Another example is acyclovir, which is active against herpes simplex virus type 1 (the cause of cold sores) as well as chicken pox and shingles, which are varicella zoster infections.

Resistance to antiviral agents involves viral mutations that alter the binding of a virion (the infectious form of a virus as it exists outside the host cell) to the host surface receptor or change the three-dimensional structure (but not the function) of the target enzyme, reverse transcriptase.

Antifungals and Antiprotozoals Antifungal compounds have been developed. Some target the production of ergosterol, a type of cholesterol that is specific to fungi. These are useful, but, as with broad-spectrum antibiotics like penicillin, come with the caution that development of resistance will become widespread in a variety of species. Other antifungal agents are more specific. One example of a targeted antifungal is griseofulvin, which is used to treat fungi that cause infections including athlete's foot, jock itch, ringworm, and nail infections. How griseofulvin acts is not yet precisely known, but it involves the blockage of formation of structures called microtubules within fungal cells. Microtubules separate chromosomes during DNA replication and cell division, so their disruption is lethal for a fungal cell. Interestingly, griseofulvin is relatively nontoxic to human cells, even though these cells also possess microtubules.

Candida albicans causes candidiasis, which can range from minor skin infections and vaginitis to life-threatening infections in people with a malfunctioning immune system. Antifungals used to treat candidiasis include diflucan and ketoconazole (which target ergosterol production), amphotericin B and nystatin (which disrupt the fungal membrane; these can be toxic to humans), and flucytosine (which mimics a nucleoside and disrupts RNA manufacture, as well as disrupting thymidylate synthase, which is crucial in DNA synthesis).

Another important and life-threatening infection affecting immunocompromised individuals is pneumonia caused by *Pneumocystis jiroveci*. The drug of choice is for this infection is pentamidine, which blocks DNA synthesis. The drug is also effective, using the same mechanism, against a group of protozoans called trypanosomes, one of which, *Trypanosoma*, causes sleeping sickness.

Other drugs active against protozoans include chloroquine, quinacrine, and primaquine in the treatment of malaria. These drugs work by inserting themselves into the DNA of *Plasmodium*. *Trypanosoma* can also be treated using a drug called suramin, which blocks the action of enzymes that degrade glucose. The lack of glucose in effect starves the protozoan, since an important energy source becomes unavailable.

Discussion of resistance to antifungal agents is limited, since little research has been done. The root of the lack of research effort is the relative unimportance of fungal infections to people in developed countries, with the important exceptions of candidiasis and *Pneumocystis* pneumonia in people who are immunocompromised. While these and fungal diseases are important in underdeveloped and developing countries, there is little profit for drug companies to develop and market drugs in these regions. Efforts have focused on developing therapies for candidiasis and *Pneumocystis* pneumonia since these infections can be chronic in immunocompromised individuals, such as those with acquired immune deficiency syndrome (AIDS).

⊕ Future Implications

The problem of antibacterial resistance is global in scope. Two related examples are multidrug-resistant tuberculosis (MDR-TB) and extensively drug-resistant tuberculosis (XDR-TB). In 2012, there were an estimated 450,000 new cases of MDR-TB, with XDR-TB present in at least 92 countries, according to the World Health Organization (WHO). A multidrug-resistant form of *Staphylococcus aureus* (methicillin-resistant *S. aureus*, or MRSA) has become common in hospitals worldwide. Antibacterial resistance has also become a widespread problem in farming, due to the practice of feeding animals antibiotic-laden feed. (See graphic on page 21.) There is evidence that the resistant bacteria or

the genetic determinants of resistance can be passed from the animals to humans.

A report published in April 2014 by the WHO, which examined antibiotic resistance in 114 countries, has revealed the global spread of antibiotic resistance. The WHO report focused on resistance to bacteria causing pneumonia, diarrhea, gonorrhea, and urinary tract infections, among others. Resistance to commonly encountered bacteria has reached levels that the WHO described as alarming, with some areas of the world now having no treatment options in their antibiotic arsenal. Resistance to carbapenem antibiotics, which have been the mainstay treatment against *Klebsiella pneumoniae*, the cause of pneumonia and infections in infants, is now global.

On March 27, 2015, the United States announced a "National Action Plan for Combating Antibiotic-Resistant Bacteria." According to the White House, the plan is intended to "enhance domestic and international capacity to prevent and contain outbreaks of antibiotic-resistant infections; maintain the efficacy of current and new antibiotics; and develop and deploy next-generation, diagnostics, antibiotics, vaccines, and other therapeutics."

The overarching goals of the plan include:

- slowing the emergence of resistant bacteria and preventing the spread of resistant infections;

- strengthening national one-health surveillance efforts to combat resistance (the "one-health" approach to disease surveillance integrates data

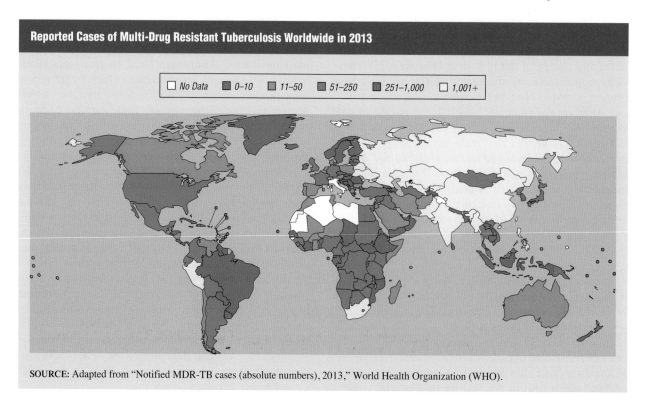

Reported Cases of Multi-Drug Resistant Tuberculosis Worldwide in 2013

☐ No Data ■ 0–10 ■ 11–50 ■ 51–250 ■ 251–1,000 ☐ 1,001+

SOURCE: Adapted from "Notified MDR-TB cases (absolute numbers), 2013," World Health Organization (WHO).

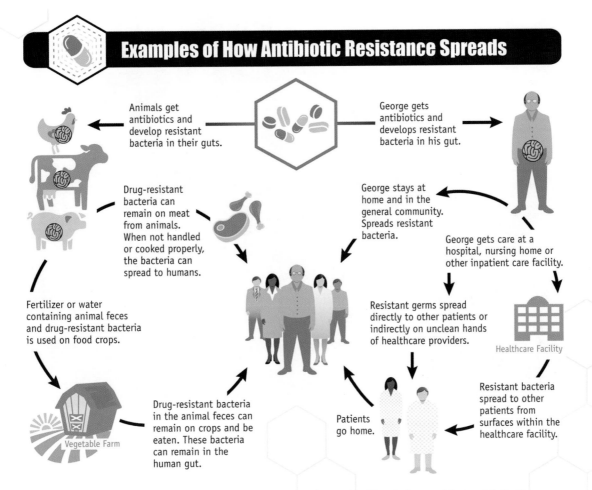

Examples of How Antibiotic Resistance Spreads

Animals get antibiotics and develop resistant bacteria in their guts.

George gets antibiotics and develops resistant bacteria in his gut.

Drug-resistant bacteria can remain on meat from animals. When not handled or cooked properly, the bacteria can spread to humans.

George stays at home and in the general community. Spreads resistant bacteria.

George gets care at a hospital, nursing home or other inpatient care facility.

Fertilizer or water containing animal feces and drug-resistant bacteria is used on food crops.

Resistant germs spread directly to other patients or indirectly on unclean hands of healthcare providers.

Healthcare Facility

Drug-resistant bacteria in the animal feces can remain on crops and be eaten. These bacteria can remain in the human gut.

Patients go home.

Resistant bacteria spread to other patients from surfaces within the healthcare facility.

Vegetable Farm

Simply using antibiotics creates resistance. These drugs should only be used to treat infections.

This infographic illustrates, in very simple terms, examples of how antibiotic resistance spreads. The takeaway message is that simply using antibiotics creates resistance, and that these drugs should be used to treat infections only. Note the important relationship between the agricultural industry and the daily lives of human beings. *Melissa Brower/U.S. Centers for Disease Control and Prevention.*

from multiple monitoring networks, according to the White House);

- advancing development and use of rapid and innovative diagnostic tests for the identification and characterization of resistant bacteria;
- accelerating basic and applied research and development for new antibiotics, other therapeutics, and vaccines; and
- improving international collaboration and capacities for antibiotic resistance prevention, surveillance, control, and antibiotic research and development.

For all the research on antibiotic resistance since the 1940s, including genetic studies described above,

resistance mechanisms may still remain to be discovered. An example includes the results of research published in September 2014. In the study, the use of fluid-filled chambers that more closely mimic environments found in the human body, rather than the typical test tube-based experiments that have been the research stalwart, has implicated genetic rearrangements that can occur quickly in response to bacterial stress, such as antibiotic exposure, in resistance. Termed accelerated evolution, this resistance mechanism is especially important since changes at the genetic level can be passed on to subsequent generations of bacteria. The WHO reported that the global spread of resistance has been driven by the overuse of antibiotics and incorrect use of antibiotics (such as

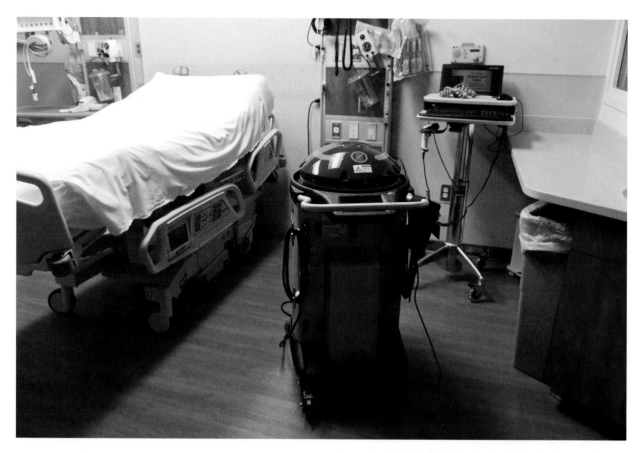

The CDC has warned that drug-resistant bacteria, including *Clostridium difficile* (*C. diff*), *Klebsiella pneumoniae*, and methicillin-resistant *Staphylococcus aureus*, better known as MRSA, have been on the rise since the beginning of the 21st century in U.S. hospitals, nursing homes, and acute care centers. One element that may be useful in the fight against the most dangerous pathogens is an ultraviolet (UV) light disinfection system, which uses UV light 25,000 times more powerful than sunlight to destroy harmful bacteria, viruses, fungi, and even bacterial spores. This can help to sterilize rooms and equipment in hospitals and reduce the number of hospital-acquired drug-resistant infections. *© Emily Rose Bennett/MLIVE.COM/Landov.*

their use to treat viral infections). At the same time, the discovery of new antibiotics has slowed. With no prospect of a variety of new antibiotics, resistance will grow more prevalent.

PRIMARY SOURCE

Antimicrobial Resistance: Global Report on Surveillance, 2014

SOURCE *"Summary," in* Antimicrobial Resistance: Global Report on Surveillance, 2014. *Geneva: World Health Organization (WHO), April 2014, p. 3. http://apps.who.int/iris/bitstream/ 10665/112647/1/WHO_HSE_PED_ AIP_2014.2_eng.pdf (accessed January 25, 2015).*

INTRODUCTION *This primary source is the summary of the World Health Organization (WHO)*

report on the growing public health danger posed by antimicrobial resistance. It presents a brief description of this global problem along with WHO's initial action plan.

Summary

Antimicrobial resistance (AMR) is an increasingly serious threat to global public health. AMR develops when a microorganism (bacteria, fungus, virus or parasite) no longer responds to a drug to which it was originally sensitive. This means that standard treatments no longer work; infections are harder or impossible to control; the risk of the spread of infection to others is increased; illness and hospital stays are prolonged, with added economic and social costs; and the risk of death is greater—in some cases, twice that of patients who have infections caused by non-resistant bacteria.

The problem is so serious that it threatens the achievements of modern medicine. A post-antibiotic era—in which common infections and minor injuries can kill—is a very real possibility for the 21st century.

Determining the scope of the problem is the first step in formulating an effective response to AMR. "Antimicrobial resistance: Global report on surveillance 2014," produced in collaboration with Member States and external partners, is WHO's first attempt to obtain an accurate picture of the magnitude of AMR and the current state of surveillance globally. The report focuses on antibacterial resistance (ABR), as the state of surveillance in ABR is not generally as advanced as it is for diseases such as tuberculosis (TB), malaria and HIV.

The most important findings of this report are:

- Very high rates of resistance have been observed in all WHO regions in common bacteria (for example, *Escherichia coli, Klebsiella pneumoniae* and *Staphylococcus aureus*) that cause common health-care associated and community-acquired infections (urinary tract infections, wound infections, bloodstream infections and pneumonia).

- Many gaps exist in information on pathogens of major public health importance. There are significant gaps in surveillance, and a lack of standards for methodology, data sharing and coordination. Overall, surveillance of ABR is neither coordinated nor harmonized.

Despite the limitations of current surveillance, it is clear that ABR has reached alarming levels in many parts of the world. There is an urgent need to strengthen and coordinate collaboration to address those gaps. Lessons learned from long-standing experience in TB, malaria and HIV programmes may be usefully applied to ABR and are discussed in the report.

WHO is developing a global action plan for AMR that will include:

- development of tools and standards for harmonized surveillance of ABR in humans, and for integrated surveillance in food-producing animals and the food chain;

- elaboration of strategies for population-based surveillance of AMR and its health and economic impact; and

- collaboration between AMR surveillance networks and centres to create or strengthen coordinated regional and global surveillance.

AMR is a global health security threat that requires action across government sectors and society as a whole. Surveillance that generates reliable data is the essential foundation of global strategies and public health actions to contain AMR.

SEE ALSO *Bacterial Diseases; Epidemiology: Surveillance for Emerging Infectious Diseases; Fungal Diseases; Methicillin-Resistant* Staphylococcus Aureus *(MRSA)*

BIBLIOGRAPHY

Books

Coates, Anthony R. M. *Antibiotic Resistance: Handbook of Experimental Pharmacology.* Heidelberg: Springer, 2012.

Drlica, Karl, and David Perlin. *Antibiotic Resistance: Understanding and Responding to an Emerging Crisis.* Upper Saddle River, NJ: FT Press, 2011.

Gillespie, S. H., and Timothy D. McHugh. *Antibiotic Resistance Protocols.* New York: Humana Press, 2010.

Mainous, Arch G., and Claire Pomeroy. *Management of Antimicrobials in Infectious Diseases Impact of Antibiotic Resistance.* Totowa, NJ: Humana Press, 2010.

Salyers, Abigail, and Dixie Whitt. *Revenge of the Microbes: How Bacterial Resistance is Undermining the Antibiotic Miracle.* Washington, DC: ASM Press, 2005.

Periodicals

Zhang, Qiucen, et al. "You Cannot Tell a Book by Looking at the Cover: Cryptic Complexity in Bacterial Evolution." *Biomicrofluidics* 8, no. 5 (September 9, 2014): 052004.

Websites

"Antibiotic Resistance Questions and Answers." *U.S. Centers for Disease Control and Prevention (CDC).* http://www.cdc.gov/getsmart/antibiotic-use/antibiotic-resistance-faqs.html (accessed February 18, 2015).

"Antimicrobial Resistance." *World Health Organization (WHO).* http://www.who.int/mediacentre/factsheets/fs194/en/ (accessed February 18, 2015).

"Combating Antibiotic Resistance." *U.S. Food and Drug Administration (FDA).* http://www.fda.gov/ForConsumers/ConsumerUpdates/ucm092810.htm (accessed February 18, 2015).

"General Background: About Antibiotic Resistance." *Tufts.edu.* http://www.tufts.edu/med/apua/about_issue/about_antibioticres.shtml (accessed February 18, 2015).

"National Action Plan for Combating Antibiotic-Resistant Bacteria." *White House.* https://www.whitehouse.gov/sites/default/files/docs/national_action_plan_for_combating_antibiotic-resistant_bacteria.pdf (accessed March 27, 2015).

Brian Douglas Hoyle

Avian (Bird) and Swine Influenzas

⊕ Introduction

The most prominent avian influenza (commonly known as "bird flu") is an infectious disease that occurs in avian (bird) populations worldwide and is caused by several subtypes of the influenza A type virus. Many species of wild migrating birds are carriers of the disease. Some avian influenza viruses cause mild disease in birds, whereas others are responsible for outbreaks of severe disease with high death rates. The avian influenza virus also can infect other animals, although far less frequently. In general, avian influenza infections seldom occur in humans, and when they do occur, usually result in mild illness. The A/H5N1 subtype (also known as the A/H5N1 or H5N1 avian influenza) is one of few exceptions: The H5N1 virus causes a highly lethal influenza in humans. H5N1 is among the variant influenza viruses that are lethal to poultry and are known as highly pathogenic (disease causing) avian influenza (HPAI).

Influenza viruses also regularly circulate in swine populations and the first definitive isolation of a swine influenza virus infecting a human was made in 1974.

H1N1

In March 2009, a novel virus with both avian and swine characteristics and ultimately officially designated as the 2009 H1N1 influenza virus (alternately, type A/H1N1) started an influenza (flu) outbreak in Mexico and the United States. Both U.S. and Canadian researchers definitively detected the novel virus as early as April 2009. Emanating initially from Mexico, the virus spread quickly around the world, and encountered little resistance to human-to-human transmission. The first official death in the United States was reported in late April 2009 and by June 2009, the World Health Organization (WHO) declared that the 2009 H1N1 influenza was officially a global pandemic (worldwide epidemic).

H5N1

H5N1-caused influenza in humans can be highly dangerous, with a global lethality (fatality) rate of approximately 59 percent. Regional lethality rates vary. In one cluster of cases in Cambodia, all eight people who contracted H5N1 influenza died. In the H5N1 outbreak in Egypt early in 2015, the lethality rate dropped to less than 40 percent.

According to the WHO, since 2003, hundreds of millions of domestic poultry have died from H5N1 infection or as a result of culls used to control outbreaks. Globally, economic losses related to H5N1 range up to $20 billion. Scientists discovered the H5N1 virus in the 1990s and trace the latest continuing outbreak to an index case (first case) reported in 2003. By July 2013, H5N1 influenza was reported in 718 confirmed human cases resulting 413 deaths. A fresh outbreak in Egypt early in 2015 gained international attention with 78 new cases of H5N1 resulting in 21 deaths in just the first two months of 2015.

H7N9

The A H7N9 avian influenza virus (usually simply called the H7N9 virus) was first detected in China in April 2013. Scientists found the novel virus in poultry and in humans almost simultaneously, and they believe that infected poultry is the source of the virus in humans, as most humans with H7N9 influenza reported recent contact with poultry.

In March 2013, Chinese health authorities officially notified the WHO of three cases of human infection of influenza A subtype H7N9, a new subtype of avian influenza. Two of the cases occurred in Shanghai and the third in Anhui Province, and two of the three patients died. In December 2013, officials reported the first case of influenza A H7N9 in Hong Kong. Chinese health officials reported a sharp increase in H7N9 cases at the beginning of 2014 but stated that the rise could be mirroring trends seen in seasonal influenza, with an

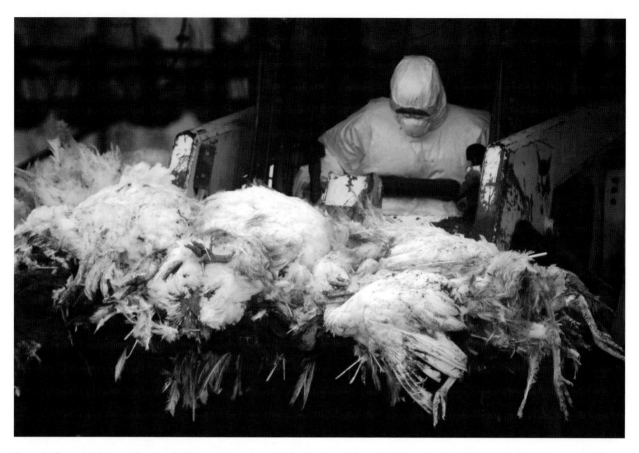

An agriculture ministry worker in a forklift carries carcasses of dead turkeys due to bird flu outbreak at Kibbutz Holit in the western Negev, Israel, on March 19, 2006. © *ChameleonsEye/Shutterstock.com.*

increase in illness during the winter months. By January 2015, the WHO and the U.S. Centers for Disease Control and Prevention (CDC) had confirmed 613 human cases of H7N9-related influenza. No cases outside China were confirmed by the WHO or CDC investigators, and H7N9-induced severe respiratory disease was officially the cause of death in about 39 percent of cases reported.

In January 2015, Canadian health officials confirmed two cases of H7N9 avian flu. A couple that had recently traveled to China together were the first reported cases of the avian influenza strain in North America. Previous incidents of H7N9 were limited to China, but Canadian health officials stated that the cases do not pose a significant health risk to the general public. Global travel provides a convenient vector (route) for infectious diseases to cross oceans and international borders.

⊕ Historical Background

In March 1976, U.S. President Gerald R. Ford (1913–2006) ordered a nationwide vaccination program to prevent a swine flu epidemic in the United States. The program was launched in response to the February 1976 death of a 19-year-old army recruit at Fort Dix, New Jersey, that was attributed to a severe case of swine influenza. Epidemiologists (scientists who study the causes, occurrence, and distribution of health and disease in populations) still debate whether the program was an overreaction to localized events or an example of swift mobilization of public health resources. Regardless, complications with the emergency vaccine caused the vaccination program to be abandoned, and the feared epidemic did not take place.

In 1988, transmission of swine flu to a woman in Wisconsin who had exposure to pigs resulted in her death. Between 2005 and the pandemic outbreak in 2009, CDC officials recorded only about a dozen cases of swine flu transmission to humans, all of whom had regular contact with pigs.

The H1N1 Pandemic

Experts usually define a viral pandemic as significant illness occurring over a large geographic area resulting from a new virus to which the general population is widely susceptible—that is, the population lacks natural immunity to the virus—and in which the virus shows the ability to spread from person to person. A virus causing a pandemic does not need to be especially lethal, although a high number of fatalities may occur depending on the number of people exposed to the virus.

The H1N1 virus—carrying a previously unencountered reassortment of genes from swine (pigs and related animals), avian (birds), and human genomes—caused a form of influenza initially described as a swine flu. The four most common viruses circulating in pigs are H1N1, H1N2, H3N1, and H3N2 viruses. However, molecular evidence showed that the novel pandemic H1N1 virus had not been immediately derived or transmitted from swine. Moreover, no evidence placed swine in the subsequent transmission chain. Accordingly, the WHO and CDC officials began to refer to the virus as 2009 H1N1 and the associated flu as H1N1 influenza. In July 2009, the WHO, CDC, and other world health authorities began to use the nomenclature "pandemic (H1N1) 2009" as a common reference for both the virus and the disease. However, the term "swine flu" continues to be used frequently, especially in media reports, to describe the illness.

Estimates of cases and deaths vary wildly from admittedly low estimates by the WHO of nearly 20,000 deaths to CDC statistics based estimates ranging up to 284,000 deaths. Because most people who die of flu-related causes are not tested for the specific virus causing death, estimates are uncertain, but official reports are acknowledged by experts to be vastly undercounted.

In January 2010, the WHO director-general Margaret Chan (1947–) characterized the H1N1 pandemic as moderate and close in scope and impact to influenza pandemics in 1957 and 1968.

H5N1

Most cases of human infection with H5N1 result from close contact with infected bird populations—for example, in situations in which people live in proximity to infected birds (mostly poultry), handle infected birds, or have contact with H5N1-contaminated surfaces. Researchers have documented that all cases involving human-to-human transmission were the result of caring for an infected patient or relative.

H5N1 has infected pigs, an animal that historically has served as the host for flu viruses that mutated into forms that more easily allow human-to-human transmission. Accordingly, the WHO has made the study and containment of H5N1 and other avian flu viruses one of its top priorities.

Avian influenza is common because migrating wild birds are natural hosts for various subtypes of influenza A, including H5N1. Most avian influenza viruses normally do not make wild birds sick, although the viruses can be transmitted through their saliva and feces. Poultry—domesticated birds such as chickens, ducks, and turkeys—can catch influenza from wild birds and, in contrast, the domesticated birds become sick. In some

cases, outbreaks of H5N1 bird flu have killed 100 percent of the birds in infected flocks.

In March 2011, a joint study by the U.S. Geological Survey, the United Nations Food and Agriculture Organization, and the Chinese Academy of Sciences established that migratory birds help spread highly pathogenic avian influenza (HPAI H5N1) by using fields shared by domestic flocks of poultry. Satellite tracking of bar-headed geese showed that the birds, known carriers of HPAI, often wintered near the sites of past H5N1 outbreaks in areas of China with high levels of poultry production.

Little can be done to stop the virus from spreading and mutating, except to reduce its host environment. Governments of affected countries often have ordered the quarantine or wholesale slaughter of sick, potentially infected, and exposed birds. In some countries, officials have directed that chickens be given vaccines—some with questionable effectiveness—against various strains of avian influenza in an attempt to reduce economic losses.

H5N8

In November 2014, health inspectors in the Netherlands detected the highly contagious influenza A (H5N8) in chickens on a poultry farm in central Netherlands. Dutch authorities immediately destroyed 150,000 chickens on the farm. European Union authorities imposed a ban on the export of poultry and eggs from the affected area. Researchers believe that the Dutch outbreak may be linked to another H5N8 outbreak at a smaller farm in northeastern Germany a few weeks prior.

Although no cases of H5N8 have ever been reported in humans, Dutch health officials warned that the disease could be transferred to humans who come into close contact with poultry. The disease is highly contagious and fatal among poultry, however, which requires culling animals with possible exposure. An outbreak of H5N8 in South Korea in early 2014 required the destruction of millions of birds.

⊕ Impacts and Issues

Three characteristics typify a new virus's potential to create a global pandemic: (1) the degree to which a virus is new genetically, (2) the transmissibility of the virus between humans, and (3) the virus's capability to cause illness to which humans have no natural immunity. As of May 6, 2009, the novel swine flu strain found in Mexico and the United States (called by some experts the H1N1 North American influenza strain) had been demonstrated to be a new strain, and human-to-human transmission was also shown, but in terms of transmissibility and lethality, experts initially concluded that the

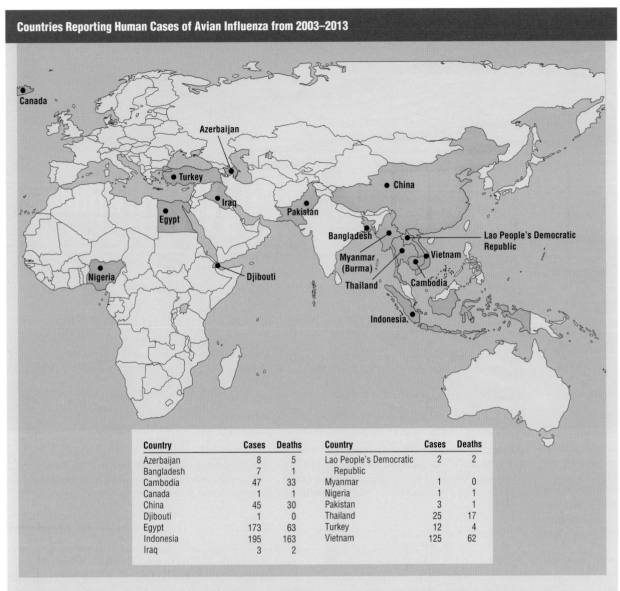

Countries Reporting Human Cases of Avian Influenza from 2003–2013

Country	Cases	Deaths	Country	Cases	Deaths
Azerbaijan	8	5	Lao People's Democratic Republic	2	2
Bangladesh	7	1	Myanmar	1	0
Cambodia	47	33	Nigeria	1	1
Canada	1	1	Pakistan	3	1
China	45	30	Thailand	25	17
Djibouti	1	0	Turkey	12	4
Egypt	173	63	Vietnam	125	62
Indonesia	195	163			
Iraq	3	2			

SOURCE: Adapted from "Areas with confirmed human cases for avian influenza A(H5N1) reported to WHO, 2003–2013," World Health Organization (WHO), January 10, 2014.

novel virus and associated flu is not significantly different from a normal seasonal flu.

The assessment of H1N1 being as deadly as a normal seasonal flu means that H1N1 influenza virus is not nearly as lethal as other existing viral threats such as the H5N1 avian flu virus or the virus responsible for severe acute respiratory syndrome (SARS). Despite the fact that H1N1 proved to have the characteristics of a seasonal flu, the WHO official argued that the pandemic alert was justified based on the susceptibility of the global population to the novel virus

In 2007, the U.S. Food and Drug Administration approved the first vaccine for humans against avian influenza in the United States. The vaccine, which several

governments have stockpiled for use during a potential H5N1 outbreak or pandemic, is generic and not specifically matched to the specific strain that may emerge to start a pandemic. Accordingly, its ultimate effectiveness in a pandemic is uncertain. In addition, scientists are watching the evolution of some H7 family of avian influenza viruses because some types are highly lethal in poultry and have shown an increasing potential to acquire the ability to spread among humans.

Because flu viruses mutate (change genetically) from year to year, novel strains of type A flu virus are not unusual. Each year, a stock of human influenza vaccine is prepared against the strains thought most likely to cause illness. However, initial assessments showed that stock

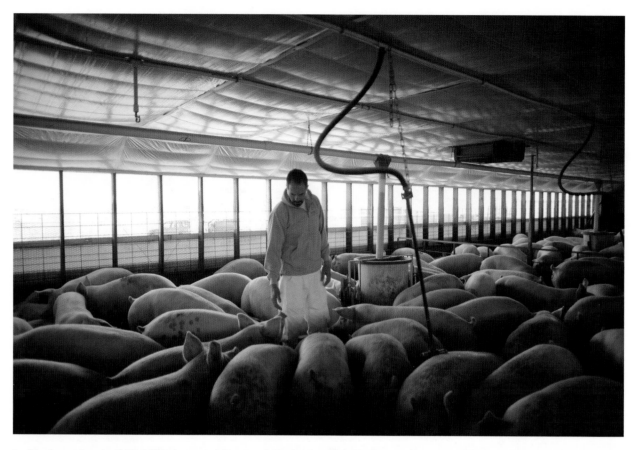

In this photo taken April 27, 2009, the general director of Granjas Carroll de Mexico stands next to pigs at one of the company's farms on the outskirts of Jicaltepec in Mexico's Veracruz State. Scientists went to La Gloria, a pig-farming village in the Veracruz mountains where Mexico's earliest confirmed case of swine flu was identified. They hoped to learn where the epidemic began by taking fresh blood samples from villagers and pigs and looking for antibodies that could suggest exposure to previous swine flu infections.
© AP Photo/Alexandre Meneghini.

vaccines may prove ineffective or have limited value in preventing unanticipated flu types. Mindful of the problems associated with preparing the 1976 emergency swine flu vaccine, both the CDC and the WHO usually recommend not rushing production of emergency vaccines to counter the initial outbreaks until such vaccines can be proven safe and effective. A notable exception to such prudent safeguards was the fast-track approval and production to combat the 2014 Ebola outbreak in West Africa. Although Ebola is totally unrelated to flu, experts noted precedent-setting decisions that could speed testing and approval of potential flu vaccines for emergency use. In general, with regard to flu, public health officials recommend incorporating protection against specific virus types into the next regular cycle of selection and production.

Bioweapons Potential and Research Issues

In May 2012, the journal *Nature* published a report that had been delayed over fears that its contents might facilitate the mutation of the deadly H5N1 avian flu virus into a more easily transmissible form capable of use as a biological weapon. The study revealed how specific H5N1 genetic mutations, including those previously unknown, affected transmissibility. In a prepared statement, University of Wisconsin–Madison researcher Yoshihiro Kawaoka (1955–), one of the authors of the report, stated, "Our study shows that relatively few amino acid mutations are sufficient for a virus with an avian H5 hemagglutinin to acquire the ability to transmit in mammals."

A review panel initially recommended withholding certain details of the original publication based on fears that information about which genes and types of mutations enhanced H5 virus transmissibility might be used by unspecified terrorist organizations to mount a biological attack. An array of scientific researchers and public health experts countered that the specific mutation and weaponization of H5N1 would be extremely difficult, even with access to advanced government research labs. Influenza experts also argued that suppression of the research constituted a far greater danger by reducing the chance that researchers around the world would detect and provide early warning of key H5N1 mutations. In his statement, Kawaoka noted that key mutations already are found in nature.

In April 2012, the Dutch government granted an export license to Ron Fouchier, a virologist at Erasmus University Medical Center, to publish his paper on the transmissibility of genetically modified H5N1. U.S. government officials objected to the publication of an unredacted version of Fouchier's study, which led Dutch authorities to block publication. Even after the U.S. government reversed course and dropped its opposition to publication, the Dutch government took the unusual step of requiring Fouchier to request an export license before submitting his paper to the journal *Science*. A year long voluntary moratorium on such research was lifted in early 2013.

⊕ Future Implications

Although human-to-human transmission is rare—and currently observed only among those having extended close contact with infected individuals—experts warn that subtle mutations in the continually evolving H5N1 virus could make it more transmissible among humans.

The specific H5N1 virus linked to human deaths is especially dangerous because it is resistant to both amantadine and rimantadine, two antiviral drugs commonly used to treat influenza. Other antiviral medications, oseltamivir (Tamiflu) and zanamivir, have shown effectiveness, but the full extent or limits of effectiveness are still subject to additional testing. In addition, it is uncertain whether any antiviral will be effective against the exact avian influenza strain that might ultimately spark a global pandemic.

By 2015, the majority of new cases of HPAI outside of Asia came from Egypt. In January 2014, however, Canadian health authorities announced the first fatality in North America linked to a confirmed case of H5N1. Canadian officials described the case as isolated, however, because the infected person contracted the disease on a visit to China.

Education, political persuasion, and changing cultural attitudes are other important ways to help build international cooperation in fighting avian influenza. In Egypt, for example, public officials reported the first avian flu case to the WHO in February 2006. Residents of Egypt are especially susceptible to H5N1 because poultry is an integral source of income and food for more than 5 million Egyptian households. In Egypt, where poultry is one of the mainstays of the diet, avian influenza in humans occurs mostly among young children. People often keep chickens on their rooftops, and children frequently are responsible for their care. Many Egyptian people are reluctant to report ill or dying chickens to local authorities for fear that their chickens and possibly those of their neighbors will be removed. Unlike those of many other countries, the Egyptian government does not compensate citizens for culled or seized poultry. Officials suggest that financial compensation to owners might provide an incentive to increase reporting when their chickens become ill or die.

UNIQUE REASSORTMENTS OF GENES

The specific genome (combination of genes) in the 2009 H1N1 virus had not previously been cataloged in infections detected in either humans or pigs. The novel virus contains a complex triple reassortment of genes previously identified in swine influenzas found in North America, Asia, and Europe as well as genes from avian and human influenzas.

The HxNx nomenclature derives from specific antigens located on the surface of type A viruses. These antigens, hemagglutinin (HA) and neuraminidase (NA), are proteins that vary in their chemical structure from year to year. This process, termed antigenic drift, results in virus particle proteins with subtle variations in structure. Currently, 15 different HA subtypes are known to exist, while there are nine different NA subtypes. These subtypes receive different number designations, and the various influenza strains are named by the specific HA (H) and NA (N) proteins on the virus. The H1N1 swine flu virus contains HA protein 1 and NA protein 1.

Of particular interest to infectious disease researchers are the genes that control hemagglutinin (H) and neuraminidase (N), two surface proteins with subtypes that are numbered (hence H1N1 flu or H5N1 avian flu virus), along with genes that control the nucleoprotein and the surrounding matrix, and three key polymerase enzymes (designated PA, PB1, and PB2) that the virus must have to reproduce. Genetically, the 2009 H1N1 presents a mixed background, with these key genes derived from human, swine, and avian sources (a triple reassortment). The hemagglutinin produced is equidistant to the swine flu sequences found in the North America, Europe, and Asia. The neuraminidase and matrix genes sequences are close to genes found in swine flu strains found in Asia. Early evidence indicates similarities to strains where the PB1 gene is of human origin and the PA and PB2 genes are from avian sources.

Proteins comprise chains of amino acids linked in a specific sequence. Genes code for (control) the sequence, and subtle changes in the genetic code can result in changes in the sequence of amino acids. Changing the genetic message can terminate transcription of a protein and create other errors that make the protein nonfunctional, or that change the way it functions. The substitution of a single amino acid for another in a long chain can alter the ultimate shape of a protein in such a way that the protein's ability to take part in complicated biochemical reactions is also altered.

When H7N9 was first detected in April 2013, there was a spike in infections and a sharp drop-off in the following months. Public health experts widely attributed the decline to quick action by Chinese health officials to shut down live poultry markets temporarily and identify cases in bird populations and humans. The ability of the H7N9 virus to spread between humans is thus far limited and less transmissible than a typical seasonal influenza virus. However, the WHO and the CDC continue to monitor the virus for its pandemic potential, especially for the ability to generate sustained person-to-person transmission. According to reports by the WHO and CDC officials, some cases of H7N9-caused influenza produce milder symptoms, but overall the influenza associated with H7N9 had a high initial case fatality rate. Accordingly, both the WHO and the CDC increased efforts to identify candidate vaccines for this potentially serious flu.

New variants continue to be detected. In December 2013 and January 2014, Chinese health officials notified the WHO of two cases of avian influenza A (H10N8), which previously had been detected only in wild and domestic birds. Both patients, one of whom died, had been in close contact with birds at poultry markets. As of mid-February 2015, the WHO reported no evidence of human-to-human transmission of H10N8.

PRIMARY SOURCE

Overview of the Emergence and Characteristics of the Avian Influenza A(H7N9) Virus

SOURCE *"Summary," in* Overview of the emergence and characteristics of the avian influenza A(H7N9) virus. *Geneva: World Health Organization (WHO), May 31, 2013, 1–2. http://www .who.int/influenza/human_animal_interface/ influenza_h7n9/WHO_H7N9_review_31May13. pdf (accessed January 25, 2015).*

INTRODUCTION *This primary source is taken from a 2013 publication of the World Health Organization (WHO) that gives an overview of a 2013 outbreak of avian influenza in China. The summary section presented here describes the symptoms of the infection, the timeline of the outbreak, and related statistics, as well as preliminary results of the WHO investigation.*

SUMMARY

This is an overview of the emergence and characteristics of avian influenza A(H7N9) virus infecting humans in China in early 2013. The public health and animal health investigations of the outbreak were facilitated by rapid sharing of information and viruses.... These activities have been essential in guiding disease control interventions and informing pandemic preparedness actions.

1. The outbreak

On 31 March 2013, the public health authorities of China reported three cases of laboratory-confirmed human infection with avian influenza A(H7N9) virus (hereafter H7N9). Two cases were detected in residents of the

city of Shanghai and one in a resident of Anhui province. The first case was an 87 year old male patient from the city of Shanghai who reported onset of influenza-like symptoms on 19 February 2013. The second and third cases had illness onset dates of 27 February and 15 March. By 29 May 2013, approximately 2 months after the initial report, the number of laboratory-confirmed H7N9 infections reached 132, with 37 deaths, originating from these locations and seven additional provinces, Shandong, Zhejiang, Henan, Hunan, Fujian, Jiangxi, and Jiangsu, and the municipality of Beijing, in addition to one case reported by Taipei, Centres for Disease Control (CDC) (with a history of recent travel from Jiangsu).

Most patients initially developed an influenza-like illness (ILI) that subsequently progressed to respiratory distress syndrome resulting in hospitalization. The case fatality proportion reached approximately 25%, which is a provisional value because many patients remain hospitalized as of 8 May 2013 and the number of mild cases remains unknown. Six patients were identified through influenza-like illness surveillance, two of them with mild symptoms not requiring hospitalization. Underlying chronic conditions were reported in most cases. The median age was 61 years with a predominance of males (2.4:1 male to female ratio). In contrast, previous infections with subtype H7 avian influenza viruses have generally been mild and associated with conjunctivitis.

Investigations of H7N9 cases have so far revealed that except for four confirmed clusters of two or more cases that were in close contact, the patients did not appear to have known exposure to each other. However, most patients had a history of recent exposure to poultry, generally at live bird markets. On April 5, 2013, the Ministry of Agriculture of China reported to the World Organization of Animal Health (OIE) the detection of low-pathogenic avian influenza A(H7N9) in a pigeon sampled at an agricultural wholesale market in the Shanghai municipality; this being the first H7N9 reported in birds in Asia since 2011.

Surveillance for ILI among people in close contact with laboratory-confirmed H7N9 cases indicated that infected individuals are not a likely source of infection. These preliminary studies suggested that despite numerous cases of H7N9 virus infection associated with poultry exposure, there is no evidence of sustained onwards virus transmission to other people.

SEE ALSO *Epidemiology: Surveillance for Emerging Infectious Diseases; Influenza; International Health Regulations, Surveillance, and Enforcement; Isolation and Quarantine; Pandemic Preparedness; Vaccine Preventable Diseases; Vaccines; Viral Diseases; Zoonotic (Animal-Borne) Diseases*

BIBLIOGRAPHY

Books

Abramson, Jon Stuart. *Inside the 2009 Influenza Pandemic.* Singapore: World Scientific, 2011.

Biehl, João Guilherme, and Adriana Petryna, eds. *When People Come First: Critical Studies in Global Health.* Princeton, NJ: Princeton University Press, 2013.

Bristow, Nancy K. *American Pandemic: The Lost Worlds of the 1918 Influenza Epidemic.* Oxford: Oxford University Press, 2012.

Crisp, Nigel. *Turning the World Upside Down: The Search for Global Health in the Twenty-First Century.* London: Royal Society of Medicine Press, 2010.

Dehner, George. *Global Flu and You: A History of Influenza.* London: Reaktion Books, 2012.

Dehner, George. *Influenza: A Century of Science and Public Health Response.* Pittsburgh, PA: University of Pittsburgh Press, 2012.

Food and Agriculture Organization of the United Nations. *Approaches to Controlling, Preventing and Eliminating H5N1 Highly Pathogenic Avian Influenza in Endemic Countries.* Rome: Food and Agriculture Organization of the United Nations, 2011.

Giles-Vernick, Tamara, Susan Craddock, and Jennifer Lee Gunn, eds. *Influenza and Public Health Learning from Past Pandemics.* London: Earthscan, 2010.

Honigsbaum, Mark. *A History of the Great Influenza Pandemics: Death, Panic and Hysteria, 1830–1920.* London: I.B. Tauris, 2014.

Humphries, Mark Osborne. *The Last Plague: Spanish Influenza and the Politics of Public Health in Canada.* Toronto: University of Toronto Press, 2013.

Jones, Esyllt Wynne, and Magdalena Fahrni, eds. *Epidemic Encounters: Influenza, Society, and Culture in Canada, 1918–20.* Vancouver: UBC Press, 2012.

Kapoor, Sanjay, and Kuldeep Dhama. *Insight into Influenza Viruses of Animals and Humans.* New York: Springer, 2014.

MacPhail, Theresa. *The Viral Network: A Pathography of the H1N1 Influenza Pandemic.* Ithaca, NY: Cornell University Press, 2014.

Matchett, Karin, Anne-Marie Mazza, and Steven Kendall. *Perspectives on Research with H5N1 Avian Influenza: Scientific Inquiry, Communication, Controversy: Summary of a Workshop.* Washington, DC: National Academies Press, 2013.

Scoones, Ian, ed. *Avian Influenza Science, Policy and Politics.* Washington, DC: Earthscan, 2010.

Spackman, Erica, ed. *Animal Influenza Virus.* 2nd ed. New York: Humana, 2014.

Van-Tam, Jonathan, and Chloe Sellwood, eds. *Pandemic Influenza.* 2nd ed. Wallingford, UK: CABI, 2013.

Webster, Robert G., Arnold S. Monto, Thomas J. Braciale, and Robert A. Lamb, eds. *Textbook of Influenza.* Chichester, UK: Wiley Blackwell, 2013.

Periodicals

Brockwell-Staats, Christy, Robert G. Webster, and Richard J. Webby. "Diversity of Influenza Viruses in Swine and the Emergence of a Novel Human Pandemic Influenza A (H1N1)." *Influenza and Other Respiratory Viruses* 3, no. 5 (2009): 207–213.

Davies, Sara E., and Jeremy Youde. "The Politics of Disease Surveillance: Special Section." *Global Change, Peace & Security* 24, no. 1 (2012): 53–107.

Institute of Biomedical Science. "A Panoply of Pathology: From Influenza to Modernisation." *Biomedical Scientist* 55, no. 3 (2011).

Kamradt-Scott, Adam. "The Politics of Medicine and the Global Governance of Pandemic Influenza." *International Journal of Health Services* 43, no. 1 (2013): 105–121.

Souza, M. J. "Influenza." *Journal of Exotic Pet Medicine* 20, no. 1 (2011): 4–8.

Suarez, David L., and Erica Spackman. "Proceedings of the Eighth International Symposium on Avian Influenza." *Avian Diseases* 56, no. 4 (2012).

Vincent, A., et al. "Review of Influenza A Virus in Swine Worldwide: A Call for Increased Surveillance and Research." *Zoonoses and Public Health* 61, no. 1 (2014): 4–17.

Websites

"Avian Influenza." Fact Sheet. *World Health Organization (WHO)*, Updated March 2014. http://www.who.int/mediacentre/factsheets/avian_influenza/en/ (accessed March 10, 2015).

"Avian Influenza A (H7N9)." *Global Early Warning System (GLEWS)*, October 21, 2013. http://www.glews.net/2013/10/avian-influenza-ah7n9-virus/ (accessed March 10, 2015).

"Influenza (Flu)." *U.S. Centers for Disease Control and Prevention (CDC).* http://www.cdc.gov/flu/index.htm (accessed March 10, 2015).

"Transboundary Animal Diseases (TADs)." *Food and Agriculture Organization of the United Nations (FAO).* http://www.fao.org/ag/againfo/programmes/en/empres/diseases.asp (accessed March 10, 2015).

"Update on Highly Pathogenic Avian Influenza in Animals (Type H5 and H7)." *World Organization for Animal Health.* http://www.oie.int/en/animal-health-in-the-world/update-on-avian-influenza/2015/ (accessed March 10, 2015).

K. Lee Lerner

Bacterial Diseases

⊕ Introduction

Bacteria are microscopic single-celled organisms, lacking a nucleus, that are capable of causing disease in humans, animals, and plants. Bacterial diseases, such as tuberculosis (TB) and cholera, have caused significant morbidity and mortality worldwide throughout history and continue to be a leading public health problem.

However, many bacterial species are entirely benign and, indeed, can be beneficial. They play a key role in food and beverage production. In addition, it is becoming increasingly apparent that the community of bacteria living in the human gut, known as the microbiome, is essential for maintaining health.

Identifying the bacterium that caused a particular infection is the key to selecting the correct drug to treat it. The traditional classification is by shape. There are the cocci, which are spherical; the bacilli, which are rod-shaped; and the spiral bacteria, which are corkscrew-shaped. These can readily be distinguished under a microscope. Bacteria can also be detected rapidly and accurately using DNA testing, but such methods may not be available in laboratories in developing countries.

An important distinction in diagnosing bacterial disease is between gram-negative and gram-positive bacteria. The classification depends upon whether the bacteria absorb a chemical called Gram's stain. Different drugs are often needed to treat gram-negative and gram-positive bacterial infections.

There are many ways in which bacteria can be transmitted to an individual and enter the body. Airborne bacteria, carried by coughs and sneezes, may be inhaled. Contaminated food and water may contain pathogenic bacteria, which can be ingested. Sexual intercourse can transmit a number of bacterial species from one person to another. Animals, when humans come into contact with them, are another source of bacterial infection. Finally, bacteria living in or on people's bodies, in their gut or on the skin, may cause infection. Such bacteria are normally harmless, or even beneficial, but may invade the bloodstream and other parts of the body if the person's immunity is undermined, as with human immunodeficiency virus (HIV) or after a bone marrow transplant or chemotherapy.

Bacterial infections can spread more quickly under conditions of poverty and poor sanitation. Thus they are more of the public health problem in developing countries, particularly where the health-care infrastructure is poor. However, bacterial disease is also a significant cause of morbidity and mortality in the hospital setting in both developed and developing nations. Invasive procedures such as the use of catheters and respirators can introduce bacteria into the body. Severely ill patients in the intensive care unit are less able to fight off these so called hospital-acquired infections because their immune systems are impaired.

There are hundreds of bacterial diseases, but only a relatively small number pose a significant public health issue. The World Health Organization (WHO) lists TB, leprosy, cholera, meningococcal meningitis, and Buruli ulcer as being particular problems in a global context. TB, which is caused by the bacterium *Mycobacterium tuberculosis*, is second only to HIV in terms of the number of deaths per year caused by a microbial disease.

TB is a good example of the damage that bacterial diseases exact in low- and middle-income countries. In these countries, health and sanitary standards can be less than optimal, and access to the medical care needed to treat the infection may be poor. TB also often displays resistance to the drugs used to treat it. Another example of antibiotic resistance is methicillin-resistant *Staphylococcus aureus* (MRSA), which is a frequent cause of infections of wounds and damaged skin. These and other types of multidrug resistant bacteria are appearing worldwide, which is complicating treatment and greatly increasing the costs of medical care.

⊕ Historical Background

Bacterial diseases are as old as humanity. Leprosy, for instance, was recognized in ancient China, Egypt, and India. The first written report of leprosy dates back to 600 BCE. Plague, which is carried by fleas living on rodents, is caused by the bacterium *Yersinia pestis*. It was the cause of the Black Death pandemic of the mid-14th century, which killed at least one-quarter of the population of the known world. Meanwhile, TB was the greatest killer of children and young adults in early industrial society, although its origins stretch back far before this period.

Science and Bacterial Disease

Microbial infections, including bacterial diseases, were originally attributed to breathing in bad air or miasma. There was a grain of truth in this, as bad air was suggestive of poor sanitation, which certainly encourages the spread of bacterial infection. However, the introduction of the microscope into scientific research in the 18th century paved the way for the germ theory of disease and the new science of bacteriology.

The French chemist Louis Pasteur (1822–1895) and the German pathologist Robert Koch (1843–1910) are generally regarded as the great pioneers of bacteriology. Pasteur showed that bacteria were involved in a disease of silkworms, while Koch identified the bacillus that causes TB, which was a landmark discovery. Koch's germ theory stated that a microbe that caused a disease should be isolated from infected animals, cultured, and then identified. Finally, it should be reinjected into healthy animals to determine if they then became ill. This established the link between specific bacteria and specific diseases.

The germ theory laid the foundations for discovering cures for bacterial diseases. Improved sanitation and hygiene, introduced in the late 19th century, undoubtedly played an important part. However, the discovery of penicillin by the Scottish bacteriologist Alexander Fleming (1881–1955) in 1928 marked the start of the antibiotic era. Pencillin was developed on a large scale in Oxford during the early years of World War II (1939–1945) by Howard Florey (1898–1968), Ernst Chain (1906–1979), and Norman Heatley (1911–2004) and was used to treat infected wounds among Allied troops.

Penicillin was isolated from a fungus. Many antibiotics are natural products, manufactured by microbes as "chemical weapons" used to protect them from competing species. The Ukrainian American biochemist Selman Waksman (1888–1973) studied bacteria that live in the soil and synthesize many compounds which can fight infection. It was Waksman who coined the term antibiotic for these compounds. He discovered streptomycin, the first effective drug against TB, in 1943. Streptomycin was isolated from the soil bacterium *Streptomyces griseus*. Waksman was awarded the Nobel Prize for his discovery in 1952.

Thus, the antibiotic era was born, and millions who would otherwise have died from bacterial diseases owed their lives to this new class of drugs. The pharmaceutical industry turned its attention to infectious disease, and soon there was a whole range of antibiotic drugs. Some were based on penicillin, streptomycin, and the sulfonamides, another of the early antibiotics. Others were entirely new classes of antibiotics, such as the quinolones and tetracylines.

Such was the success of the administration of antibiotics that by the 1960s, TB was presumed to be under control and destined for eradication. Yet physicians already were reporting cases of *M. tuberculosis* resistant to the antibiotics being used in treatment. In 1993, the WHO declared TB a "global emergency." Long prevalent in underdeveloped and developing countries, multidrug-resistant TB is now becoming a problem in the United States. One source is the entry of infected individuals from other countries. In 2001, 106 of the 124 reported cases of multidrug resistant TB in the United States were from individuals entering from countries where TB is prominent, such as Mexico. In 2014, the number was 85 of the 95 reported multidrug-resistant cases.

⊕ Impacts and Issues

Of all the bacterial diseases, TB is probably the one that has the most global impact. It is the second-leading cause of death from infectious disease, after HIV/AIDS, and the fifth-most-important cause of death worldwide. It mainly affects those between the ages of 15 to 64. In 2013, there were 9 million cases of TB and 1.5 million deaths from the disease.

TB is found everywhere in the world, and it is largely a disease of poverty. In 2013, the South-East Asia and Western Pacific WHO Regions accounted for 56 percent of the world's cases of TB. The African region had around 25 percent of cases and the highest rates of cases and deaths relative to the population. Rates of new cases of TB vary widely between countries, reflecting the fact that it is a disease of poverty. The lowest rates are found in high-income countries, including most countries in Western Europe, Canada, the United States, Japan, Australia, and New Zealand.

HIV infection increases susceptibility to TB infection. Part of the resurgence of TB since the late 1990s can be attributed to the spread of HIV. Around 1.1 million of the 9 million people who developed TB in 2013 were HIV positive. At least one-third of the 35 million people living with HIV worldwide are infected with latent TB. If active TB develops and diagnosis and treatment are delayed, HIV patients are at high risk of dying from drug-resistant TB.

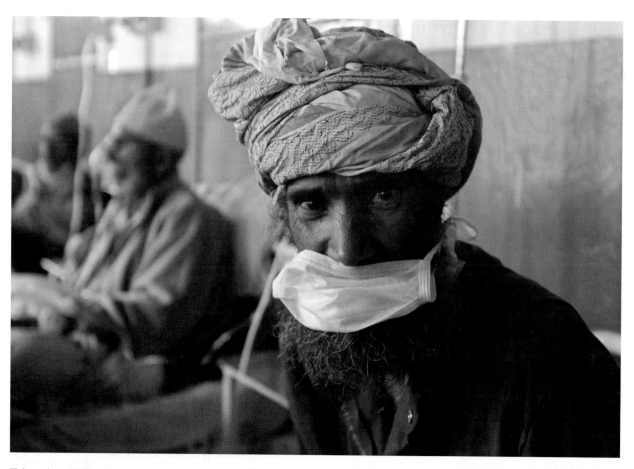

Tuberculosis (TB) patients receive treatment at a ward in Chest Diseases hospital in Srinagar, the summer capital of Indian Kashmir, March 24, 2012. Strains of TB that are becomingly increasingly resistant to antibiotic treatment are putting thousands of lives at risk in Africa, Asia, and even in Europe, according to Médecins sans Frontières (MSF). The group said that multidrug-resistant forms of the disease are a growing threat to patients in developing countries in Africa, where crippled health-care systems mean that the daily treatment required to treat resistant strains can be hard to come by. In 2010, 1.4 million people died as a result of TB; 95 percent of those deaths were in developing countries such as Nigeria, the Central African Republic, and Swaziland.   © *Farooq Khan/epa european pressphoto agency b.v. / Alamy*

Tackling TB

The Stop TB, End TB Strategy is aligned with Millennium Development Goal (MDG) 6, which is to combat HIV/AIDS, malaria, and other diseases. The MDGs were formulated in 2000 at the United Nations Millennium Summit. There are eight MDGs, all related directly or indirectly to global health. The TB-specific target within MDG 6 is to have reversed the incidence of TB by 2015. The world has largely achieved this, although incidence is falling very slowly. End TB strategies intensified existing efforts in 2015, and aim to reduce deaths from tuberculosis by 95 percent by 2035.

Central to the Stop TB Strategy is an approach to drug administration known as directly observed therapy (DOT). The drug combination used is isoniazid, rifampicin, pyrazinamide, and ethambutol for two months, then isoniazid and rifampicin for the next four months. This is a lengthy and complex regimen. The key to DOT is that a local care provider dispenses the medication and observes it being taken by the patients, thus supporting them through the treatment.

The success of DOT depends upon the existence of a political commitment to a national TB program, which requires advocacy work from the WHO and other stakeholders. Access to a quality-assured diagnostic service is also needed. Once an active case is identified, then a supply of the drugs needed for the six-month treatment is required. The direct observation component is needed to ensure the patient takes the whole course of medication. The observers can be health-care workers, nongovernmental organization staff, teachers, religious leaders, or other respected community figures. The drugs needed for DOT are cheap. However, for the program to achieve and be cost effective, a regular supply of quality-assured medication is needed, which is why the Stop TB, End TB campaign set up its Global Drug Facility to ensure this.

Cholera

Cholera remains a serious global health concern, as it thrives wherever sanitation and clean drinking water are lacking. Cholera is caused by a bacteria called *Vibrio cholerae*, which lives in aquatic environments, including salty or brackish waters. In highly developed countries, cholera cases are sporadic and are almost always traced to eating raw or undercooked shellfish contaminated with the bacteria. In the rest of the world, cholera often goes undetected and causes severe diarrhea and sometimes-fatal dehydration. The WHO estimates that 3 million to 5 million cases of cholera occur each year, but only a small fraction (about 10 percent) of those are reported.

Outbreaks of cholera have occurred after natural disasters (Haiti after the major 2010 earthquake), in developing countries (Vietnam in 2008), and in areas of conflict (Sudan in 2014). Although there are two different vaccines available against cholera, they are generally reserved for children or for use during outbreaks, as they require repeated doses and provide only short-term protection. Health officials stress that a more effective long-term strategy against cholera would be to invest in sanitation and water purifying measures to eliminate exposure to *Vibrio cholerae*.

Leprosy

Leprosy is a chronic infection caused by *Mycobacterium leprae*. It affects the skin, nerves, upper respiratory tract, and the eyes. Leprosy is transmitted by droplets emitted from the nose and mouth of an infected person. However, it is not a highly infectious disease, and it is also curable. Untreated leprosy can cause permanent damage to the limbs and eyes.

WHO data from 115 countries show that there were an estimated 189,018 existing cases of leprosy at the end of 2012, while 232,857 new cases were reported. Nearly 16 million persons with leprosy have been cured since the mid-1990s. Leprosy is a good example of how a bacterial disease that is a public health threat can be tackled. It is treated with multidrug therapy (MDT), which involves giving the patient a combination of three drugs, namely dapsone, rifampicin, and clofazimine.

Having effective drugs against a bacterial disease is only part of the answer. They must be cheap, or free, and made widely available to those who need them. Since 1995, the WHO has provided free leprosy MDT all around the world. Initially, the funding for this came from the Nippon Foundation and later from the Novartis Foundation for Sustainable Development. Leprosy control has improved significantly because of national and local campaigns against the disease in countries where it is endemic. Integration of primary leprosy services into existing general health service has been key to this control.

The prevalence of leprosy has dropped by 90 percent since 2000, and it has been eliminated from 119 countries out of 122 countries where it was a public health problem in 1985. Thus far, no resistance to MDT has

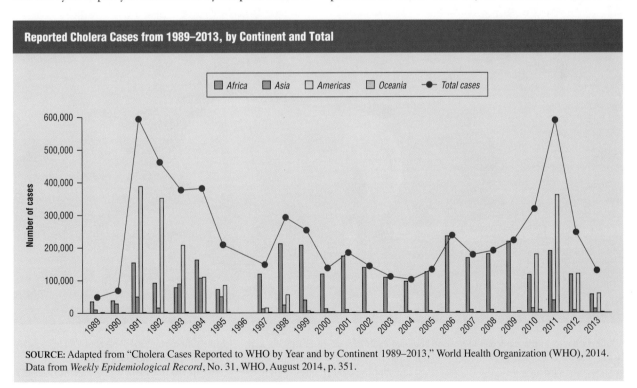

Reported Cholera Cases from 1989–2013, by Continent and Total

SOURCE: Adapted from "Cholera Cases Reported to WHO by Year and by Continent 1989–2013," World Health Organization (WHO), 2014. Data from *Weekly Epidemiological Record*, No. 31, WHO, August 2014, p. 351.

Bacterial diseases spread quickly in areas where sanitation is an issue. Diseases such as cholera become bigger public health issues in developing countries as well as in areas experiencing catastrophic environmental disasters, where sanitation is poor.

BRUCELLOSIS AND RAW MILK

Some bacterial diseases can be transferred from person to person, while others can spread from a nonhuman to a human. The latter type of disease is termed a zoonosis. An example of a zoonotic disease is brucellosis, caused by bacteria in the genus *Brucella*. The disease infects animals such as swine, cattle, and sheep. Humans are infected by contact with infected animals or their milk that is contaminated with *Brucella* (typically, this involves drinking unpasteurized milk or eating unpasteurized cheese).

In the United States, most farm animals are vaccinated against the bacteria, however the bacteria can be passed from nondomesticated animals, such as elk, to domesticated animals, such as cattle.

Brucellosis in humans is caused by *Brucella melitensis*, which infects goats; *B. abortis*, which infects cattle (if the animal is pregnant, the infection causes abortion of the fetus, hence its name); and *B. suis*, which infects pigs. Other than in pregnant cattle, animals usually are not affected unduly by the infection,

and they soon become healthy. However, for days or several weeks after recovery, they can continue to excrete the bacteria in urine and milk.

Brucella are hardy bacteria. Once outside of the animal, they may survive in the environment for weeks. So even if a person does not have direct contact with the animal, the disease still can be transmitted by coming into contact with bacteria-laden soil or water. Transfer of bacteria through a cut in the skin is a common route of infection. The bacteria first invade lymph node cells, then spread to the spleen, bone marrow, and liver. About three weeks after the initial contact with the bacteria, weakness and fatigue develops. An infected person may also have muscle aches, fever, and chills.

In humans, brucellosis caused by *B. abortus* is mild and usually does not require treatment. But brucellosis due to *B. melitensis* can cause severe and long-lasting fevers and anemia. Brucellosis is treated by a combination of antibiotics that can enter host cells.

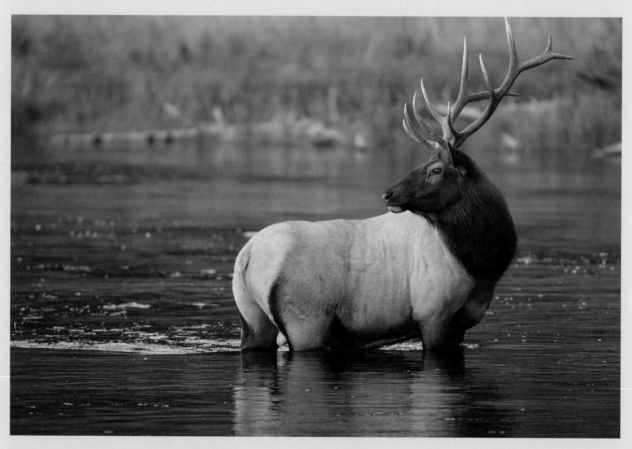

A bull elk stands in the water at Yellowstone National Park. Brucellosis in wild elk in the Greater Yellowstone Area (parts of Wyoming, Idaho, and Montana) has been linked to the transmission of *Brucella abortus* to cattle herds near the park. Wild elk and bison are the last reservoirs of *B. abortus* in the United States, and controversy surrounds plans to try to eliminate the disease in wildlife. © *Mary Ann McDonald/Shutterstock.com.*

been detected, which makes tackling the disease much easier. Efforts are now focusing on eliminating the disease from currently underserved and inaccessible areas. Pockets of leprosy are currently found in certain areas of many countries, including Angola, India, Bangladesh, Brazil, and Sudan.

Food Poisoning

Many bacterial diseases are caused by consuming contaminated food or water. Such infections are often known as food poisoning. One example is campylobacteriosis, a disease of the intestinal tract of humans. The infection, which typically results in diarrhea, is caused most often in the United States by *Campylobacter jejuni*. The U.S. Centers for Disease Control and Prevention (CDC) estimates that 2 million cases of campylobacteriosis occur in the country each year. Globally, 5 to 14 percent of all diarrhea may be due to campylobacteriosis. In underdeveloped countries, where recovery from diarrhea may be harder because of more limited medicine and lack of freshwater, campylobacteriosis is a significant health threat. The WHO works to improve water quality in an effort to decrease the incidence of waterborne campylobacteriosis.

Another significant food-borne and waterborne bacterial disease is caused by *Escherichia coli*. *E. coli* is a gram-negative bacterium that lives in the intestinal tract of humans and other warm-blooded animals. Of the many subtypes, or strains, of the organism, strain O157:H7 (named based on an antigen on the bacterial surface and on the flagella, which move to propel the bacterium) is especially important. Most *E. coli* live naturally in the human intestinal tract, except for O157:H7, which resides in cattle. When present in the human intestinal tract, as usually occurs by the ingestion of contaminated food or water, O157:H7 causes a severe, and potentially life-threatening, disease called hemorrhagic colitis, which involves the destruction of the cells lining the intestinal tract.

Hemorrhagic colitis begins with severe abdominal pain accompanied by watery diarrhea. As damage to the epithelial cells lining the intestinal tract occurs, the diarrhea becomes bloody. Vomiting also can occur. These symptoms usually pass between one and two weeks as the body's immune defenses become able to overcome the infection, usually resulting in no permanent damage. However, in people whose immune system is faulty and in children whose immune system has yet to mature fully, the disease can spread body-wide, particularly to the kidney. The latter damage can be so extensive that kidney function is lost. About 10 to 15 percent of those infected develop hemolyticanemia, which is the leading cause of sudden-onset kidney failure in children. As well, the elderly can develop thrombocytopenic purpura, which results in fever, excessive bruising, and bleeding. In the elderly, this kills nearly half of those who become infected.

Scientists first recognized strain O157:H7 in 1982, when an outbreak of severe diarrhea in the midwestern United States was traced to a batch of undercooked hamburgers. This remains the most common cause of disease, hence the nickname "hamburger disease." However, there are other sources of the disease, which include alfalfa sprouts, unpasteurized apple juice, lettuce, cheese curds, and raw milk. A common reason for contamination of produce is the agricultural practice of irrigation with sewage-containing water. Inadequately washed produce can pose a danger. Organically grown produce might not be washed adequately, given the incorrect assumption that such foods are free from bacteria.

Meat can become contaminated with feces during slaughter. The bacteria are distributed throughout the meat when the meat is ground. Thorough cooking is necessary to kill the bacteria buried in the ground meat. Eating as many as 10 surviving O157:H7 bacteria can be enough to cause disease. In another infamous example, contamination of the water supply of Walkerton, Ontario, Canada, by run-off from a neighboring cattle farm in the summer of 2000 sickened thousands and killed seven people.

Antibiotic Resistance

One line of defense against bacterial diseases is antibiotics. However, resistance to antibiotics is an increasing global health problem that means that the weapons that were once so effective against bacterial diseases are rapidly losing their power. Infections that do not respond to standard treatment cause prolonged illness, higher health-care costs, and increased mortality. For example, patients with MRSA, a particularly common hospital-acquired infection, are 64 percent more likely to die than those with a nonresistant form of the infection.

The WHO's 2014 report on global surveillance of antibiotic resistance contains some alarming findings. For instance, resistance to the carbapenem antibiotics, which are the last resort treatment for life-threatening intestinal infections, has now spread to all regions of the world. Furthermore, several countries report treatment failure for the last resort drug for gonorrhea, the third-generation cephalosporins. This threatens to reverse the gains made in the treatment of this common sexually transmitted infection. Untreated gonorrhea causes infertility and neonatal blindness.

Bacteria multiply very rapidly and, each time they do, they copy their DNA. The copying process introduces mutations into the DNA sequence. Some of these mutations enable the bacterium to become resistant to an antibiotic. There are various ways in which this can happen. The resistant bacterium may become able to break down the antibiotic molecules, rendering them ineffective, or may pump them out through its cell wall.

Another way bacteria can acquire resistance to antibiotics is by growing as a biofilm. They may grow adhered to a nonliving surface (e.g., a catheter inserted in the body during a medical procedure or a heart pacemaker) or to a surface of living cells in the body, encased in a sticky, sugar-based coating that is produced by the adherent bacteria. It is hard for the antibiotic to penetrate the biofilm in sufficient concentration to kill the bacteria. Because the concentration of the antibiotic within the biofilm is lowered, the bacteria can develop tolerance to the compound, often determined by the genetic changes discussed above. An important example is the lung infection in cystic fibrosis that develops due to infection with *Pseudomonas aeruginosa*. The lung infection can damage lung tissue progressively, as the body's immune system repeatedly tries unsuccessfully to get rid of the infection. This progressive damage can kill the infected person.

Antibiotic resistance is promoted by the way in which health-care professionals and patients use these drugs. They are often prescribed inappropriately. Many bacterial infections clear up on their own and do not require antibiotic treatment, but the doctor prescribes such treatments because the patient expects to be given a prescription. Antibiotics are sometimes prescribed for viral infections, even though they only work against bacteria. In some countries, antibiotics are even available over the counter, so the patient can take antibiotics even when they are not indicated. Finally, a patient often fails to complete the course of antibiotics, which encourages the stronger, most resistant bacteria to thrive. In short, the overuse of antibiotics creates an environmental pressure that encourages the emergence of resistant bacteria.

⊕ Future Implications

Bacterial diseases have always been a part of the human experience, and this will continue. With an aging global population, bacterial diseases may have a greater impact in the future, as natural immunity declines with age. This trend will be exacerbated by the burgeoning resistance of many bacteria to antibiotics that once were effective in killing them. As with many diseases, those who live in underdeveloped or developing countries, where access to quality medical care is not as reliable as in developed countries, will be disproportionately affected.

Urgent and coordinated action on antibiotic resistance is needed. The WHO has developed a draft global action plan to combat resistance to both antibiotics and other antimicrobial drugs. This aims to improve awareness and understanding and strengthen surveillance and research. It will also work to optimize the use of existing antimicrobial drugs. Crucially, the plan will also encourage investment in new medicines, vaccines, and diagnostic tools. Thus far, many pharmaceutical companies have tended to neglect infection as a therapeutic area, focusing instead upon noncommunicable diseases. The plan

was initiated by the WHO's World Health Assembly in 2015. If it does not succeed, the prospect of returning to a previous time as in the pre-antibiotic era, where common infections cause death and disability, could become a reality.

Meanwhile, research is showing that the microbiome plays an important role in establishing health and in disease. For example, the intestinal microflora of those who suffer from Crohn's disease has disproportionately more harmful bacteria, including *Salmonella* and *E. coli*, and less beneficial bacteria, including *Bifidobacterium*. Many people now take probiotic supplements, live bacteria that are beneficial for the digestive system, in an effort to maintain a healthy microbiome in the digestive tract. The microbiome may also play a role in various chronic diseases, including diabetes and obesity.

SEE ALSO *Cholera and Dysentery; Epidemiology: Surveillance for Emerging Infectious Diseases; Fungal Diseases; Parasitic Diseases; Prion Diseases; Sanitation and Hygiene; Viral Diseases; Water Supplies and Access to Clean Water; Waterborne Diseases; Zoonotic (Animal-Borne) Diseases*

BIBLIOGRAPHY

Books

Brachman, Philip S., and Elias Abrutyn, eds. *Bacterial Infections of Humans: Epidemiology and Control.* 4th ed. New York: Springer, 2009.

Faruque, Shah M., ed. *Foodborne and Waterborne Bacterial Pathogens: Epidemiology, Evolution, and Molecular Biology.* Norfolk, UK: Caister Academic Press, 2012.

Maczulak, Anne E. *Allies and Enemies: How the World Depends on Bacteria.* Upper Saddle River, NJ: FT Press, 2011.

Spellberg, Brad. *Rising Plague: The Global Threat from Deadly Bacteria and Our Dwindling Arsenal to Fight Them.* Amherst, NY: Prometheus Books, 2009.

Zourob, Mohammed, Souna Elwary, and Anthony Turner, eds. *Principles of Bacterial Detection Biosensors, Recognition Receptors, and Microsystems.* New York: Springer, 2008.

Periodicals

Oosten, Marlene van, et al. "Real-Time In Vivo Imaging of Invasive- and Biomaterial-Associated Bacterial Infections Using Fluorescently Labelled Vancomycin." *Nature Communications* 4 (October 5, 2013): 2584.

Websites

"Antimicrobial Resistance: Global Report on Surveillance." *World Health Organization (WHO)*, 2014. http://apps.who.int/iris/bitstream/10665/

112642/1/9789241564748_eng.pdf?ua=1 (accessed February 10, 2015).

"Bacterial Infections." *U.S. National Institutes of Health.* http://www.niaid.nih.gov/topics/bacterialinfections/Pages/default.aspx (accessed February 10, 2015).

"Division of Bacterial Diseases." *U.S. National Center for Immunization and Respiratory Diseases (NCIRD), U.S. Centers for Disease Control and Prevention (CDC).* http://www.cdc.gov/ncird/DBD.html (accessed February 10, 2015).

"Invasive Bacterial Vaccine Preventable Diseases Laboratory Network." *World Health Organization (WHO).* http://www.who.int/immunization/monitoring_surveillance/burden/laboratory/IBVPD/en/ (accessed February 10, 2015).

Brian Douglas Hoyle

Body Image and Eating Disorders

⊕ Introduction

Body image is the way a person perceives how his or her own body looks. It may or may not be an accurate perception, and it can affect and change the way one feels about one's body and the way the person behaves. Body image discussions are increasingly frequent in the health profession, social sciences, and feminist theory, as well as around the role of ethical advertising.

Positive body image builds self-worth, promotes physical health, and protects the person from developing eating disorders, whereas a negative body image can cause a person to suffer from low self-esteem, and can affect social, mental, and physical health. In addition to leading to the development of eating disorders, a poor body image can contribute to depression, anxiety, problems in relationships, and the development of substance use disorders. Consequently, this can cause various health problems. People can be internally influenced by their family, friends, teachers, and the media to feel negatively about the way their bodies look, and this feeling can be exacerbated if they receive negative feedback from individuals that they hold in high esteem. It is important that role models such as parents promote positive and realistic beauty ideals.

How you see your own body is called your "perceptual body image," whereas how you feel about that perception is called your "affective body image." How people feel about their own bodies can change their way of thinking about themselves as a whole, in a positive or a negative way, and influence behaviors. If an individual thinks that he or she is overweight, regardless of the factual accuracy, that person might choose to change eating habits or dress differently to fit what feels appropriate. The ways that perceptual body image and affective body image make people think about their bodies is called cognitive body image. The changes in actions that people would not otherwise make were it not for feelings about their body are called behavioral body image.

The media can be a constant source of external contribution to a negative body image because of its constant presence in 21st-century society. Television, movies, and the Internet are able to create images and edit them in a way that obscures the actual images. People's bodies are edited in ways that create "perfect" bodies that are unobtainable. People who feel they need to compare themselves to persons they see in media can experience deep psychological and physical harm. Since the mid-1960s, body consciousness has increased internationally, affecting people from every age group. This is concerning because it reflects a movement toward defining one's self-worth as dependent upon attaining an unattainable physical ideal.

Negative body issues can affect anyone, but certain factors can increase the likelihood that some individuals develop dissatisfied feelings about their bodies more than others. Having close relationships with people such as family and friends who express their own feelings of negativity about themselves can pass on the negativity to the people who consider them role models. Long-term body image is shaped most frequently during late childhood and adolescence, and the impressions that are developed early can persist long into adulthood. This is especially true for girls, and most prevalently teenage girls, although negative body image issues in boys is increasing rapidly to almost the same rate. If a person is bullied, has a larger body type, or has otherwise "perfectionist" standards, these factors all increase the likelihood of a person internalizing common beauty ideals and developing a negative body image.

A person who has a negative body image is more likely to diet, get plastic surgery, or develop eating disorders. There are ways to prevent and treat negative body image, including positive thinking, setting health-focused rather than weight-focused goals, and remembering that those persons featured by the media are the physical minority and may have been artificially enhanced or perfected using computer editing techniques.

⊕ Historical Background

All societies in the world throughout history have prized physical appearance, but the standard for the ideal body is drastically different across cultures and changes constantly over time. Beauty includes weight but also ritual, and voluntary body modification such as body piercing or plastic surgery. The standards for women fluctuate frequently and are markedly more pervasive than those for men across every culture. This is not to say that standards for male beauty do not, or have not existed; however, society holds women to a more rigid standard more frequently for a variety of reasons.

The most drastic of changes has been the concentration the 21st century has put specifically on weight. In the 1500s, standards existed for women to be "pear-shaped," with a large lower half emphasized by an enormous bell skirt and a tiny waist and flat chest, an almost complete opposite from that of the 21st century, in which the word Rubenesque is a polite but slightly derogatory term for a woman who is heavy or overweight. However, the term derives from the style of the painter Peter Paul Rubens (1577–1640), whose paintings often contained representations of large, voluptuous, and usually nude women who were the feminine ideal during his lifetime. Until the early 1900s, for a person to have extra weight on the body and look voluptuous was a sign of good health and wealth. The only people able to eat well and frequently, and refrain from performing physical labor, were the wealthy. In the 21st century the balance is inverted: healthful food is increasingly more expensive, and having the spare time and money for physical activity has become a luxury.

Twenty-first-century standards, particularly in Western countries, are focused primarily on thinness. The waif-like figure, which came to popularity most notably with the supermodel Twiggy (1949–) in the United States during the 1970s, is particularly detrimental to the women who try to achieve this standard. This was the first time in history that a woman who was objectively underweight for her height became an ideal beauty standard. A person who is underweight has a body weight that is too low to be considered healthy, as determined by the body mass index, or BMI. Lifetime prevalence of eating disorders has been found to be consistently 1.75 to 3 times as high among women as men.

Many women struggle with the difference between how their bodies look as compared to these standards. Eating disorders, dieting, plastic surgery, and diet aids often are the "answer" chosen to try to modify their bodies to meet the standards of society's "ideal." Dieting and weight-loss efforts are common and often unsuccessful ways to try to combat a negative body image when people feel they do not have the perfect body. Eating disorders such as anorexia nervosa, bulimia nervosa, and binge eating are extreme behaviors that are the result of people being unable to control the way they think, feel,

BODY MASS INDEX

Body mass index (BMI) is a number calculated from a person's weight and height. In metric units the formula is: BMI = weight in kilograms / [height in meters]². In the United States, or Imperial measurements, the formula is: BMI = weight in pounds / [height in inches]² x 703.

According to the U.S. Centers for Disease Control and Prevention (CDC), BMI provides a dependable gauge of body fatness for most people and is used to screen for weight categories that may lead to health problems. It does not measure body fat directly, and is not a diagnostic tool but a good standardizing measure of comparison, especially between persons of the same age. According to the CDC, "for adults 20 years old and older, BMI is interpreted using standard weight status categories that are the same for all ages and for both men and women. For children and teens, on the other hand, the interpretation of BMI is both age- and sex-specific." BMI calculation is inexpensive and easy to use for clinicians and for the general public, as it requires only height and weight. It also allows individuals to make a comparison between their own weight and that of the general population.

Once measurements have been added to the BMI equation, the number falls within a range between 18.5 and 40. Any number between 16 and 18.5 is considered underweight, and anything below 16 is considered severely underweight. People suffering from anorexia nervosa have a BMI under 18.5. A normal weight is considered between 18.5 and 24.9. Persons who are overweight have a number between 25 and 29.9, whereas any number higher than 30 classifies as obesity.

There are limitations to using BMI as an indicator of health. A person may have a high BMI and still be within a healthy range, and it especially overestimates body fat in athletes and other people who have a muscular build. Muscle is denser and weighs more than fat, so BMI is unreliable for persons with a large amount of muscle mass. Also, people lose muscle mass as they age, and BMI does not take this into account. Therefore it is possible that BMI underestimates how much body fat has replaced muscle mass in an older person. The CDC notes that more accurate assessments to pinpoint body fat percentage, and whether weight is detrimental, might include skinfold thickness measurements and evaluations of diet, physical activity, and family history, as well as other appropriate health screenings.

Not maintaining a body weight within the 18.5–24.9 normal range can cause detrimental health effects. People who are underweight can be at risk of bone loss and osteoporosis, as well as become anemic. Also, it is difficult for their bodies to heal from sickness and even minor cuts and scrapes. Women can miss months of menstruation at a time or stop completely. Finally, being severely underweight can cause heart palpitations, heart attack, and heart failure. People who are overweight are at risk of heart disease because excess plaque in the arteries builds up, reducing blood flow to the heart muscle. Being overweight or obese additionally can cause high blood pressure, stroke, and type 2 diabetes.

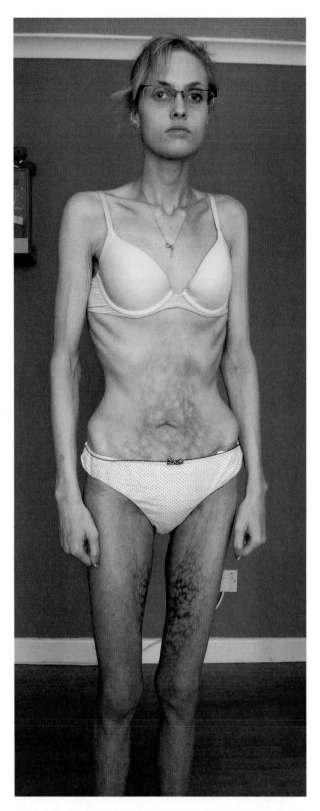

After seeing pictures of herself, Lauren Brudenell became anorexic. She lost more than half her body weight, dropping from over 230 pounds (105 kilograms) to a life-threatening 84 pounds (38 kilograms). She later recovered and weighed a healthy 112 pounds (50 kilograms). *© Worldwide Features/Barcroft Media/Getty Images*

and act as a result of their own negative body image. However much someone may try, the actions taken to create the perfect body when suffering from one of these disorders will never make a person feel better about his or her body image.

⊕ Impacts and Issues

People with positive body images feel comfortable within their skin and tend to think about their bodies as products of nature, but human bodies are also the product of culture. When one's body does not align with cultural ideals, a person might choose extreme behavioral measures to "correct" it. Body image disorders, bulimia in particular, increased dramatically in the latter half of the 20th century, and research suggests that it continues to be on the rise. There is evidence to suggest that advertising and media play the largest role in this increase. As with most things, the media does not affect everyone in the same way. Cross-cultural studies on body image suggest that consumers' gender, race, and age can affect how strongly they identify with the people in advertising.

Body Dysmorphic Disorder

People with body dysmorphic disorder (BDD) perceive their looks to be different than they actually are and can spend hours each day thinking about, and camouflaging, the perceived imperfections. People with BDD can dislike any part of their body, although they often find fault with their hair, skin, nose, chest, or stomach. Hard to resist or control, these obsessions make it difficult for people with BDD to focus on anything other than their bodies and can lead to low self-esteem, avoidance of social situations, and problems at work or school. BDD and the body image issues that accompany anorexia and bulimia usually occur together, but BDD can exist independently of weight concerns, instead causing the person to concentrate on things such as the length of the legs, or the shape of the hairline. BDD also is associated with obsessive compulsive disorder, social anxiety, and depression.

Anorexia

The most commonly known eating disorder is anorexia nervosa. People suffering from anorexia are obsessed with being thin and have a severely distorted body image that makes them believe they are fat, regardless of reality. In order to decrease their weight, they severely restrict their food intake and may exercise obsessively. In 1952, anorexia was the first eating disorder to be classified as an illness by the psychological community. However, physicians have been describing the disease for centuries as a "wasting disease," which at the time was indistinguishable from other physiological conditions that caused extreme weight loss, such as endocrine disorders. In the 1970s, doctors starting seeing an obvious increase in patients diagnosed with anorexia, and in 1983 the singer Karen Carpenter (1950–1983) of the Carpenters died as a result of heart failure related to the disease. Her death brought the disorder into the public consciousness, and discussions around body image and anorexia became increasingly frequent.

Someone suffering from anorexia continues to lose weight even after what may be an healthy weight for body height and shape has been attained. The person continues to diet until his or her body weight is far below what is in an ideal range. This can lead to severe health complications that are common with starvation: the hair and nails become brittle, the skin dries out, menstrual periods cease in females, blood pressure lowers, and heart and brain function may be impacted. Death can result if the symptoms are not treated and the underlying causes of the anorexia are not addressed.

Bulimia

Another well-known eating disorder is bulimia nervosa. The symptoms of bulimia are closely related to those of anorexia; however, persons suffering from bulimia binge on food, causing themselves to overeat drastically. Sufferers then compensate by using laxatives, diuretics, or vomiting, also called purging. The disorder first was categorized in 1980 as bulimia, and then the name was modified to bulimia nervosa in 1987 so as to associate it more closely with anorexia. Like anorexia, bulimia has been known for centuries and in some cultures even promoted. In ancient Rome, wealthy patricians would go to

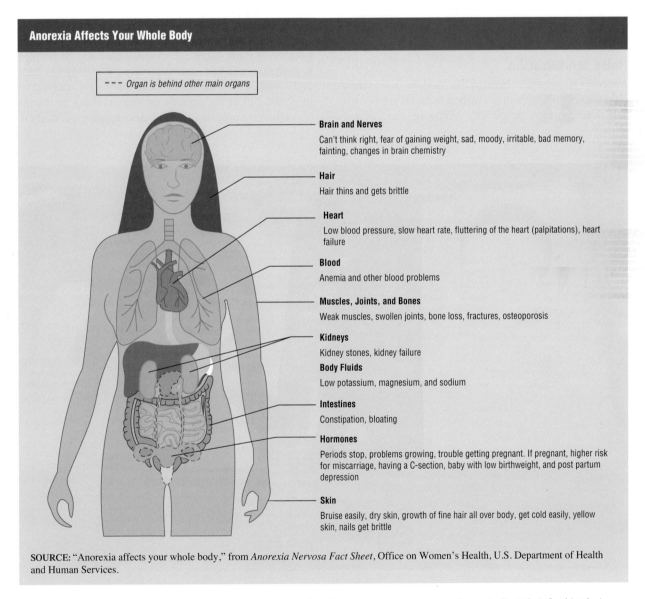

Anorexia Affects Your Whole Body

- - - *Organ is behind other main organs*

Brain and Nerves
Can't think right, fear of gaining weight, sad, moody, irritable, bad memory, fainting, changes in brain chemistry

Hair
Hair thins and gets brittle

Heart
Low blood pressure, slow heart rate, fluttering of the heart (palpitations), heart failure

Blood
Anemia and other blood problems

Muscles, Joints, and Bones
Weak muscles, swollen joints, bone loss, fractures, osteoporosis

Kidneys
Kidney stones, kidney failure

Body Fluids
Low potassium, magnesium, and sodium

Intestines
Constipation, bloating

Hormones
Periods stop, problems growing, trouble getting pregnant. If pregnant, higher risk for miscarriage, having a C-section, baby with low birthweight, and post partum depression

Skin
Bruise easily, dry skin, growth of fine hair all over body, get cold easily, yellow skin, nails get brittle

SOURCE: "Anorexia affects your whole body," from *Anorexia Nervosa Fact Sheet*, Office on Women's Health, U.S. Department of Health and Human Services.

An individual with a distorted body image can develop an eating disorder such as anorexia nervosa. Anorexics limit their food intake in order to lose weight. Excessive weight loss seen in anorexics affects the whole body and can cause permanent damage.

a specially designated room called a "vomitorium" after gorging themselves on food to purge so that they could continue eating.

Binge Eating and Eating Disorders Not Otherwise Specified

There are a variety of other eating disorders, such as binge eating (without purging); pica, in which a person regularly consumes nonnutritional substances such as chalk or paper; and rumination disorder in which a person regurgitates food into the mouth to continue chewing it. However, these eating disorders are not related directly to the perception of one's own body image in the same way as anorexia nervosa and bulimia nervosa. According to the National Eating Disorders Association, what all these conditions have in common is "serious emotional and psychological suffering and/or serious problems in areas of work, school, or relationships."

Body Modification

Anorexia nervosa and bulimia nervosa are two extreme ways that people try to modify their outward appearance, and both can have devastating effects on the sufferer's health. Body modification, practiced virtually all over the world, also is used to align one's own body image with a cultural ideal. Tanning, piercing, tattooing, and hair dying are relatively innocuous types of body modification popular in Western culture. However, examples of more extreme body modifications from around the world include body building in North America, neck elongation in Thailand and Africa, henna tattooing in Southeast Asia and the Middle East, lip and earlobe stretching in Africa, and foot binding in China. Some of these practices can be highly detrimental to the person's health.

Foot binding, a practice started during infancy on Chinese girls, was practiced up until the middle of the 20th century. After breaking the child's toes, the feet were kept under constant pressure by being wrapped in fabric, resulting in the feet growing only a few inches over the course of their lifetime, sometimes crippling them completely. Similarly, tight corseting that began during a woman's adolescence in Europe and the United States was an attempt to make the waist as small as possible, sometimes as little as 12 inches. Eventually the body grew and adapted to its shape, but at the expense of women being unable to stand for long periods and sometimes fainting. All of these

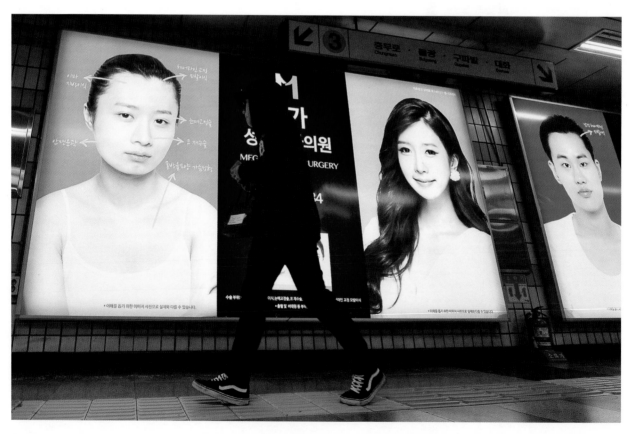

A pedestrian walks past advertisements for plastic surgery clinics at a subway station in Seoul on March 26, 2014. The South Korean capital Seoul is to restrict the use of plastic surgery advertisements on public transport, officials said, after complaints that they were fueling an unhealthy obsession with body image. *© Jung Yeon-Je/AFP/Getty Images.*

practices are ways in which the body is modified in order to align with the ideals of a particular culture, and accordingly to improve one's own body image.

Reconstructive or plastic surgery procedures, originally developed to restore facial symmetry after combat injuries in World War 1 (1914–1918), have since become among the fastest-growing elective medical procedures. According to the International Society of Aesthetic Plastic Surgery, more than 23 million cosmetic and nonsurgical procedures are performed annually worldwide. Botox injections are the most popular procedure, followed by breast surgery, liposuction, eyelid surgery, lipostructure, and rhinoplasty (nose surgery).

Race, Body Image, and Eating Disorders

When research on body image and eating disorders first began, the studies were concentrated primarily on Caucasian women. Very little research had been conducted on persons of color. However, one study done at a New York City hospital indicated that African American women preferred heavier body types compared with their white counterparts and were less likely to develop eating disorders despite having a higher incidence of obesity.

In 2004, a report indicated that African American and Hispanic women had more positive feelings about their looks compared to white Caucasian women aged 20–65 years. Fifty-nine percent of African Americans and 60 percent of Hispanics liked the way they looked, compared to 51 percent of white women.

This suggests that the role culture plays in body image can be a strong preventive measure in the fight against eating disorders and the prevalence of negative body image, but since those studies that influence has decreased. A study by Savita Bakhshi, "Women's Body Image and the Role of Culture: A Review of the Literature," indicated that, as with other races/ethnicities, eating disorders among black women are also on the rise as a result of assimilating beauty standards. The study showed that an increasing number of women of different ethnicities reported that they did not like their body shape and had resorted to dieting to change the way they felt about themselves. In India, the prevalence of eating disturbances rarely is reported, perhaps due to the traditional Indian culture that encourages plumpness as a symbol of feminine beauty. However, the effect non-Western cultures previously had in supporting larger, more realistic body ideals continues to decrease. A thinner body ideal has become more standardized across various cultures and ethnicities, leading to increasing body dissatisfaction.

The National Eating Disorders Association notes that researchers, clinicians, and educators should make efforts to increase their awareness of factors affecting minority populations, such as stress triggers in minority communities. Understanding the factors that might make a person more or less susceptible to these disorders such as worldviews, values, and beliefs; patterns of acculturation, assimilation, and immigration; and effects of oppression and ethnic identity will improve the quality of psychological care and success of prevention.

⊕ Future Implications

It should be stressed that every human body is different, and internalizing and accepting differences is healthier than internalizing social ideals. Preventing the internalization of ideals projected by society and the media should be systematic and should reduce the factors that contribute to negative body image. There are two main types of ways to prevent negative body image issues and the development of eating disorders: universal prevention and targeted prevention.

Universal prevention applies to the general public regardless of whether they have indicators of body issue disorders. An example of universal prevention would be when a major clothing retailer intentionally changes its advertising to show models that have bodies closer to those seen in reality because of the effect that abnormal body representations have on society. Another example would be a public awareness campaign on the prevalence of body image disorders and eating disorders. These actions affect the community as a whole, without directing influence to specific people in the way that targeted prevention does. Targeted prevention is when a person is already exhibiting dissatisfaction with his or her body, and measures are taken to make sure that dissatisfaction does not evolve into an eating disorder. Both targeted and universal prevention have been helpful in leading to positive change.

As has been discussed, body image dissatisfaction and eating disorders have increased drastically since the mid-1960s. However, there has been backlash on the standards of beauty that advertising and media play in this trend, and more people are discussing these issues. A study on advertising used different body types within advertisements to assess whether the body types changed an ad's effectiveness. The first utilized traditional, thin models, and the second employed average-sized models or none at all, yet both were equally effective. The implication of this study is that businesses could choose to use average-sized models without that choice being detrimental to business interests. Further work should be done to universally target the things that influence people's body perceptions to prevent the rise of connected eating disorders and the related health effects.

SEE ALSO *Malnutrition; Mental Health Treatment Access; Noncommunicable Diseases (Lifestyle Diseases); Nutrition; Obesity; Stigma*

BIBLIOGRAPHY

Books

Agras, W. Stewart, ed. *The Oxford Handbook of Eating Disorders.* Oxford: Oxford University Press, 2010.

American Psychiatric Association. *Diagnostic and Statistical Manual of Mental Disorders: DSM 5.* Washington, DC: American Psychiatric Association, 2013.

Cash, Thomas F., ed. *Encyclopedia of Body Image and Human Appearance.* Amsterdam: Elsevier/Academic Press, 2012.

Cash, Thomas F., and Linda Smolak, eds. *Body Image: A Handbook of Science, Practice, and Prevention.* New York: Guilford Press, 2011.

Fox-Kales, Emily. *Body Shots: Hollywood and the Culture of Eating Disorders.* Albany: Excelsior Editions, State University of New York Press, 2011.

Greene, Sophia B., ed. *Body Image: Perceptions, Interpretations and Attitudes.* New York: Nova Science, 2011.

Latzer, Yael, Joav Merrick, and Daniel Stein, eds. *Understanding Eating Disorders: Integrating Culture, Psychology and Biology.* New York: Nova Science, 2011.

Periodicals

Bakhshi, Savita. "Women's Body Image and the Role of Culture: A Review of Literature." *Europe's Journal of Psychology* 7, no. 2 (December 2010): 374–394. Available online at http://ejop.psychopen.eu/article/download/135/pdf (accessed April 7, 2015).

Hudson, James I., Eva Hiripi, Harrison G. Pope, and Ronald C. Kessler. "The Prevalence and Correlates of Eating Disorders in the National Comorbidity Survey Replication." *Biological Psychiatry* 61, no. 3 (February 2007): 348–358.

Levinson, Cheri A., et al. "Social Appearance Anxiety, Perfectionism, and Fear of Negative Revaluation: Distinct or Shared Risk Factors for Social Anxiety

and Rating Disorders?" *Appetite* 67, no. 1 (August 2013): 125–133.

Striegel-Moore, Ruth H., et al. "Gender Difference in the Prevalence of Eating Disorder Symptoms." *International Journal of Eating Disorders* 42, no. 5 (December 2009): 471–474.

Thomas, Jennifer J., et al. "Do DSM-5 Eating Disorder Criteria Overpathologize Normative Eating Patterns among Individuals with Obesity?" *Journal of Obesity* 2014, no. 1 (June 2014): 320–328.

Websites

"Body Image." *Office of Women's Health, U.S. Department of Health and Human Services.* http://womenshealth.gov/body-image/ (accessed November 16, 2014).

"Diseases and Conditions: Eating Disorders." *Mayo Clinic.* http://www.mayoclinic.org/diseases-conditions/eating-disorders/basics/definition/con-20033575 (accessed November 16, 2014).

"Healthy Weight, It's not a Diet It's a Lifestyle!" *U.S. Centers for Disease Control and Prevention (CDC).* http://www.cdc.gov/healthyweight/assessing/bmi/adult_bmi/index.html (accessed November 16, 2014).

Mallick, Nadira, Subha Ray, and Susmita Mukhopadhyay. "Eating Behaviours and Body Weight Concerns among Adolescent Girls." *Advances in Public Health* 2014 (2014). Available online at http://www.hindawi.com/journals/aph/2014/257396/ (accessed March 31, 2014).

"Media, Body Image, and Eating Disorders." *National Eating Disorders Association.* http://www.nationaleatingdisorders.org/media-body-image-and-eating-disorders (accessed November 16, 2014).

"NEDC Fact Sheets and Other Resources." *National Eating Disorders Collaboration.* http://www.nedc.com.au/ (accessed November 16, 2014).

Margaret Loraine Scott

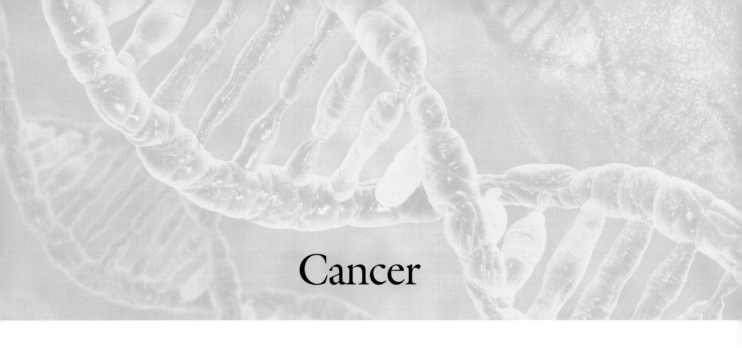

Cancer

⊕ Introduction

Cancer is a broad term for a group of diseases that can affect people of all ages and ethnicities. It arises when abnormal cells begin to grow uncontrollably anywhere on the body. Other words for cancer include neoplasm and malignancy. As one of the leading causes of illness and death worldwide, access for everyone to cancer screening, diagnosis, and treatment is a top priority in global health development. Many cancers occurring today can be successfully treated or cured with surgery, chemotherapy, or radiation, provided it is detected early. Some cancers are preventable; many societies engage in cancer prevention activities by minimizing exposure to risk factors like tobacco smoke and alcohol, by enacting environmental and industrial regulations, and by promoting a healthy lifestyle through diet and physical activity.

The term cancer denotes abnormally fast growth of cells. It also refers to the mechanism that determines the rate at which cells grow and divide being defective and the capability of some cancer cells to migrate from their site of uncontrolled growth and division to other sites in the body. The latter process is called metastasis.

When cells grow and divide in one site they can form an aggregate that is called a tumor. Cells from fast-growing tumors that metastasize can threaten health and life. But metastasis is not a universal feature of cancer cells. An example is benign tumors, in which the cells grow relatively slowly compared to cancerous cells and do not migrate. Benign tumors are not cancerous, and unless their growth impinges on blood vessels or other important structures in the immediate vicinity, they are not considered dangerous and may even not require surgery to remove them. Instead, a physician will adopt an increasingly popular strategy, termed watchful waiting, in which nothing is done until it is determined action should be taken, with the patient monitored frequently.

Cells that make up tumors that grow in size and from which cells migrate to other body sites are a concern.

Early signs of cancer can, but do not always, involve development of a lump, a cough that persists, a weight loss that is not the result of a known event such as a diet, and/or a change in bowel movements. Other common conditions can also cause these symptoms, so these are first ruled out when the cause of the symptoms is being evaluated.

⊕ Historical Background

Cancer has been a fact of life for millennia. The American Cancer Society (ACS) details in its "History of Cancer" that early recorded history includes references to cancer, and examination of fossilized bone has revealed damage consistent with cancer. Geologists have found growths suggestive of bone cancer (osteosarcoma) in mummies.

The earliest recorded description of what was probably cancer dates to about 3000 BCE in an ancient Egyptian textbook on trauma surgery. The text describes cases of tumors or ulcers of the breast.

According to the ACS, historians credit the origin of the word cancer to the Greek physician Hippocrates (c. 460–c. 377 BCE) who called tumors either *carcinos* and *carcinoma*, depending on whether they were non-ulcer-or ulcer-forming. These words refer to a crab, possibly because the shape presented by the spread of the cancer visually resembles the legs sprouting from the body of a crab. These terms were translated into the Latin word *cancer* by the Roman physician Celsus in the 2nd century CE.

Hippocrates believed that the body had four humors (bodily fluids): blood, phlegm, yellow bile, and black bile. He associated health with a balance in the four humors; an imbalance caused disease. Cancer was thought to be the result of too much black bile. This theory of cancer was accepted by another Greek physician, Galen (129–c. 199 CE), whose theories formed the basis for medical treatment for more than a millennium.

Galen's word for cancer, *oncos*, Greek for "swelling," is now the prefix for the English word for the study of cancer: oncology. However, Galen's humeral theory was eventually discarded as scientific thought progressed during the Renaissance and Enlightenment periods and more evidence-based scientific methods and tools, including autopsies and microscopes, came into use.

In 1838, German pathologist Johannes Müller (1801–1858) demonstrated that cancer is made up of cells, but he did not accept that cancer cells originated from normal cells. However, his student Rudolf Virchow (1821–1902), a famous German pathologist, proved this to be correct. Yet Virchow incorrectly surmised that cancer spread like a liquid. In the 1860s, German surgeon Karl Thiersch (1822–1895) demonstrated that liquid was not involved, but rather that cancers metastasize by the spread of malignant cells.

Though there were continued advances in the understanding of cancer during the 19th and 20th centuries, misconceptions regarding its causes (and whether it was contagious) remained widespread into the early 1900s. People now know that cancer itself is not contagious. Yet, as noted by the ACS, some microorganisms, such as viruses, that are linked with development of cancer are transmissible. In addition, it is now known that some inherited genetic mutations that are linked to cancer may appear within families. It is also known that genetic damage can be caused by exposure to carcinogens such as chemicals and radiation. However, there are many questions that continue to perplex researchers and doctors who study and treat cancer.

⊕ Impacts and Issues

Despite the advances in cancer detection and treatment, cancer remains a prevalent killer. In 2012, there were more than 14 million new cases of cancer diagnosed worldwide, with more than 8 million people dying of cancer. Annually, cancer-related deaths represent around 15 percent of all human deaths. In men, lung, prostate, colorectal, and stomach cancers are most prevalent. The list for women includes breast, colorectal, lung, and cervical cancers. Skin cancer is also prevalent in both genders, accounting for about 40 percent of all cancers annually. Some cancers are more prevalent in children; these include acute lymphoblastic anemia and malignant brain tumors. The risk of cancer increases with age, and some cancers are associated with developed countries. These statistics are further evidence of the strong link between lifestyle and cancer.

Aside from its toll on human lives, cancer is an expensive drain on health care. In the United States, researchers estimated the direct medical costs of cancer diagnosis, treatment, and care in 2011 to be nearly US$89 billion. Of this, 50 percent is for hospital

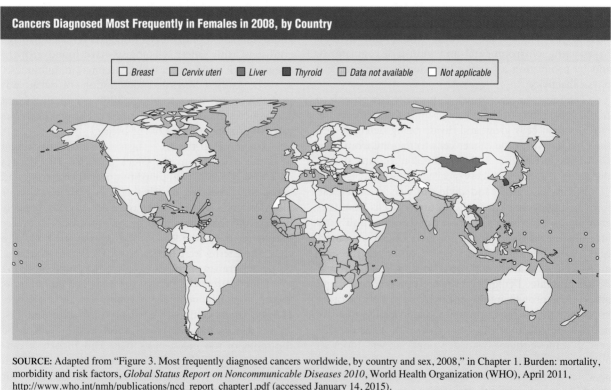

Cancers Diagnosed Most Frequently in Females in 2008, by Country

☐ Breast ☐ Cervix uteri ◼ Liver ◼ Thyroid ☐ Data not available ☐ Not applicable

SOURCE: Adapted from "Figure 3. Most frequently diagnosed cancers worldwide, by country and sex, 2008," in Chapter 1. Burden: mortality, morbidity and risk factors, *Global Status Report on Noncommunicable Diseases 2010*, World Health Organization (WHO), April 2011, http://www.who.int/nmh/publications/ncd_report_chapter1.pdf (accessed January 14, 2015).

According to a World Health Organization (WHO) report, breast cancer is by far the most often diagnosed cancer in females worldwide.

Cancers Diagnosed Most Frequently in Males in 2008, by Country

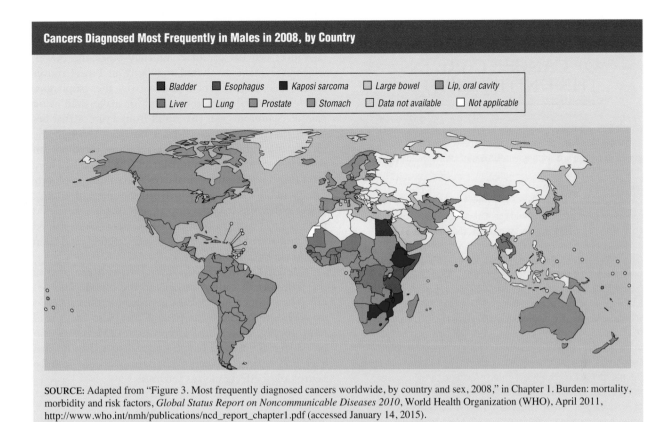

SOURCE: Adapted from "Figure 3. Most frequently diagnosed cancers worldwide, by country and sex, 2008," in Chapter 1. Burden: mortality, morbidity and risk factors, *Global Status Report on Noncommunicable Diseases 2010*, World Health Organization (WHO), April 2011, http://www.who.int/nmh/publications/ncd_report_chapter1.pdf (accessed January 14, 2015).

According to a World Health Organization (WHO) report, prostate and lung cancers are the most often diagnosed cancers in men worldwide.

outpatients doctor visit costs. Prevention strategies that lessened outpatient and personal physician care would potentially save tens of billions of dollars annually. About 10 percent of the direct medical cost is for prescription drugs. Drug therapy of cancer is expensive but can be cost-effective in the longer term for those individuals in whom cancer is permanently prevented.

According to a 2010 report from the ACS, the global economic toll from cancer is estimated at US$895 billion annually. This does not include direct medical costs. Cancer is the leading health-related cause of economic loss, followed by heart disease (US$753 billion annually).

Treatment of cancer can involve use of radiation, surgery to remove the cancerous tissue and often some of the immediately surrounding tissue, pharmaceutical drugs (chemotherapy), and more recently, therapies including monoclonal antibodies that exclusively target the cancerous tissue. Even as recently as the 1960s, a diagnosis of cancer was a death sentence. Enormous strides in cancer prevention and treatment were made in the intervening decades. Now, in the developed world, the five-year survival rate for some cancers is high if the cancer is diagnosed early, though other cancers may not be detected until they have progressed too far for

effective treatment. As of 2011, according to the U.S. National Cancer Institute, the five-year survival rate (for all stages of cancer combined) for breast, prostate, lung and bronchus, colorectal, and bladder cancer—the five most common cancers—were 90 percent, 99 percent, 18 percent, 65 percent, and 77 percent, respectively.

The high cost of cancer treatment and follow-up patient care can be prohibitive for nations that are less affluent than, for example, the United States. But, even within the United States, disparities of cancer care exist, with those who are less affluent and lack private health insurance being at risk of diminished opportunities of cancer care. According to figures from the U.S. Census Bureau, about 48 million Americans, representing 15 percent of the population, lacked health insurance in 2012. Other contributors to the disparity in cancer care include cultural issues (i.e., risk promoting lifestyle) and differing access to cancer screening technologies.

Decades of research have established some common features of cancer. Cancer cells generate and respond to their own signals concerning growth. Their growth is not regulated by other cells. Cancer cells do not respond to the chemical signals that in normal cells trigger cell growth to stop. Cancer cells have the ability to escape from the process of self-destruction that

THE STAGGERING COST OF CANCER CARE IN THE UNITED STATES

As the U.S. population continues to grow and age, the costs of cancer care will continue to rise. A study released in January 2011 by the U.S. National Institutes of Health predicts that medical expenditures for cancer in 2020 will top $158 billion (in 2010 dollars), a 27 percent increase over 2010. The projections were based on the most recent data available on cancer incidence, survival, and costs of care. In 2010, medical costs associated with cancer were projected to reach $124.6 billion, with the highest costs associated with breast cancer (about $17 billion), followed by colorectal cancer ($14 billion), lymphoma ($12 billion), lung cancer ($12 billion), and prostate cancer ($12 billion). If the incidence of cancer, survival rates, and costs remained about the same as those in 2010, and the U.S. population ages as predicted, direct cancer care expenditures would reach $158 billion in 2020. The advances being made against cancer are not cheap. If these expensive options continue, the cancer care cost could climb even higher—to an estimated $207 billion. Another factor adding to the costs is the growing proportion of obese Americans: Thirty-five percent of Americans are obese. This will drive new cases of cancer and contribute to other maladies, such as diabetes, which will exact even more health-care costs.

is known as apoptosis. These features can essentially make cancer cells immortal, capable of endless rounds of growth and division. Along with this, cancer cells can induce and maintain the formation of new blood vessels (angiogenesis), which is vital in supplying nourishment to the growing tumor. Finally, cancer cells can undergo metastasis, the movement from one body location to another. This can also involve the invasion of host tissue in the new site. These features often do not arise at the same time. Rather, the process from normal cells to cells that form a tumor to cells that migrate from the tumor occurs in steps. The process is referred to as malignant progression.

Cancer symptoms vary, depending on the site of metastasis. Many cancers have few if any symptoms in their early stages. Or, symptoms such a persistent cough might not be recognized as being indicative of cancer. Symptoms tend to appear as the cancer grows. The growing tumor occupies more room and requires more nutrients. Both come at expense of other organs and body parts. The symptoms tend not to be specific in the early stages, and people will tend to be treated for other ailments. When the cancer is finally recognized and diagnosed, it has progressed further.

Symptoms that appear initially at the origin of a tumor typically can be due to the size and weight of the tumor. A lung cancer mass can block the bronchus, causing a persistent cough or leading to pneumonia. Colorectal cancer can narrow or completely block the bowel, which is evident as altered regularity in bowel movements. Esophageal cancer can narrow the esophagus, which can impede swallowing and/or make swallowing painful. Symptoms can also result from a tumor that lies below the surface of a cell layer breaking through the surface (ulcerating tumor). The resulting bleeding can occur in the lung, the intestinal tract (the blood loss here can cause anemia), the urinary tract (resulting in bloody urine), and in the uterus (which causes vaginal bleeding). Other symptoms may develop at sites that are unrelated to the cancer's origin or sites of metastasis. Unexplained and unplanned weight loss, fever, fatigue, and skin changes are examples.

Metastasis can occur in several ways. It can involve the transport of cancerous cells in the blood. This so-called hematogenous spread can distribute the cancer to many sites throughout the body. Cancer also can spread more focally, to regional lymph nodes. Metastasis can be evident as enlarged lymph nodes, larger than normal liver, and enlarged spleen. Metastasis may also produce neurological effects such as seizures.

Causes

Chemicals that have been linked to the development of cancer are termed carcinogens. Cigarettes are a concentrated source of carcinogens. Analysis of cigarette smoke has detected more than 50 carcinogens. The carcinogenic brew is responsible for more than 30 percent of all cancer deaths in the developed world and about 20 percent of all global cancer deaths worldwide. In the United States, the patterns of tobacco use and lung cancer have been similar. Although this does not prove smoking causes cancer, it is more evidence that strongly links smoking as a cause of cancer. Another probable cause of cancer is excessive and long-term alcohol consumption. The progressive damage to the liver from the alcohol stress likely spawns liver cancer. Environmental exposure in the workplace to compounds including asbestos and benzene has been linked with cancer. Workplaces containing these and other hazardous compounds are mandated to have safety measures in place, such as the wearing of protective face masks when in a potentially hazardous environment.

Another probable correlation with cancer is obesity, which is often combined with a poor diet and little or no physical activity. According to the U.S. Centers for Disease Control and Prevention, as of 2014, 70 million Americans (35 percent of the population) are classified as obese. This is an important statistic because it indicates that in subsequent decades, the prevalence of cancer in the United States will likely continue to increase, along with other obesity-related diseases such as diabetes.

Some cancers can also be caused by certain infections. Viruses and their associated cancers include human papillomavirus (cervical cancer), Epstein-Barr virus (B-cell lymphoproliferative disease and nasopharyngeal carcinoma), Kaposi's sarcoma herpesvirus, hepatitis B and C viruses (hepatocellular carcinoma), and human T-cell leukemia virus. Bacteria associated with cancer include *Helicobacter pylori*, which, when residing in the stomach, can lead to ulceration or cancer development.

Yet another cause of cancer is radiation exposure. This link makes straightforward sense because radiation damages cell DNA. In medicine, an emphasis over the past few decades has been to reduce the amount of radiation people receive via x-ray examination and magnetic resonance imaging (MRI). In a similar fashion, excessive exposure to sunlight can cause skin cancer (melanoma). High-energy components of the spectrum of sunlight, in particular ultraviolet B, can break DNA strands, which increases the risk that the genetic damage will fuel development of cancer.

Our own bodies can also be involved in cancer. Certain hormones that function normally to trigger growth and development of cells can drive the development of cancer if the body does not regulate their activity properly. Researchers have linked higher-than-normal levels of estrogen and progesterone in women with breast cancer. Men with elevated levels of testosterone may be at greater risk of prostate cancer. Hormone replacement therapy used by some postmenopausal women has been linked with increases in endometrial cancer.

The various causes of cancer all unite in a common feature: they ultimately affect growth regulation. At the genetic level, regulation involves two sets of genes. Tumor suppressor genes act to prevent cell growth and division. Oncogenes function to spur cell growth and division. Normally, the two systems are in balance and allow cell growth when growth is needed. Enhanced oncogene activity and/or diminished tumor suppressor gene activity causes the uncontrolled growth that is the hallmark of cancer.

Normally, according to the American Society of Clinical Oncology (ASCO), tumor suppressor genes "suppress (limit) cell growth by monitoring how quickly cells divide into new cells, repairing mismatched DNA (which is often a cause of mutations), and controlling when a cell dies." Damage to a tumor suppressor gene may be due to heredity (inherited mutations) or environmental factors (acquired mutations). Both types of mutation can lead to cells growing uncontrollably and possibly forming a tumor.

According to ASCO, it is the oncogenes that transform a healthy cell into a cancerous cell. Oncogenes have a variety of functions, including controlling cancer cell growth and spread, cell communication pathways, cell growth, and cell death. Mutations in oncogenes almost always are acquired.

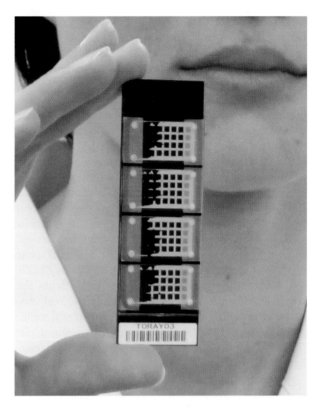

Research continues on a chip to gauge the levels of microRNAs in the blood of cancer patients. A group composed of Japan's National Cancer Center, private companies, and universities in Japan said in August 2014 they will begin a five-year project to enable the detection of 13 kinds of cancer via blood sample. © *Kyodo/AP Images.*

DNA repair genes fix mistakes that can occur during the process where DNA is copied prior to cell division. An error in a DNA repair gene can prevent the normal repair of genetic mistakes. The persistent mistakes are mutations. Some can lead to cancer, particularly if the mutations reside in a tumor suppressor gene or oncogene.

The genetic changes underlying cancer can be major, involving addition or removal of large stretches of DNA. Or the changes can be minor, involving a change in one or a few of the genetic building blocks of DNA. Even a small change to DNA can have a profound effect if the change affects a critical enzyme or other protein.

Research

Despite this underlying genetic basis, all cancers are not alike, and so there is no single cure for all cancers. Just as no one antibiotic kills all bacteria (and they ultimately would become resistant anyway), similarly there is no one cure for cancer. Once it was thought that a common cure could be found. One promising candidate included compounds that inhibit angiogensis—the establishment of new blood vessels in tumors. However, this hope has not held up in the face of cancer research reality. In 2014 research involved angiogenesis inhibitors being used along with other compounds in combinations tailored to the target cancer.

Cancer research is a huge enterprise that involves hundreds of thousands of scientists worldwide (scientists who study cancer are called oncologists). Among the research they conduct is testing the effectiveness and safety of new and known drugs used in different combinations. Some research involves testing the drugs against cancer cells grown in laboratory conditions. But ultimately, the drugs need to be tested in people in clinical trials. Clinical trials are designed to maximize participant safety and seek to test the candidate drug(s) against either a known drug (a head-to-head trial) or to test the new drugs against the effect of applying nothing. The "nothing" is disguised so that patients and researchers do not know who is getting the real drug and who is getting the placebo. This type of trial, called a double-blind trial, can yield a very convincing depiction of the candidate drug's beneficial effects or lack of benefit.

Despite the value of clinical trials for cancer, the information being produced may not be applicable to all patients. Trials have criteria that patients must meet to be included and other factors that can be used to exclude patients. The intent of the exclusion criteria is to eliminate patients with other conditions that might confuse the result and make it difficult to judge if the effect seen was from the cancer agent being tested.

A study done by the University of Texas Southwestern Medical Center has reported that many lung cancer patients are excluded from trials because of a past history of cancer. But this good intent may go too far: this exclusion removes an important real-world subset of patients because many patients being treated for lung cancer have had cancer in the past. Of the cancer trials examined by the researchers, more than 80 percent excluded patients with a history of cancer. In many of the cases, prior cancer was the sole reason for exclusion, even though a prior bout with cancer likely would not have interfered with the trial findings.

Researchers examined lung cancer trials conducted by the Eastern Cooperative Oncology Group, a prominent National Cancer Institute-funded organization that designs and conducts cancer clinical trials. Even within this organization, prior cancer eligibility criteria varied widely. Forty-three percent of trials excluded patients with prior cancer diagnosed within five years of study enrollment, 16 percent of trials excluded those with active cancer, 14 percent excluded those with any history of cancer, and 7 percent excluded patients who had cancer within the past two to three years.

Less than 2 percent of adults participate in clinical trials, partially due to the tough enrollment criteria.

Other reasons include limited access to clinical trials and lack of patient interest.

⊕ Future Implications

There are more than 100 different types of cancer, yet the list of causes is short. Most—about 20 percent—result from tobacco use, either the inhalation of tobacco in the form of cigarettes or as smokeless tobacco, which is chewed or applied to the gums. Smokeless tobacco is especially high in nicotine, the physically addictive component of tobacco. Nicotine has been implicated in high rates of oral, esophageal, and pancreatic cancer among smokeless tobacco users. Scientists have linked an estimated 10 percent of cancers to a number of factors including obesity, an unhealthy diet, a sedentary lifestyle, and excessive alcohol drinking (the latter being particularly associated with cancer of the liver). Other causes include infection with the hepatitis B virus, hepatitis C virus, or human papilloma virus (HPV), radiation exposure, and environmental exposure to chemicals that damage genetic material. Virus-related cancer is a substantial cause of cancers in developed countries. Viral infection of human cells also can alter the genetic composition of the cells.

Future cancer therapies are being driven by increasing knowledge of the molecular biology of cancer cells and the processes of cancer. Examples of potential therapies include lessening the tendency of cancer cells to becomes resistant to treatment, refinements in the specific targeting of cancerous cells (such as exploiting the presence of certain proteins on the surface of cancer cells to target delivery of cancer-toxic drugs), use of viruses to target cancer cells that lack a protein called p53, blocking the blood supply to cancer cells, prevention of activation of oncogenes, vaccines, and therapies tailored to the genetic constitution of individual patients.

Given the association of a variety of cancers with lifestyle-related factors, it is understandable that researchers have linked improving lifestyle changes—such as weight loss, quitting smoking, eating a healthy and balanced diet, exercise, and protecting from excessive exposure to sunlight—to cancer prevention. Another prudent action, particularly for cervical and colorectal cancer, is having a screening test done. Screening can detect cancer at earlier stages, which can be more readily treatable. Screening for breast cancer using mammograms can also be an effective tool in early discovery of cancer. It is recommended by some health organizations annually starting at age 40 and others at age 50. However, the use of annual mammograms in women between 40 and 49 years is more contentious, with the efficiency of screening in breast cancer detection in younger women having been questioned by some researchers due to the number of false positive results.

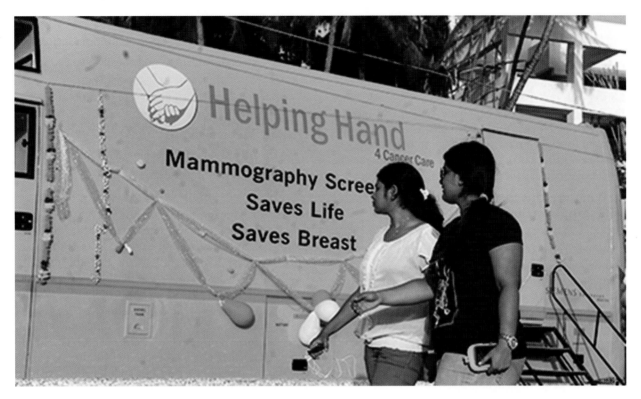

A mobile mammography screening bus is set up to reach women in areas where such exams may not be easily accessible. © *STR/AFP/Getty Images.*

PRIMARY SOURCE

National Cancer Institute Fact Sheet

SOURCE *"Cancer Staging" from* National Cancer Institute Fact Sheet, *National Cancer Institute at the National Institutes of Health, May 3, 2013. http://www.cancer.gov/cancertopics/factsheet/ Detection/staging (accessed January 25, 2015).*

INTRODUCTION *This primary source is one of a series of fact sheets produced by the National Cancer Institute at the National Institutes of Health. It covers the topic of staging, or describing the extent of the patient's cancer.*

CANCER STAGING

Key Points

- Staging describes the extent or severity of a person's cancer. Knowing the stage of disease helps the doctor plan treatment and estimate the person's prognosis.
- Staging systems for cancer have evolved over time and continue to change as scientists learn more about cancer.

- The TNM staging system is based on the size and/ or extent (reach) of the primary tumor (T), whether cancer cells have spread to nearby (regional) lymph nodes (N), and whether metastasis (M), or the spread of the cancer to other parts of the body, has occurred.
- Physical exams, imaging procedures, laboratory tests, pathology reports, and surgical reports provide information to determine the stage of a cancer.

1. What is staging?

Staging describes the severity of a person's cancer based on the size and/or extent (reach) of the original (primary) tumor and whether or not cancer has spread in the body. Staging is important for several reasons:

- Staging helps the doctor plan the appropriate treatment.
- Cancer stage can be used in estimating a person's prognosis.
- Knowing the stage of cancer is important in identifying clinical trials that may be a suitable treatment option for a patient.
- Staging helps health care providers and researchers exchange information about patients; it also gives them a common terminology for evaluating the results of clinical trials and comparing the results of different trials.

Staging is based on knowledge of the way cancer progresses. Cancer cells grow and divide without control or order, and they do not die when they should. As a result, they often form a mass of tissue called a tumor. As a tumor grows, it can invade nearby tissues and organs. Cancer cells can also break away from a tumor and enter the bloodstream or the lymphatic system. By moving through the bloodstream or lymphatic system, cancer cells can spread from the primary site to lymph nodes or to other organs, where they may form new tumors. The spread of cancer is called metastasis.

2. What are the common elements of staging systems?

Staging systems for cancer have evolved over time. They continue to change as scientists learn more about cancer. Some staging systems cover many types of cancer; others focus on a particular type. The common elements considered in most staging systems are as follows:

- Site of the primary tumor and the cell type (e.g., adenocarcinoma, squamous cell carcinoma)

- Tumor size and/or extent (reach)

- Regional lymph node involvement (the spread of cancer to nearby lymph nodes)

- Number of tumors (the primary tumor and the presence of metastatic tumors, or metastases)

- Tumor grade (how closely the cancer cells and tissue resemble normal cells and tissue)

3. What is the TNM system?

The TNM system is one of the most widely used cancer staging systems. This system has been accepted by the Union for International Cancer Control (UICC) and the American Joint Committee on Cancer (AJCC). Most medical facilities use the TNM system as their main method for cancer reporting.

The TNM system is based on the size and/or extent (reach) of the primary tumor (T), the amount of spread to nearby lymph nodes (N), and the presence of metastasis (M) or secondary tumors formed by the spread of cancer cells to other parts of the body. A number is added to each letter to indicate the size and/or extent of the primary tumor and the degree of cancer spread.

Primary Tumor (T)

- TX: Primary tumor cannot be evaluated

- T0: No evidence of primary tumor

- Tis: Carcinoma in situ (CIS; abnormal cells are present but have not spread to neighboring tissue; although not cancer, CIS may become cancer and is sometimes called preinvasive cancer)

- T1, T2, T3, T4: Size and/or extent of the primary tumor

Regional Lymph Nodes (N)

- NX: Regional lymph nodes cannot be evaluated

- N0: No regional lymph node involvement

- N1, N2, N3: Degree of regional lymph node involvement (number and location of lymph nodes)

Distant Metastasis (M)

- MX: Distant metastasis cannot be evaluated

- M0: No distant metastasis

- M1: Distant metastasis is present

For example, breast cancer classified as T3 N2 M0 refers to a large tumor that has spread outside the breast to nearby lymph nodes but not to other parts of the body. Prostate cancer T2 N0 M0 means that the tumor is located only in the prostate and has not spread to the lymph nodes or any other part of the body.

For many cancers, TNM combinations correspond to one of five stages. Criteria for stages differ for different types of cancer. For example, bladder cancer T3 N0 M0 is stage III, whereas colon cancer T3 N0 M0 is stage II. Question 6 describes sources of additional information about staging for specific types of cancer.

4. Are all cancers staged with TNM classifications?

Most types of cancer have TNM designations, but some do not. For example, cancers of the brain and spinal cord are staged according to their cell type and grade. Different staging systems are also used for many cancers of the blood or bone marrow, such as lymphomas. The Ann Arbor staging classification is commonly used to stage lymphomas and has been adopted by both the AJCC and the UICC. However, other cancers of the blood or bone marrow, including most types of leukemia, do not have a clear-cut staging system. Another staging system, developed by the International Federation of Gynecology and Obstetrics (FIGO), is used to stage cancers of the cervix, uterus, ovary, vagina, and vulva. This system is also based on TNM information. Additionally, most childhood cancers are staged using either the TNM system or the staging criteria of the Children's Oncology Group (COG), which conducts pediatric clinical trials; however, other staging systems may be used for some childhood cancers.

Many cancer registries, such as those supported by NCI's Surveillance, Epidemiology, and End Results (SEER) Program, use "summary staging." This system is used for all types of cancer. It groups cancer cases into five main categories:

- In situ: Abnormal cells are present only in the layer of cells in which they developed

- Localized: Cancer is limited to the organ in which it began, without evidence of spread

- Regional: Cancer has spread beyond the primary site to nearby lymph nodes or tissues and organs

- Distant: Cancer has spread from the primary site to distant tissues or organs or to distant lymph nodes

- Unknown: There is not enough information to determine the stage

5. What types of tests are used to determine stage?

The types of tests used for staging depend on the type of cancer. Tests include the following:

- Physical exams are used to gather information about the cancer. The doctor examines the body by looking, feeling, and listening for anything unusual. The physical exam may show the location and size of the tumor(s) and the spread of the cancer to the lymph nodes and/or to other tissues and organs.

- Imaging studies produce pictures of areas inside the body. These studies are important tools in determining stage. Procedures such as x-rays, computed tomography (CT) scans, magnetic resonance imaging (MRI) scans, and positron emission tomography (PET) scans can show the location of the cancer, the size of the tumor, and whether the cancer has spread.

- Laboratory tests are studies of blood, urine, other fluids, and tissues taken from the body. For example, tests for liver function and tumor markers (substances sometimes found in increased amounts if cancer is present) can provide information about the cancer.

- Pathology reports may include information about the size of the tumor, the growth of the tumor into other tissues and organs, the type of cancer cells, and the grade of the tumor. A biopsy may be performed to provide information for the pathology report. Cytology reports also describe findings from the examination of cells in body fluids.

- Surgical reports tell what is found during surgery. These reports describe the size and appearance of the tumor and often include observations about lymph nodes and nearby organs.

6. How can a patient find more information about staging?

The doctor most familiar with a patient's situation is in the best position to provide staging information for that person. For background information, PDQ®, NCI's comprehensive cancer information database, contains cancer treatment summaries that describe the staging of adult and childhood cancers.

SEE ALSO *Alcohol Use and Abuse; Genetic Testing and Privacy Issues; Life Expectancy and Aging Populations; Noncommunicable Diseases (Lifestyle Diseases); Nutrition; Radiation Exposure; Tobacco Use; Viral Diseases*

BIBLIOGRAPHY

Books

Bapat, Sharmila, ed. *Cancer Stem Cells: Identification and Targets.* Hoboken, NJ: Wiley, 2009.

Bunz, Fred. *Principles of Cancer Genetics.* Baltimore, MD: Springer, 2008.

Fialho, Arsenio M., and Ananda M. Chakrabarty, eds. *Emerging Cancer Therapy: Microbial Approaches and Biotechnological Tools.* Hoboken, NJ: Wiley, 2010.

Georgakilas, Alexandros, ed. *Cancer Biomarkers.* Boca Raton: Taylor & Francis/CRC Press, 2013.

Johnson, George. *The Cancer Chronicles: Unlocking Medicine's Deepest Mystery.* New York: Knopf, 2013.

Keating, Peter, and Alberto Cambrosio. *Cancer on Trial: Oncology as a New Style of Practice.* Chicago: University of Chicago Press, 2012.

Klawiter, Maren. *The Biopolitics of Breast Cancer: Changing Cultures of Disease and Activism.* Minneapolis: University of Minnesota Press, 2008.

Krishnan, Shobha S. *The HPV Vaccine Controversy: Sex, Cancer, God, and Politics: A Guide for Parents, Women, Men, and Teenagers.* Westport, CT: Praeger, 2008.

Lawman, Michael J. P., and Patricia D. Lawman, eds. *Cancer Vaccines: Methods and Protocols.* New York: Springer, 2014.

Moorland, Margarite T., ed. *Cancer in Female Adolescents.* New York: Nova Science, 2008.

Mukherjee, Siddhartha. *The Emperor of All Maladies: A Biography of Cancer.* New York: Scribner, 2011.

National Cancer Institute (U.S.). *What You Need to Know about Breast Cancer.* Bethesda, MD: National Institutes of Health, 2012.

National Cancer Institute (U.S.). *What You Need to Know about Cervical Cancer.* Bethesda, MD: National Institutes of Health, 2012.

National Cancer Institute (U.S.). *What You Need to Know about Prostate Cancer.* Bethesda, MD: National Institutes of Health, 2012.

Ochs, Michael F., John T. Casagrande, and Ramana V. Davuluri, eds. *Biomedical Informatics in Cancer Research.* New York: Springer, 2010.

Oldham, Robert K., and Robert O. Dillman, eds. *Principles of Cancer Biotherapy,* 5th ed. Dordrecht, Netherlands: Springer, 2009.

Pelengaris, Stella, and Michael Khan, eds. *The Molecular Biology of Cancer.* Chichester, UK: Wiley, 2009.

Sarkar, Amita. *Cytology of Cancer.* New Delhi: Discovery Pub. House, 2009.

Periodicals

Thakor, Avnesh S., and Sanjiv S. Gambhir. "Nanooncology: The Future of Cancer Diagnosis and Therapy." *CA: A Cancer Journal for Clinicians* 63 (November/December 2013): 395–418.

Yoo, Christine B., and Peter A. Jones. "Epigenetic Therapy of Cancer: Past, Present and Future." *Nature Reviews Drug Discovery* 5 (January 2006): 37–50.

Websites

"Cancer." *MedlinePlus.* http://www.nlm.nih.gov/medlineplus/cancer.html (accessed January 15, 2015).

"Cancer." *World Health Organization (WHO).* http://www.who.int/cancer/en/ (accessed January 15, 2015).

"Cancer Prevention and Control." *U.S. Centers for Disease Control and Prevention (CDC).* http://www.cdc.gov/cancer (accessed January 15, 2015).

"Cancer: Rogue Cells." *National Geographic.* http://science.nationalgeographic.com/science/health-and-human-body/human-diseases/cancer-article.html (accessed January 15, 2015).

"The Genetics of Cancer." *American Society of Clinical Oncology (ASCO).* http://www.cancer.net/navigating-cancer-care/cancer-basics/genetics/genetics-cancer (accessed April 20, 2015).

"The History of Cancer." *American Cancer Society.* http://www.cancer.org/cancer/cancerbasics/thehistoryofcancer/index (accessed April 20, 2015).

"Human Papillomavirus (HPV) and Cervical Cancer," Fact Sheet No. 380. *World Health Organization (WHO),* November 2014. http://www.who.int/mediacentre/factsheets/fs380/en/ (accessed January 15, 2015).

National Cancer Institute. http://www.cancer.gov/ (accessed January 15, 2015).

"SEER Cancer Statistics Review (CSR) 1975–2012." *National Cancer Institute,* April 23, 2015. http://seer.cancer.gov/csr/1975_2012/ (accessed April 27, 2015).

Brian Douglas Hoyle

Cardiovascular Diseases

⊕ Introduction

Cardiovascular diseases (CVDs) affect the heart and blood vessels, including arteries, capillaries, and veins. Either the heart or the blood vessels can be involved, or both simultaneously. The World Health Organization (WHO) estimates that CVDs are the number one killer of people worldwide; 17.5 million people died of CVDs in 2012, with the number anticipated to rise to more than 23 million annually by 2030.

More than 75 percent of the global deaths due to CVDs are in low- and middle-income countries. In these countries, the exposure to cardiovascular risk factors such as tobacco can be greater than in developed countries. In developed nations, smoking cessation has become more ingrained, whereas low- and middle-income countries often do not have prevention programs. People in poorer regions also have less access to health-care services that are readily available and affordable, including early detection of CVDs. As a result, many people in low- and middle-income countries die at a younger age from CVDs compared to those in more developed nations.

The death of wage earners is bad for the economies of nations that are hard-pressed financially. As with other debilitating events, it is the poorest segment of the population in underdeveloped and developing nations that is affected disproportionately by CVDs. The WHO has estimated that noncommunicable diseases (conditions not transmitted from person to person), including CVDs and diabetes, reduce the gross domestic product by about 7 percent in low- and middle-income nations that are undergoing rapid economic growth, due to the early death of active members of the workforce.

This grim news is at least somewhat balanced by the knowledge that some of the risk factors—which include tobacco smoking, unhealthy eating habits, and lack of physical activity—can be changed for the better. Physicians have linked 30 minutes of physical activity per day to lessened risk of heart attack and stroke, along with adopting a diet that is reduced in sodium and includes daily helpings of vegetables and fruit.

⊕ Historical Background

More than 2,000 years ago, Chinese physicians argued that the heart was a pump that pushed blood through the body via blood vessels. The influential Greek physician Galen (129–c. 199), however, did not believe that blood circulated; he thought it was produced in the liver and then sent out to the various parts of the body through veins, where it was absorbed and utilized. Though many of his theories about the human body were later disproven, Galen was a prolific writer, and his views about the human body were the standard of medical knowledge for over a millennium. However, through a series of experiments on animals and humans, William Harvey (1578–1657) made the discovery that blood is conserved and circulated through the body via the veins and arteries. He published his theory in 1628.

While medical science advanced throughout the following centuries, in many ways the heart remained enigmatic, considered a part of the body that could never be fully explored or improved surgically, but a revolution in surgical treatments for heart disease occurred in the 20th century. Blocked coronary arteries now can be bypassed using new tissue, and failing hearts can be replaced with transplants. As the mechanisms of the vascular system become better understood, it became recognized that most CVDs are linked to lifestyle, such as tobacco use and unhealthy diets that lead to overweight or obesity. Many of the millions of deaths from CVDs each year can be prevented with simple changes in diet, regular exercise, and limiting or stopping tobacco and alcohol use.

⊕ Impacts and Issues

In the United States alone, about 600,000 people die of heart disease every year, according to the U.S. Centers for Disease Control and Prevention (CDC), representing 25 percent of all deaths annually. Heart disease is the leading killer of American men and women, and the leading cause of death for most ethnicities. Nearly 400,000 of the deaths are due to coronary heart disease, in which coronary arteries become reduced in diameter due to the buildup of plaque. Globally, the WHO estimates that in 2012, 7.4 million deaths were due to coronary heart disease.

The buildup of plaque in coronary arteries is called atherosclerosis. The plaque changes blood flow through the arteries, increases the pressure needed to pump blood, and, if plaque dislodges and travels to the heart, can cause a heart attack. If the altered blood flow affects the brain, the result is stroke.

In a heart attack, the blood flow to a part of the heart is blocked by a blood clot. The blood clot can originate from plaque that sloughs off the wall of a coronary artery. The clot can act like a dam across a river, cutting off blood flow completely. If this occurs, then the affected portion of the heart muscle begins to die. A first heart attack usually is not a killer. But it definitely is a warning that the individual requires lifestyle changes to curb atherosclerosis. As well, because the heart has been weakened, the degree of physical activity may need to be curbed in some people. Others will resume a near-normal life.

According to WHO estimates, 6.7 million deaths in 2012 were due to strokes. A stroke, most commonly an ischemic stroke, occurs when the blockage is to a blood vessel that supplies blood to the brain. The resulting brain damage can cause disabilities including impaired walking and speech. The extent of the disability over time depends on the length of time the brain cells were deprived of oxygen. If the cells are damaged but still living, some repair can occur, with at least a partial restoration of function. If the cells have died from oxygen deprivation, other brain cells can assume some of the missing functions. The recovery will not be absolute, but movement, speech, and memory can improve with time after a stroke.

Another type of stroke, called hemorrhagic stroke, is caused by the bursting of a blood vessel in the brain. The rupture usually is the result of increased vessel pressure caused by hypertension, and often is fatal. Treatment for stroke is directed at freeing the blockage and must be started as soon as possible to avoid prolonged oxygen deprivation. The treatment, termed thrombolytic therapy (popularly known as clot-buster therapy), is given by injection into a vein, because that delivers the drug to the site of the clot as quickly as possible; this therapy is best given within three hours of the first appearance of symptoms. This therapy also can be

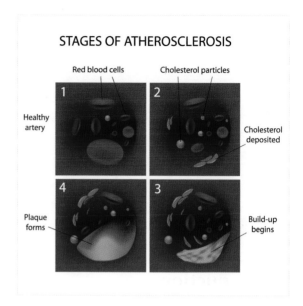

STAGES OF ATHEROSCLEROSIS

Cholesterol forms plaque in an artery. The buildup of plaque causes atherosclerosis, which eventually can lead to heart attack.
© *Alila Medical Media/Shutterstock.com.*

used for treatment of heart attack. Thrombolytic drugs include tissue plasminogen activator, tenecteplase, alteplase, urokinase, reteplase, and streptokinase. Another treatment option used when the plaque blockage involves one of the common carotid arteries in the neck is cardiac endarterectomy. During surgery, the physician makes an insertion at the artery and physically clears out the plaque.

Transient ischemic attack, commonly termed mini-stroke, occurs when an artery becomes blocked for a short time (one to five minutes) by a blood clot. The clot is washed away, normal blood flow resumes, and often there is no permanent damage to the brain. However, this does not lessen the seriousness of a ministroke, which should serve as a warning of a dire outcome if the individual does not take steps to lessen the risk of stroke. Lifestyle and diet changes can be useful.

There are a number of CVDs that specifically involve the heart. One is heart failure (also termed congestive heart failure). The word failure does not indicate a total stop in activity; rather, it indicates a deficiency in function: The heart is pumping but not optimally. As a result, the supply of blood and oxygen to the body is insufficient. If left untreated, and even with treatment, congestive heart failure can worsen with time. Another heart-associated CVD is arrhythmia, or an irregular heartbeat. Normally the heart beats at a constant pace, about 100,000 beats daily. In arrhythmia, the heart can beat at a constant rate, but a rate that is too fast (more than 100 beats per minute, which is termed tachycardia) or too slow (less than 60 beats per minute, known as bradycardia).

Male Cardiovascular Disease (CVD) Mortality Rates

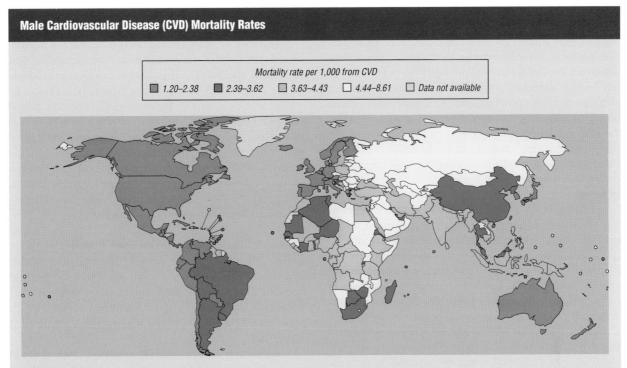

Mortality rate per 1,000 from CVD

☐ 1.20–2.38   ■ 2.39–3.62   ☐ 3.63–4.43   ☐ 4.44–8.61   ☐ Data not available

SOURCE: Adapted from "Figure 6. World map showing the global distribution of CVD mortality rates in males (age standardized, per 100,000)," *Global Atlas on Cardiovascular Diseases Prevention and Control*, World Health Organization (WHO), in collaboration with the World Heart Federation and the World Stroke Organization, 2014, p. 5, http://whqlibdoc.who.int/publications/2011/9789241564373_eng .pdf?ua=1 (accessed January 14, 2015).

Female Cardiovascular Disease (CVD) Mortality Rates

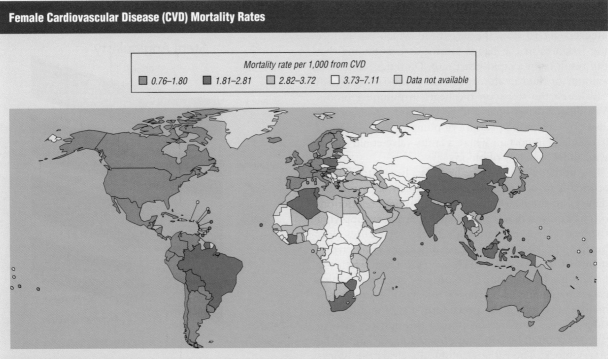

Mortality rate per 1,000 from CVD

☐ 0.76–1.80   ■ 1.81–2.81   ☐ 2.82–3.72   ☐ 3.73–7.11   ☐ Data not available

SOURCE: Adapted from "Figure 7. World map showing the global distribution of CVD mortality rates in females (age standardized, per 100,000)," *Global Atlas on Cardiovascular Diseases Prevention and Control*, World Health Organization (WHO), in collaboration with the World Heart Federation and the World Stroke Organization, 2014, p. 5, http://whqlibdoc.who.int/publications/2011/9789241564373_eng .pdf?ua=1 (accessed January 14, 2015).

Another CVD is malfunctioning heart valves. Normally the heart valves open and close in a synchronized manner that enables blood to exit the heart while preventing backflow of blood into the heart chambers. In a condition known as stenosis, the heart valves fail to open fully, which restricts the proper flow of blood. The valves also may not close properly, and the improper seal allows blood to leak. This condition is termed regurgitation. Another malfunction can be due to the bulging of the valve into the upper chamber of the heart. In this condition, which is termed mitral valve prolapse, closing of the valve can be impaired, leading to the backward flow of blood.

Treatment of heart-related CVDs varies depending on the condition. Heart valves may need surgical correction. Alternatively, the problem may not be debilitating and/or urgent enough to warrant surgery. Physicians can prescribe an angiotensin-converting enzyme inhibitor as a means to open a blood vessel more fully, which reduces high blood pressure. Anti-arrhythmic drugs can restore a proper heartbeat. In more severe cases, or when arrhythmia does not respond to drug treatment, cardiac defibrillation or the surgical installation of a pacemaker may be required. In defibrillation, a short pulse of electrical energy is applied to the heart. This can force the heartbeat back into a normal rhythm. A pacemaker supplies electrical energy as needed to maintain a normal heart rhythm. Anticoagulants, commonly known as blood thinners, can lessen the risk of blood clot formation due to faulty flow of blood in the vicinity of malfunctioning valves. Beta blockers act to slow the heartbeat, which can reduce the jerkiness in the hands known as palpitations that can result from a rapid heart rate. Diuretics reduce the amount of fluid in the tissue and bloodstream, which can lessen the stress on the heart in pumping blood. Vasodilator drugs open and relax blood vessels, which also can reduce the pressure of pumping blood. This is particularly important where a faulty valve could otherwise allow backflow of blood.

Another assault on the heart is a heart attack (also termed a myocardial infarction), which is permanent damage to the heart muscle due to oxygen restriction, often because a blood clot lodges in an artery supplying the heart. Drug treatment for a heart attack uses clot-busters in an attempt free the blockage. Other treatments of heart attack usually are performed when the patient has been stabilized. Coronary angioplasty (also called percutaneous coronary intervention) does not involve surgery. In the procedure, a thin and flexible tube called a catheter is inserted through the skin in the upper thigh or arm, and directed to the site of the artery block. The catheter physically clears the blockage. It also can be equipped to put in place a cylindrical meshlike object called a stent, which keeps that section of artery from collapsing. A surgical option is coronary artery bypass grafting: a healthy artery from elsewhere in the body is used to bypass the blocked section, and then becomes the new route for blood flow.

Yet another heart-related CVD is pericardial disease, an inflammation of the pericardium (the membrane that surrounds the heart). The disease can occur suddenly (acute pericarditis) in which case it usually is caused by a viral infection, or can build up over time and persist (chronic pericarditis). Normally the acute form dissipates as the infection resolves. However, sometimes fluid accumulates in the space between the pericardium and the heart, which can impair heart function; it can be fatal unless the fluid is removed. In chronic form, the inflammation gradually thickens the pericardium and progressively interferes with the heart's ability to function.

Vascular disease is a CVD that affects the blood vessels. It results from the impaired function of endothelial cells that line the vessels. The altered function begins when the cells become activated due to infection and other causes. This activation causes a series of reactions that thicken the wall of the blood vessels, which impedes blood flow and can lead to the formation of blood clots.

According to the WHO, a person with a CVD involving the blood vessels may not display symptoms until a heart attack or stroke occurs. Symptoms of a heart attack include pain or discomfort (for some people, a crushing sensation) in the center of the chest, and pain or discomfort in the arms, left shoulder,

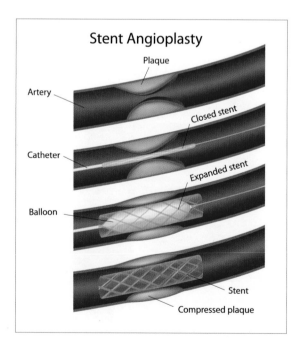

Stent angioplasty is a procedure in which a catheter is inserted into an artery that is partially blocked by plaque; a small balloon is opened to push out a mesh net, which compresses the plaque and opens the artery to increased blood flow. *© Alila Medical Media/ Shutterstock.com.*

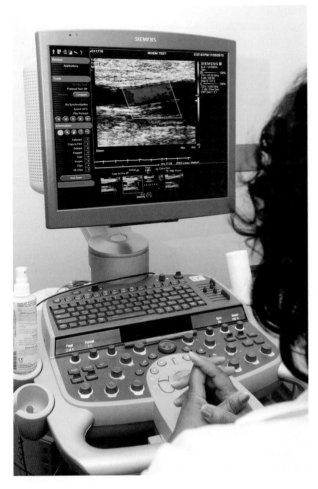

A registered diagnostic sonographer monitors a sonogram of the brachial artery of a participant in the Jackson Heart Study (JHS) at their Jackson, Mississippi, facility. JHS is receiving funds from the American Heart Association for vascular heart research and may expand their involvement with the Framingham Heart Study at Boston University, which is the longest-running, large-scale analysis of cardiovascular disease in the United States. *© Rogelio V. Solis/AP Photo.*

elbows, jaw, or back. Other symptoms include difficulty in breathing or shortness of breath, nausea or vomiting, feeling light-headed or faint, profuse sweating in the absence of exercise, and becoming pale. Women are more likely than men to experience shortness of breath, nausea, vomiting, and back or jaw pain. Stroke manifests most commonly as a sudden weakness of the face, arm, or leg, usually on one side of the body. Other symptoms include sudden onset of numbness of the face, arm, or leg, especially on one side of the body; mental confusion and difficulty speaking or understanding speech; difficulty seeing with one or both eyes; difficulty walking, dizziness, loss of balance or loss of coordination; severe headache; and fainting or unconsciousness. These symptoms signal the need for immediate medical attention.

Rheumatic heart disease occurs when heart valves and muscle are damaged due to inflammation and scarring associated with rheumatic fever. Rheumatic fever is an infection caused in children by streptococcal bacteria. The infection begins relatively mildly, usually as a sore throat. Tonsillitis can occur. Early treatment of the sore throat will prevent the development of rheumatic fever. If someone has had rheumatic fever, regular and long-term treatment with penicillin can be effective in preventing another bout of rheumatic fever, which could prelude rheumatic heart disease. A repeat occurrence is serious because the heart valves may already have been damaged. Rheumatic fever and rheumatic heart disease are prevalent in children in developing countries, where health can be poorer and health care less available.

According to statistics from the WHO, nearly 2 percent of global deaths from CVDs are due to rheumatic heart disease, with slightly more than 40 percent of CVD-related deaths due to ischemic heart disease and about 35 percent caused by cerebrovascular disease.

⊕ Future Implications

Many CVDs are associated with risk factors that can be modified. These behavioral risk factors—which underlie about 80 percent of cases of cerebrovascular disease (CVD that involves the brain) and coronary heart disease—include unhealthy diet, physical inactivity, tobacco use, and the excessive and long-term consumption of alcohol. Those whose diet is unhealthy and who shun physical inactivity can be overweight (defined by the CDC as a body mass index of 25–29.9) or obese (body mass index of 30 or higher), have raised blood pressure, and have glucose and lipid concentrations in the blood that are elevated. These are risk factors for heart attack, stroke, heart failure, and other complications.

Lifestyle changes known to reduce the risk of CVDs include stopping tobacco use, reducing salt in the diet, altering a diet to include more servings of fruits and vegetables, regular physical activity, and avoiding excessive use of alcohol. Other options to reduce risk that an individual can take with the advice of a health-care provider include preventing or treating hypertension, diabetes, and elevated levels of blood lipids.

Smoking is the most preventable risk factor for cardiac and lung disease. Scientists have predicted there will be upward of 1 billion smoking-related deaths occurring during the 21st century. The development and marketing of electronic cigarettes as a safer way for smokers to indulge their need for smoking-related pleasure, has resulted in several million people worldwide using electronic cigarettes.

THE MICROBIOME AND CARDIOVASCULAR DISEASE

Research published in the *FASEB Journal*, published by the Federation of American Societies for Experimental Biology, suggests that the intestinal microbiome—the collective types and numbers of bacteria in the intestines—may one day be used as a way of predicting the likelihood of heart attack. Manipulating the composition of the microbiome by increasing or decreasing the relative proportions of certain bacteria (this area of research is known as probiotics) could lower the risk of heart attack. The research findings could lead to new diagnostic tests and therapies used to prevent and treat heart attacks. In addition, findings indicate that probiotics with demonstrated positive effects in other areas of the body, such as the vagina in women with vaginal infections, may be able to protect the heart in patients undergoing heart surgery and angioplasty.

The study was conducted using rats. Researchers used three groups of rats: one group was fed a standard diet, another group received the antibiotic vancomycin in their drinking water, and a third group was given a probiotic supplement containing *Lactobacillus plantarum*, a bacterium that suppresses the production of leptin. Leptin is a hormone that is important in appetite and metabolism. The rats treated with the antibiotic had less leptin, displayed less severe heart attacks, and showed improved recovery of mechanical function compared to the group that had been fed a standard diet. However, the antibiotic also had other effects: the total bacterial numbers in the intestines were reduced and the numbers of specific types of bacteria and fungi that live in the gut were altered. This alteration offset the protection bestowed by the antibiotic. The third group of rats had both the advantage of leptin in reducing heart attack severity and improving recovery, and had an intestinal composition of bacteria that was healthier.

Smoking an electronic cigarette simulates the effect of smoking a regular cigarette with an inhaled vapor rather than smoke. An electronic cigarette consists of a battery, a liquid-containing cartridge, and a heating element that warms and evaporates the liquid. The liquid is less toxic than smoke from regular cigarettes. According to research by Konstantinos Farsalinos and colleagues presented to the European Society of Cardiology (ESC) in 2012, nitrosamines—a toxic component of cigarette smoke—were not found in previous studies of electronic cigarettes or were present in levels 500–1,400 times less than the amount present in one tobacco cigarette. Based on the nitrosamine level, electronic cigarettes would have to be used daily for 4 to 12 months to equal the nitrosamines present in a single tobacco cigarette.

Farsalinos and other researchers studied the influence of electronic cigarettes on heart function compared to the use of regular cigarettes. The rationale for the study was the knowledge that heart disease is the main cause of morbidity and mortality in smokers; 40 percent of deaths in smokers are caused by coronary artery disease alone. Inhaling regular cigarette smoke impairs the heart. Thus, apparently healthy young smokers are likely to have heart damage already that is as yet clinically undetectable using typical examination tools. The study sought to determine whether these signs of preclinical disease would be present in a similar population using electronic cigarettes. The researchers measured myocardial function using ultrasound (cardiac ultrasound also is known as echocardiography) in 20 healthy young (25–45 years of age) individuals who smoked every day before and after smoking one tobacco cigarette. The measurements also were taken of 22 individuals of similar age and health who used electronic cigarettes before and after using the device for seven minutes. The commercially available e-cigarette liquid had a nicotine concentration of 11 milligrams per milliliter but did not contain nitrosamines or polycyclic aromatic hydrocarbons.

Smoking one tobacco cigarette produced immediate impairment of heart function, whereas the e-cigarette did not. The tobacco cigarette immediately increased systolic blood pressure (the pressure associated with pumping of blood through the arteries), diastolic blood pressure (the pressure in the arteries when the heart rests in between beats), and the rate at which the heart was pumping. "In contrast, electronic cigarettes produced only a slight elevation in diastolic blood pressure," according to the presentation to the ESC. The findings indicated that the body absorbs nicotine from an electronic cigarette more slowly, compared to a conventional cigarette.

The echocardiography examination focused on the left ventricle of the heart. This is the part of the heart that receives oxygenated blood from the lungs during the filling (diastolic) phase and delivers the blood to the body during the pumping (systolic) phase. Smoking a single cigarette produced an appreciable impairment in the filling of the left ventricle. In contrast, none of the echocardiographic parameters worsened appreciably in any of the subjects using the electronic cigarettes.

The research needs to be corroborated. Nonetheless, it offers hope that smokers may be able to lessen their self-inflicted cardiovascular damage at the same time as they are embarking on a path that could wean them entirely from the cardiovascular damage caused by smoking.

PRIMARY SOURCE

Heart Disease and Stroke: The Nation's Leading Killers

SOURCE *"Heart Disease and Stroke Prevention: Addressing the Nation's Leading Killers." National Center for Chronic Disease Prevention and Health Promotion, 2011, 2–3. http://www.*

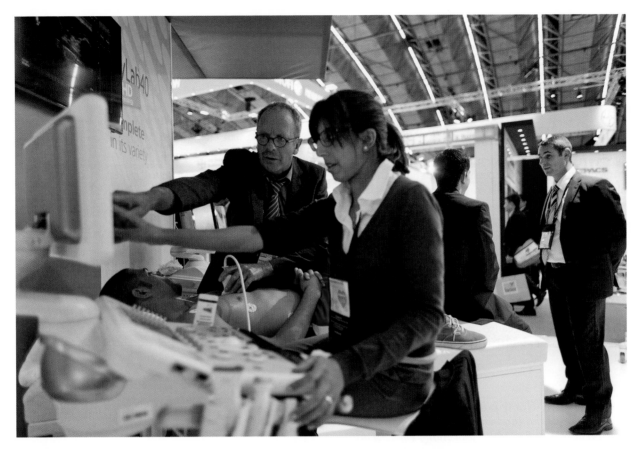

A volunteer receives a 3-D heart scan at the European Society of Cardiology meeting venue in Amsterdam in 2013. The future of cardio-vascular treatment was the main talking point for some 30,000 medics gathered in Amsterdam for the European Society of Cardiology annual congress. Cardiovascular disease remains the number one killer worldwide and doctors fear a renewed epidemic of heart problems in 20 to 30 years time as a new generation of overweight and obese youngsters reaches middle age. *© Cris Toala Olivares/Reuters.*

cdc.gov/chronicdisease/resources/publications/ aag/pdf/2011/heart-disease-and-stroke- aag-2011.pdf (accessed January 25, 2015).

INTRODUCTION *The following primary source is an information sheet published by the National Center for Chronic Disease Prevention and Health Promotion, a division of the U.S. Centers for Disease Control and Prevention (CDC). The fact sheet describes the CDC's response to the public health challenge presented by cardiovascular disease, and presents relevant statistics.*

Heart disease and stroke, the first and third leading causes of death for men and women, are among the most widespread and costly health problems facing our nation today, yet they also are among the most preventable. Cardiovascular diseases, including heart disease and stroke, account for more than one-third (33.6 percent) of all U.S. deaths.

In 2007, of all Americans who died of cardiovascular diseases, 150,000 were younger than age 65. Heart disease and stroke also are among the leading causes of disability in the United States, with nearly 4 million people reporting disability from these causes.

The Costs of Disease Are Staggering

Death rates alone cannot describe the burden of heart disease and stroke. In 2010, the total costs of cardiovascular diseases in the United States were estimated to be $444 billion. Treatment of these diseases accounts for about $1 of every $6 spent on health care in this country. As the U.S. population ages, the economic impact of cardiovascular diseases on our nation's health care system will become even greater.

Overall, death rates for heart disease and stroke have decreased in the United States in recent decades. However, rates for incidence and death continue to be high, especially among some populations, including members of certain racial and ethnic groups, people with low socioeconomic status, and those living in the southeastern United States.

For example, age-adjusted death rates for cardiovascular disease are 37 percent higher among African Americans than among whites. The risk of having a first-ever stroke is nearly two times higher among African Americans than among whites. In addition, about 55,000 more women than men have a stroke each year. Recent studies show that the prevalence of heart disease and the percentage of associated premature deaths are higher among American Indians and Alaska Natives than among any other U.S. racial or ethnic group.

Prevention Saves Lives

Leading a healthy lifestyle—not using tobacco, being physically active, maintaining a healthy weight, and making healthy food choices—greatly reduces a person's risk of developing heart disease or stroke. Preventing and controlling high blood pressure and high cholesterol also play a significant role in cardiovascular health. For example, a 12–13 point reduction in average systolic blood pressure over 4 years can reduce heart disease risk by 21 percent, stroke risk by 37 percent, and risk of total cardiovascular death by 25 percent. Public health strategies and policies that promote healthy living, encourage healthy environments, and promote control of blood pressure and cholesterol levels are vital to improving the public's health and saving lives. Ensuring that all Americans have access to early, affordable, and appropriate treatment also is essential to reducing disability and costs.

SEE ALSO *Global Health Initiatives; Health-Related Education and Information Access; High Blood Pressure; Life Expectancy and Aging Populations; Noncommunicable Diseases (Lifestyle Diseases); Obesity; Tobacco Use*

BIBLIOGRAPHY

Books

Bonow, Robert O., et al. *Braunwald's Heart Disease: A Textbook of Cardiovascular Medicine,* 9th ed. Philadelphia, PA: Saunders, 2012.

Kokkinos, Peter. *Physical Activity and Cardiovascular Disease Prevention.* Sudbury, MA: Jones and Bartlett, 2010.

Mancini, Mario, et al., eds. *Nutritional and Metabolic Bases of Cardiovascular Disease.* West Sussex, UK: Wiley-Blackwell, 2011.

Mieszczanska, Hanna, and Gladys P. Velarde, eds. *Management of Cardiovascular Disease in Women.* London: Springer, 2014.

Shaheen, Ghazala, Tahira Shamim, and Zareena Yasmeen. *Cardiovascular Diseases.* New York: Lambert Academic, 2011.

Sutton, Amy L., ed. *Cardiovascular Disorders Sourcebook,* 4th ed. Detroit, MI: Omnigraphics, 2010.

Watson, Ronald R., and Victor R. Preedy, eds. *Bioactive Food as Dietary Interventions for Cardiovascular Disease.* San Diego, CA: Academic Press, 2013.

Periodicals

Lam, Vy, et al. "Intestinal Microbiota Determine Severity of Myocardial Infarction in Rats." *FASEB Journal* 26, no. 4 (April 2012): 1727–1735. Available online at http://www.fasebj.org/content/26/4/1727.full (accessed April 21, 2015).

Lim, Stephen S., et al. "A Comparative Risk Assessment of Burden of Disease and Injury Attributable to 67 Risk Factors and Risk Factor Clusters in 21 Regions, 1990–2010: A Systematic Analysis for the Global Burden of Disease Study." *The Lancet* 380, no. 9859 (December 15, 2012): 2224–2260.

Websites

"Cardiovascular Disease Terms." *World Heart Federation.* http://www.world-heart-federation.org/press/fact-sheets/cardiovascular-disease-terms/ (accessed February 10, 2015).

"Cardiovascular Diseases (CVDs)." *World Health Organization (WHO).* http://www.who.int/mediacentre/factsheets/fs317/en/ (accessed February 10, 2015).

"Electronic Cigarettes Do Not Damage the Heart." *European Society of Cardiology (ESC),* August 25, 2012. http://www.escardio.org/The-ESC/Press-Office/Press-releases/Last-5-years/Electronic-cigarettes-do-not-damage-the-heart (accessed April 8, 2015).

"Heart Disease." *Mayo Clinic.* http://www.mayoclinic.org/diseases-conditions/heart-disease/basics/definition/con-20034056 (accessed February 10, 2015).

"Heart Diseases." *National Institutes of Health.* http://www.nlm.nih.gov/medlineplus/heartdiseases.html (accessed February 10, 2015).

Brian Douglas Hoyle

Centers for Disease Control and Prevention (CDC)

⊕ Introduction

The Centers for Disease Control and Prevention (CDC) is a federal agency of the United States in charge of protecting the country against health threats and improving national security regarding this matter. Its headquarters are located in DeKalb County, Georgia, just miles from the center of Atlanta. There, and in other locations throughout the United States, the CDC employs 15,000 people, from engineers to veterinarians, including professionals of all health areas. The CDC functions under the Department of Health and Human Services of the U.S. government and has an annual budget that in 2014 totaled $6.9 billion.

This agency has three main priorities: to improve health security in the United States and around the world; to help prevent the leading causes of illnesses, injury, disability, and death; and to strengthen the collaboration between public health and health-care institutions. To comply with these objectives, the CDC conducts and funds science research, monitors diseases, and can respond against health emergencies, among other actions.

Because of the possibility of these emergencies, the CDC works 24 hours per day, seven days per week. Its actions reach outside of the United States, collaborating with foreign governments, researchers, and international organizations, thus working to prevent new diseases from spreading into the country. It had an active role, for example, in coordinating help against the 2014 Ebola outbreak in West Africa, but it also has a fundamental importance in the battle against illnesses that are seen in daily American life, such as influenza. It also covers non-infectious diseases and health concerns such as obesity. The issues that are relevant to the CDC are as wide as the possible threats to human health.

⊕ Historical Background

Although the range of action of the CDC is vast, this has not always been the case. Its origin was in a very specific context and with a very specific mission. After World War II (1939–1945) started, the United States prepared its armed forces for a possible conflict. Most of the military camps and maneuver areas were located in the south of the country, and the Department of War was worried about illnesses that could affect the troops. Malaria, present in those areas, could be a large risk for those soldiers.

In 1940, the Department of War asked the Public Health Service (PHS) for help in organizing public health activities in the areas surrounding the camps and, in the spring of 1941, the PHS assigned their chief malariologist to work with the U.S. Army in Atlanta to control malaria. On December 7 of that year, Japan attacked Pearl Harbor, and early in 1942 the PHS started an independent malaria control program in military bases and industries related to war. The Malaria Control in War Areas program (MCWA) was established in Atlanta and initially operated in 15 southeastern states, plus the Virgin Islands, Puerto Rico, and other Caribbean areas. Engineers, entomologists, and physicians worked together to control mosquitoes in those regions. Although there was laboratory work involved, the main efforts were draining ditches (mosquitoes thrive in still waters) and the application of larvicides.

Before the war was over, the MCWA expanded its activities to other problems, such as controlling the mosquito *Aedes aegypti*, the vector of yellow fever and dengue, as well as controlling typhus. The organization started preparing for the return of the troops from tropical regions, as well, and provided education on tropical diseases. "MCWA also began to respond to states' calls for help with infectious disease problems, such as an outbreak of amoebic dysentery in a mental institution in Alabama," medical historian John Parascandola (1941–) explains.

After the war, the need for a permanent institution such as the MCWA became obvious. On July 1, 1946, the Communicable Disease Center (CDC) began operations, continuing the role of the MCWA. Although at first most of its efforts were in malaria control, it soon began expanding. In 1947 a Veterinary Public Health

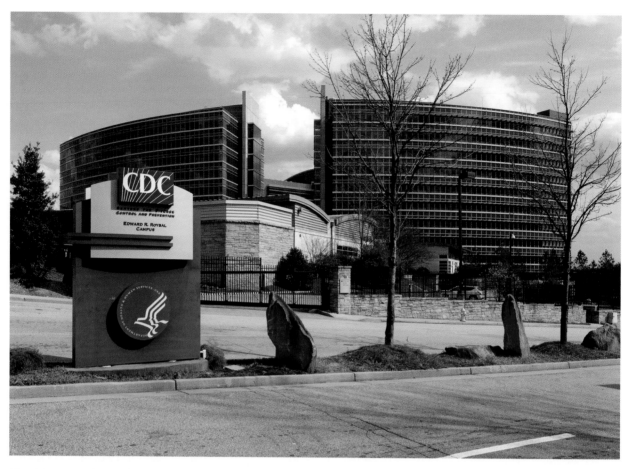

The U.S. Centers for Disease Control and Prevention (CDC) headquarters in Atlanta, Georgia. The CDC focuses on health promotion; prevention of disease, injury, and disability; and preparedness for new health threats in the United States. © *Katherine Welles/Shutterstock.com.*

division was created and the CDC took over the Plague Laboratory of the PHS in San Francisco. In 1951, motivated by concerns about biological warfare during the Cold War (1945–1991), the CDC added an Epidemic Intelligence Service. "CDC also soon was engaged in work relating other public health problems, such as diarrheal diseases and polio," Parascandola adds.

These expansions would continue over the years, adding areas as nutrition, environmental health, and chronic diseases. Reflecting different changes such as this, the CDC adapted its name several times: In 1967 it became the National Communicable Disease Center; in 1970, the Center for Disease Control; and in 1981 the word "Center" was changed to the plural "Centers." The current designation as Centers for Disease Control and Prevention originated in 1992, but despite the changes in the formal name, the abbreviation of CDC has stuck through the years.

As both a research center and an organization where medical innovations are applied into the field, the CDC has not only been a health agency but an innovation hot spot. "A magnet for gifted scientists and other professionals looking to serve in public health, CDC has attracted

an exceptional cadre of talent over the years," researchers Tanja Popovic and Dixie E. Snider write in a paper for the medical journal *Emerging Infectious Diseases.*

"In this climate of idealism and dedication, the achievements have been many and span all areas," Popovic and Snider continue, "CDC scientists, typically working with like-minded colleagues, identified and characterized several infectious agents and emerging infectious diseases; invented devices, tools, and stains for diagnoses and systems for surveillance; demonstrated the value of combining laboratory practices and epidemiology; and through vision and leadership, worked closely with state and local health departments to increase their effectiveness as public health organizations."

In 1976, a CDC laboratory scientist discovered the cause of Legionnaires' disease, a form of pneumonia with a high fatality rate. Thirty years later, researchers identified the genome of the smallpox virus, and more recently another group of scientists at the CDC re-created the 1918 influenza A (H1N1) virus, which helped to understand why it was so deadly.

The agency has made fundamental contributions to creating vaccines and controlling diseases such as polio and rabies. But there are sad episodes in the history of CDC too. In 1932, before the creation of the CDC, the PHS began a study to record the natural history of syphilis. It was called the Tuskegee Study of Untreated Syphilis in the Negro Male, and it lasted until 1972. It involved 600 black men—399 with syphilis and 201 healthy men—who were told they were treated for "bad blood." Actually, they were being monitored for syphilis. "The study was conducted without the benefit of patients' informed consent," the CDC has explained, "they did not receive the proper treatment needed to cure their illness. In exchange for taking part in the study, the men received free medical exams, free meals, and burial insurance. Although originally projected to last six months, the study actually continued for 40 years."

During the latter years, the CDC supported and funded the Tuskegee experiment. In 1972, an article by the news agency the Associated Press denounced the experiment and its ethical practices. In 1973 the participants and their families filled a lawsuit and reached a $10 million settlement. In 1997, President Bill Clinton (1946–) issued an apology on behalf of the nation. Afterward, the CDC contributed funding to Tuskegee University to create a center for bioethical research.

Since the mid-1990s, the CDC has continued its commitment to bioethics, with a strong emphasis in its global role. In 2003, when the first case of severe acute respiratory syndrome (SARS) was reported in Asia, it gave guidance and helped in the clinical and laboratory evaluation. During 2014, it participated in monitoring and fighting Ebola both in Africa as well as in the United States.

⊕ Impacts and Issues

CDC's Role in Emergencies

One of most known roles of the CDC is what the organization defines as "public health preparedness and response." This consists of being able to deploy quickly the required disease detectives, vaccines, medicines, and other kinds of support in health emergencies such as natural disasters, disease outbreaks, or possible attacks on the United States.

For this, the CDC has an Emergency Operations Center that works 24/7. Also, it keeps a repository of medicine and medical supplies called the Strategic National Stockpile. In case it is needed, the CDC can get lifesaving medication from this supply and have it anywhere in the United States in 12 hours or less. This repository is updated constantly. During the 2014 Ebola crisis, the CDC spent $2.7 million in new protective gear for hospitals.

Another relevant aspect of the CDC's functions is detecting outbreaks, as well as tracking, eliminating, and preventing them. This is the area that the CDC calls "Emerging and Zoonotic Infectious Diseases," which focuses on a range of infectious diseases. Zoonotic

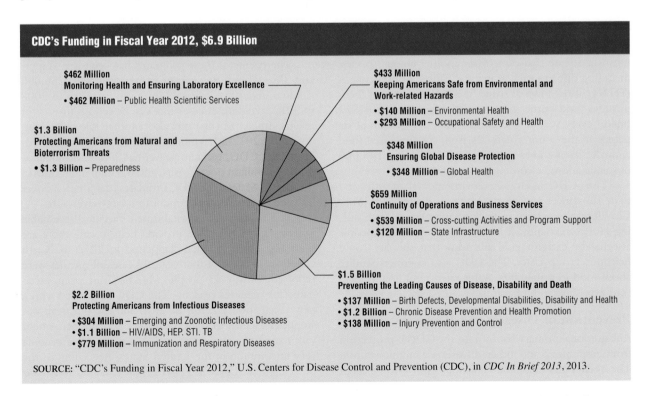

CDC's Funding in Fiscal Year 2012, $6.9 Billion

$462 Million
Monitoring Health and Ensuring Laboratory Excellence
• **$462 Million** – Public Health Scientific Services

$1.3 Billion
Protecting Americans from Natural and Bioterrorism Threats
• **$1.3 Billion** – Preparedness

$2.2 Billion
Protecting Americans from Infectious Diseases
• **$304 Million** – Emerging and Zoonotic Infectious Diseases
• **$1.1 Billion** – HIV/AIDS, HEP. STI. TB
• **$779 Million** – Immunization and Respiratory Diseases

$433 Million
Keeping Americans Safe from Environmental and Work-related Hazards
• **$140 Million** – Environmental Health
• **$293 Million** – Occupational Safety and Health

$348 Million
Ensuring Global Disease Protection
• **$348 Million** – Global Health

$659 Million
Continuity of Operations and Business Services
• **$539 Million** – Cross-cutting Activities and Program Support
• **$120 Million** – State Infrastructure

$1.5 Billion
Preventing the Leading Causes of Disease, Disability and Death
• **$137 Million** – Birth Defects, Developmental Disabilities, Disability and Health
• **$1.2 Billion** – Chronic Disease Prevention and Health Promotion
• **$138 Million** – Injury Prevention and Control

SOURCE: "CDC's Funding in Fiscal Year 2012," U.S. Centers for Disease Control and Prevention (CDC), in *CDC In Brief 2013*, 2013.

Though the Centers for Disease Control (CDC) has a strong international presence, a breakdown of its federal funds show that the primary focus of the CDC is to keep Americans safe from infectious diseases.

EUROPEAN CDC

By 2003, the European Union (EU) was consolidated as more than a community of countries. It had a new common currency, the euro, and it was planning a European constitution. Going from one member country to another one was easy, as in most cases customs had been lifted. This was great for commercial and cultural exchange, but it presented a health challenge. An outbreak was no longer the problem of one country but of all of the members.

At that time, the SARS pandemic had started growing in Asia. The EU had funded disease surveillance networks since 1999, but they were uncoordinated efforts, and they could be weak against a major threat. Plus, there were 10 new members coming to the union. All of these factors led to the creation of the European Centre for Disease Prevention and Control (ECDC).

The legal process to approve this agency was conducted in a record time for the EU. It was proposed in July 2003; in December Sweden was chosen as the host for the center, and in May 2005 it was operational in the city of Solna, near Stockholm. The established mission for the ECDC was "to identify, assess and communicate current and emerging threats to human health posed by infectious diseases."

Unlike the American CDC, similar health agencies in Europe had already existed but on a national level. This meant that one of the big differences in the European case is that it has to work in partnership with other health protection bodies all across the continent to develop and strengthen surveillance systems. Among the specific objectives of this center, it was established that it would have to search, collect, and disseminate relevant scientific and technical data; provide scientific assistance and training; provide information to the EU and its members; coordinate the European networking of bodies in this field; and facilitate the development and implementation of joint actions.

As of late 2014, the ECDC had a staff of approximately 300 people and a budget of 58.3 million euros (2013). Its range of action reaches the 28 EU member states (Austria, Belgium, Bulgaria, Croatia, Cyprus, the Czech Republic, Denmark, Estonia, Finland, France, Germany, Greece, Hungary, Ireland, Italy, Latvia, Lithuania, Luxembourg, Malta, Netherlands, Poland, Portugal, Romania, Slovakia, Slovenia, Spain, Sweden, and the United Kingdom), plus three other non-EU countries (Iceland, Liechtenstein, and Norway).

This center has a strong focus on research. In 2013 it produced 211 scientific publications with high-impact levels. The ECDC also publishes *Eurosurveillance*, a peer-reviewed scientific journal that is free to access and covers topics such as epidemiology, prevention, and control of infectious diseases and health surveillance. It also publishes reports on different illnesses and threats, such as its Annual Epidemiological Report, which gives advice on the actions that Europe should take in this matter.

Through all these actions, the ECDC constantly is monitoring and evaluating different risks. Just as for the American CDC, Ebola was one of their biggest concerns in 2014, and they are permanently researching it and publishing guidelines and updates regarding the outbreak's status.

means a disease that came from another animal species, including diseases such as malaria, rabies, or influenza A (H1N1, also known as swine flu). Another area of focus includes food-borne diseases, a problem that costs $77 billion every year in the United States. One out of six people in the country gets sick from contaminated food annually. That comes to 48 million people and 128,000 hospitalizations, according to the CDC.

The CDC addresses environmental health and toxic substances too. For example, it helped New York City develop a system to track weather events and, during Hurricane Sandy, it identified an increase of people affected by extreme cold and ways that the city could help this group faster. The CDC also conducts studies about food in restaurants, water safety, and how to prevent exposures to biohazards.

Prevention of Diseases and Research

An additional primary concern for the CDC is protection from respiratory and other diseases via immunization. The agency has launched enormous efforts to research vaccines and launch programs to apply solutions. In 2013, for example, the CDC designated $679 million of its budget toward these diseases.

The results of these programs has been very important throughout the country. Approximately 250,000 children under five years old were vaccinated from 2008 to 2012, avoiding diseases that can be serious threats for infants. Influenza (flu) was also another relevant target: during the 2012-2013 influenza vaccine program, according to the CDC, vaccines prevented 79,000 hospitalizations, 3.2 million doctor visits, and 6.6 million flu cases in the United States. The CDC estimates that for each dollar invested in vaccinations, American society saves $10.

The CDC also has established Vaccine-Preventable Diseases Centers, which provide help in case there are outbreaks, such as what happened in 2013 in North Carolina. In April of that year, 23 cases of measles were reported, mostly in people who had not been vaccinated for religious reasons. The CDC responded with a new vaccination plan in the area, and the outbreak was stopped. Thanks to these responses and the permanent vaccination plans, diseases such as measles have become very uncommon in the United States. According to the book *Epidemiology and Prevention of Vaccine-Preventable Diseases* (also known as "the Pink Book"), in 1950 there were more than 300,000 cases of measles, but in 2009 there were only 71.

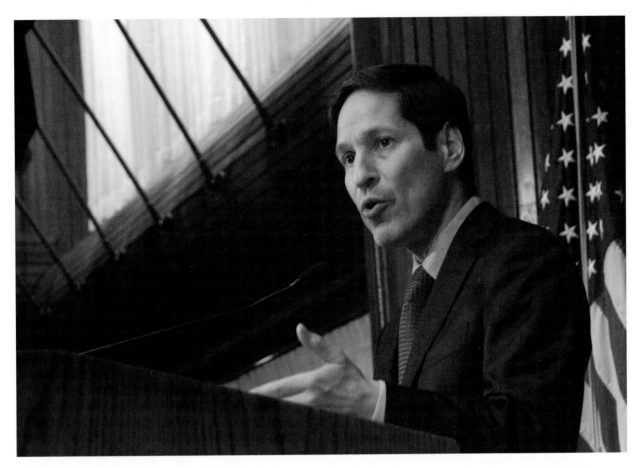

Dr. Thomas Frieden, director of the U.S. Centers for Disease Control and Prevention, speaks to the National Press Club in Washington, D.C., in 2013.   © *Albert H. Teich/Shutterstock.com.*

In terms of sexually transmitted diseases, the CDC works to fight HIV (human immunodeficiency virus), hepatitis B, and others. In regard to tuberculosis, the agency has helped reduce cases from 25,103 in 1993 to 9,945 in 2012. The CDC also gives attention to developmental disabilities, chronic disease prevention, occupational safety, injury prevention, and health promotion in general.

An Institution with Global Reach

Because borders are rarely a defense against diseases, the CDC has decided to have an important role in global health. According to the agency's data, it has responded to more than 288 global disease outbreaks and has trained more than 3,000 disease detectives from 47 countries. "Real health threats usually look innocuous. They arrive every day, along with millions of people and millions of tons of cargo that enter the U.S. from all parts of the globe," CDC director Thomas R. Frieden (1960–) wrote in the *Atlantic*. "With the globalization of travel and trade of foods and drugs, dangerous pathogens that arise anywhere in the world are just a plane ride away. U.S. national health security depends on global health security, because a threat anywhere is a threat everywhere."

Collaborating with other countries and international organizations is a key part of this objective. "No single country can achieve global health security by itself. Ensuring national health security means working with international partners," Frieden says. The battle against polio has been a good example of what global health efforts can achieve: The CDC and its foreign equivalents have eradicated this illness almost totally from the world. In 1998, 350,000 cases in 125 countries were reported. By 2013 there were only 416 cases reported in three countries.

It is not unusual to see CDC experts traveling around the world. The President's Emergency Plan for AIDS Relief (PEPFAR), which attempts to identify, treat, and prevent HIV, had taken 1,800 CDC staff to more than 44 countries by 2013. According to the CDC, this has meant treating 6.7 million people and preventing 1 million babies from being infected with HIV.

Although this international role is very important for the CDC, it is a federal agency and, according to this qualification, it has the responsibility to support state, tribal, local, and territorial health departments too. More than 800 specialists of the CDC work with local institutions, and approximately two-thirds of CDC's funding supports state and local health departments.

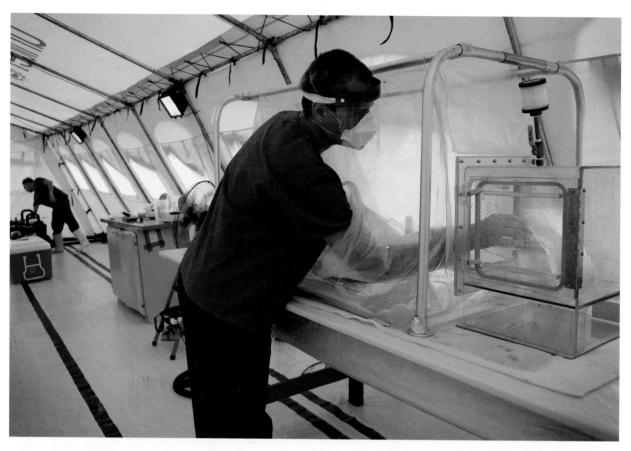

Virologist Heinrich Feldman handles blood samples while testing them for the Ebola virus in a "glove box" at a mobile laboratory for Ebola testing opened in August 2014, near Monrovia, Liberia. The U.S. Centers for Disease Control and Prevention (CDC), opened the lab next to the Médecins Sans Frontières (Doctors Without Borders) Ebola treatment facility to test the surge of patients being admitted with Ebola symptoms. The lab tested dozens of blood samples in its first two days and expected the number to increase drastically. The facility was shipped to Liberia as a joint project between the CDC, the U.S. National Institutes of Health, and the Global Outbreak Alert and Response Network, and constitutes one of the U.S. government's major contributions to containing the Ebola epidemic in Liberia.   *© John Moore/Getty Images.*

For all of these partners, inside and outside the United States, there is another relevant role: keeping track of information, in other words, health statistics. The CDC organizes surveys and measures and tracks data that is fundamental to plan and project needs. It has promoted the use of electronic medical records, which had a 315 percent increase of use from 2003 to 2012, and it has connected the different systems of 34 states. "This provided information for clinical and public health decisions so more children get only the vaccines they need, and get them on time," a 2013 CDC report explains.

⊕ Future Implications

As with any government agency, the CDC always is subject to the judgment of the public. But due to its role in areas as sensitive as health and safety, this is even more emphasized in the mid-2010s. The Ebola pandemic is one of many examples of this increased relevance. The CDC constantly has been visible in the media regarding

this subject, sometimes to explain the situation, sometimes to give guidelines, and also sometimes to receive criticisms.

After a nurse was infected with Ebola in a hospital in Dallas, Texas, the CDC was criticized publicly by experts. Bonnie Castillo, a disaster relief expert of the organization National Nurses United, explained to Reuters news agency that the instructions to handle this disease were insufficient and that hospitals "post something on a bulletin board referring workers and nurses to the CDC guidelines. That is not how you drill and practice and become [an] expert."

One of the challenges for the CDC is to respond to a growing number of concerns in a fast and effective way. This is why it is an agency that must constantly evaluate its own responses and improve its standards. After this negative experience in Texas, for example, the CDC modified its guidelines. "Under new protocols, Ebola health-care workers also must undergo special training and demonstrate competency in using protective equipment. Use of the gear, now including coveralls, and single-use, disposable hoods, must be overseen by a supervisor to ensure proper procedures are followed when caring for patients with Ebola, which is transmitted through direct contact with bodily fluids but is not airborne," the CDC explained.

There was also self-criticism. "Even a single health-care worker infection is unacceptable," CDC director Frieden said to the press after the presentation of the new guidelines.

Similar evaluation processes have been done after natural disasters. Hurricane Katrina, in 2005, was described by the CDC as "a lesson like no other." In this case, around 700 CDC experts were deployed from nearly every area of the agency. After the disaster, the experts reviewed their work, preparing for a future similar situation. "We took a multi-disciplinary approach to identifying both strengths and opportunities for improvement to CDC's all-hazards preparedness and response so immediate steps could be taken," the director of the Division of Emergency Operations, Phil Navin, explained. The corrective actions that were put in place went from improving management standards to adding pets as an issue of concern for which to plan.

But not all the new problems are pandemics or natural disasters. The CDC also is addressing changes in the society, such as the dangerous trend of avoiding vaccinations, especially in infants. The agency is keeping a close eye on other new phenomena too, such as the use of electronic cigarettes. In the 2014 Youth Tobacco Survey, which the CDC conducts, the organization warned about the rising amount of high school students who are smoking with these devices. In 2014, 13.4 percent of high school students had used an e-cigarette in the past 30 days, triple the number who used them in 2013 (4.5 percent) and almost nine times the number who used them in 2011 (1.5 percent), according to the survey.

Finally, the CDC is making extra efforts abroad in response to globalization. In February 2014 it announced plans to commit $40 million in 10 new countries for programs to improve rapid response and increase global health security. These investments hope to address what the CDC director has explained to be the three threats to global health: emerging diseases, drug-resistant infections, and the intentional or accidental dissemination of genetically altered infectious agents. "Why now?" Frieden wrote in the *Atlantic*, "because not only are the threats greater than ever, our chances of stopping them are better than ever too. There is unprecedented political commitment around the world. We have exciting new technologies. And we've seen encouraging successes to build on."

SEE ALSO *Antibiotic/Antimicrobial Resistance; Cancer; Cardiovascular Diseases; Child Health; Cholera and Dysentery; Climate Change: Health Impacts; Dengue; Diabetes; Drug and Substance Abuse; Ebola Virus Disease; Epidemiology: Surveillance for Emerging Infectious Diseases; Global Health Initiatives; High Blood Pressure; HIV/AIDS; Influenza; Insect-Borne Disease; International Health Regulation, Surveillance, and Enforcement; Isolation and Quarantine; Malaria; Methicillin-Resistant* Staphylococcus aureus *(MRSA); Neglected Tropical Diseases; Noncommunicable Diseases (Lifestyle Diseases); Pandemic Preparedness; Parasitic Diseases; Pneumonia and Pneumococcal Diseases; Poliomyelitis (Polio); Prion Diseases; SARS, MERS, and the Emergence of Coronaviruses; Smallpox Eradication and Storage of Infectious Agents; Tobacco Use; Tuberculosis (TB); Vaccine-Preventable Diseases; Viral Hepatitis; Waterborne Diseases; World Health Organization: Organization, Funding, and Enforcement Powers; Zoonotic (Animal-Borne) Diseases*

BIBLIOGRAPHY

Books

Atkinson, William, et al., eds. *Epidemiology and Prevention of Vaccine-Preventable Diseases* ("The Pink Book"), 13th ed. Washington, DC: Public Health Foundation, 2014.

Periodicals

Parascandola, John. "From MCWA to CDC—Origins of the Centers for Disease Control and Prevention." *Public Health Reports* 111, no. 6 (November–December 1996): 549–551.

Popovic, Tanja, and Dixie E. Snider. "60 Years of Progress—CDC and Infectious Diseases." *Emerging Infectious Diseases* 12, no. 7 (July 2006): 1160–1161.

"Regulation (EC) No 851/2004 of the European Parliament and of the Council of 21 April 2004 Establishing a European Centre for Disease Prevention and Control." *Official Journal of the European Union* (April 30, 2004): L 142/1.

Websites

"CDC Issues New Protocols for Health Care Workers Treating Ebola Patients." *Christian Science Monitor*, October 20, 2014. http://www.csmonitor.com/USA/Latest-News-Wires/2014/1020/CDC-issues-new-protocols-for-health-care-workers-treating-Ebola-patients (accessed January 27, 2015).

"CDC Learns from Katrina, Plans for Pandemic." *U.S. Centers for Disease Control and Prevention (CDC).* http://www.cdc.gov/news/2006_11/katrina.htm (accessed January 27, 2015).

"CDC: Saving Lives. Protecting People. *U.S. Centers for Disease Control and Prevention (CDC)*, August 2014. http://www.cdc.gov/about/report/2013/docs/cdcreport_2013.pdf (accessed January 27, 2015).

"CDC Tightened Guidance for U.S. Healthcare Workers on Personal Protective Equipment for Ebola." *U.S. Centers for Disease Control and Prevention (CDC)*, October 20, 2014. http://www.cdc.gov/media/releases/2014/fs1020-ebola-personal-protective-equipment.html (accessed January 27, 2015).

"E-cigarette Use Triples among Middle and High School Students in Just One Year." *U.S. Centers for Disease Control and Prevention (CDC)*, April 16, 2015. http://www.cdc.gov/media/releases/2015/p0416-e-cigarette-use.html (accessed May 21, 2015).

Frieden, Thomas R. "Why Global Health Security Is Imperative." *Atlantic*, February 13, 2014. http://www.theatlantic.com/health/archive/2014/02/why-global-health-security-is-imperative/283765/?single_page=true (accessed November 23, 2014).

Steenhuysen, Julie. "U.S. CDC Head Criticized for Blaming 'Protocol Breach' as Nurse Gets Ebola." *Reuters*, October 13, 2014. http://www.reuters.com/article/2014/10/13/us-health-ebola-usa-nurse-idUSKCN0I206820141013 (accessed January 27, 2015).

Stein, Rob. "Big Measles Outbreaks Worry Federal Health Officials." *National Public Radio*, September 12, 2013. http://www.npr.org/blogs/health/2013/09/12/221737535/big-measles-outbreaks-worry-federal-health-officials (accessed January 27, 2015).

"Strategic National Stockpile (SNS)." *U.S. Centers for Disease Control and Prevention, Office of Public Health Preparedness and Response.* http://www.cdc.gov/phpr/stockpile/stockpile.htm (accessed January 27, 2015).

"U.S. CDC Boosts National Stockpile of Ebola Protective Gear." *Reuters*, November 7, 2014. http://www.reuters.com/article/2014/11/07/us-health-ebola-usa-gear-idUSKBN0IR1UQ20141107 (accessed January 27, 2015).

"U.S. Public Health Service Syphilis Study at Tuskegee." *U.S. Centers for Disease Control and Prevention (CDC)*. http://www.cdc.gov/tuskegee/ (accessed January 27, 2015).

Juan Pablo Garnham

Child Health

⊕ Introduction

Child health spans the continuum, beginning with promoting adequate nutrition and self-care in women before pregnancy; through prenatal, antenatal, and postnatal care and home visits; to managing diseases and infections of infancy and childhood. Other aspects include providing viable ways of accessing clean water for drinking and cooking, preventing child abuse and maltreatment, instituting appropriate sanitation and hygiene programs, protecting and enhancing the environment to make it as hospitable for human life as possible, timely and effective immunizations and dental care, creating safety in areas where children may be used as soldiers or unskilled workers, and ensuring that the environment is conducive to continuing health.

Common causes of death during the first five years of life are severe acute malnutrition (SAM), pneumonia or acute respiratory illnesses, diarrheal illnesses including dysentery, malaria, or a mix of illnesses. While all are potentially treatable, they are associated with high mortality rates because they often occur in regions where there is minimal medical care and support. The World Health Organization (WHO) created a guidebook for local level outpatient treatment based on the Integrated Management of Childhood Illness rubric for ill babies, toddlers, and children in outpatient settings in 2005, which was updated in 2012 based on changes in WHO guidelines.

⊕ Historical Background

In September 1978, an International Conference on Primary Health Care took place in Alma-Ata, Kazakhstan, and an urgent concern was raised regarding the health, safety, and well-being of the world's population, particularly infants and young children. At that time, some 15 million children below the age of five were dying annually from preventable, inexpensively controllable,

curable diseases. By 2007, the rate had decreased by 27 percent to 9.2 million infants and young children annually, with 5.5 million more children surviving annually. By 2013, the rate had declined to 8 million deaths annually. Despite improvements in mortality rates, the highest number of deaths, some 80 percent, remains concentrated in sub-Saharan Africa and South Asia and the causes remain unchanged: malaria, measles, pneumonia, and diarrheal diseases. Malnutrition, especially SAM, remains a significant contributing factor.

Infectious, communicable diseases such as pneumonia, malaria, measles, and diarrheal diseases have been leading causes of infant and young childhood death throughout history, frequently exacerbated by SAM. Breathing issues are worsened by indoor air pollution caused by cooking within a dwelling without sufficient ventilation. Immunizations, vaccinations, availability and correct usage of supplemental oxygen, accessibility of antibiotics, and breast-feeding are keys to prevention and treatment of respiratory illnesses.

Historically, children are at the greatest mortality risk during their first month. There is a chronic shortage of skilled childbirth attendants worldwide, resulting in a high percentage of women worldwide delivering babies at home, under unsanitary conditions, and without trained assistance in case of emergent complications. Infant mortality rates drop by as much as 60 percent when certain conditions are met: (1) women receive prenatal care, including nutritional guidance or supplementation; (2) deliveries are attended by trained birthing assistants; (3) mothers are given immediate postnatal care. This last condition includes making certain that the infant is breathing, using hygienic measures to care for the umbilical cord stump, utilizing infant skin care to prevent infections, teaching the importance of keeping the infant warm through skin-to-skin contact immediately after birth and throughout the neonatal period, and providing instruction on immediate, exclusive breastfeeding for at least the first six months of life.

Breast-feeding has always led to increased infant survival. Initially, a mother provides her newborn with immune-boosting nutrients. Continuing to breast-feed exclusively for the first six months of life increases the likelihood of survival dramatically, in part by reducing the occurrence of SAM and diarrheal diseases through inadequate nutrition or ingestion of contaminated formulas. The WHO recommends supplementation with safe foods beginning at six months and continuing to breastfeed for at least two years. Malnutrition is a significant contributing factor to mortality in young children. When children do get diarrheal diseases, the WHO and the United Nations Children's Emergency Fund (UNICEF) recommend effective treatment with zinc supplementation and oral rehydration salts.

Mosquito infestation occurs in areas with poor sanitation, stagnant water, or lack of refrigeration. Mosquitos carry malaria, another leading cause of childhood deaths. The WHO reports that a child dies every minute as a result of infection with malaria. Using nets treated with insecticide in sleeping areas is an inexpensive and highly effective means of preventing disease transmission.

Human immunodeficiency virus (HIV) and acquired immune deficiency syndrome (AIDS) have been recognized as a major cause of disease and death since the early 1980s. When a mother has inadequately treated HIV/AIDS, the likelihood of transmission to her children before or during birth is greater than 90 percent. Prenatal care, including treatment with antiretroviral medications, dramatically reduces transmission rates, enhanced by assisted deliveries and teaching about safer feeding methods.

Child abuse, neglect, and maltreatment have always occurred; physical, emotional/psychological, and sexual abuse are the most commonly reported. What is considered abuse in a developed, first world, highly educated, or high-income country may be an accepted cultural practice in a developing, impoverished, or poorly educated country. Sexual abuse is particularly prevalent in areas where there are high population concentrations with little privacy, such as refugee camps or military settings.

Throughout history, another significant health and mortality risk for children and adolescents has been their use as soldiers. They are used in direct combat, as spies, messengers, decoys, carriers of explosives, unskilled workers, laborers, and sex workers. Although the United Nations (UN) has a treaty prohibiting child soldiers that has been ratified in more than 125 countries, it is estimated by UNICEF that 250,000 to 300,000 child soldiers are active in armed conflicts worldwide at any given time.

⊕ Impacts and Issues

According to the WHO 2012 *Recommendations for Management of Common Childhood Conditions,* each year around 8 million children (about 1,000 every hour) who live in developing countries perish before they reach five years of age. (See map on page 75.) Of those 8 million, roughly 80 percent die as neonates, defined by the WHO as infants in the first four weeks of life. The most common causes of death during the first month in developing countries are preterm birth, birth asphyxia, and infections. Birth asphyxia occurs when a baby's brain and vital organs fail to get sufficient oxygen either right before, during, or shortly after birth. Severe, prolonged oxygen deprivation can lead to death, typically within the first week after birth. For asphyxia survivors, there may be mild to severe neurological or organ system damage, cerebral palsy, seizure disorder, or global developmental delays.

The WHO and UNICEF report that 350,000 women die of preventable complications of pregnancy and childbirth annually. Millennium Development Goal 4 (MDG 4) set a target of decreasing mortality rates in children less than five years of age by two-thirds by 2015. Millennium Development Goal Five (MDG 5) called for a three-fourths reduction in mortality among mothers before, during, and after childbirth. MDG 5 also specifies that all women should have access to reproductive health care. The goal is to prevent unwanted pregnancies, to provide good care and monitoring during pregnancy and delivery, and to follow-up with home visits during the most critical seven-day period after birth.

Children often die of a combination of factors, with food insecurity and malnutrition most commonly associated with communicable diseases and infections. It is estimated that malnutrition is a significant contributing factor or underlying cause in almost half of the infant and young child deaths in developing or low-income countries.

Contraception and Family Planning

In order to reduce the rate of unintended or unwanted pregnancies, women and their partners must first have understandable education about family planning and pregnancy choices, delivered in appropriately leveled and colloquial language by trusted and respected individuals.

In addition, they need reliable low- or no-cost access to effective methods of contraception. When women are given choice about pregnancies, the rates of unwanted pregnancies decrease and incidence of maternal and infant deaths related to unintended pregnancies also goes down. Women who make informed choices about reproduction are more economically stable because they are able to pursue scholastic and occupational opportunities they might not otherwise have been able to. Women in the workforce are able to contribute positively to their families and communities, leading to increased physical and psychological health as well as improved financial conditions.

Mortality Rates for Children Younger than Age 5 by Country in 2013

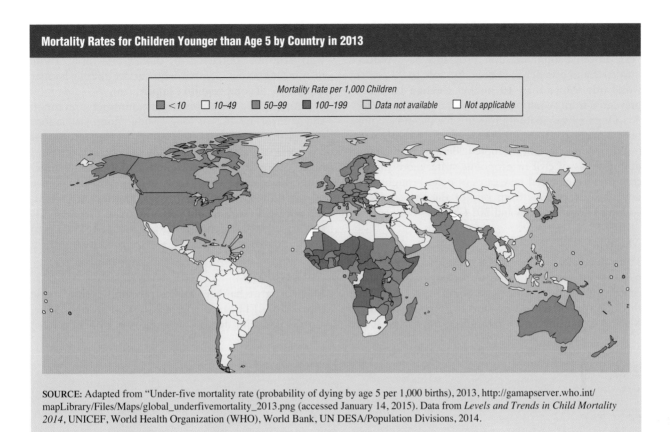

SOURCE: Adapted from "Under-five mortality rate (probability of dying by age 5 per 1,000 births), 2013, http://gamapserver.who.int/ mapLibrary/Files/Maps/global_underfivemortality_2013.png (accessed January 14, 2015). Data from *Levels and Trends in Child Mortality 2014*, UNICEF, World Health Organization (WHO), World Bank, UN DESA/Population Divisions, 2014.

Women and girls in developing, low-income countries typically lack access to modern forms of contraception. The Bill & Melinda Gates Foundation estimates that, in 2012, more than 220 million women in developing countries who wished to avoid pregnancy were unable to obtain modern contraception, resulting in at least 80 million unintended pregnancies and 20 million medically risky abortions.

Immunizations and Vaccinations

UNICEF is the world's largest purchaser of vaccines and immunizations, helping to increase global immunization rates by more than 400 percent from 1980 to 2015. Local vaccination and immunization efforts have decreased infant and young child deaths from preventable illnesses by more than 3 million annually. UNICEF makes a public record of the price paid for each vaccine purchased, a very effective means of cost containment.

Vaccinations save lives, yet millions of children, especially in developing, impoverished, war-torn countries or those experiencing significant civil unrest, do not receive them. UNICEF estimates that 1.5 million children die from vaccine-preventable diseases every year, with pneumonia and diarrheal diseases prominent among them. Many thousands of children who survive vaccine-preventable diseases are left with significant, permanent disabilities.

Measles is a potentially life-threatening communicable disease entirely preventable through vaccination. UNICEF reports that more than 100,000 unvaccinated children die as a result of contracting measles each year. Many survivors experience long-term impacts such as deafness, blindness, or neurological damage. By the middle of the second decade of the 21st century, more than 1 billion children had been vaccinated against measles. Measles deaths were decreased by more than 74 percent between 2000 and 2014.

Acquisition of sufficient quantities of high-quality vaccines can be cost prohibitive for impoverished or developing countries. Many areas lack adequate storage and refrigeration systems for vaccines or may not have reliable means of moving the immunization supplies and equipment from storage facilities to the field for use.

Poliomyelitis (Polio)

Polio, once a disease of global epidemic proportions, particularly in infants and young children, has been largely eradicated in all but three countries (Nigeria, Pakistan, and Afghanistan) as a result of worldwide immunization and vaccination programs. The number of cases in those three countries decreased from 650 reported cases in 2011 to fewer than 250 cases in 2012.

The WHO's World Health Assembly launched the Global Polio Eradication Initiative in 1988. At that time, the disease was widespread in 125 countries, resulting in paralysis and permanent disabling conditions in more than 350,000 individuals, mostly young children, every year. Effective immunization programs have reduced incidence and prevalence of polio by close to 99 percent worldwide. More than 10 million children have been prevented from acquiring polio.

Ongoing vaccination programs for the disease must be maintained, as the disease tends to flourish when health systems become disrupted. Because of migration during times of civil or economic strife, more than 20 countries experienced new cases of polio brought in by unvaccinated persons from one of the three endemic countries between 2008 and 2014.

Malaria

More than 200 million people contracted malaria and 627,000 died in 2012, with 90 percent of cases occurring in sub-Saharan Africa and South Asia. More than three-fourths of those who died were young children. Malaria is transmitted by mosquitos and causes severe illness, even in the milder cases. It is particularly devastating for infants, young children, and pregnant women who have not contracted the disease previously. Those infants and young children who survive the illness may experience lifelong cognitive impairment.

Among the most effective measures for prevention and control are use of long-lasting, nontoxic, indoor insecticides, netting to surround sleeping areas that has been saturated with the same insecticides, development of rapid, reliable diagnostic tools and pharmaceutical advances. These tools may be cost-prohibitive in many low-income, developing countries. At present, the disease is evolving and parasitic strains that are resistant to current insecticides have developed, leading to medication-resistant cases.

Tuberculosis

Much progress has been made in the efforts to decrease tuberculosis (TB) incidence and related mortality during the past four decades, leading to a global decrease

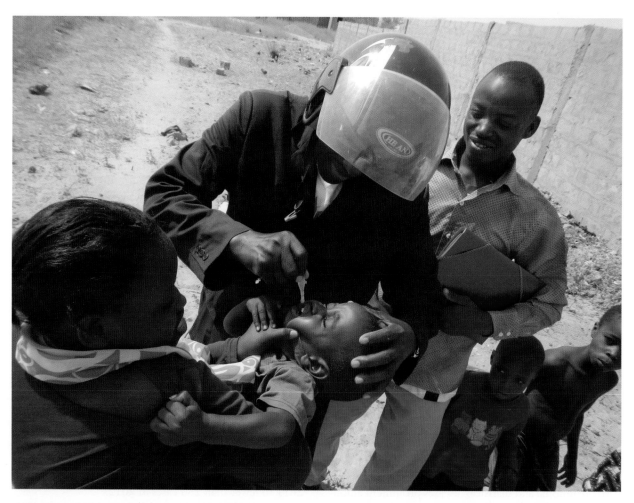

Photographed in the West African country the Republic of Niger, a young boy receives two drops of oral polio vaccine. The boy had not received the vaccine during the country's mass polio eradication campaign, so vaccinators went back the next day on his behalf, in order to make sure he would be protected into the future. *McKenzie Andre, M.D., M.P.H./U.S. Centers for Disease Control and Prevention.*

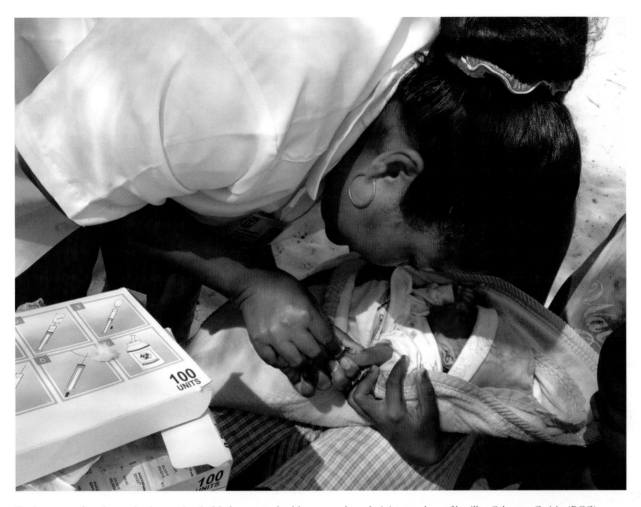

During an outdoor immunization session in Madagascar, a health-care worker administers a dose of bacillus Calmette-Guérin (BCG) vaccine to a newborn infant using a very small syringe and needle to administer the miniscule dose of vaccine. Based on World Health Organization (WHO) recommendations, BCG vaccine is used once at birth in most developing countries with high TB rates to reduce the severe consequences of tuberculous meningitis and miliary disease in infants and children. *Dr. Carolyn Sein/U.S. Centers for Disease Control and Prevention.*

in mortality of nearly 50 percent. A protocol called directly observed therapy, short-course (DOTS), developed in the 1980s, is the global standard and has led to the successful treatment of nearly 60 million individuals and saved more than 20 million lives since 1995.

Tuberculosis remains a significant global threat, with 1.3 million deaths and 8.6 million new cases reported during 2012. Two particularly dangerous new strains of TB, multidrug resistant (MDR-TB) and extensively drug-resistant (XDR-TB) have been reported. MDR-TB does not respond to frontline drugs; XDR-TB does not respond to frontline drugs and is also resistant to many second-line drugs. MDR-TB has been reported in nearly every country in the world, with 450,000 new cases reported in 2012.

In order to effectively stem the rate and incidence of TB worldwide, it is necessary to improve prevention, diagnosis, and treatment protocols. Current vaccines for

infants and young children have limited utility and are ineffective against the pulmonary TB strains in adults. Diagnostic tools need to be streamlined and modernized in order to maximize rapid and accurate diagnosis. In regions where there is a shortage of trained health-care workers, treatment may not be adequately overseen, leading many to stop treatment prior to completion. An effective and durable vaccine must be developed and implemented globally.

Diarrheal and Enteric Diseases

Diarrheal and gut diseases are very prevalent in the developing world, causing more than 500,000 deaths in infants and young children annually. Multiple and repeated infections are common, often leading to life-long gastrointestinal issues in children who survive them. When gut function is affected, it is difficult for the body to adequately process and absorb available nutrients. The body is weakened, affecting the immune system

THE ENVIRONMENT AND CHILD HEALTH: HYGIENE, SANITATION, AND WATER

Approximately 3 million young children die every year due to environmentally-related causes. Chief among these are respiratory, gastrointestinal, and diarrheal diseases. Nearly all are related to exposure to contaminated food; unsafe housing resulting in avoidable injuries; indoor air pollution resulting from cooking inside homes with inadequate ventilation and use of solid fuel; air, water, and ground pollution outdoors; exposure to toxic substances and hazardous wastes in the local community; lack of clean, safe, potable water for drinking, bathing, and cooking; insufficient access to sanitary facilities and proper hygiene; and inappropriate treatment and disposal of human excrement and waste.

In much of the world, there is no formalized system for disposal of human waste and excrement. Public urination and defecation are commonly practiced, often resulting in contaminated waste flowing into ground water or left in the open. Where there are indoor or communal toilets, there may not be adequate sewage or waste treatment, leading to soil and water contamination. Lack of adequate sanitation leads to proliferation of diarrheal diseases, some fatal, especially in infants and young children.

Technological advances in the treatment of sludge and solid waste, more effective means of emptying and disposing of waste from emptying pit latrines, and the development of advanced toilet systems will all contribute to the development of appropriate sanitation systems for developing countries. Key components of workable large scale and public systems will be sustainability and cost-effectiveness. There is a stepwise process involved in the sanitation system: (1) development and employment of waste collection systems such as toilets and sanitary latrines; (2) safe means of emptying those containers—septic systems and latrine pits—when full, (3) movement of the collected waste to facilities created for its treatment; (4) sustainable treatment of waste with the intention to safely and hygienically reduce, re-use, and recycle all possible returnable materials; and (5) environmentally safe disposal of non-reusable materials.

In addition to the creation of new technologies for improving environmental health, it is most financially and logistically efficient to build new systems and improve existing systems. Part of supporting and developing systems involves the creation of policy and procedure to support infrastructure expansion and to assure sustainability over time.

Disease prevention is critical, and more efficacious than treatment. By examining the causes of diseases at their environmental origins, it is possible to create more impactful and lasting prevention programs. By managing the environment, it is possible to reduce disease exposure and incidence rates. Children who are never exposed to potentially lethal diseases have a far better long-term outcome than those who become ill, are treated, and may experience long-term adverse consequences of the illness.

The Global Plan of Action for Children's Health and the Environment was designed "to provide a road map for WHO, governments, intergovernmental, and nongovernmental organizations, all concerned stakeholders, to contribute to the attainment of the Millennium Development Goals (MDGs) and other internationally agreed development declarations, commitments, and goals, in particular those related to reducing infant mortality (MDG 4) and ensuring environmental sustainability (MDG 7)."

and leading to incomplete response and uptake of orally administered vaccines, as well as to stunted growth, cognitive impairment, and global developmental delays.

Effective vaccines exist for some gastrointestinal and diarrheal diseases, such as rotavirus and cholera. WHO guidelines suggest that rotavirus vaccine be incorporated into national vaccine plans worldwide. By 2025, Gavi, the Vaccine Alliance, anticipates using the rotavirus vaccine in more than 30 low-income and developing countries. The WHO licensed a cholera vaccine called Shanchol in India in 2011 and created a significant stockpile of the vaccine for rapid deployment during acute outbreaks and epidemics. Other vaccines currently in development are targeted to treat *E. coli*, *Shigella*, and typhoid fever.

Diarrheal diseases have multiple etiologies and can rapidly lead to death in the youngest and frailest. Treatment with oral rehydration and zinc supplementation has been widely implemented and is responsible for a nearly 70 percent decrease in mortality since the mid-1980s. Antibiotics aid in the treatment of children with dysentery. When mothers are given nutritional instruction and access to a balanced diet and then encouraged to exclusively breast-feed for the first six months, the incidence of diarrheal diseases decreases by as much as two-thirds. When hygiene programs are utilized for hand washing and provision is made for safe and potable water for drinking, cooking, and bathing as well as sanitation systems for processing human waste, rates of diarrheal diseases further decrease.

Pneumonia

Although worldwide deaths from pneumonia have dropped by half during since the mid-1990s, pneumonia continues to be the leading cause of death in children under the age of five. In 2011, nearly 1.5 million young children died of pneumonia. Close to one-fifth of all deaths in infants and young children were attributable to pneumonia in 2011; the majority were in sub-Saharan Africa and South Asia.

Pneumonia often has multiple viral and bacterial causes, requiring a broad base of treatment approaches. There are effective vaccines available for pneumococcal forms of pneumonia, particularly streptococcus pneumonia and pneumonia caused by *Haemophilus influenza* type B (HiB), which are the most prevalent forms of bacterial pneumonia in children older than one month.

In countries with widespread poverty and acute shortage of health workers and medical facilities, mortality rates are very high. The WHO and UNICEF report 1 million annual young child deaths from pneumococcal diseases, including pneumonia and pneumococcal meningitis. The highest incidence of case reports and fatalities occur in the Western Pacific region, Southeast Asia, and sub-Saharan Africa. Widespread infant immunization programs using conjugate vaccines are key to prevention and reduction in mortality rates in the most widely affected countries. A number of public and private sector partnerships provide low-cost immunization and vaccine systems and train workers to administer immunizations.

Oral Health and Dental Care

According to 2012 WHO data, between 60 and 90 percent of school-aged children worldwide have at least one dental cavity. Cavities are preventable through the use of fluoride, either in drinking water or by application to the tooth surfaces. Cavities are most prevalent in low-income and developing countries, where access to oral care is most limited, diets tend to be least enriched,

and oral hygiene is not a consistent priority. Dental cavities are painful, may lead to infection and abscesses in the mouth, and can result in tooth loss if untreated. Young children with HIV/AIDS exposure or infection may experience oral health issues such as thrush, bacterial, or viral infections of the mouth. A potentially lethal oral health condition called noma affects children living in extreme poverty, most often in sub-Saharan Africa and South Asia. Lip and chin lesions consisting of dying (necrotic) tissue appear and can lead to death from resulting gangrene if not promptly treated. Noma is most prevalent in children who have a concomitant infection or condition such as HIV/AIDS or measles.

The WHO, in its Global Oral Health Programmme, has proposed that oral treatment facilities be combined with health centers dedicated to treatment and prevention of chronic diseases or incorporated into national public health protocols.

Food Security and Nutrition

Malnutrition or SAM are implicated in nearly half of all deaths occurring in young. When children fail to obtain adequate nutrition, they are physically smaller and more frail, their immune systems are weakened,

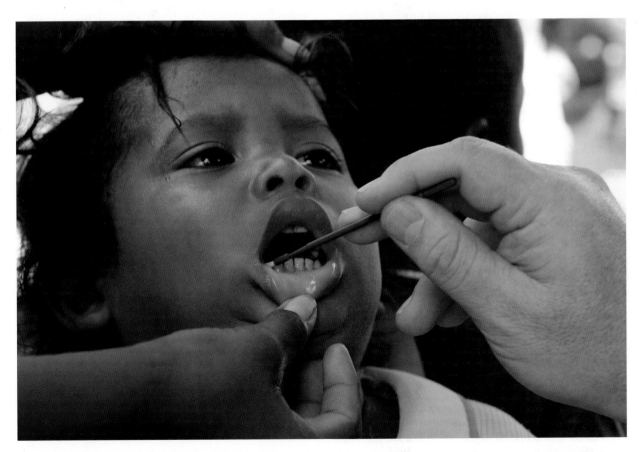

U.S. Public Health Service (USPHS) Lieutenant Commander Gary Brunette cleans and applies fluoride to the teeth of a young Nicaraguan child in Betania, Nicaragua, so that over time, the enamel of his teeth is strengthened. *U.S. Navy Photographer/U.S. Centers for Disease Control and Prevention/ Lt. Cmdr. Gary Brunette*

cognitive and physical growth may be stunted, and they have a diminished capacity to fight off infections.

Since 1990, UNICEF has had a program targeting prevention and treatment of malnutrition during the first three years of life, which has impacted close to 100 million infants and young children. Because the high prices of some staple foods such as rice, wheat, salt, sugar, oil, and maize make them unaffordable for many, UNICEF has initiated a program involving ingestion of a micronutrient-rich peanut-based paste that is tasty, easily and inexpensively packaged, readily shipped, and does not need refrigeration.

Millions of children in the world do not get enough to eat. In impoverished and developing areas, diarrheal diseases are endemic, often resulting in long-lasting gastrointestinal disorders. Malnutrition significantly contributes to early childhood deaths. Just over one-third of all infant and early childhood deaths are either directly or indirectly caused by issues related to nutrition. Many children who survive will have lasting physical and cognitive impacts. Malnutrition is especially dangerous during pregnancy, leading to significantly increased likelihood of mother, baby, or both dying during childbirth. Babies who survive are often of low birth weight, have a diminished ability to fight off infections, and may be left with chronic diseases.

The most cost-effective, beneficial means of protecting infants from undernutrition is to supplement the diets of mothers and then encourage exclusive breast-feeding for the first six months of life, followed by safe and highly nutritious complementary food addition, with continuing breast-feeding for at least the first two years of life. It is important to ensure supplementation with vitamins, minerals, and micronutrients in women and children at risk of malnutrition or undernutrition.

Child Maltreatment

Child maltreatment is defined as any type of abuse or neglect occurring in individuals less than 18 years of age. It encompasses all forms of neglect; commercial or other types of exploitation; coercion; physical, emotional, or sexual abuse; and negligence that results in actual or potential harm to the child's well-being, health, survival, dignity, ability to thrive, or safety. It occurs within the context of a relationship of trust, authority, or inequality in power. Child maltreatment in any form leaves lasting impacts, often lifelong, on physical and psychological development, wellness, and resiliency.

In areas of armed conflict, civil unrest, natural disasters, or forced migrations, resulting in crowded or refugee living conditions with loss of personal privacy, the incidence of sexual abuse, violence, or exploitation, particularly perpetrated on girls, rises steeply.

Adults with reported history of childhood maltreatment are more likely to become perpetrators as adults. They may develop mood disorders, particularly depression. They are more prone to addictions and substance abuse, including smoking, illicit drugs, and alcohol; they are more likely to experience eating disorders and obesity; they have higher incidence of risky sexual behaviors and unwanted pregnancies; and they are more likely to be revictimized than the general population.

Those most likely to be victimized are infants or nonverbal children, children less than four years of age, adolescents, children in institutional or correctional settings, those who are disabled or who have cognitive differences, those who are not physically appealing, and those who cry or whine persistently.

Adults who engage in child maltreatment may have been victimized as children; they may be dealing with an unintended or unwanted child; they may abuse substances, either currently or during the pregnancy; they may have unrealistic expectations of child behavior due to a lack of developmental understanding; they may be under excessive financial or emotional stress; they may be victims of abuse in current intimate partner relationships; or they may be engaging in criminal or socially discouraged behaviors.

The incidence and prevalence of child maltreatment often increases, according to WHO data, in cultures where there is significant gender or social inequality; where there is lack of available housing or lack of privacy in dwelling areas; where the poverty and unemployment rates are exceptionally high and access to illicit drugs and alcohol is widespread; where interpersonal violence, physical punishment and exploitation is considered acceptable; where there are few social or legal protections to prevent abuse and exploitation; where there are rigid gender roles and expectations; and where children are undervalued as human beings.

Child maltreatment is entirely preventable, and a number of evidence-based culturally sensitive programs have been developed and supported by the WHO and its partners. Education and widespread programming are key. Home visits during the neonatal period, particularly during the first week after birth, in which the health-care worker is able to share information about typical infant behavior and ways to safely respond to excessive or stressful crying in the infant are critical in preventing incidences of abusive head trauma or shaken baby syndrome. Prenatal education and community programming are also effective prevention tools. Creation and implementation of parenting groups in local communities broaden the group's knowledge base and shared experience of safe parenting practices and developmentally appropriate behavior. Where there is access to childcare, available preschool settings, and parent education, the incidence of child maltreatment is significantly decreased.

Child Soldiers

According to UN data, hundreds of thousands of children serve in areas of armed conflict. Some volunteer in order to escape poverty or intolerable living situations, others are recruited, coerced, or abducted. Some serve as armed soldiers and some serve as porters, where they are put at great risk by being made to carry wounded soldiers or ammunition in the field. Although many serve standard military support functions such as cooking, cleaning, messenger, or reconnaissance duties, girls are often used as sex slaves and repeatedly abused. In modern scenarios, children are sometimes used as suicide bombers or decoys to draw fire. Children are routinely subjected to physical and emotional stressors and are frequently left with lifelong physical and emotional scars. It is very difficult for them to return to civilian life, and a number of programs have been created in order to facilitate healing and reintegration.

Near the end of the 20th century, the United Nations Security Council mandated that children be released from active duty and prevented from conscription during times of armed conflict. Since 2000, thousands of children have been released. The UN publishes an annual report in which it lists names of countries recruiting child soldiers; this public scrutiny has led to steadily decreasing child conscription and recruitment. As of early 2015, seven national security forces were listed as recruiting and utilizing child soldiers: Yemen, Myanmar, the Democratic Republic of the Congo, South Sudan, Afghanistan, Sudan, and Somalia. In March 2014, UNICEF and the Special Representative of the Secretary-General for Children and Armed Conflict launched a campaign called Children, Not Soldiers, aimed at engendering worldwide support to eradicate the recruitment and use of children as soldiers.

⊕ Future Implications

In order to continue achieving momentum toward MDG 4 and MDG 5 beyond 2015, with the UNICEF-led goals of improving maternal and child health while continuing to reduce and eventually ameliorate preventable maternal, infant, and child deaths, the UN, through UNICEF, has created a Global Strategy for Women's and Children's Health, designed to bring together the world community in order to improve the lives and dramatically decrease the mortality rates of women and children.

The partnering agencies involved in this program propose to lower overall neonatal and early childhood mortality rates to not more than 20 deaths per 1,000 live births by 2035 by mobilizing five priority goals: (1) Prevention and increased survival efforts will be targeted to the countries with the highest infant and early childhood mortality rates; (2) underserved populations around the globe will receive increased focus on achieving access to quality, appropriate, evidence-based health care; (3) increased focus will be given to

the major, historical, and unchanged causes of infant and child mortality: complications related to preterm birth, acute issues arising during the labor and birthing process, diarrheal diseases, malaria, and pneumonia. These medical conditions lead to nearly two-thirds of global infant and early childhood deaths. (4) Human rights issues will be addressed, particularly as related to the self-actualization of women, especially as they relate to economic stability, job development, education, access to family planning information, and safe and effective forms of contraception; and (5) provisions will be made to use evidence-based and best clinical and medical practice, share data, use consistent and valid measurement techniques and tools to evaluate outcomes.

The most cost-effective, simplest ways to reduce infant mortality involve training local workers to provide accessible prenatal care within their communities, assist with the birthing process, and provide close follow-up care immediately after birth. Whenever possible, the provision of home visits by a local maternal and infant care worker on the first, third, and seventh day after birth are associated with significantly increased survival rates.

The WHO and UNICEF report that more than 2.5 million lives are saved every year by vaccination programs, with more than 100 million children immunized against vaccine preventable diseases annually. Worldwide, children are increasingly receiving vaccines that protect them from polio, measles, tetanus, pertussis, tuberculosis, diphtheria, hepatitis B, HiB, and yellow fever. A program called the Global Vaccine Action Plan (GVAP) aims to provide fair and affordable access to proven, current vaccines worldwide by 2020. GVAP has been endorsed by the 194 World Health Assembly member countries. It is estimated that this program will save more than 20 million lives.

PRIMARY SOURCE

Facts for Life

SOURCE *"Essential Messages" in* Facts for Life, *4th ed. UNICEF, WHO, UNESCO, UNFPA, UNDP, UNAIDS, WFP and the World Bank. New York: UNICEF, April 2010, x–xii. Copyright © 2010 UNICEF. http://www.unicef. org/publications/index_53254.html (accessed January 25, 2015).*

INTRODUCTION *This primary source is a publication of the United Nations Children's Fund (UNICEF) that provides information on childbearing and early childhood for parents and caregivers. The information it contains is based on medical science and also on human rights.*

GUIDE FOR USING FACTS FOR LIFE

Using *Facts for Life* can increase people's knowledge and change their practices and behaviour to improve and save children's lives. This can lead to positive changes in social beliefs and norms (what is considered normal by society) concerning the survival, growth, learning, development, protection, care and support of children.

Facts for Life is both a practical source of information for individuals and an essential tool for empowering individuals, young people, families and communities. Its messages and information can promote dialogue, learning and communication among children, youth, families, communities and social networks.

People from all walks of life can drive social change in favour of children's rights. Working together can make it possible to find diverse, relevant, interesting and constructive ways of using and communicating *Facts for Life* messages far and wide.

This guide for using *Facts for Life* provides:

- some conceptual thinking on the process of behavioural and social change
- information on using formative research and assessment to measure behaviour change
- research determines 'baseline' behaviours for use in helping to design and plan an intervention or campaign aimed at changing behaviours
- assessment measures behaviour changes against the 'baseline' behaviours during or following implementation of an intervention or campaign
- practical guidance on how to use *Facts for Life* to promote behaviour and social change that favours children's right to survive, grow, learn, develop and achieve their full potential in life.

Changing behaviours

Knowledge alone is insufficient for behaviour change

It is often assumed that if people are provided with information, products (such as vaccines or handpumps) and services (such as health or education), they will adopt healthier behaviours. However, information, products and services are often not enough to ensure adoption of new behaviours.

It is important to go beyond giving people information. *Facts for Life* should be used in consultation with children, families, communities and social networks. Their participation is vital to influencing behavioural and social change in favour of children's rights. Using *Facts for Life* as a tool in communication and development interventions involves:

- listening to the concerns of children, families and communities about the topics in *Facts for Life*

- communicating the messages and supporting information in *Facts for Life* in interesting and constructive ways that are relevant to a particular context
- stimulating dialogue among all concerned
- supporting actions with children, families and communities that improve behaviours related to the topics in *Facts for Life*
- assessing the actions to determine behaviour change and outcomes.

Stages of behaviour change

As individuals, we go through different stages in changing our behaviour. These stages include:

- not being aware
- becoming aware
- becoming motivated to try something new
- adopting a new behavior
- sustaining and 'internalizing' a new behaviour so that it becomes part of our normal everyday practice.

First, we have to become aware that a particular behaviour may not be healthy for us or our children. We then learn that there are other choices or alternative behaviours. We decide to try a new behaviour. If we are satisfied that the new behaviour is beneficial we may repeat it. Ultimately, we may adopt it. Then we may advocate or promote it with others, encouraging them to adopt it too.

Learning a new behaviour takes place in this continual cycle of awareness, experimentation and repetition. For example, a father may be persuaded through talking with the local religious leader to have his children sleep under insecticide-treated mosquito nets. He then sees that the nets prevent mosquito bites and that his children do not get malaria. He becomes an advocate for sleeping under insecticide-treated mosquito nets, sharing his experience with friends and urging them to use the nets.

Sometimes people who appear to have adopted a new behaviour eventually reject it and return to their former behaviour. For example, the father who was promoting use of mosquito nets may start to feel that they are too much trouble, so he and his family members stop using them. Returning to this old behaviour can harm the health of his family.

Ensuring the adoption of a new behaviour that benefits children and families requires an integrated and sustained communication and development strategy. This involves using different messages and methods to support the "change continuum" of adopting the new behaviour by individuals and families. The new behaviour may gradually be adopted by the whole community so that, for example, everyone is using insecticide-treated mosquito nets.

Behaviour change creates a dynamic that may result in social change

Individuals rarely change all by themselves. Their behaviour often depends on and is influenced by the views and practices of their families, friends and communities. Sometimes these are positive, as when everybody washes their hands with soap and water after using the toilet or latrine. Other times they may be harmful, as when parents have their daughters undergo genital cutting or refuse to have their children vaccinated.

To change social behaviour means changing the everyday views and practices of families and communities. What parents, other caregivers, children and adolescents decide to do is often influenced by what others are doing around them.

Resistance can be expected when social norms are challenged. This is because change involves shifting the dynamics of a group on fundamental issues related to gender roles, power relations and many other factors within the family or community.

But acceptance can become contagious when society begins to see the economic and social benefits of adopting a new behaviour. An example is when families using mosquito nets no longer have to cope with sickness or death caused by malaria. Their energies can be directed to sustain their children's learning and the family's productivity. People begin to see and hear about the change, and interest spreads, prompting others to adopt the new behaviour that can benefit their lives. Eventually, the behaviour is considered normal practice by everyone.

SEE ALSO *Malnutrition; Maternal and Infant Health; Nutrition; Pneumonia and Pneumococcal Diseases; Water Supplies and Access to Clean Water; Waterborne Diseases*

BIBLIOGRAPHY

Books

Child Soldiers International. *Louder than Words: An Agenda for Action to End State Use of Child Soldiers.* London: Child Soldiers International, 2012.

International Labour Office. *Marking Progress against Child Labour: Global Estimates and Trends 2000–2012.* Geneva: Labour Office, International Programme on the Elimination of Child Labour (IPEC), 2013.

United Nations. *Global Strategy for Women's and Children's Health.* New York: UNICEF, 2010.

United Nations Children's Fund. *Paris Principles and Guidelines on Children Associated with Armed Forces or Armed Groups, 2007.* New York: UNICEF, 2007.

World Health Organization. *Recommendations for Management of Common Childhood Conditions: Newborn Conditions, Dysentery, Pneumonia, Oxygen Use and Delivery, Common Causes of Fever, Severe Acute Malnutrition and Supportive Care.* Geneva: WHO Press, 2012.

Periodicals

Bhutta, Zulfiqar A., and Robert E. Black. "Global Maternal, Newborn and Child Health—So Near and Yet So Far." *New England Journal of Medicine* 369 (December 5, 2013): 2226–2235.

Cabral, S. A., A. T. Soares de Moura, and J. E. Berkelhamer. "Overview of the Global Health Issues Facing Children." *Pediatrics* 129, no. 1 (January 2012): 1–3. doi:10.1542/peds.2011-2665.

Golubnitschaja, O., et al. "Birth Asphyxia as the Major Complication in Newborns: Moving towards Improved Individual Outcomes by Prediction, Targeted Prevention and Tailored Medical Care." *EPMA Journal* 2, no. 2 (2011): 197–210.

Loaiza, E., T. Wardlaw, and P. Salama. "Child Mortality 30 Years after the Alma-Ata Declaration." *The Lancet* 372, no. 9642 (2008): 874–876.

Lokuge, K., et al. "Mental Health Services for Children Exposed to Armed Conflict: Médecins Sans Frontières' Experience in the Democratic Republic of Congo, Iraq and the Occupied Palestinian Territory." *Paediatrics and International Child Health* 33, no. 4 (November 2013): 259–272.

Websites

Ban Ki-moon. "Global Strategy for Women's and Children's Health." *Partnership for Maternal, Newborn & Child Health (PMNCH)*, 2010. http://www.who.int/pmnch/activities/advocacy/fulldocument_globalstrategy/en/ (accessed February 17, 2015).

"A Call for Global Citizens: What We Do." *Bill & Melinda Gates Foundation.* http://www.gatesfoundation.org/ (accessed March 20, 2015).

"Celebrating 25 Years of the Convention on the Rights of the Child." *World Health Organization (WHO).* http://www.who.int/maternal_child_adolescent/topics/child/en/ (accessed February 17, 2015).

"Child Health." *World Health Organization (WHO).* http://www.who.int/topics/child_health/en/ (accessed February 17, 2015).

"Child Survival: Nutrition and Food Security." *UNICEF Children First.* http://www.unicefusa.org/mission/survival/nutrition (accessed March 21, 2015).

"Convention on the Rights of the Child." *United Nations Human Rights, Office of the High Commissioner for Human Rights.* http://www.ohchr.org/EN/ ProfessionalInterest/Pages/CRC.aspx (accessed March 21, 2015).

"Global Plan of Action for Children's Health and the Environment (2010–2015)." *World Health Organization (WHO).* http://www.who.int/ceh/ceh-planaction10_15.pdf?ua=1 (accessed March 21, 2015).

"International Standards." *Child Soldiers International.* http://www.child-soldiers.org/international_ standards.php (accessed February 17, 2015).

"Oral Health," Fact Sheet No. 318. *World Health Organization (WHO),* April 2012. http://www.who .int/mediacentre/factsheets/fs318/en/ (accessed March 21, 2015).

Stewart, Christopher. "Global Children's Health and Mortality Tutorial." *Kaiser Family Foundation,* 2013. http://kff.org/interactive/global-childrens-health-and-mortality-tutorial/ (accessed February 17, 2015).

"Vaccines and Immunizations." *U.S. Centers for Disease Control and Prevention (CDC).* http://www .cdc.gov/vaccines/vac-gen/default.htm (accessed February 17, 2015).

"We Are Children, Not Soldiers." *UNICEF Office of the Special Representative of the Secretary-General for Children and Armed Conflict.* https:// childrenandarmedconflict.un.org/childrennot-soldiers/ (accessed March 21, 2015).

Pamela V. Michaels

Cholera and Dysentery

⊕ Introduction

Cholera and dysentery are diseases caused by poor sanitary conditions and the lack of access to clean drinking water. These illnesses spread through water and food contaminated with feces. Both provoke intense diarrhea. When this and other symptoms are not assessed properly, they can lead to severe dehydration and have fatal consequences, especially in infants and the elderly.

The U.S. Centers for Disease Control and Prevention (CDC) defines dysentery as "diarrhea with visible blood." It can be caused by viral, bacterial, or parasitic infections. Among the causes, two of the most common are the amoeba *Entamoeba histolytica* and bacteria of the genus *Shigella*. Cholera is caused by the bacteria *Vibrio cholerae*. All of these microorganisms attack the intestine, reaching the digestive system through contaminated water or food. To avoid these outbreaks, clean sanitary conditions and proper systems for waste sewage waters are fundamental.

These diseases tend to present themselves as epidemics and are a serious public health concern, especially in Africa, South Asia, and some countries in the Caribbean. Every year there are between 1.4 million and 4.3 million cases of cholera-type disease, mostly undiagnosed, according to researchers' estimates at the International Vaccine Institute, and 28,000 to 142,000 people die worldwide because of this illness. Due to good water quality and sewage treatment infrastructure, cholera cases have been extremely rare in industrialized countries over the last century. However, there have been large outbreaks in places such as Haiti, Vietnam, and Zimbabwe since 2005.

⊕ Historical Background

The History of Cholera

Waterborne diseases always have been part of human life, though they have not always been recognized as such. As a paper published in the medical journal the *The Lancet* by David Sack, explains, cholera "has been endemic in South Asia, especially the Ganges delta region, since the beginning of recorded history. It was always much feared because it regularly occurred in epidemics with high mortality rates." As a matter of fact, in the city of Calcutta (now Kolkata) there is a temple to the divinity of Ola Bebee, meaning "our lady of the flux." The disease began expanding to other countries through trade routes. In 1817, the first epidemic of cholera reached as far as southern Russia. As part of a second pandemic in the early 1830s, most European cities had been affected by the illness.

In 1831, cholera arrived in the United Kingdom. Here, one of the biggest steps toward understanding it would be achieved. "The authorities at that time didn't fully understand the connection between waste and disease. Many of them subscribed to the then prevailing 'miasma' theory," author Steven Johnson explains in his book *How We Got to Now*. Cholera, among other diseases, was believed to be transmitted through poisonous vapors, also known as the "deadly fogs."

During an outbreak in 1854, in the London neighborhood of Soho, physician John Snow (1813–1858) found the miasma theory to be wrong. He believed that the disease was not in the air but rather in the water. His problem was that early microscopes were not advanced enough to see bacteria. Snow had to come up with another plan. He mapped the fatalities in the area and discovered a relationship with a particular source of water, which was contaminated. Although his theories were resisted at first, his findings eventually would lead to separating clean and sewage waters, thus contributing to the fight against cholera and dysentery.

Snow's discoveries, while fundamental for the rise of epidemiology, did not stop the disease, and three more pandemics spread cholera to Africa, Australia, and the Americas. In 1885, the bacteria *Vibrio cholerae* was identified as the agent that caused the disease. In 1886, an epidemic in New York led to the first board of health in the United States. Cholera became the first reportable disease, meaning that hospitals were required to inform authorities of any cases that they saw.

A Total of 26 Countries Reported Cholera Deaths in 2013

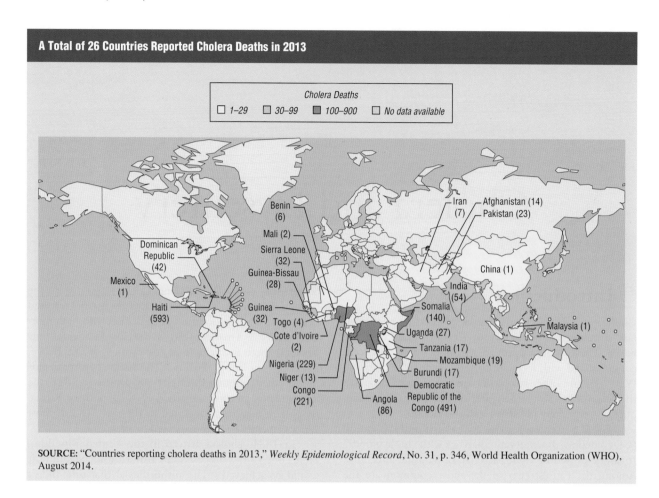

SOURCE: "Countries reporting cholera deaths in 2013," *Weekly Epidemiological Record*, No. 31, p. 346, World Health Organization (WHO), August 2014.

The pandemic of the early 21st century has been the seventh that eventually spread all over the world. This strain was first isolated in a quarantine station in Egypt in 1905 from a group of Indonesian pilgrims that were traveling to Mecca. Later it would reach India in 1964, Africa and Southern Europe in 1970, and South America in 1991. A similar strain has been found since 1973 along the Gulf of Mexico. That has caused sporadic outbreaks associated with seafood, specifically in summer.

A new kind of *Vibrio cholerae* was identified in 1992 and caused outbreaks in India and Bangladesh. This one is, according to experts, likely to be the cause of a next pandemic. In the spring of 2002, 30,000 people reportedly contracted it in Dhaka, the capital of Bangladesh. This exceeds the number estimated to have been reached by the 1905 strain.

The History of Dysentery

Just as with cholera, dysentery has a history as long as humankind's. Books portray it as the cause of death of numerous historical figures, including King John of England (1166–1216), the philosopher Erasmus of Rotterdam (1466–1536), Sir Francis Drake (c. 1540–1596), and the explorer David Livingstone (1813–1873).

Dysentery also has been a major cause of deaths among armies, sometimes taking more lives than war itself. Unhealthy conditions among troops create a perfect environment for the spread of dysentery. There are records of its importance in conflict as far back as the Peloponnesian War in 431 BCE. "Dysentery accompanied the Crusades and had a decisive effect on the Crusade led by Louis XI when it decimated the French crusaders camped near Carthage," R. S. Bray writes in the book *Armies of Pestilence: The Impact of Disease on History*. It weakened the Norman troops in 1107; it stopped Prussian intervention in the French Revolution; and it killed 44,558 during the American Civil War (1861–1865). It was present in the Second Boer War (1899–1902) in South Africa; in Gallipoli during World War I (1914–1918), where it killed 120,000 soldiers; and in the concentration camps during World War II (1939–1945).

One of the milestones in understanding what caused dysentery occurred in 1897 in Japan. During an epidemic that had reached 90,000 people and killed nearly 30 percent of them, a 26-year-old physician named Kiyoshi Shiga (1871–1957) discovered a microorganism that turned out to be one of the main causes of the disease. This bacteria would be named *Shigella* in his honor.

As with cholera, changes in Western society during the 19th and 20th centuries also contributed to the battle against dysentery. Along with discoveries such as Shiga's, the rise of antibiotics, the creation of modern sewage systems, and the popularization of cleaning methods had a huge impact in seeing fewer and fewer cases of dysentery. Modern capitalism also was an important ally. By the 1920s, advertising communicated throughout the modern world the importance of using soap and other hygiene products to avoid diseases such as dysentery and cholera.

Whereas in the developed world dysentery and cholera are not a major issue, they remain a fundamental problem for developing countries. According to the WHO, diarrhea causes up to 7.7 percent of the deaths in Africa. In Southeast Asia, that percent is 8.5.

⊕ Impacts and Issues

The microorganisms that can cause dysentery are various, as previously mentioned, but the result is similar, whether the causative agent is a virus, a parasite, or a bacterium. After entering the human body through contaminated water or food, or oral contact with contaminated hands or objects, the pathogens reach the large intestine and cause inflammation. This process can provoke fever, abdominal pain, and diarrhea with blood, the latter being the main characteristic of this illness. There can be vomiting and sometimes muscle aches. However, the biggest consequence—and the most dangerous—is dehydration. In extreme cases, it can lead to the collapse of the circulatory system and consequently death.

In the case of cholera, dehydration also is the main enemy. The critical problem with cholera is that dehydration can be fast and extremely effective. After entering the human body through water or food contaminated with feces that have the bacteria, symptoms start suddenly. The period of incubation can be as short as 12 hours and as long as five days. The patient can defecate between 10 to 20 liters of diarrhea per day. Cholera has very particular characteristics: people infected with the disease produce a very liquid diarrhea of white color. It is described as "rice water" and can smell like fish.

Due to this extreme process, several effects can be seen on the body. These include lethargy, sunken eyes, dry mouth, difficulty breathing, low blood pressure,

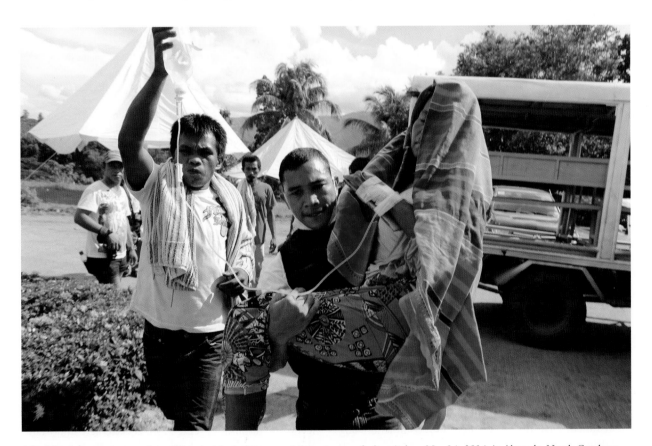

A health worker carries a woman afflicted with cholera toward the entrance of a hospital on May 14, 2014, in Alamada, North Cotabato, Philippines, an area where villagers still depend on mineral springs and deep wells for their sources of water. At least eight people died and hundreds were hospitalized that month due to a cholera epidemic that hit the village. Cholera is an acute intestinal infection that causes severe vomiting and diarrhea, which can lead to serious dehydration and prove fatal if not properly treated. © *Jeoffrey Maitem/Getty Images.*

CHOLERA IN NATURAL DISASTERS

An earthquake or a tropical storm can have a devastating effect on services such as drinking water or sewage systems. Natural disasters are not only a direct risk to human lives themselves, but they can have a broader effect on health months and even years after the catastrophe.

On January 12, 2010, Haiti experienced an earthquake that reached 7.0 on the Richter scale. More than 100,000 people died, and at least 52 aftershocks affected this country of 9 million, the poorest in the Americas. But beyond this huge toll, the earthquake had a profound impact on the country's already weak infrastructure. The presidential palace in Port-Au-Prince was razed completely, schools and hospitals were damaged severely, and roads and sewage systems were destroyed. In the heat of the Caribbean, finding clean drinking water became a significant problem.

In spite of not having a developed water system, Haiti had never experienced cholera until 2010. But in mid-October of that year, in a rural area 62 miles (100 kilometers) from the capital, people started coming down with the symptoms of cholera. The source, apparently, was the Artibonite River, from which most affected people drank water. Some have speculated that the bacteria was brought by the United Nations (UN) peacekeepers from Nepal, which the UN has denied repeatedly. In 10 weeks, cholera spread throughout the country. By December, Haiti was registering 2,300 hospitalizations and 40 deaths per week. The outbreak triggered panic and confusion.

The lack of good distribution of health supplies and other logistical problems did not help. But according to international organizations such as the Pan American Health Organization, the main problem was access to clean water. This has become the worst epidemic of cholera in recent history, according to the U.S. Centers for Disease Control and Prevention (CDC). By the end of 2013, it had killed more than 8,000 Haitians and hospitalized almost 400,000 in total. It also expanded to the neighboring country of the Dominican Republic, where there were 31,070 cases and 458 deaths as of November 2013. Additionally, cholera affected people from Cuba, Mexico, Venezuela, and the state of Florida in the United States.

The crisis continued into 2014. According to an article in the *New York Times* in April 2014, Haiti was less equipped than it was three years earlier to face the outbreak. The UN had problems raising money toward this issue: it achieved only a quarter of the $38 million needed to provide supplies such as water purification tablets at the time of the article. Hospitals lacked enough oral rehydration solutions to treat diarrhea and, with aid groups leaving the country, some health centers in the countryside had to close down.

By early 2015, the UN estimated that 8,600 had died and 707,000 had been sickened from the outbreak. Human rights groups tried to sue the United Nations to receive compensation for the victims of the outbreak. In January 2015 a U.S. judge ruled that the United Nations could not be held legally responsible by victims for the outbreak, as it has immunity from such lawsuits. However, this judgment was expected to be appealed.

Since the earthquake, the U.S. Department of State has maintained a travel warning advising people to avoid traveling to Haiti. The CDC has explained that travelers are not at high risk of contracting cholera, but due to the problems in the access to health care, they should bring their own supplies, including water purification tablets, oral rehydration salts, and antibiotics.

Haiti's experience with cholera shows how countries and international organizations need to think ahead and be prepared for the domino effect that a natural disaster can spur, especially with waterborne epidemic diseases such as cholera.

---

and general weakness. Seizures and comas can happen also. The skin might change its color to a bluish-gray, thus giving cholera the nickname "the blue death." If it is not treated properly, cholera can cause death within hours.

Prevention and Treatment

Preventing waterborne diseases such as cholera and dysentery comes down to hygiene. The CDC and the World Health Organization (WHO) have prepared a series of recommendations for prevention, and most of them have to do with water and food and the way these are handled. First, the health agencies recommend using and drinking safe water. If in doubt, one should defer to bottled water and canned or bottled carbonated beverages rather than drinking from the tap or other sources. If this is not an option, water should be boiled (allowing it to boil for at least a minute) or treated with chlorine. This includes the water used when brushing one's teeth and for cooking.

Another recommendation is always washing hands with soap and clean water, especially before eating, preparing food, feeding children, cleaning, and after going to the bathroom. In cholera and dysentery prone regions, food must be handled with care. It must be cooked well, kept covered, and eaten hot, and fruits and vegetables always should be peeled. Bathrooms and kitchens must be cleaned properly and constantly.

Finally, because this disease is transmitted through feces, the disposal of fecal waste is extremely important. While in most of the developed world clean water and sewage water are separated, in situations where this is not the case precautions must be taken. If there are latrines or chemical toilets, those should be cleaned constantly

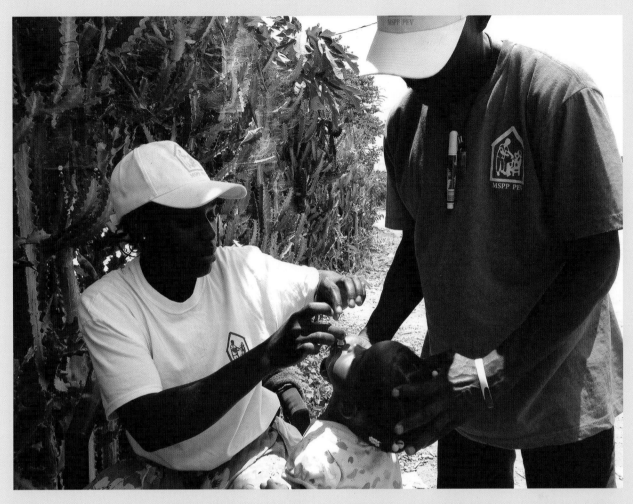

During an August 2013 cholera vaccination campaign on the island country of Haiti, two health-care workers work as a team to administer a dose of cholera vaccine to a young Haitian girl. *Rania A. Tohme, M.D., M.P.H./U.S. Centers for Disease Control and Prevention.*

with bleach. If there are no latrines, people should defecate at least 100 feet (about 30 meters) away from water sources and then bury the fecal matter.

If symptoms of cholera or dysentery are seen, it is important to act quickly and go immediately to the nearest health center. Because the biggest danger is dehydration, the person that is affected needs to drink water. The most successful option for this is to drink oral rehydration solution (ORS), a fluid consisting of water mixed with sugar, salt, and in extreme cases, zinc. If ORS is not available, it can be made at home easily, by mixing six teaspoons of sugar, half a teaspoon of salt, and a liter of clean water. Experts also stress the importance, in cases to which it applies, that mothers not stop breastfeeding children if they have diarrhea.

Because dehydration also leads to the loss of electrolytes, it is recommended to consume food that is high in potassium, such as bananas or green coconut water. There also are antibiotic treatments against cholera although reports have shown that in some places of the world antibiotic resistance is growing. Additionally, there is vaccine treatment, but that takes two separate doses and weeks to protect. Thus, the CDC recommends that this not replace prevention and control measures.

When treatment comes quickly, cholera's mortality rate is less than 1 percent. But if it goes untreated, between 50 to 60 percent of patients die, so it is very important to take measures immediately after symptoms begin.

Surveillance and the Role of Governments

For many reasons, the role of government and international organizations is extremely important in the fight against diseases such as cholera and dysentery. Because they are highly contagious epidemical illnesses, many of

A SARI CAN SAVE LIVES

Women are key in the fight against waterborne diseases. Mothers learn and teach hygiene education to their children and are usually the ones in charge of the nutrition of children, one of the most affected groups when it comes to cholera and dysentery. In some villages in Bangladesh, women also have learned how to produce their own homemade oral rehydration solutions, a cheap and fast remedy against dehydration. But scientists have found another possibility for women to contribute in South Asia: their traditional clothing can act as a water filter.

Saris are five- to nine-yard-long (4.6- to 8.2-meter-long) drapes that women in India, Bangladesh, and Sri Lanka wear as their traditional garment. They wrap this long cloth around their waist, with one end over the shoulder. Traditionally made out of silk, saris vary enormously in color and decorations depending on the region of South Asia. They are part of a long tradition. Though there are more than 80 recorded ways of wearing a sari, there is only one that could help against cholera.

Rita Colwell (1934–), a professor at both the University of Maryland and Johns Hopkins University, discovered that a sari can be an efficient filter for removing cholera from water. When folded four times, it can stop 99 percent of the bacteria. This conclusion is the result of a three-year study that involved around 50 villages and 150,000 people. "By having women filter their water collected from the ponds and rivers every day, we showed about a 50 percent decrease in cholera. A very simple step, and very important," Colwell explained to CNN.

But how can a piece of cloth stop a minuscule bacterium? The key is another finding by Colwell: she discovered that cholera is tied to plankton. It is part of the natural flora of plankton, a photosynthetic microorganism. When water goes through a four-time folded sari, plankton stays in the sari, and attached to the plankton is most of the cholera bacteria.

The fieldwork of Colwell's project was conducted in 2007, and it included a team of people going to the villages every week. They would meet with the villagers, explain why it was good to filter the water, how they could do it, and the difference it would mean for their health and their children's health. "With this constant reinforcement, we found that indeed, they did filter because they found that their children didn't get sick. And that, of course, was a big incentive," Colwell told CNN. A group of scientists subsequently went back to see the villages and analyze if the habit was still in place. They came back happy: 75 percent of the women were still filtering water with their saris.

the preventive and remedial actions can be achieved only through national and global efforts. Creating sewage systems and water treatment plants, for example, are public works projects that are too expensive for individuals or small communities to put in place.

There also is an important role for education, both in preventing and solving crises. Governments and international organizations are key in explaining how to avoid risks and assessing cholera and dysentery before it is too late. Simple actions, such as explaining to parents how to make homemade ORS, can save lives without the need to spend a lot of money or reach a hospital. In Bangladesh, for example, a very successful program is doing exactly that, thereby improving health of families in poor villages.

Finally, governments and international organizations have a fundamental role in monitoring these diseases, thus planning responses and controlling outbreaks before it is too late. This is the reason that cholera became the first reportable disease in the United States. To this day, the WHO publishes periodic reports with very precise information about the cases and deaths reported country by country.

⊕ Future Implications

Any step forward in the battle against cholera and dysentery is related directly to water quality. According to the WHO, since 1990 more than 2 billion people have gained access to improved sources of drinking water, thus taking an important step toward avoiding new epidemics of cholera and dysentery. Nevertheless, it remains a big challenge, especially in developing countries. Of the more than 700 million people who do not have access to improved sources of drinking water, nearly half are in sub-Saharan Africa. "More than one third of the global population—some 2.5 billion people—do not use an improved sanitation facility, and of these one billion people still practice open defecation," the UN's Deputy Secretary-General Jan Eliasson (1940–) explained in a 2014 report on the subject.

As access to clean water has become more common, mortality from waterborne diseases has decreased. During the early 1990s, 5 million children under five years old died annually from diarrhea. In 2004, the yearly number had gone down to 1.5 million deaths in children under five; in 2009 it accounted for 800,000 deaths, and, according to the WHO, in 2013 it had decreased to 760,000 deaths. Still, diarrhea remains a major challenge for children's health. According to the WHO and UNICEF, nearly one in five child deaths is due to this illness. It is the second cause of deaths after pneumonia. These casualties are extremely focalized in specific areas of the world: 80 percent of child deaths caused by diarrhea occur in Africa and South Asia. "Just 15 countries account for almost three quarters of all deaths from diarrhea among children under five years of age annually," UNICEF/WHO explains in a 2009 report.

In the specific case of cholera, the WHO attempts to keep a detailed track of reported cases and deaths, however, it also reports in a 2012 bulletin that such cases and deaths are seriously underreported—the numbers reported each year may represent only 5 to 10 percent

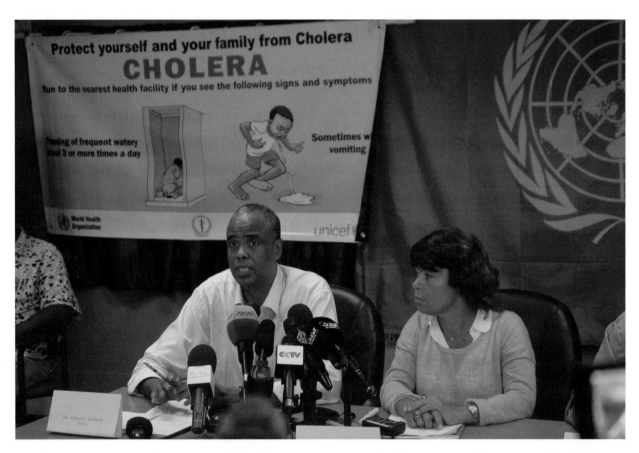

Dr. Abdinasir Abubakar, of the WHO South Sudan, left, and Ariane Quentier, United Nations Mission in South Sudan spokesperson, right, at a press conference at the office of emergency programs for UNICEF South Sudan on May 27, 2014. Juba, the capital of South Sudan, recorded more than 600 cases of cholera and the related deaths of 23 people between when the outbreak began in April and the conference. UNICEF pledged to help citizens avoid and fight the disease. © *Samir Bol/ZUMA Press, Inc./Alamy.*

of all cases and deaths. According to the WHO in 2013, 47 countries reported a total of 129,064 documented cholera cases, including 2,102 deaths. This represented a 47 percent decrease compared to 2012. From the 26 countries that reported deaths, 17 were in Africa. Other foci of deaths were in the Dominican Republic and Haiti. These two Caribbean countries reported 635 deaths, 30 percent of the global total.

These numbers portray clearly the heavy burden that these diseases represent for some of the poorest countries in the world. Governments have carried out important efforts to prevent and respond to outbreaks, but for the international organizations, major improvements are needed to overcome this problem significantly. "Many concerns remain about the high proportion of people living in unsanitary conditions who are at risk of cholera and other diarrhea diseases," a WHO report comments, "There is a need to scale up prevention measures in order to avert cholera and other water borne diseases by expanding access to improved sources of drinking water and improved sanitation, and by working with communities to encourage behavioral change to reduce the risks of infection."

PRIMARY SOURCE

Notes from the Field: Identification of *Vibrio cholerae* Serogroup O1, Serotype Inaba, Biotype El Tor Strain—Haiti

SOURCE *"Notes from the Field: Identification of* Vibrio cholerae *Serogroup O1, Serotype Inaba, Biotype El Tor Strain—Haiti, March 2012," from Morbidity and Mortality Weekly Report (MMWR) 61, no. 17, May 4, 2012: 309. Centers for Disease Control and Prevention (CDC). http://www.cdc.gov/mmwr/preview/mmwrhtml/ mm6117a4.htm (accessed January 25, 2015).*

INTRODUCTION *This primary source is an article from a weekly publication of the U.S. Centers for Disease Control and Prevention (CDC). The article describes in detail the strain of cholera identified in the Haiti epidemic and touches on the public health implications of the outbreak.*

Notes from the Field: Identification of *Vibrio cholerae* Serogroup O1, Serotype Inaba, Biotype El Tor Strain—Haiti, March 2012

Weekly

May 4, 2012 / 61(17);309–309

On October 20, 2010, an outbreak of cholera was confirmed in Haiti for the first time in more than a century. As of April 10, 2012, a total of 534,647 cases, 287,656 hospitalizations, and 7,091 deaths have been reported in Haiti as a result of the outbreak (*1*). The *Vibrio cholerae* strain that caused the Haiti epidemic has been characterized as toxigenic *V. cholerae*, serogroup O1, serotype Ogawa, biotype El Tor (*2*).

Recently, two *V. cholerae* isolates collected on March 12 and 13, 2012, in Anse Rouge, Artibonite Department, were characterized at the National Public Health Laboratory in Haiti as non-Ogawa serotypes. The isolates subsequently were confirmed by CDC to belong to the Inaba serotype. By molecular analyses (pulsed-field gel electrophoresis, multilocus variable number of tandem repeat analysis, and virulence gene sequencing [*ctxB* and *tcpA*]), these two isolates are indistinguishable from the currently circulating *V. cholerae* serotype Ogawa strain in Haiti. The molecular analyses conducted to date suggest that they arose from serotype switching, which is a commonly observed phenomenon in cholera epidemics, often driven by population immunity to the circulating serotype. Further characterization efforts are ongoing. Finding these two isolates does not change current clinical management guidelines (*3*).

Ogawa and Inaba serotypes do not appear to differ in the severity or duration of illness they cause; most persons infected with *V. cholerae* of either serotype will not develop clinically apparent disease. Type-specific immunity is induced by infection; however, cross-protective immunity between the two serotypes is incomplete (*4*). Previous studies have indicated that the Ogawa serotype offers less protective immunity than Inaba from reinfection with the heterologous serotype (*5*). Thus, if the Inaba strain becomes established in Haiti, persons who previously were infected with the Ogawa serotype of *V. cholerae* might be relatively more susceptible to reinfection with the Inaba serotype than with the Ogawa serotype because there tends to be stronger serotype-specific protective immunity. Immunologically naïve persons are equally susceptible to both serotypes. Because the Inaba strain is also biotype El Tor, its ability to survive outside of a host is likely the same as that of the Ogawa strain.

The two World Health Organization prequalified vaccines provide protection against the Ogawa and Inaba serotypes. In addition, the cholera rapid diagnostic tests detect all O1 serogroup infections, including Ogawa and Inaba serotypes.

This serotype conversion illustrates the increasing diversity of *V. cholerae* in Haiti (*2*) and emphasizes the importance of continued public health surveillance by the National Public Health Laboratory and CDC, which are partnering to establish a laboratory-enhanced sentinel surveillance system for a range of infectious diseases, including cholera and other diarrheal diseases. The system will provide data to determine the burden of diarrheal disease attributable to cholera and to help direct prevention efforts and programs to reduce morbidity and mortality from cholera in Haiti.

SEE ALSO *Sanitation and Hygiene; Vulnerable Populations; Water Supplies and Access to Clean Water; Waterborne Diseases*

BIBLIOGRAPHY

Books

Bray, R. S. *Armies of Pestilence: The Impact of Disease on History.* Cambridge, UK: James Clark, 2004.

Johnson, Steven. *How We Got to Now: Six Innovations That Made the Modern World.* New York: Riverhead Books, 2014.

Krasner, Robert I., and Teri Shors. *The Microbial Challenge: A Public Health Perspective*, 3rd ed. Burlington, MA: Jones & Bartlett Learning, 2013.

UNICEF and World Health Organization. *Diarrhoea: Why Children Are Still Dying and What Can Be Done.* New York: UNICEF and WHO, 2009. Available online at http://www.who.int/maternal_child_adolescent/documents/9789241598415/en/ (accessed January 6, 2015).

World Health Organization. *Global Annual Assessment of Sanitation and Drinking-Water (GLAAS): The Challenge of Extending and Sustaining Services.* Geneva: WHO, 2012. Available online at http://www.who.int/water_sanitation_health/publications/glaas_report_2012/en/ (accessed January 6, 2015).

World Health Organization. *Guidelines for the Control of Shigellosis, Including Epidemics Due to Shigella Dysenteriae Type 1.* Geneva: WHO, 2005. Available online at http://www.who.int/maternal_child_adolescent/documents/9241592330/en/ (accessed January 6, 2015).

World Health Organization and UNICEF. *Progress on Drinking Water and Sanitation: 2014 Update.* New York: WHO and UNICEF, 2014. Available online at http://www.who.int/water_sanitation_health/publications/2014/jmp-report/en/ (accessed January 6, 2015).

Periodicals

Ali, Mohammad, et al. "The Global Burden of Cholera." *Bulletin of the World Health Organization* 90, no. 3 (March 24, 2012): 209–218A. doi: 10.2471/BLT.11.093427. Available online at http://www.who.int/bulletin/volumes/90/3/11-093427/en/ (accessed February 13, 2015).

Sack, David A., et al. "Cholera." *The Lancet* 363, no. 9404 (January 17, 2004): 223–233.

Sack, David A., et al. "Getting Serious about Cholera." *New England Journal of Medicine* 355, no. 7 (August 17, 2006): 649–651.

Trofa, Andrew F., Hannah Ueno-Olsen, Ruiko Oiwa, and Masanosuke Yoshikawa. "Dr. Kiyoshi Shiga: Discoverer of the Dysentery Bacillus." *Clinical Infectious Diseases* 29, no. 5 (November 1999): 1303–1306.

World Health Organization. "Cholera, 2013." *Weekly Epidemiological Record* 31 (August 1, 2014): 89: 345–356.

Websites

Archibold, Randal, and Somini Sengupta. "U.N. Struggles to Stem Haiti Cholera Epidemic." *New York Times*, April 19, 2014. http://www.nytimes .com/2014/04/20/world/americas/un-struggles-to-stem-haiti-cholera-epidemic.html?_r=0 (accessed February 13, 2015).

"Cholera in Haiti." *U.S. Centers for Disease Control and Prevention (CDC)*. http://wwwnc.cdc.gov/travel/ notices/watch/haiti-cholera (accessed January 6, 2015).

"Cholera—*Vibrio cholerae* Infection." *U.S. Centers for Disease Control and Prevention (CDC)*. http://www.cdc. gov/cholera/index.html (accessed January 6, 2015).

Mason, Margie. "'Poor Man's Gatorade' Could Save Kids from Diarrhea Death." *USA Today*, June 5, 2013. http://usatoday30.usatoday.com/news/health/2010-05-01-diarrhea-kids_N.htm (accessed February 13, 2015).

Murray, Kelly. "The Link between Saris and Cholera." Interview with Rita Colwell. *CNN Health*, May 5, 2010. http://www.cnn.com/2013/06/05/health/ lifeswork-colwell-cholera/ (accessed January 6, 2015).

"Water-Related Diseases." *World Health Organization (WHO)*. http://www.who.int/water_sanitation_ health/diseases/diarrhoea/en/ (accessed January 6, 2015).

Juan Pablo Garnham

Climate Change: Health Impacts

🌐 Introduction

Climate change refers to a set of changes in the global climate that result from the rise in average global temperature, including changes in precipitation patterns, increased occurrence of droughts, heat waves, and other extreme weather. Climatologists generally attribute this change to human-made emissions of carbon dioxide and other greenhouse gases that have accompanied economic development since the Industrial Revolution. Climate change affects many social and environmental factors that determine human health, including air quality, drinking water, food supplies, and shelter. Therefore, changes in the patterns of health and disease can be expected to occur throughout the world in the future.

It has been clear for some time that sea levels are rising, glaciers are melting, and weather patterns are changing. Extreme weather events, such as hurricanes and flooding, are becoming more common. Scientists predict that during the 21st century, the average temperature of Earth's surface will rise by at least 3.6 degrees Fahrenheit (2 degrees Celsius), compared with preindustrial temperatures, with higher rises likely in high latitude areas such as northern Canada, Greenland, and Siberia. Although there may be a few benefits arising from a warmer climate, such as fewer winter deaths and increased food production, the overall impact of climate change on human health is likely to be overwhelmingly negative.

There is a wide range of possible health consequences of climate change. These include direct effects from natural weather-related disasters, such as the destruction of homes and contamination of the water supply. There are also likely to be changes in the geographical range and transmission season of insects, which will increase cases of vector-borne disease, such as malaria.

It is hard to predict the precise impact of climate change on human health. All populations probably would be affected to some extent. However, some will be more vulnerable than others, and it is here that prevention and support efforts should be targeted. These groups include people living in coastal regions, in very large cities, and in mountainous or polar regions. Children, especially those in low-income countries, will be particularly at risk. The elderly, and those with preexisting medical conditions, also will be more at risk of the health-damaging effects of climate change. Finally, people living in countries where the health infrastructure is weak will be less able to respond and cope with the impact of climate change on their populations. Overall, those living in poorer countries, which have contributed least to global warming but have less access to the resources to deal with its problems, are likely to bear the greatest burden in health terms. However, no country will be immune to the impact of a changing climate; extreme weather events such as Hurricane Katrina in 2005 have affected the United States, and heat waves have caused thousands of deaths in Europe.

There are plans to reduce the level of global warming and alleviate its effects at international, national, and local levels. These efforts have focused upon decreasing the amount of greenhouse gases entering the atmosphere. Many countries also have strengthened their defenses against natural disaster and put emergency plans in place. There are many approaches, from developing alternatives to fossil fuels to persuading individuals to be less reliant on their cars.

In 2009, scientists at the University College of London Institute for Global Health, writing in a special issue of *The Lancet* medical journal, stated "Climate change is the biggest threat to global health." They noted that both health-care professionals and the public remain largely unaware of what a changing climate will do to people's health around the world. More action is urgently needed in the areas of advocacy, research, and preparedness planning.

🌐 Historical Background

The idea that human activity could change the climate is not new: the ancient Greeks suspected that cutting down forests might increase rainfall. Irish scientist John Tyndall (1820–1893) first carried out experiments demonstrating

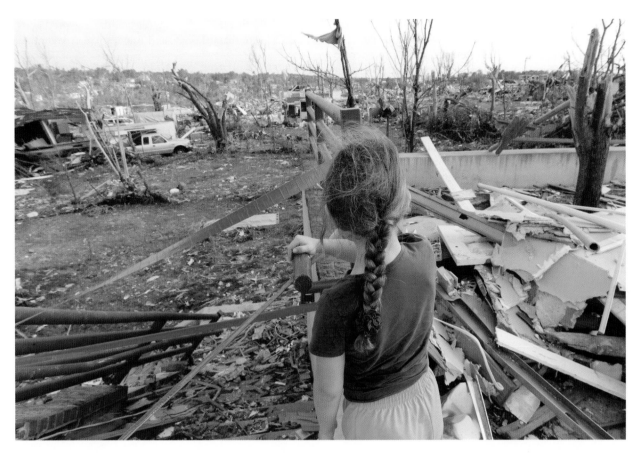

A girl surveys the damage after a tornado ripped through Joplin, Missouri, in May 2011, cutting a path of destruction that resulted in the deaths of 160 people. In 2011, more than 1,500 tornadoes were recorded in the United States, killing 533 people and causing billions of dollars worth of damage. As global temperatures rise, many climate scientists predict that destructive storms like hurricanes and tornadoes will increase in number. *© Dustie/Shutterstock.com.*

the greenhouse effect. In 1896, Swedish chemist Svante Arrhenius (1859–1927) published a paper that outlined the basic science of global warming, warning that human activity could warm Earth by adding carbon dioxide to the atmosphere.

The global average temperature increased by 1.53 degrees Fahrenheit (0.85 degrees Celsius) between 1880 and 2012. However, it was not until the 1950s that scientists began to look in detail at a potential link between carbon dioxide emissions from fossil fuels and global warming. In the 1970s, concern rose with the spread of environmentalism. Computer models began to predict how the climate might change in future years. It was notable that summers were becoming hotter. In 1988, the hottest summer on record at the time, the Intergovernmental Panel on Climate Change (IPCC) was established, marking the start of international efforts to understand the issue.

Action on Climate Change

Concern about the impact of climate change on human health has always been a prime focus of the work of the IPCC. In 2001, the IPCC produced a scientific consensus confirming the reality of climate change, although there were—and still are—dissenters. Since then, research driven by improved computer models and data has strengthened the conclusion that emissions from human activity are very likely to cause climate change, with the accompanying impact upon human health.

In parallel with scientific progress on climate change, there has also been political and social change. In 1992, there was the Rio Summit on the environment, which produced the United Nations Framework Convention on Climate Change. Then in 1997, the Kyoto Protocol set targets for greenhouse gas emissions for industrialized nations. This came into effect in 2005. However, there are many challenges involved in fulfilling these targets, and it is still very much a work in progress. Meanwhile, evidence for climate change and its impacts on human health continues to accumulate.

⊕ Impacts and Issues

High temperatures and hot summers can cause increased mortality from heart and lung disease, particularly among older people. During the heat wave experienced in Europe in the summer of 2003, there were 70,000 deaths more than expected, mainly from lung and heart disease. High temperatures also encourage the formation of ground-level ozone, a potent air pollutant that has adverse effects on lung health. Meanwhile, levels of pollen and other airborne allergens increase in hot weather, which puts those with asthma and other allergies at risk of attacks.

According to the World Health Organization (WHO), the number of weather-related natural disasters, such as floods, droughts, monsoons, and hurricanes, has increased more than threefold since the 1960s and further increases of such events can be expected. Every year, such disasters cause more than 60,000 deaths, most of them in developing countries. These events immediately impact human health and claim lives by destroying homes, hospitals, and other services. Flooding, and the accompanying disruption, is a particular concern, because more than half of the world's population lives within 37 miles (approximately 60 kilometers) of the sea. There are many cities in the world that are at risk of floods or sea-level

rise in the future, including Alexandria, Egypt; Lagos, Nigeria; Mombasa, Kenya; and Buenos Aires, Argentina.

Impact on Water Supplies Access to fresh, clean water and sanitation already are restricted in many parts of the world. Climate change is likely to exacerbate this problem. Rainfall is predicted to increase in some places, which could benefit areas where water has been scarce, but only if they develop the capacity to store runoff water. Decreased waterfall is predicted to affect the Mediterranean, central and southern Africa, southern United States, and parts of Europe. Research has shown that by the 2090s, climate change will increase the area of the world affected by drought, double the frequency of extreme droughts, and increase their duration by sixfold. Rising temperatures and unpredictable rainfall also will decrease food production, leading to malnutrition, particularly in Africa.

Meanwhile, one-sixth of the world's population is dependent on water from glaciers. The melting of the glaciers that already has occurred will lead inevitably to water shortages for these populations. Flooding of rivers

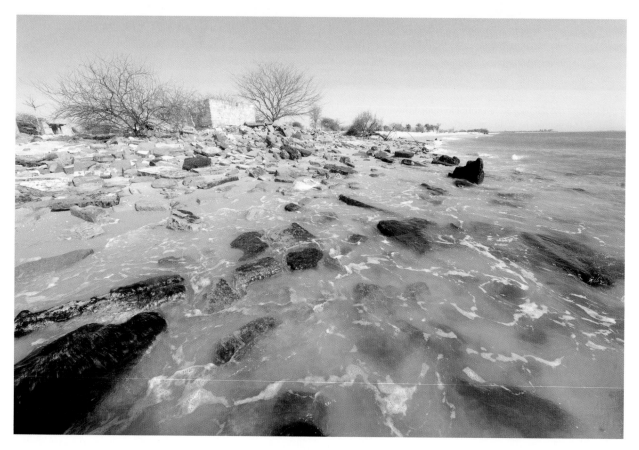

Ruins of a house are seen on May 7, 2013, on the beach of the village of Doun Baba Dieye, northern Senegal. Doun Baba Dieye, settled by the Normans in 1364, was the first casualty among many districts of the Senegalese city of Saint-Louis, the former colonial capital of French West Africa, which, little by little, is disappearing underwater. In 2008, Alioune Badiane of the United Nations' Habitat agency designated Saint-Louis as "the city most threatened by rising sea levels in the whole of Africa," citing climate change and a failed 2003 canal project as the cause. The city is plagued by flooding during the rainy season when the river overflows and scientists say climate change is exacerbating the problem with increasingly heavy rain and a rise in the sea level. *© SEYLLOU/AFP/Getty Images.*

VECTOR MIGRATION

Vectors are organisms such as insects and snails that carry infectious agents such as bacteria, viruses, and protozoa. Ticks, mosquitoes, and fleas are among the most significant vectors of human infectious disease. According to a fact sheet from Physicians for Social Responsibility, malaria is probably the most important vector-borne disease, having the greatest disease burden with 350 million to 500 million cases occurring annually around the world. Other parasitic vector-borne diseases include leishmaniasis and Chagas disease. Insect vectors also carry arboviral diseases, such as dengue fever, yellow fever, West Nile virus, Rift Valley fever, and tick-borne encephalitis. Bacterial and rickettsial diseases carried by vectors include Lyme disease (borreliosis), tularemia, and plague.

Disease vectors are cold-blooded, so they must live in relatively warm places to function. Changes in global temperature and rainfall therefore affect their development, reproduction, behavior, and survival. These changes may be expected to increase the geographic range of these vectors, as well as the seasonal period of disease risk. Moreover, temperature changes will affect how the pathogen develops within its vector. Rainfall will affect the availability of breeding sites for the vector. Finally, migration brought about by climate change will affect the location of their human host, perhaps bringing people into contact with a vector for the first time.

The malaria parasite is carried by the *Anopheles* mosquito. Mosquitoes are very sensitive to temperature: a higher temperature will increase their reproduction rate, lengthen their breeding season, and also increase the frequency with which they bite their human hosts. It also shortens the time in which the malaria parasites inside them mature to the infectious stage. Finally, increased temperature will expand the range of mosquitoes to higher elevations and more northern latitudes. This will put previously unexposed people at risk of malaria.

Some specific observations and predictions about changes in disease patterns brought about by vector migration already have been made. A study from researchers at the University of Michigan and the London School of Hygiene and Tropical Medicine focused upon cases of malaria occurring in the highland regions of Ethiopia and Colombia. Traditionally, prevalence of malaria in these regions is low. People there have no immunity, so the disease will hit them hard. The researchers found that in warm years, the median altitude of malaria was higher than in cooler years. Thus, the mosquito literally is climbing the mountain when the temperature rises. This is firm evidence of the beginning of migration in a disease-carrying vector.

Meanwhile, scientists in China have developed a biology-driven model to look at how climate change may affect the range of schistosomiasis. This disease is caused by a group of parasitic flatworms, and is second only to malaria as a parasitic disease in terms of health and economic impact. The parasites are carried by the snail *Oncomelania hupensis*. The researchers found that its optimum developmental temperature was 59.7 degrees Fahrenheit (15.4 degrees Celsius). Given that China's mean temperature will increase by 1.62 degrees Fahrenheit (0.9 degrees Celsius) by 2030, and by 2.88 degrees Fahrenheit (1.6 degrees Celsius) by 2050, this means an expansion in the range of the snail vector. This study predicts that schistosomiasis will spread to previously unaffected areas of northern China, affecting nearly an extra 308,881 square miles (800,000 square kilometers), which is 8.1 percent of China's land surface.

and coastal areas also will deplete the supply of freshwater and affect sanitation. A lack of safe water will increase the risk of diarrheal disease, which kills around 600,000 children under five each year. It will also increase the risk of insect-borne and rodent-borne diseases, such as malaria and cholera.

Patterns of Infection Malaria, which is transmitted by the *Anopheles* mosquito, kills almost 800,000 people per year. Climate change is likely to expand the range of the mosquito to previously unaffected areas. Dengue is another mosquito-borne disease. This viral illness, which causes severe flulike symptoms, is sometimes called "breakbone" fever because of the extreme aches and pains it causes. Research at the University of East Anglia, England, suggested that climate change may make dengue more common in Europe. Specifically, dengue-carrying mosquitoes are expected in the Po Valley, Italy; the Spanish Mediterranean; and southern Spain.

The dengue study used data from Mexico, where dengue is common, and notes how its incidence related to climatic factors such as temperature and rainfall. The researchers then modeled their findings using climate data from European countries. Indeed, there has been an increase in the number of travelers returning to England with dengue, from 343 in 2012 to 541 in 2013, which is a rise of 58 percent. Most were returning from India or Thailand, but there has been an increase in dengue among travelers coming back from Barbados.

Climate change also is likely to result in new infectious diseases, known as emerging or reemerging diseases. These include West Nile fever and leishmaniasis. The WHO has stated that emerging and reemerging diseases are causing one-third of deaths around the world. Changes in temperature and humidity are changing the ecology and transmission dynamics of pathogens, vectors, and their reservoirs. Unfortunately, these changes are poorly understood, so improved surveillance and research are urgently needed to counter these new threats.

A study by French researchers sheds light on the link between climate change and Buruli ulcer, an emerging disease affecting Latin America. The methods used may be applicable to the study of other emerging diseases. The researchers compared changes in rainfall in French Guyana since 1969 with cases of Buruli ulcer recorded in the region. Decreasing rainfall has led to an increase in residual stagnant water, allowing *Mycobacterium ulcerans*, the bacteria that causes Buruli ulcer, to flourish. Human access to the organism's swampy habitat, for hunting and fishing, has expanded over the years, increasing outbreaks of the disease. The researchers warn that changes in climate, such as decreased rainfall, are likely to encourage the emergence of other infectious organisms.

Undernutrition Hunger and undernutrition are major global health issues, affecting more than 1 billion people, with children under the age of five being particularly affected. Undernutrition refers to being underweight and of short stature for one's age. It might have been expected that the economic growth occurring in many countries may be able to alleviate hunger and undernutrition, although hard evidence for this is lacking. There is growing concern that climate change may reverse any trend toward alleviating hunger and undernutrition by impacting food security. Undernutrition is caused by many factors, a primary one being a lack of food; it is linked directly to risk of poor health and death.

Global food security depends upon many components, one of which is cereal production. The world per capita cereal production reached a plateau during the 1980s, and has since been in decline. It is too soon to say whether climate change has contributed to this reduction, and if so, by how much. Scientific assessments indicate that warming of the climate will reduce cereal yields in low latitude areas, but could increase them in some high latitude areas.

Projection studies conducted in the 1990s suggested that climate change may place an additional 5 million to 170 million people at risk of hunger and undernutrition by the 2080s. A more recent study by researchers at the London School of Hygiene and Tropical Medicine estimated undernutrition (measured as stunting of growth) resulting from the impact of climate change on crop productivity. The estimates were calculated for five regions of Africa and Asia for 2050. The study showed that, even

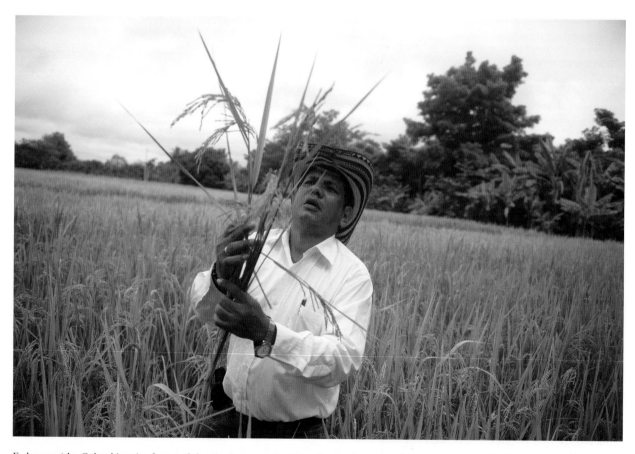

Fedearroz (the Colombian rice farmers federation) agronomist Cristo Perez selects rice plants at La Victoria research center in Monteria, Cordoba department, northern Colombia, on September 18, 2014. In Colombia, where more than 200 communities live off of growing rice in a surface of 1,111,970 acres (450,000 hectares), in the previous five years the yield per hectare decreased one ton due to climate change. © *Eitan Abramovich/AFP/Getty Images.*

Estimated Mean Number of Deaths Attributable to Climate Change in 2030 Based on Five Global Climate Model Runs

Region	Undernutrition (Children < 5 years)	Malaria	Dengue	Diarrheal disease (Children < 15 years)	Heat (Adults > 65 years)
Asia Pacific, high income		0	0	1	1,488
		(0 to 0)	(0 to 0)	(0 to 2)	(1,208 to 1,739)
Asia, central	473	0	0	111	740
	(−215 to 1,161)	(0 to 0)	(0 to 0)	(49 to 150)	(364 to 990)
Asia, east	1,155	0	39	216	8,010
	(−5,313 to 7,622)	(0 to 0)	(23 to 48)	(95 to 298)	(5,710 to 9,733)
Asia, south	20,692	1,875	197	14,870	9,176
	(−39,019 to 80,404)	(1,368 to 2,495)	(101 to 254)	(6,533 to 20,561)	(7,330 to 10,620)
Asia, south-east	3,348	550	0	765	2,408
	(−2,635 to 9,331)	(398 to 779)	(0 to 0)	(336 to 1,105)	(1,629 to 3,192)
Australasia		0	0	0	93
		(0 to 0)	(0 to 0)	(0 to 0)	(58 to 151)
Caribbean		12	3	72	117
		(12 to 12)	(3 to 3)	(31 to 104)	(73 to 148)
Europe, central		0	0	1	880
		(0 to 0)	(0 to 0)	(0 to 1)	(570 to 1,523)
Europe, eastern		0	0	3	1,974
		(0 to 0)	(0 to 0)	(1 to 4)	(1,325 to 2,904)
Europe, western		0	0	2	2,625
		(0 to 0)	(0 to 0)	(1 to 13)	(1,152 to 5,279)
Latin America, Andean	445*	17	2	49	181
	(−327 to 1,218)	(6 to 37)	(0 to 4)	(21 to 69)	(119 to 241)
Latin America, central	859**	39	6	109	878
	(−837 to 2,554)	(32 to 47)	(−1 to 9)	(48 to 156)	(540 to 1,113)
Latin America, southern	14	0	0	1	421
	(−49 to 76)	(0 to 0)	(0 to 0)	(0 to 2)	(303 to 686)
Latin America, tropical		95	5	19	739
		(87 to 113)	(4 to 5)	(9 to 27)	(623 to 954)
North America, high income		0	0	2	2,990
		(0 to 0)	(0 to 0)	(0 to 2)	(2,297 to 3,287)
North Africa/Middle East	1,617	14	0	1,323	2,058
	(−2,030 to 5,264)	(14 to 14)	(0 to 0)	(582 to 1,850)	(1,381 to 2,342)
Oceania		44	0	22	13
		(44 to 44)	(0 to 0)	(10 to 32)	(9 to 20)
Sub-Saharan Africa, central	14,385	56,705	0	6,326	344
	(−27,448 to 56,217)	(34,908 to 112,719)	(0 to 0)	(2,774 to 8,946)	(281 to 389)
Sub-Saharan Africa, eastern	27,999	143	6	10,997	1,212
	(−8,701 to 64,699)	(142 to 143)	(5 to 7)	(4,811 to 15,585)	(1,064 to 1,552)
Sub-Saharan Africa, southern	1,245	0	0	489	254
	(−1,505 to 3,994)	(0 to 1)	(0 to 0)	(215 to 685)	(163 to 313)
Sub-Saharan Africa, western	22,944	597	1	12,737	987
	(−31,728 to 77,616)	(597 to 597)	(1 to 1)	(5,581 to 18,110)	(712 to 1,214)
World	95,176	60,091	258	48,114	37,588
	(−119,807 to 310,156)	(37,608 to 117,001)	(136 to 331)	(21,097 to 67,702)	(26,912 to 48,390)

Note: The first line is the mean estimate and the numbers in parentheses are the lowest and highest estimates.
*Undernutrition estimate for Andean Latin America and tropical Latin America combined.
**Undernutrition estimate for central Latin America and Caribbean combined.

SOURCE: Adapted from "Table 1.2. Additional deaths attributable to climate change, under A1b emissions and the base case socioeconomic scenario, in 2030," in *Quantitative Risk Assessment of the Effects of Climate Change on Selected Causes of Death, 2030s and 2050s*, World Health Organization (WHO), 2014, p. 7.

Global health will be impacted by climate change. According to the WHO, weather-related natural disasters have increased threefold since the 1960s.

taking economic growth into account, climate change will lead to a 62 percent increase in stunting of growth in South Asia and a 55 percent increase in east and south sub-Saharan Africa. The authors conclude that efforts to improve socioeconomic conditions, to protect people—and children in particular—from undernutrition should be redoubled in order to offset the negative impact of climate change

Action to Reduce Health Impacts

There are many policies, and many options for individual choices, that could reduce, but likely not stop, climate change. If effective, these actions could mitigate the predicted impact on human health. If carbon emissions are reduced, climate change may be reduced. Cleaner energy systems and reduced traffic also will have direct benefits on health by improving air quality.

In 2009, the World Health Assembly of the WHO launched a new work plan on climate change and health. This plan calls for raising awareness of the threat that climate change poses to health. Another goal is to set up partnerships with the appropriate agencies in the United Nations to ensure that health is given due attention on the climate change agenda. More science and evidence is needed to learn more about the impacts on health. It is particularly important to improve the models used to assess the specific impacts on health, so these can be made more accurate. Detailed estimates on which to base effective policy measures are necessary. Finally, health systems need to be strengthened in those places where people are known to be most at risk from the health effects of global warming.

The WHO also is placing a new emphasis on research into climate change and health, because there are some significant information gaps. In a six-point plan, the agency states that it is essential that this research is placed firmly in the context of overall global health. Risk assessment needs to be made relevant to policy, so that effective action can be taken. It is also necessary to strengthen health surveillance systems, so that early warnings of health impacts, including the incidence of emerging diseases, can be noted and acted upon. It is particularly important that risk assessments are localized because regions vary greatly in how climate change will affect them. All of this will require a multidisciplinary approach because the impact of a changing climate on human health is such a complex issue.

⊕ Future Implications

The WHO has produced some estimates for the impact of climate change on human health in 2030 and 2050. These take into account the impact of economic growth, which might be expected to mitigate the mainly negative health impacts arising from a changing climate. In 2030, it is estimated that there will be around 65,000 deaths due to heat exposure among the elderly, and 95,000 children will die from undernutrition. An additional 48,000 people will die from diarrhea and 60,000 from malaria.

By 2050, the picture is expected to have changed again. Child mortality is likely to decline overall between 2030 and 2050, so there will be fewer deaths from diarrhea and undernutrition. However, due to the aging population, deaths from heat exposure will rise to 100,000 by 2050. Overall, assuming base case (most likely) socioeconomic growth, climate change will claim 250,000 additional lives per year between 2030 and 2050.

The above figures are an underestimate because it is not possible to quantify all the potential health impacts, such as water shortage, river or coastal flooding, and major heat wave events. Nor does the WHO model predict the impact of climate change on human security, which could cause migration and conflict, both of which are likely to increase morbidity and mortality. Moreover,

merely assessing mortality does not give a complete picture of the total impact of climate change on human health. It does not estimate the economic damage, for instance. Nor does it predict morbidity from diseases such as dengue, which may not actually be fatal.

The Role of Economic Growth

High economic growth and adaptation to a changing climate could go a long way toward mitigating the adverse effects on health. Low economic growth will make them worse. Thus, a major concern is that climate change is likely to exacerbate preexisting health inequities between rich and poor. This can, however, be alleviated if climate change is used as a catalyst to accelerate sustainable economic development in the poorest nations, thereby lifting billions of people out of poverty. These actions should include strengthening health-care systems and scientific research capacity in the poorest nations.

Strengthened public health measures, properly targeted, could help people adapt to the risk of global warming. Increased food production and improved flood defenses will also be needed. Climate change is now clearly a threat to global development. Therefore, development policy must, increasingly, take on board environmental risks. The strong impact of socioeconomic development found in these studies underlines the need to be more aware of the links between climate, health, and wider sustainable development objectives, particularly with respect to the poorest and most vulnerable populations. All of this will require unprecedented international cooperation between policy makers, scientists, and a wide range of other stakeholders.

PRIMARY SOURCE

A Human Health Perspective on Climate Change

SOURCE *"Executive Summary: Highlights" from* A Human Health Perspective on Climate Change. *The Interagency Working Group on Climate Change and Health (IWGCCH). Research Triangle Park, NC: Environmental Health Perspectives and the National Institute of Environmental Health Sciences, April 2010, vi–vii. U.S. Department of Health and Human Services. http://www.niehs.nih.gov/ health/materials/a_human_health_perspective_ on_climate_change_full_report_508. pdf (accessed January 25, 2015).*

INTRODUCTION *This primary source is the Highlights section of the Executive Summary appearing in a report published by Environmental Health Perspectives and the U.S. National Institute of Environmental Health Sciences.*

It outlines "the research needs on the human health effects of climate change."

Highlights:

Asthma, Respiratory Allergies, and Airway Diseases—Respiratory allergies and diseases may become more prevalent because of increased human exposure to pollen (due to altered growing seasons), molds (from extreme or more frequent precipitation), air pollution and aerosolized marine toxins (due to increased temperature, coastal runoff, and humidity) and dust (from droughts). Mitigation and adaptation may significantly reduce these risks. Research should address the relationship between climate change and the composition of air pollutant mixtures (e.g., how altered pollen counts and other effects of climate change affect the severity of asthma) to produce models to identify populations at risk. Such tools support the use of science in understanding disease risks and as such, are an integral component of developing effective risk communication and targeting the messages to vulnerable populations.

Cancer—Many potential direct effects of climate change on cancer risk, such as increased duration and intensity of ultraviolet (UV) radiation, are well understood; however the potential impact of changes in climate on exposure pathways for chemicals and toxins requires further study. Science should investigate the effects of mitigation and adaptation measures on cancer incidence so that the best strategies can be developed and implemented; for example, research to inform understanding of the benefits of alternative fuels, new battery and voltaic cells, and other technologies, as well as any potential adverse risks from exposure to their components and wastes. Better understanding of climate change impacts on the capacity of ocean and coastal systems to provide cancer curative agents and other health-enhancing products is also needed.

Cardiovascular Disease and Stroke—Climate change may exacerbate existing cardiovascular disease by increasing heat stress, increasing the body burden of airborne particulates, and changing the distribution of zoonotic vectors that cause infectious diseases linked with cardiovascular disease. Science that addresses the cardiovascular effects of higher temperatures, heat waves, extreme weather, and changes in air quality on health is needed, and this new information should be applied to development of health risk assessment models, early warning systems, health communication strategies targeting vulnerable populations, land use decisions, and strategies to meet air quality goals related to climate change. In some areas, cardiovascular and stroke risks resulting from climate change could be offset by reductions in air pollution due to climate change mitigation.

Foodborne Diseases and Nutrition—Climate change may be associated with staple food shortages, malnutrition, and food contamination (of seafood from chemical contaminants, biotoxins, and pathogenic microbes, and of crops by pesticides). Science research needs in this area include better understanding of how changes in agriculture and fisheries may affect food availability and nutrition, better monitoring for disease-causing agents, and identification and mapping of complex food webs and sentinel species that may be vulnerable to climate change. This research could be used to prepare the public health and health care sectors for new illnesses, changing surveillance needs, and increased incidence of disease, as well as development of more effective outreach to affected communities.

Heat-Related Morbidity and Mortality—Heat-related illness and deaths are likely to increase in response to climate change but aggressive public health interventions such as heat wave response plans and health alert warning systems can minimize morbidity and mortality. Additional science should be focused on developing and expanding these tools in different geographic regions, specifically by defining environmental risk factors, identifying vulnerable populations, and developing effective risk communication and prevention strategies.

Human Developmental Effects—Two potential consequences of climate change would affect normal human development: malnutrition—particularly during the prenatal period and early childhood as a result of decreased food supplies, and exposure to toxic contaminants and biotoxins—resulting from extreme weather events, increased pesticide use for food production, and increases in harmful algal blooms in recreational areas. Research should examine the relationship between human development and adaptations to climate change, such as agriculture and fisheries changes that may affect food availability, increased pesticide use to control for expanding disease vector ranges, and prevention of leaching from toxic waste sites into floodwaters during extreme weather events, so that developmental consequences can be prevented.

Mental Health and Stress-Related Disorders—By causing or contributing to extreme weather events, climate change may result in geographic displacement of populations, damage to property, loss of loved ones, and chronic stress, all of which can negatively affect mental health. Research needs include identifying key mental health effects and vulnerable populations, and developing migration monitoring networks to help ensure the availability of appropriate health care support.

Neurological Diseases and Disorders—Climate change, as well as attempts to mitigate and adapt to it, may increase the number of neurological diseases and disorders in humans. Research in this area should focus on identifying vulnerable populations and understanding the mechanisms and effects of human exposure to neurological hazards such as biotoxins (from harmful algal blooms), metals (found in new battery technologies and compact fluorescent lights), and pesticides (used in response to changes in agriculture), as well as the potentially exacerbating effects of malnutrition and stress.

Vectorborne and Zoonotic Diseases—Disease risk may increase as a result of climate change due to related expansions in vector ranges, shortening of pathogen incubation periods, and disruption and relocation of large human populations. Research should enhance the existing pathogen/vector control infrastructure including vector and host identification; integrate human with terrestrial and aquatic animal health surveillance systems; incorporate ecological studies to provide better predictive models; and improve risk communication and prevention strategies.

Waterborne Diseases—Increases in water temperature, precipitation frequency and severity, evaporation-transpiration rates, and changes in coastal ecosystem health could increase the incidence of water contamination with harmful pathogens and chemicals, resulting in increased human exposure. Research should focus on understanding where changes in water flow will occur, how water will interact with sewage in surface and underground water supplies as well as drinking water distribution systems, what food sources may become contaminated, and how to better predict and prevent human exposure to waterborne and ocean-related pathogens and biotoxins.

Weather-Related Morbidity and Mortality—Increases in the incidence and intensity of extreme weather events such as hurricanes, floods, droughts, and wildfires may adversely affect people's health immediately during the event or later following the event. Research aimed at improving the capabilities of healthcare and emergency services to address disaster planning and management is needed to ensure that risks are understood and that optimal strategies are identified, communicated, and implemented.

In addition to the research needs identified in the individual research categories, there are crosscutting issues relevant to preventing or avoiding many of the potential health impacts of climate change including identifying susceptible, vulnerable, and displaced populations; enhancing public health and health care infrastructure; developing capacities and skills in modeling and prediction; and improving risk communication and public health education. Such research will lead to more effective early warning systems and greater public awareness of an individual's or community's health risk from climate change strategies. For example, health communications research is needed to properly implement health alert warning systems for extreme heat events and air pollution that especially affects people with existing conditions such as cardiovascular disease. Such a risk communication pilot project might demonstrate communication practices that are effective in multiple areas, and contribute to a comprehensive strategy for addressing multiple health risks simultaneously.

Other tools are needed and should be applied across multiple categories to close the knowledge gaps, including predictive models to improve forecasting and prevention, evaluations of the vulnerability of health care and public health systems and infrastructure, and health impact assessments. Trans-disciplinary development would help to ensure tools such as improved baseline monitoring that will be more widely applicable, and thus more efficient and cost effective than those currently available. In fact, many of the identified science needs will require trans-disciplinary responses. For example, to study how heat waves alter ambient air pollution and the resulting combined impact of heat and pollution on human illness and death, will require expertise in atmospheric chemistry, climate patterns, environmental health, epidemiology, medicine, and other science fields. Given the complexity of the science needs and the potential overlap of research questions across disciplines, promoting trans-disciplinary collaboration among and within federal agencies would be a logical approach and should be a high priority.

Recently, the National Research Council issued a report addressing how federal research and science could be improved to provide support for decision and policy making on climate change and human health.4 Specifically, the report calls for a more complete catalogue of climate change health impacts, increasing the power of prediction tools, enhancing integration of climate observation networks with health impact surveillance tools, and improving interactions among stakeholders and decision makers. The IWGCCH approached this research needs assessment with these goals in mind. The next step will be for federal agencies to discuss the findings of this white paper with stakeholders, decision makers, and the public as they work to incorporate and prioritize appropriate research needs into their respective science agendas and collaborative research efforts. A coordinated federal approach will bring the unique skills, capacities, and missions of the various agencies together to maximize the potential for discovery of new information and opportunities for success in providing key information to support responsive and effective decisions on climate change and health.

SEE ALSO *Air Pollution: Urban, Industrial, and Transborder; Dengue; Insect-Borne Diseases; Malaria*

BIBLIOGRAPHY

Books

Butler, Colin, ed. *Climate Change and Global Health.* Wallingford, UK: CABI International, 2014.

Epstein, Paul, and Dan Ferber. *Changing Planet, Changing Health: How the Climate Crisis Threatens Our Health and What We Can Do about It.* Berkeley: University of California Press, 2011.

Hales, Simon, Sari Kovats, Simon Lloyd, and Diarmid Campbell-Lendrum. *Quantitative Risk Assessment of the Effects of Climate Change on Selected Causes of Death, 2030s and 2050s.* Geneva: World Health Organization, 2014.

Stocker, Thomas, et al., eds. *Climate Change 2013: The Physical Science Basis: Working Group I Contribution to the Fifth Assessment Report of the Intergovernmental Panel on Climate Change.* New York: Cambridge University Press, 2014.

Periodicals

Costello, Anthony, et al. "Managing the Health Effects of Climate Change." *The Lancet* 373, no. 9676 (May 16, 2009): 1693–1733.

Robine, Jean-Marie, et al. "Death Toll Exceeded 70,000 in Europe during the Summer of 2003." *Les Comptes Rendus/Série Biologies* 331, no. 2 (February 2008): 171–178.

St. Louis, Michael E., and Jeremy J. Hess. "Climate Change: Impacts on and Implications for Global Health." *American Journal of Preventive Medicine* 35, no. 5 (August 2008): 527–538. Available online at http://www.ajpmonline.org/article/S0749-3797(08)00688-0/fulltext (accessed March 31, 2015).

Zhou, Xiao-Nong, et al. "Potential Impact of Climate Change on Schistosomiasis Transmission in China." *American Journal of Tropical Medicine and Hygiene* 78, no. 2 (February 2008): 188–194.

Websites

"Climate Change and Health." Fact Sheet No. 266, *World Health Organization (WHO)*, August 2014. http://www.who.int/mediacentre/factsheets/fs266/en/ (accessed January 15, 2015).

"Climate and Health." *U.S. Centers for Disease Control and Prevention (CDC).* http://www.cdc.gov/climateandhealth/default.htm (accessed March 31, 2015).

"Climate Impacts on Human Health." *U.S. Environmental Protection Agency (EPA).* http://www.epa.gov/climatechange/impacts-adaptation/health.html (accessed January 15, 2015).

"Health Implications of Global Warming: Vector-borne and Water-borne Disease." *Physicians for Social Responsibility.* http://www.psr.org/assets/pdfs/vector-borne-and-water-borne.pdf (accessed January 15, 2015).

"The Impacts of Climate Change on Health." *Climate and Health Council.* http://www.climateandhealth.org/health_impacts.html (accessed January 15, 2015).

Susan Aldridge

Complementary and Alternative Medicine

⊕ Introduction

There are many definitions of complementary and alternative medicine (CAM), none of which is able to encompass succinctly the variety of methods and opinions that inhabit the field. "Complementary" and "alternative" frequently are used interchangeably despite having very different meanings. The difference between the way science uses these terms versus the way they are used in marketing and advertising further complicates the issue.

The U.S. National Center for Complementary and Integrative Health (NCCIH; formerly the National Center for Complementary and Alternative Health) defines CAM modestly: CAM is a group of diverse medical and health care interventions, practices, products, or disciplines that are not generally considered part of conventional medicine. Conventional medicine also is referred to as Western, or allopathic, medicine. The parameters of CAM are changing constantly, as some practices that once may have been considered unconventional become more widely accepted.

Generally, "complementary" medicine includes a nontraditional approach that is used together with conventional tactics to treat symptoms or diagnosis. Alternative medicine refers to nontraditional approaches when used instead of any traditional medicine. As evidenced by the name change from NCCAM to NCCIH, some complementary medicine is being integrated into the modern medical system and will be part of the medical curriculum and the teaching programs of medical institutions. Issues of efficacy and safety of complementary medicine increasingly have become contested because they generally lack long scientific histories. To understand what alternative medicine looks like, it is necessary to understand how conventional medicine, as it is thought of in the mid-2010s, became the dominant approach.

⊕ Historical Background

Perhaps the ancient home of what is thought of as conventional medicine was in ancient Greece. A physician named Hippocrates, who lived in the 4th century BCE, was the first to list and describe a series of medical conditions and diseases, and to teach students about his findings. He is considered the founder of Western medicine and is the creator of the Hippocratic oath. The Hippocratic oath is an oath, still used, that requires new physicians to swear to uphold the ethical standards of medical practice. There is no legal obligation of medical students to swear this oath, but upon graduating 98 percent of students in the United States and 50 percent of British students choose to do so.

Medical practice advanced in fits and starts until the Age of Enlightenment in the 18th century, when people started to rely heavily on research and science to advance the field. That reliance on science paved the way for the rise of modern medicine in the 19th century, compounded by the discovery of germ theory, vaccinations, and equipment sterilization practices. These advances evolved into the conventional medicine that includes cancer therapy, antibiotic use, organ transplants, and pharmacology. Conventional medicine seems to have reached critical mass, and the population it serves has started to return to some ancient and traditional medicines to complement their treatment. In the United States about 4 out of 10 adults use some form of alternative therapies, and they are used by people from all different backgrounds. Herbal medicine, also called natural remedies; breathing exercises; meditation; chiropractic work; and massage and yoga are the most common CAM practices in the United States.

Most patients continue to rely on their doctors to know what is best for them, but the growing trend is for patients/clients to take responsibility for their own care in a collaborative effort by seeking out information on what other options exist. Turning to the Internet looking for help, sometimes desperate people are especially vulnerable to sham cures and treatments that may at be benign at best and dangerous at worst.

Homeopathy

German physician Samuel Hahnemann (1755–1843) established homeopathy in 1796. Based on the postulate *similia similibus curentur* or "like cures like," homeopathic remedies are created using combinations of mineral, herbal, or animal substances. While observing the effects treatments had on patients, Hahnemann noticed that large doses of particular solutions could cause symptoms similar to the illnesses they were intended to treat. Using this reasoning, he concluded that smaller, diluted doses of substances should have greater effectiveness.

Hahnemann's premise for treating disease is quoted as: "We should imitate nature, which sometimes cures a chronic affliction with another supervening disease, and prescribe for the illness we wish to cure, especially if chronic, a drug with power to provoke another, artificial disease, as similar as possible, and the former disease will be cured: fight like with like." In some circumstances, the homeopathic solutions are diluted so much that it is impossible to identify any of the original raw material. Hahnemann published the entire medical system for homeopathy in *The Organon of the Healing Art* in 1921; it is still in use by practitioners in the mid-2010s.

Naturopathy

American physician Benedict Lust (1872–1945) developed naturopathy in 1902. Naturopathic treatments include herbal medicines, vitamins, minerals, dietary supplements, hydrotherapy, therapeutic massage, and lifestyle counseling. Naturopathy is based on the underlying principle that an intelligence force—present throughout the entire universe and human body—can be called upon and directed to heal the body intrinsically without requiring drugs or surgery. Practitioners focus on a holistic approach to health, taking into account their patients' physical, mental, spiritual, and environmental circumstances.

Touch as a Complementary or Alternative Medicine

The healing power of touch also could be considered a form of CAM. Chiropractic adjustment, clinical massage, and yoga are ways in which body movements and human touch can be used to complement or replace conventional medicine. The touch from acupuncture also crosses over into this category. Chiropractic adjustment is a procedure in which specialists (chiropractors) use their hands or small instruments to manipulate the spine to correct poor positioning. Originally, chiropractic manipulation was thought to improve neurological dysfunction, though that effect came to be considered only speculative in nature. However, spinal manipulations are shown to relieve pain, increase a person's range of movement, and help strengthen muscle strength. Similar to chiropractic adjustment, massage is the manipulation of the muscles and the connective tissues to increase blood flow, decrease depression, and assist in relaxation. A variety of massage techniques exist that range from recreational to clinical in intensity.

Chiropractic

Chiropractic combines the Greek root words *cheir* (hand) and *praxis* (practice) to mean literally "done by hand." Daniel David Palmer (1845–1913) developed the principal tenets of chiropractic medicine after allegedly restoring hearing in a man who was partially deaf. Originally from Canada, Palmer established the first chiropractic college, the Palmer School of Chiropractic, in Davenport, Iowa. According to the central premise, human diseases and pathologies are the result of structural spinal dysfunctions, called subluxations. The core treatment

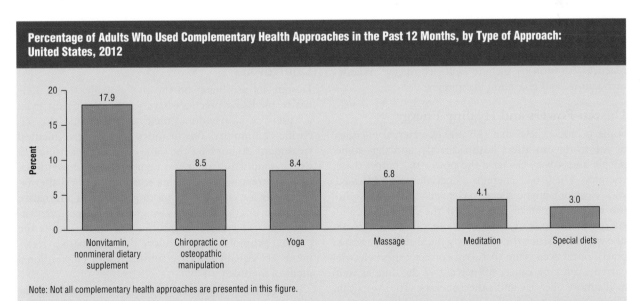

Percentage of Adults Who Used Complementary Health Approaches in the Past 12 Months, by Type of Approach: United States, 2012

Note: Not all complementary health approaches are presented in this figure.

SOURCE: Peregoy, Jennifer A., et al., "Figure 1. Percentage of adults who used complementary health approaches in the past 12 months, by type of approach: United States, 2012," in *NCHS Data Brief*, No. 146, U.S. Centers for Disease Control and Prevention/National Center for Health Statistics, April 2014. Data from CDC/NCHS, National Health Interview Survey, 2012.

EFFICACY

Supporters claim that the reason evidence is lacking for alternative medicine is due to the poor availability of funding for these treatments. Government-sponsored medical research customarily is required to gain approval from an ethical review board. The Helsinki Declaration, the governing set of principles regarding the proper use of human subjects in research, states that withholding effective treatments for scientific purposes is unethical. This guideline creates a problematic funding landscape for alternative therapies if an existing conventional medical treatment exists.

In the United Kingdom, German physician Edzard Ernst (1948–) has become a widely known critic of alternative medicine after conducting research for 15 years as the world's first professor of alternative medicine. In 2008, Ernst addressed an open letter to Great Britain's Royal Pharmaceutical Society regarding his concerns over the sale of homeopathic remedies in pharmacies. The letter urged the organization to take action in ensuring their ethical standards are upheld. Dr. Ernst stated that homeopathic treatments "are biologically implausible and the clinical tests have shown they don't do anything at all in human beings." In an interview published the same year, Ernst was also quoted saying, "there is no such thing as alternative medicine. There is either medicine that is effective or not, or medicine that is safe or not."

Steven Novella (1964–), an American neurologist at Yale University and the founder of Science-Based Medicine, an organization "dedicated to evaluating medical treatments and products of interest to the public in a scientific light" also has criticized researching alternative medicine. Novella claims that investigations into medical treatments and modalities whose underlying theories are contrary to established scientific theories are futile. Despite the numerous results demonstrating the inability of these methods to produce a treatment effect, public interest in these products and practices continues to grow.

In a time when health-care costs continue to rise, socio-economic conditions can limit access to conventional medicine, making alternative medicines the only option for certain populations. However, these increases in demand and worldwide Internet availability have also made these products a growing part of the economic development in some countries.

The Cochrane Collaboration is an international non-profit organization that regularly evaluates medical claims and provides guidance to the WHO. Their systematic reviews provide medical professionals, policy makers, and consumers with comprehensive summaries of medical treatments and products. Cochrane conducts systematic reviews using explicit, peer-reviewed, and transparent methodologies. The Cochrane reviews have been an invaluable resource for reducing bias and errors in planning research and selecting appropriate treatments. The Cochrane Collaboration has stated that all treatments should be held to the same standards of science, alternative or not.

As of 2014, the Cochrane Collaboration had produced nearly 700 reviews of complementary and alternative medicine, and more than 200 reviews of complementary and alternative medical protocols. The systematic reviews on the efficacy of alternative medical treatments and protocols tend to lack well-defined methodology, making them prone to bias.

method for chiropractors is manual manipulation and adjustment of the spinal column. Additional chiropractic practices occasionally include heat, ice, dietary recommendations, and relaxation techniques.

Unseen Powers and Healing Energy

Some people believe that the unseen external energies of the world can affect health directly, and that some people and substances have the power to control these energies. These bad energies sometimes are addressed with electromagnetic therapy. Generally, therapists who use electromagnetism believe that the frequencies and energy of the body can become out of balance, cause disease, and disrupt the body's chemical makeup. Some practitioners even claim that used correctly these electric currents can cure cancer 80 percent of the time as well as diagnose allergies and other diseases. The American Cancer Society has urged cancer patients not to seek this treatment as complementary or alternative cures for any illness because there is no evidence to suggest that such cures exist.

⊕ Impacts and Issues

Controversy

Despite its use being on the rise globally, some alternative medicine practices have received criticism from a variety of conventional medical groups and the scientific community. The majority of alternative medical treatments do not have the same degree of scientific evidence supporting their use compared to conventional medical treatments. For this reason, critics of alternative medicine consider promoting the use of alternative medicine unethical. They also claim the term *alternative medicine* creates misinformation and misleads the public, promoting the notion that alternative treatments are equally effective substitutes for conventional medical methods.

Supporters of alternative medicine argue that individuals should have the freedom to choose their own therapies, conventional or otherwise. Over-the-counter medicines, supporters contend, can be just as toxic or harmful as alternative medical products.

The Placebo Effect

Critics claim that alternative medicine works through the placebo effect. Derived from the Latin words meaning "I shall please," placebos are inactive substances given in experimental studies designed to control for or reinforce the patient's expectation to get better. When designing a clinical trial, researchers often test the efficacy of a new treatment against a placebo by randomly assigning participants into each group. Placebo treatments are designed to mimic every aspect of the treatment being tested (psychological, surgical, etc.), but are physiologically inert. Because many alternative medical remedies are unable to demonstrate a specific treatment effect, opponents have suggested that much of the perceived effectiveness is a result of the patient's subjective experience with the practitioner and environment. Supporters of alternative medicine counter that any treatment resulting in an improvement of a patient's psychological well-being is worth investigating.

Safety and Regulation

Concerns about the safety of some alternative medicine methods have arisen from the medical community due to the limited amount of regulations and governmental oversight. In the United Kingdom, critics of alternative medicine claim that regulatory bodies, such as the General Chiropractic Council (GCC), have little to no effect on quality control in their field. This accusation partially stems from a court case in which the British Chiropractic Association attempted to sue a journalist for claiming that chiropractic treatments were useless and ineffective. The GCC initially rejected a majority of the ensuing claims made against chiropractors, before finally issuing a statement in 2010 that denounced "vertebral subluxations," a major component of chiropractic theory. In an article published in the *Scottish Universities Medical Journal*, professor David Colquhoun (1936–) stated that the GCC was "there to protect chiropractors, not to protect the public."

Future Implications

Although alternative medicine use has gained global popularity, the most rapid increases have occurred in developed countries. As developed countries continue to expand their individual health systems, several policy makers and public health officials have recommended that alternative medical practices be integrated into their local health delivery strategies.

Research and general public awareness confirms that interest in CAM is increasing in the United States and throughout the world. As CAM continues to grow, it likely will become increasingly integrated in the conventional Western medical system, and eventually not be considered outside existing health-care structure but rather a vital part of it. Doctors, nurses, and other health care providers are becoming more knowledgeable of medicine and CAM options, and even beginning to advertise their services as "holistic." With the establishment of the National Center for Complementary and Alternative Medicine (NCCAM in 1998), CAM received a nod of legitimacy by the U.S. government. With the change in name to NCCIH, the government hoped to signal its "commitment to studying promising health approaches already in use by the American public." There is still resistance to commit any more funding toward study, or toward any provisions that would decrease the costs of CAM for the consumer.

Increased funding for clinical trials will go a long way toward finding CAM that is effective and being able to safely integrate those practices into the existing health structure, in the similar ways India and China maintain parallel medical options. With the passage of the Affordable Care Act (ACA), the United States is in the process of enrolling millions of people in publicly supported health care with great political difficulty. ACA does not include CAM within the coverage provisions, despite its many advocates. It is possible that the interest in CAM will decrease in the United States with the increase of people enrolled in affordable, conventional health care, but that remains to be seen.

SEE ALSO *Cultural and Traditional Medicine; Health as a Human Right and Health-Care Access; Health-Related Education and Information Access; Pharmaceutical Research, Testing, and Access; Universal Health Coverage; World Health Organization: Organization, Funding, and Enforcement Powers*

BIBLIOGRAPHY

Books

Balch, Phyllis, and Stacey J. Bell. *Prescription for Herbal Healing*, 2nd ed. New York: Avery, 2012.

Baran, George R., Mohammad F. Kiani, and Solomon P. Samuel. "Science, Pseudoscience, and Not Science: How Do They Differ?" In *Healthcare and Biomedical Technology in the 21st Century: An Introduction for Non-science Majors*, 19–58. New York: Springer, 2013.

Bauer, Brent, et al. *Mayo Clinic Book of Alternative Medicine*, 2nd ed. New York: Time Inc. Home Entertainment Books, 2010.

Beinfield, Harriet, and Efrem Korngold. *Between Heaven and Earth: A Guide to Chinese Medicine*. New York: Ballantine Books, 1991.

Cotter, Ann C., Samuel C. Shiflett, and David Kuo. "Complementary and Alternative Medicine." In *Physical Medicine & Rehabilitation: Principles and Practice*, 4th ed., Joel L. DeLisa and Bruce M. Gans, eds., vol. 1, chapter 19. Philadelphia: Lippincott Williams & Wilkins, 2005.

Dikötter, Frank *The Cambridge History of Science,* Vol. 4: *18th Century Science.* New York: Cambridge University Press, 2008.

Haehl, Richard. *Samuel Hahnemann: His Life and Work: Based on Recently Discovered State Papers, Documents, Letters, &c.* New Delhi: B. Jain, 1922; reprint 1995.

Horstmanshoff, H. F. J., Martin Stol, and C. R. van Tilburg, eds. *Magic and Rationality in Ancient Near Eastern and Graeco-Roman Medicine.* Leiden, Netherlands: Brill, 2004.

Leach, Robert. *The Chiropractic Theories: A Textbook of Scientific Research,* 4th ed. Philadelphia: Lippincott, Williams and Wilkins, 2004.

O'Reilly, Wenda, ed. *The Organon of the Healing Art by Dr. Samuel Hahnemann,* 6th ed. Redmond, WA: Birdcage Press, 2010.

Schultz, Andrea M., Samantha M. Chao, and J. Michael McGinnis. *Integrative Medicine and the Health of the Public: A Summary of the February 2009 Summit.* Washington, DC: National Academies Press, 2009.

Sointu, Eeva. *Theorizing Complementary and Alternative Medicines: Wellbeing, Self, Gender, Class.* New York: Palgrave Macmillan, 2012.

Stux, Gabriel, Brian Berman, and Bruce Pomeranz. *Basics of Acupuncture,* 5th ed. New York: Springer, 2003.

Yang, Yifan. *Chinese Herbal Medicines: Comparisons and Characteristics,* 2nd ed. New York: Elsevier, 2010.

Periodicals

Ernst, Edzard. "The Public's Enthusiasm for Complementary and Alternative Medicine Amounts to a Critique of Mainstream Medicine." *International Journal of Clinical Practice* 64, no. 11 (October 2010): 1472–1474.

Gorski, David H., and Steven P. Novella. "Clinical Trials of Integrative Medicine: Testing Whether Magic Works?" *Trends in Molecular Medicine* 20, no. 9 (September 2014): 473–476.

Juckett, Gregory. "Cross-Cultural Medicine." *American Family Physician* 72, no. 11 (December 1, 2006): 2267–2274. Available online at http://www.aafp.org (accessed January 18, 2015).

Kupferschmidt, Kai. "Scourge of Snake Oil Salesmen Bids an Early Farewell." *Science* 333, no. 6043 (August 5, 2011): 687.

Lee, Myeong Soo, M. H. Pittler, and Edzard Ernst. "Effects of Reiki in Clinical Practice: A Systematic Review of Randomized Clinical Trials." *International Journal of Clinical Practice* 62, no. 6 (June 2008): 947–954.

Linde, Klaus, Michael M. Berner, and Levente Kriston. "St John's Wort for Major Depression." *Cochrane Database of Systematic Reviews* 4, no. CD000448 (October 8, 2008). Available online at http://summaries.cochrane.org/CD000448/DEPRESSN_st.-johns-wort-for-treating-depression (accessed January 18, 2015).

Marcus, Donald M., and Arthur P. Grollman. "Science and Government: Review for NCCAM Is Overdue." *Science* 313, no. 5785 (July 21, 2006): 301–302.

Oumeish, Oumeish Youssef. "The Philosophical, Cultural, and Historical Aspects of Complementary, Alternative, Unconventional, and Integrative Medicine in the Old World." *Archives of Dermatology* 134, no. 11 (November 1998): 1373–1386.

Saper, Robert B., Russell S. Phillips, Anusha Sehgal, et al. "Lead, Mercury, and Arsenic in US- and Indian-Manufactured Medicines Sold via the Internet." *JAMA* 300, no. 8 (August 2008): 915–923.

Servick, Kelly. "Outsmarting the Placebo Effect." *Science* 345, no. 6203 (September 19, 2014): 1446–1447.

Wieland, L. Susan, Eric Manheimer, and Brian M. Berman. "Development and Classification of an Operational Definition of Complementary and Alternative Medicine for the Cochrane Collaboration." *Alternative Therapies in Health and Medicine* 17, no. 2 (March/April 2011): 50–59.

Websites

"Acupuncture: Definition." *Mayo Clinic.* http://www.mayoclinic.org/tests-procedures/acupuncture/basics/definition/prc-20020778 (accessed January 21, 2015).

"Benchmarks for Training in Ayurveda." *World Health Organization (WHO),* 2010. http://apps.who.int/medicinedocs/en/m/abstract/Js17552en/ (accessed January 18, 2015).

"Benchmarks for Training in Naturopathy." *World Health Organization (WHO),* 2010. http://apps.who.int/medicinedocs/en/m/abstract/Js17553en/ (accessed January 18, 2015).

"Benchmarks for Training in Traditional Chinese Medicine." *World Health Organization (WHO),* 2010. http://apps.who.int/medicinedocs/en/m/abstract/Js17556en/ (accessed January 18, 2015).

Brown, David. "Critics Object to 'Pseudoscience' Center." *Washington Post,* March 17, 2009. http://www.washingtonpost.com/wp-dyn/content/article/2009/03/16/AR2009031602139.html (accessed January 18, 2015).

"Chinese Herbal Medicine." *American Cancer Society.* http://www.cancer.org/treatment/treatmentsandsideeffects/complementaryandalternativemedicine/herbsvitaminsandminerals/chinese-herbal-medicine (accessed January 18, 2015).

Cochrane Collaboration. http://www.cochrane.org/ (accessed November 15, 2014).

Colquhoun, David. "Regulation of Alternative Medicine—Why It Doesn't Work." *Scottish Universities Medical Journal,* July 2012. http://sumj.dundee.ac.uk/data/uploads/epub-article/016-sumj.epub.pdf (accessed June 16, 2015).

"Complementary, Alternative, or Integrative Health: What's in a Name?" *National Center for Complementary and Integrative Health.* http://nccih.nih.gov/health/integrative-health (accessed January 18, 2015).

"Funding Strategy." *National Center for Complementary and Integrative Health.* http://nccih.nih.gov/grants/strategy (accessed January 18, 2015).

"NCCIH Facts-at-a-Glance and Mission." *National Center for Complementary and Integrative Health.* http://nccih.nih.gov/about/ataglance (accessed January 18, 2015).

"Quality Control Methods for Herbal Materials." *World Health Organization (WHO).* http://apps.who.int/medicinedocs/en/m/abstract/Jh1791e/ (accessed November 15, 2014).

"Research Funding Priorities." *National Center for Complementary and Integrative Health.* http://nccIH.nih.gov/grants/priorities (accessed November 15, 2014).

"Safety Issues in the Preparation of Homeopathic Medicines." *World Health Organization (WHO),* 2010. http://apps.who.int/medicinedocs/en/m/abstract/Js16769e/ (accessed January 18, 2015).

"Traditional and Complementary Medicine Policy. (MDS-3: Managing Access to Medicines and Health Technologies, Chapter 5)." *World Health Organization (WHO),* 2012. http://apps.who.int/medicinedocs/en/m/abstract/Js19582en/ (accessed January 18, 2015).

"Traditional Medicines: Definitions." *World Health Organization (WHO),* 2000. http://www.who.int/medicines/areas/traditional/definitions/en/ (accessed January 18, 2015).

"WHO Guidelines on Basic Training and Safety in Chiropractic." *World Health Organization (WHO),* 2005. http://apps.who.int/medicinedocs/en/m/abstract/Js14076e/ (accessed January 18, 2015).

"WHO Traditional Medicine Strategy: 2014–2023." *World Health Organization (WHO),* 2013. http://apps.who.int/medicinedocs/en/m/abstract/Js21201en/ (accessed January 18, 2015).

Martin Frigaard

Margaret Loraine Scott

Conflict, Violence, and Terrorism: Health Impacts

⊕ Introduction

The direct effects of war, terrorism, conflict, and general violence on collective human health are readily apparent. Military combatants and personnel are subject to casualties, and civilians, persons in proximity to the fighting, but otherwise uninvolved, may be intentionally targeted or unintentional victims of violence. Witnessing violence and destruction causes less obvious, but potentially as devastating, psychological trauma. These are all direct health effects on a population.

There also are indirect effects of war and violence that may cause additional collateral damage. A hospital may be unable to operate because of conflict in the area, supply lines may be disrupted, or there may be a critical lack of human resources to perform medical services during war. People who would otherwise have received lifesaving treatment may be unable to gain access to it. Worse still, devastated infrastructure can effect sanitation and food availability, and prevent timely treatment of communicable diseases, especially in the displaced populations of a war-torn environment.

Sometimes the outcome of conflicts is decided not by overwhelming force, or superior firepower, but by sanitation levels and adequate food sources. During war, contact between different populations is made that otherwise would never occur, facilitating the spread of disease to new populations without acquired immunity. Infectious or "communicable" diseases, those passed from one person to another, may be spread more easily as populations attempting to escape violence are forced into crowded conditions. Epidemics may begin as unsanitary conditions intensify as a result of crowding in refugee camps or the breakdown of health-care systems as infrastructure weakens or is destroyed.

After the destruction of infrastructure, people may lack adequate shelter, and they may become particularly susceptible to insect-borne illnesses, such as malaria. When sanitation and hygiene suffer, there may be increased rates of food-borne and waterborne illnesses. Diseases such as cholera and dysentery, which are primarily caused by a lack of clean drinking water, occur routinely when large groups of people live together without access to adequate clean water and hygiene. Both are preventable with clean drinking water and adequate medical facilities, but in times of war, when access to these necessities is limited, people may be left to die slow deaths from dehydration.

Terrorism as it is thought of today has a direct impact on civilians. Terrorists may use the deliberate targeting of civilians to cause the greatest amount of damage and fear within a population. Acts of terrorism are sometimes, but not always, associated with an ongoing conflict. For example, a violent attack like the Oklahoma City bombing has nothing to do with international warfare, but the health effects may be the same. Terrorists may target civilians and military personnel equally when biohazardous weapons are deployed. Over the course of history, sometimes the greatest impacts of war have been the unintended consequences on the physical and mental health of the surrounding populations.

⊕ Historical Background

The history of conflict is the history of humanity, culture, and civilization. With war came the adoption and obliteration of whole civilizations, and the government participants primarily drove these changes. Traditionally, when a military force invaded, they brought with them not only new languages, culture, and art but also new diseases. Soldiers brought sexually transmitted diseases like syphilis that spread rapidly through populations. Some of these conflict-related issues, such as sanitation problems and diseases attributable to dietary deficiencies such as scurvy (caused by a deficiency of vitamin C), are preventable, while others, such as a statistically higher increase in birth defects in the children of victimized populations, occur with no obvious cause.

The Plague of Athens

War bringing plague is nothing new or exclusive to modern warfare, or even documented history. The plague of ancient Greece is a prime example of how a powerful civilization and military force can be devastated by the health consequences of conflict. During the second year of the Peloponnese War, 430 BCE, a plague of unknown medical origin swept through Athens, driven by poor hygiene and close quarters. It is not known which disease crippled the city; it may have been bubonic plague, smallpox, or measles. Documentation from Thucydides (460–395 BCE) indicating that the disease was of African origin and was brought to the city by returning soldiers also suggests that the disease may have been an earlier form of the Ebola virus. Thucydides claimed it took almost 15 years for the city to recover from the deaths of up to two-thirds of the population. Before the epidemic, an Athenian victory would have been possible, afterward it was unthinkable.

The 1918 Influenza Pandemic

Jumping forward two millennia, another war spurred a pandemic of epic proportions that likely decided the outcome of the war. In 1918 a pandemic of flu swept through the world, killing more people than were lost in combat during World War I (1914–1918). Fear of an influenza epidemic recurring still exists today and has huge implications for contemporary global health policy. The majority of deaths during this epidemic occurred in a four-month period during the third quarter of 1918, but between that fall and the next year somewhere between 50 million and 100 million people from every populated continent succumbed to the disease. That the war ended in November 1918, just as the deadliest weeks of the pandemic were coming to a close, is not a coincidence.

This flu strain, now known as H1N1, has also been called avian flu, swine flu, and Spanish flu. Though it was most certainly of avian origin, studies to precisely determine its origin were inconclusive. One widely accepted theory is that the outbreak started in a town in Kansas approximately 300 miles out of what is now Fort Reilly. There had been an outbreak there in the local population of a particularly virulent type of flu, which was reported to public health officials by one of the treating physicians. At the time, army recruits were reporting to the nearby base where family and friends would visit. The recruits from the nearby areas would return home for the weekends.

In early March the first soldier fell ill, and within three weeks 1,100 soldiers were hospitalized with the disease. Thousands more fell ill but did not require hospitalization. The virus spread predictably into most of the remaining army camps in the United States, and the majority of major cities had mortality (deaths) spikes from flu and pneumonia. As soldiers left for Europe from the base, they took the virus with them to the entry points for the U.S. troops. Without the massive migration of people caused by the troop movements, the virus still might have reached Europe but at a considerably slower rate. The spread of this flu is an important example of how even epidemics that start in sparsely populated regions like the Midwest of the United States are exponentially more dangerous during conflict.

Typhus Fever during World War I

The influenza pandemic was not the only disease to ravage civilians and soldiers alike during World War I. Typhus fever broke out on the Eastern European front during the early days of conflict. Typhus is common among populations that live in close quarters with poor sanitation because it is spread by lice that infest infrequently washed hair as well as by fleas, mites, and ticks. Serbian refugees began to flee the conflict in Belgrade in the winter of 1914, and the surrounding army started reporting cases of typhus. Northern Serbia was heavily damaged by the war despite having successfully resisted Austrian invasion, but the destruction created a breeding ground for ideal typhus conditions. Within six months 200,000 people, almost half of which were Serbian troops, had died. By the end of the war, the destruction of infrastructure and lack of medical care ultimately resulted in the death of 10 million people. This initial epidemic, which contributed to the inability of Serbia to mount a successful countercampaign against Austria, likely changed the outcome of the war.

⊕ Impacts and Issues

As history demonstrates, conflict and war act to severely compromise infrastructure, social structure, and security, all of which contribute to the overall decline of public health. Civilians and military personal are physically and mentally affected, and the violence has far-reaching social implications.

Casualties

A casualty of war is a person who has been killed or injured during the conflict. Casualties are the most direct illustration of the connection between conflict and health. Throughout most of history, and particularly before the discovery of penicillin in 1928, the association between lack of proper sanitation and infection was particularly important. Today, every wound on a battlefield or caused by a terrorist event is now presumed to be infected and is treated with antibiotics and sterile dressings, but that was not always the case.

Tetanus, a bacterial infection also known as lockjaw, was held at bay for the first time during World War I, when soldiers were injected with a form of the tetanus vaccine before going to war. Penicillin was used to combat infection of war wounds for the first time in 1943. The need for penicillin for combat soldiers was so high that it lessened the supply to civilians. Because

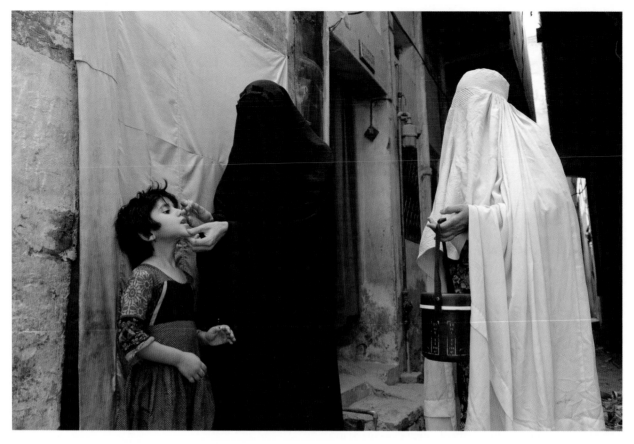

A Pakistani health worker administers the polio vaccine to a child during a vaccination campaign in Bannu, Pakistan. Pakistan launched a polio vaccination drive in its restive tribal belt in May 2014, but officials warned that nearly 370,000 children were likely to miss out because of security problems. Pakistan's seven semiautonomous tribal areas along the Afghan border are the epicenter of the country's polio cases, and the government has set up checkpoints to ensure anyone leaving the belt is immunized.   © A Majeed/AFP/Getty Images.

about 85 percent of the nation's supply went directly to the military, and the demand for the drug was so great, the scientific community was incentivized to develop mass-production techniques. Using these techniques, the drug supply tripled between 1944 and 1945 and the number of deaths from the war was dramatically decreased.

Refugees and Epidemics

During conflict, combatants and civilians may be injured or killed. When war tears apart the infrastructure of a city or town, or the area becomes too dangerous for them to remain, civilians may flee the area, creating large masses of refugees. In many instances, civilians flee the combat zones, but the places to which they flee are not any safer. Refugee camps spring up with makeshift shelters or in nearby areas that are also devastated by fighting. Today, there are hundreds of thousands of refugees who fled their homes because of violence in the Middle East and North Africa. The United Nations reports that serious food shortages, lack of clean water, and poor sanitation turn these refugee camps into ideal breeding grounds for a variety of life-threatening diseases. The threats of cholera, malaria, scurvy, jaundice, and malnutrition replace the threats of bombs and crossfire.

In South Sudan military conflict forced thousands of people into camps that are now rampant with hepatitis E, a viral disease spread through contaminated water and sometimes food, which is otherwise easily prevented. Unfortunately, hepatitis E generally affects the healthiest people the hardest. Persons between ages 15 and 40 are usually the caretakers of the very young and the elderly. When this population is infected with hepatitis E, there is no one to care for the weaker and more vulnerable members of the population who cannot care for themselves. Additionally, South Sudan, Sierra Leone, and Nigeria have all reported cases of severe cholera. Cholera effects the ability for people to absorb water. Hours after infection, an affected individual may be unable to retain any fluids and may waste away from severe dehydration.

With proper sanitation, prevention of diseases like cholera and dysentery is possible, but people have to be educated about how to effectively prevent such diseases. Proper disinfecting techniques can help to prevent the spread of cholera. The United Nations

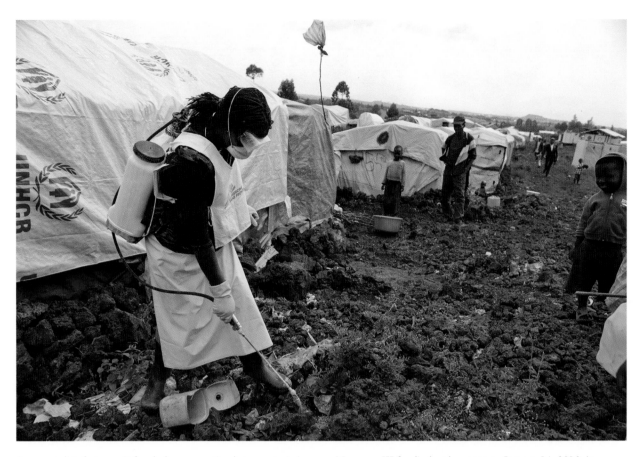

A woman disinfects vomit for cholera prevention between tents in camp Mugunga III for displaced persons on January 14, 2013, in Goma, Democratic Republic of the Congo. The war in the Congo, which has pitted government forces supported by Angola, Namibia, and Zimbabwe against rebels and militias supported by Rwanda and Uganda, has dragged on for years and claimed millions of lives. © *Thomas Lohnes/Getty Images.*

Children's Fund (UNICEF) and many nonprofit organizations provide water purification tablets and health clinics in refugee camps to help refugees remain safe from disease. Experts continue to warn that bacterial, viral, and parasitic diseases could become deadly epidemics and even pandemics (worldwide epidemics) if these camps remain.

Another devastating effect on those in conflict or in refugee camps is a lack of food, which can be caused by a curtailed ability to grow or harvest food in areas where combat is ongoing or disruption of supply lines in conflict zones. In 2015, UNICEF estimates that 400,000 children under age five across the globe will require treatment for severe malnutrition. Conflict areas make a significant contribution to this number. When people suffer from malnutrition, their immune systems are severely debilitated.

Refugees, especially women, are susceptible to additional risks. For example, during the second civil war in Liberia (1999–2003), an estimated 40 percent of all Liberian women had been raped. Many rape victims were exposed to sexually transmitted diseases such as HIV, infections with long-term health consequences.

Noncommunicable Effects of Conflict

Sometimes the public health consequences of conflict are less apparent than disease and injury. For as yet unknown reasons, some research has shown that the rate of birth defects in children born in Iraq has steadily risen since the late 1990s. According to a study published in the *Bulletin of Environmental Contamination and Toxicology* in 2012, between 1994 and 2003, the rate increased 17-fold in one hospital in Al Basrah.

There is evidence that suggests the heavy bombardment of Iraqi cities such as Al Basrah and Fallujah and the environmental contamination caused by the heavy metals generated by military bases are likely to be linked to the observed increase in birth defects. Exposure during pregnancy to heavy metals like lead can cause some of the neurodevelopmental disorders that have been observed. Samples taken from parents of children born with birth defects and the children themselves also have been found to have unusually high levels of uranium, lead, and mercury within their bodies. However, the Iraq Ministry of Health released a preliminary report on September 11, 2013, stating that their analysis of data from 18 districts in Iraq "provides no clear evidence to suggest an

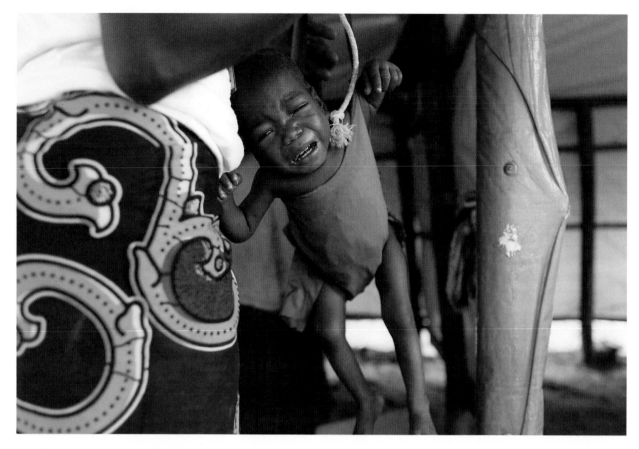

A child is weighed at a malnourishment clinic run by Médecins Sans Frontières (Doctors Without Borders) at the Makpandu refugee camp on January 14, 2011, outside of the town of Yambio, South Sudan. At the time, the camp housed nearly 4,000 people from both the Congo and the Central African Republic (CAR) who fled violence from the Lord's Resistance Army (LRA) outside of Yambio, a poor and isolated town near the borders of CAR and the Congo. The LRA has terrorized much of the population along the border regions of the three countries. South Sudan is one of the world's poorest regions, where over 2 million people were killed in the north-south civil war that began in the 1950s.   *© Spencer Platt/Getty Images.*

unusually high rate of congenital birth defects in Iraq." A full report was to be published after more detailed analysis.

Soldiers and civilians in Iraq and Afghanistan were also exposed to open-air burn pits that destroyed everything from batteries and electronic items to the remains of animals and humans. Some of those who were exposed to the pits state that the toxins in the smoke caused both short- and long-term health consequences, including severe lung and respiratory conditions. The U.S. Department of Veterans Affairs (VA) initiated the Airborne Hazards and Open Burn Pit Registry in 2014 for veterans exposed to fumes in Iraq, Afghanistan, Djibouti after 2001, or during the 1991 Persian Gulf War. Though the VA states that exposure to some of the toxins possibly in the smoke is known to cause "long-term effects to the skin, respiratory system, eyes, liver, kidneys, central nervous system, cardiovascular system, reproductive system, peripheral nervous system, and gastrointestinal tract," it also states that there is not enough medical or scientific evidence that the burn pits created such exposure and

that research was ongoing. Lawsuits by U.S. soldiers who served in Iraq and Afghanistan against the contractors operating the pits continued into 2015. In addition to the soldiers, there is the lasting environmental impact to the regions where the pits operated. The closing of the burn pits and the establishment of a more effective waste disposal systems would go a long way toward halting or reducing some of the health and environmental effects.

Health Care Shortages

The civil war in Syria, which began in March 2011 and is ongoing in 2015, has created one of the largest refugee crises in history. Nearly 450,000 people fled the country by July 2013. Lebanon hosts the most people from Syria who were escaping the conflict, followed closely by Jordan. As the crisis continues, neighboring countries have become increasingly reluctant to allow Syrians to cross into their borders, knowing that they may bring disease with them along with increased pressure on already struggling health-care delivery systems. As an indirect consequence, there is a chronic shortage of adequate health care in Syria and in the countries that host its refugees. By 2014, more than half of Syria's hospitals were completely nonfunctional, and about 70 percent of health-care professionals had fled the country. Less than half of the once high functioning health-care facilities in operation in Syria are still open and operational. Access to health services is severely limited, and many facilities require patients to pay for their services up-front, a practice that is impossible for most people.

In 2014, the WHO reported more than 6,500 cases of typhoid and 4,200 cases of measles in Syria. In addition, cases of polio, an almost eradicated disease, have been reported, as are deaths from diseases and injuries that would have been preventable. In Lebanon, refugees live with up to 30 Syrians in one home, and the influx of people has obligated the government of Lebanon to appeal to the international community for medical aid because the health-care burden of the refugees exceeds the capacity of the infrastructure in Lebanon. In order for Syria to restore a functioning health-care system, the country must first return to a state of peace and rebuild its infrastructure. Lebanon and Jordan need the support of the international community to help care for the refugees.

Terrorism and Biological Agents

Even bioterrorism, a threat that many consider new, has its roots in history. In a particularly grotesque account of the 1364 Siege of Caffa, Black Plague victims were said to have been catapulted over the city walls in what is now part of Ukraine with the express purpose of causing a plague. Although it is possible that this account is accurate, it is likely that the resulting plague would have occurred regardless of the catapult victims, because of the already close contact between the city and the soldiers. During World War II (1939–1945) the Japanese are said to have purposefully infected fleas with plague and released them over Manchurian cities and to have experimented heavily with human subjects to gain information about biological warfare. It is impossible to know if all of these claims are true, or are merely legends to explain the numerous human plague cases that were documented during the war. During the Vietnam War (1954–1975), a vaccine for the plague had been developed and administered to the members of the U.S. Armed Services. Only eight cases were reported among U.S. troops in Vietnam, while the surrounding, unvaccinated population suffered 330 times more cases.

Not every disease can be weaponized to inflict biological warfare on a population. Anthrax, however, is considered ideal for this purpose. Anthrax occurs naturally in soil, and therefore does not have to be produced in a laboratory, and once acquired, it can be easily cultured. The anthrax spores are easily aerosolized, to produce a maximum amount of dispersion and damage. Following the anthrax attacks on the United States in 2001, the possibility of the intentional release of biological agents by

LONG-TERM HEALTH EFFECTS OF 9/11

More than 71,000 people who were affected by the terrorist attacks on the New York City World Trade Center in 2001 have been tracked by a health Registry was created in 2002. The World Trade Center Health Registry is comprehensive and confidential and tracks through the use of questionnaires those most directly exposed to the environmental and psychological events of 9/11. No blood tests or health tests are used for health tracking, and completion of the survey questionnaire is entirely voluntary.

In 2014 the registry reported that 9/11-related dust exposure had decreased the lung function of affected individuals even eight to nine years after the attacks. People who had sustained physical injuries from the attacks, such as broken bones and burns, were found to be at an increased risk of chronic diseases such as heart disease, diabetes, and cancer. Those who had suffered multiple injuries and post-traumatic stress disorder (PTSD; an anxiety disorder that can develop after exposure to a terrifying event or ordeal) symptoms reported heart disease at three times the expected rate. The greater the exposure and physical proximity to the towers' collapse, the more detrimental the long-term health effects have been.

A total of 343 New York City firefighters died on 9/11, and on September 11, 2014, three additional firefighters died from illnesses related to their duties as first responders to the scene that day. As of 2014, 92 firefighters who served on 9/11 had died, and 850 active, on duty, or retired firefighters who survived the initial attacks have been diagnosed with 9/11-related illnesses.

Other health effects suffered by direct victims of 9/11 include higher rates of PTSD and higher rates of binge drinking directly related to the extent of exposure to the event. The occurrence of diabetes is also higher in persons exposed to the attacks.

The most likely explanation for much of the illness suffered by 9/11 survivors is the toll that the chronic stress of the trauma has taken on their immune systems, the body's natural defenses. For example, stress hormones can cause cells to become resistant to insulin and cause blood sugar to spike, triggering full-blown diabetes. It is evident from these findings that the long-term health effects of terrorism and the stress and trauma of war change the public health of a conflict area and its residents years after the initial events take place.

At the time of 9/11 first responders had no way to know that their contributions to the rescue mission would have such devastating health consequences. The close tracking of their health conditions enables researchers and health professionals to anticipate and prepare for these types of health consequences should a devastating occurrence of this kind happen again. For example, first responders will know to wear gas masks and protective clothing to shield them from inhalants and debris. All findings from the World Trade Center Health Registry and detailed guidelines are shared with health professionals worldwide to help them to research and effectively prevent and treat disease occurrences in victims of terrorism.

combatants began to receive urgent attention. The immunization of the military became the greatest shield against the use of these threats. The World Health Organization estimated that 110 pounds (50 kilograms) of anthrax in aerosolized form could produce up to 125,000 infections and 95,000 fatalities in the correct environmental conditions. Improvement of the anthrax vaccines for use by civilians to prevent infection are currently underway.

⊕ Future Implications

With the exception of lasting world peace, the most effective way to mitigate the damages done by conflict, war, and terrorism is through preventive health measures such as vaccines and the rapid deployment of emergency aid. Sanitation in refugee camps is critical to halting the onset and spread of preventable diseases and infection. The international medical community is working to develop drugs to combat antibiotic resistant strains of disease, and vaccines like those created to prevent anthrax infection will become vital components of plans to mitigate the health risks of biological warfare.

Governments also have a critical role to play in the future of combating the ill health effects of conflict and war on their people. Using history as a guide, it is possible to anticipate the consequences of war and conflict and use best practices in war zones and refugee situations.

It is important to consider that while thorough preparation, research, and preventive measures will increase the survival rate for civilians and military personnel alike, the trauma of war will remain with the survivors for long after the conflicts have subsided. Coordinated strategies that include psychological therapies and supportive care to assist with the long-term consequences of conflict could dramatically improve the long-term health outcomes for victims, survivors, and affected countries.

PRIMARY SOURCE

UNHCR News Stories

SOURCE *Dunmore, Charlie. "Displaced at Two Weeks Old, Rahav Finds Safety in Iraq's Newest Camp." United Nations High Commissioner for Refugees (UNHCR) online, September 3, 2014. Copyright © 2014 United Nations High Commissioner for Refugees. http://www.unhcr.org/540727ac6.html (accessed January 25, 2015).*

INTRODUCTION *This primary source is an article released by the office of the United Nations High Commissioner for Refugees (UNHCR). It tells the story of one Iraqi family displaced by fighting in their village, and describes their dire circumstances living in a refugee camp.*

Displaced at two weeks old, Rahav finds safety in Iraq's newest camp

KHANKE VILLAGE, Iraq, September 3 (UNHCR)—One-month-old Rahav has spent most of her short life on the move. A fortnight after she was born, her parents joined thousands of other families from the Yazidi ethnic minority fleeing their homes after armed groups captured the northern Iraqi city of Sinjar in early August. Wrapped in a headscarf and sleeping peacefully in a broken wooden cradle, she appears blissfully unaware of the ordeal her family has been through. But as her mother Chenar watches over the baby and recounts their flight, the strain of the past several weeks is apparent.

"At 2a.m. they started attacking our village," she tells visitors from UNHCR, as she sits on the concrete floor of an old building where her family has been living since the middle of August. "So we escaped. We left our homes and ended up here."

Chenar and her husband Naif are among the latest to find shelter in the Kurdish region of northern Iraq. They will soon move to a new camp, currently home to 650 families and one of nine set up to provide safety and shelter to the 1.8 million people displaced inside Iraq this year. As more and more Iraqis flee worsening violence in the country, another six such camps are planned.

Chenar had a harrowing journey. After deciding to flee, she and Naif loaded Rahav and two young sons into their car, together with her father-in-law. They spent the next week driving from town to town in search of safety. At one point, their battered vehicle broke down and Chenar was forced to sell her jewellery to pay for the repairs so they could continue their escape.

"We had a very difficult journey. For three days we had no water and no food," she says. "The whole way until I ended up here I used to use an empty tomato crate for my baby to sleep in."

They finally reached the village of Khanke in Iraq's Kurdistan region, safe but destitute. Since then they have been living in the courtyard of a local public building with several other Yazidi families. They spend their days huddled under a corrugated iron awning to protect them from the fierce summer heat.

"When we arrived in Khanke, there was no one to help us," she says. "We slept on the bare floor, there were no toilets and we did not have water. We had to bathe in neighbours' houses."

Life in the courtyard has been a struggle. As a result, Chenar is pleased to learn that they have been allocated a place at a new camp in Khanke where they will receive a tent, mattresses, blankets and other essentials provided by UNHCR.

Work is under way to provide each tent with electricity and families with their own drinking water supply and sanitary facilities, but for now the camp at least offers more privacy than the courtyard.

"I'm not sure how life there will be, but I'm sure that it's going to be better than this place," says Chenar. Her biggest worry is how the family will cope during the coming winter, when temperatures plunge and heavy rainfall is common. Work has already begun a few hundred metres away to construct new tent foundations with concrete floors and walls that will offer greater protection during winter.

Later, after the family has moved with their few possessions into the new tent, Chenar busies herself, settling Rahav down and sprinkling water outside to keep the dust from blowing in. But her father-in-law sits cross-legged in a corner, buries his face in his hands and begins to weep.

"We all have the same pain, but my father-in-law is really heartbroken," she says. "Every time he looks around and sees us in this situation and in this place, he starts crying."

By Charlie Dunmore in Khanke Village, Iraq

SEE ALSO *Epidemiology: Surveillance for Emerging Infectious Diseases; Health-Care Worker Safety and Shortages; Médicins Sans Frontières; NGOs and Health Care: Deliverance or Dependence; Post-Traumatic Stress Syndrome; Vulnerable Populations*

BIBLIOGRAPHY

Books

Barry, John M. *The Great Influenza: The Epic Story of the Deadliest Plague in History.* New York: Viking, 2004.

Crenshaw, Martha. *Explaining Terrorism: Causes, Processes, and Consequences.* London: Routledge, 2011.

Farb, Daniel. *Bioterrorism Hemorrhagic Viruses.* Los Angeles: University of Health Care, 2004.

Fong, I. W., and Kenneth Alibek, eds. *Bioterrorism and Infectious Agents: A New Dilemma for the 21st Century.* New York: Springer, 2009.

Johnstone, R. William. *Bioterror: Anthrax, Influenza, and the Future of Public Health Security.* Westport, CT: Praeger Security International, 2008.

Kahn, Laura H. *Who's in Charge?: Leadership during Epidemics, Bioterror, Attacks, and Other Public Health Crises.* Santa Barbara, CA: Praeger Security International, 2009.

Langwith, Jacqueline. *Population, Resources, and Conflict.* Detroit: Greenhaven Press, 2011.

Radest, Howard B. *Bioethics: Catastrophic Events in a Time of Terror.* Lanham, MD: Lexington Books, 2009.

Zinsser, Hans. *Rats, Lice and History.* Boston: Little, Brown, 1935 (reprinted 1996).

Zubay, Geoffrey, et al., eds. *Agents of Bioterrorism Pathogens and Their Weaponization.* New York: Columbia University Press, 2010.

Periodicals

Al-Sabbak, M. "Metal Contamination and the Epidemic of Congenital Birth Defects in Iraqi Cities." *Bulletin of Environmental Contamination and Toxicology* 89, no. 5 (November 16, 2012): 937–944. Available online at http://link.springer.com/article/10.1007%2Fs00128-012-0817-2 (accessed April 8, 2015).

Websites

"Bioterrorism Agents/Diseases." *U.S. Centers for Disease Control and Prevention (CDC).* http://emergency.cdc.gov/agent/agentlist.asp (accessed January 14, 2015).

"Bioterrrorism Overview." *U.S. Centers for Disease Control and Prevention (CDC).* http://www.bt.cdc.gov/bioterrorism/overview.asp (accessed March 5, 2015).

"Burn Pits Fact Sheet." *U.S. Department of Veterans Affairs.* http://www.warrelatedillness.va.gov/education/factsheets/burn-pits.pdf (accessed April 8, 2015).

"Disasters and Conflicts." *United Nations Environment Programme (UNEP).* http://www.unep.org/disastersandconflicts/ (accessed January 14, 2015).

"The Health Crisis That's Plaguing War-Torn Syria." *Think Progress.* http://thinkprogress.org/health/2014/12/19/3605820/syria-conflict-health-crisis/ (accessed March 28, 2015).

Iraq Ministry of Health. "Summary of the Prevalence of Reported Congenital Birth Defects in 18 Selected Districts in Iraq." *World Health Organization (WHO), Eastern Mediterranean Region (EMRO).* http://www.emro.who.int/images/stories/iraq/documents/Congenital_birth_defects_report.pdf?ua=1 (accessed April 8, 2015).

"War and Public Health." *Health Alliance International.* http://www.healthallianceinternational.org/advancing-global-health/war-and-public-health/ (accessed March 30, 2015).

Wheelis, Mark. "Biological Warfare at the 1346 Siege of Caffa." *Emerging Infectious Diseases* 8, no. 9. September 2002. http://wwwnc.cdc.gov/eid/article/8/9/01-0536_article (accessed January 15, 2015).

"WTC Health Registry." *Office of the Mayor, New York City.* http://www.nyc.gov/html/doh/wtc/html/registry/registry.shtml (accessed January 15, 2015).

Margaret Loraine Scott

Cultural and Traditional Medicine

⊕ Introduction

Cultural and traditional medicine practices health care that is most closely associated with a specific national, ethnic, or racial identity. Cultural medicine often is made up of treatments that have been developed by a culture in isolation that is unique to that racial, national, or ethnic identity. Ayurvedic practices in India and traditional Chinese medicine (TCM) are examples of cultural medicine that could be considered as complementary or alternative to conventional Western medicine.

Culture influences not only the treatments that people seek but also the way people interact with conventional medicine. Even people from outside a culture may use a cultural medicine such as TCM to supplement conventional medicines for a variety of reasons. As the world has become more interconnected, information regarding cultural medicine has become more widely available and cultural medical options also have increased. Additionally, as more people turn to cultural medicine for treatment, the need for reliable data on these topics drives funding for scientific studies. Most funding for research on cultural medicine is provided through government grants.

Andrew Weil (1942–), a prominent American physician and director of the Arizona Center for Integrative Medicine at the University of Arizona, states on his website, "If our healthcare system is to achieve greatness, our medicine needs to return to its roots. It must focus again on the natural healing power of human beings. This means investing more in research that will help us understand the body's ability to defend itself from harm, regenerate damaged tissue and adapt to injury and loss."

Despite the increasing acceptance of some cultural medicine into conventional Western treatments, the outcomes used for examining the effectiveness of cultural medicine often are subjective or difficult to quantify and can vary across practices and region. These discrepancies also make replication of the study results challenging for researchers. Even with these barriers, cultural medical techniques receive the majority of their research funding from governmental agencies. Private industry research

funding is difficult for culturally based medical practices because of the inability to hold patents or intellectual property rights. In the United States the majority of public funding comes from the National Center for Complementary and Integrative Health (NCCIH; formerly the National Center for Complementary and Alternative Medicine, or NCCAM), a government agency responsible for the study and funding of both cultural medicine and alternative treatments that have arisen outside the bounds of conventional Western medicine.

Despite ongoing major advances in conventional Western medicine, many people turn to cultural medicine when they find themselves disappointed in either the outcome or practice of their conventional treatments. The increased number of patients seeking other options is changing the way conventional practices and doctors are approaching their treatment.

People from other cultures turn to traditional or cultural medicine for a variety of reasons, all deeply personal and individualized. Some of those reasons are:

- the failure of more conventional medical treatments to provide results
- a connection with the complementary and alternative medicine treatment chosen
- a desire to be actively involved in their own treatment
- the high costs associated with conventional medicine

Doctors have recognized the possibility for abuse, which is one of the reasons why they have begun to embrace cultural medicine—so that during treatment the patient has adequate supervision. Perhaps, with the integration of cultural and conventional medicine, new advancements will be made to improve general health and medical treatments.

⊕ Historical Background

The history of cultural medicine is much longer than the history of the medical practices many in the West consider conventional. Humans have likely been treating their

NATIONAL CENTER FOR COMPLEMENTARY AND INTEGRATIVE HEALTH (NCCIH)

The National Center for Complementary and Integrative Health (NCCIH; formerly the National Center for Complementary and Alternative Medicine, or NCCAM) is the government agency responsible for the scientific research and dissemination of information regarding complementary and alternative medicine (CAM) in the United States. NCCIH categorizes CAM into two separate domains: natural products (herbs, vitamins, minerals, probiotics, etc.) and mind-body interventions (acupuncture, mindfulness meditation, spinal manipulations, yoga, tai chi or qi gong, and massage therapies).

NCCIH's goals outlined in its strategic plan include: (1) advancing the science and practice of symptom management, (2) developing effective, practical, and personalized strategies for promoting health and well-being, and (3) enabling better evidence-based decision making regarding CAM use and its integration into health care and health promotion.

Originally established as the Office of Alternative Medicine in 1991, NCCIH operates under the U.S. National Institutes of Health (NIH). Research priorities for NCCIH include basic and translational investigations into the underlying biological effects and mechanisms of CAM therapies and observational and/or clinical studies on their effectiveness in "real-world" settings. Chronic pain management, reduction of inflammatory responses, and improved health and wellness are considered special research interests of NCCIH research.

NCCIH also is invested in creating well-trained clinical researchers in various CAM fields of expertise. Combining the experience of knowledgeable CAM practitioners with well-trained biomedical and behavioral scientists, NCCIH's strategic plan includes fostering and creating interdisciplinary partnerships that can expand the evidence base for CAM therapies.

Since 2004, NCCIH has funded research for more than 2,500 projects, resulting in the publication of more than 3,000 articles in peer-reviewed scientific journals. Published reports and national survey responses suggest that NCCIH research influences American consumer choices of CAM products. For example, fish oil and omega-3 fatty acid use increased between 2003 and 2007 after evidence emerged supporting health benefits of the dietary supplement. Conversely, the use of echinacea and St. John's wort declined following reports of dangerous drug interactions, ineffectiveness, and harmful side effects.

In 2014, the peer-reviewed journal *Nutrition* published a collection of findings from the Botanical Research Centers program. The special edition outlined how certain herbs—specifically *Artemisia dracunculus*—can be used to slow the progression of factors related to the development of metabolic syndrome (a set of conditions that usually include obesity centered around the waist, high blood pressure, abnormal cholesterol levels, and insulin resistance). Located in Louisiana State University's Pennington Biomedical Research Center and Rutgers University's Department of Plant Biology and Pathology, the Botanical Research Center receives the majority of its funding from NCCIH and NIH's Office of Dietary Supplements. Established in 1998, this center is a cornerstone for the collaborative approach to investigating the use of herbs and botanicals in medicine. The center also studies supplements that have a high potential for being translated into benefits for human health.

In October 2014, NCCIH's director, Dr. Josephine Briggs (1947–), issued a statement regarding the funding of several research projects related to the nondrug management of pain and related conditions among military veterans. A disproportionate number of veterans in United States suffer from chronic pain, post-traumatic stress disorders, depression, anxiety, and sleep disturbances. NCCIH-funded projects are aimed at developing self-management techniques, new technologies, and analytic methods for conducting needs assessments into who is suffering from chronic pain and what remedies they are currently seeking.

own, as well as others', ailments for long before recorded time. The earliest recordings of plants and herbs in medicine can be traced to the Third Dynasty of Ur in about 2000 BCE. Written in Sumerian, these texts indicate that most herbal remedies were used to treat gastrointestinal, dermatological, and respiratory ailments. Common herbs used in medicine include ginseng, hoodia, yohimbe, and valerian root.

Healing techniques also were recorded by the ancient Egyptians, Babylonians, and ancient Indians. The oldest medical system known to humans is Siddha medicine, reported to have been created more than 10,000 years ago. The practice of Indian Ayurvedic medicine has its roots in this ancient branch of a three-part Indian medicine, which was not recorded until the early Iron Age somewhere between 1200 to 300 BCE. According to H. F. J. Horstmanshoff and others, in *Magic and Rationality in Ancient Near Eastern and Graeco-Roman Medicine*, the Babylonians were recording medicinal texts by the first half of 2000 BCE. The most extensive Babylonian medical text is the *Diagnostic Handbook*, which contains methods of therapy and etiology as well as the practices of diagnosis, prognosis, and physical examination, already established by the Egyptians, Babylonians, and Indians. The Egyptians furthered medical care with the creation of an extensive tradition of a public health care system and doctor specialization that in many ways mirrors the conventional medicine that is practiced in the 21st century.

In China, traditional medicine holds a place of great importance in the health-care system and boasts a long history, having started somewhere between the 3rd and 5th centuries CE, according to Frank Dikötter in *The Cambridge History of Science*. During the Tang dynasty, the standard practice of medicine was revised, and now can be considered the most accurate foundation for the TCM that still exists. Like Ayurvedic medicine, TCM has a strong foothold in its country of origin.

⊕ Impacts and Issues

Traditional Chinese Medicine

TCM is a broad set of treatment practices including acupuncture, herbal medicine, dietary therapy, massage, and various forms of meditation and exercise (called tai chi or qi gong). The earliest documentation of TCM practices occurred during the Shang dynasty (1600–1046 BCE). Two seminal publications during the Qin and Han dynasties (221 BCE–220 CE) established the theoretical and clinical systems upon which TCM is built. The first text, *The Classic of Internal Medicine*, introduced the concept of qi, described as the human body's, "vital energy force." Qi travels through the body via channels called meridians, forming an interconnected pathway between human organs and their functions. The second publication, *The Treatise on Exogenous Febrile Diseases and Miscellaneous Diseases*, outlined the diagnosis and treatment recommendations for various ailments and pathologies.

According to TCM methodology, an imbalance between life's two energy forces, yin and yang, is used to explain human illnesses, maladies, and affliction. Treatment often involves identifying the source of energy imbalance and prescribing a variety of possible treatments. The Chinese *Materia Medica* is the pharmacological reference for TCM herbal remedies.

TCM and Herbal Medicine   In TCM, herbs are prescribed according to the patient's individual condition and not only on the basis of acute current symptoms. Herbal medicines are used to regulate the natural balance of the body and restore health. They come in the form of pills or powders, as tea and raw herbs taken internally, or as balms for external use. Chinese herbal medicine has been used for centuries to treat most health conditions and as a preventive dietary supplement. This same idea has made its way into mainstream western culture, with mixed results. Supplements such as St. John's wort, which is used to stabilize a person's mood, or *Ginkgo biloba*, used to enhance mental functioning, are used commonly by traditionally Western culture. Clinically, it has been found that St. John's wort performs better than placebos in clinical trials, as detailed in an article published in 2008 by Klaus Linde, Michael M. Berner, and Levente Kriston.

Acupuncture   TCM also has brought the practice of acupuncture to the West, and the practice has grown dramatically since the mid-1990s. According to TCM, stimulating specific points in the body channels the flow of qi through organized channels in the body, in order to restore internal balance. Qi is translated roughly as

"breath," "air," or "gas," but interpreted to mean the "life force" of a person. The balance of qi is the underlying principle of TCM. Acupuncture is the practice of inserting long, thin needles into a person's skin at specific pressure points to help direct qi onto the correct channels. Some scientific research seems to suggest that acupuncture can provide a positive effect in the treatment of chronic pain. It is noted in Harriet Beinfield and Efrem Korngold's *Between Heaven and Earth: A Guide to Chinese Medicine* that it also is used for conditions such as insomnia, nausea, migraines, and fertility. Most studies suggest that the positive effects are due mainly to the placebo effect. The placebo effect is the phenomenon that occurs when ineffective medicine is administered to an unknowing patient, but the mere administration of it provides whatever effect was desired by the patient.

Reiki, Qi Gong, and Meditation   Reiki and qi gong are techniques developed by the Chinese and adopted by the Japanese to channel the same energies acupuncture seeks to direct, and they often are used together. Reiki is a technique that is performed by others or on oneself to

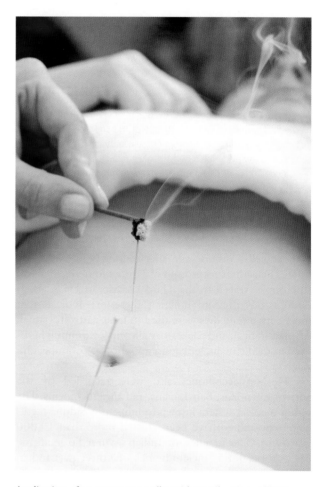

Application of acupuncture needles with moxibustion, a TCM therapy that uses the burning of mugwort, a dried herb, to facilitate healing. © *Neeila/Shutterstock.com.*

heal the internal imbalances of qi. When used on others, the practitioner places his or her hands in specific areas of the body to transfer energy through the practitioner's palms to allow for self-healing. Many medical organizations, including the American Cancer Society and NCCIH, concur that there is no benefit from Reiki when used as a medical treatment, as detailed by Myeong Soo Lee, M. H. Pittler, and Edzard Ernst in a 2008 article in the *International Journal of Clinical Practice*. Similarly, qi gong is the practice of aligning the body, breath, and mind to balance the qi. Qi gong typically involves moving meditation, similar to yoga, in which breathing and focus on body help to calm the mind. The effectiveness of qi gong is yet unknown, and past clinical trials have been unclear, but no harmful effects have been found.

Finally, most practitioners of conventional medicine know how important the power of a healthy mind is over physical health. Meditation, hypnosis, and sensory stimulation (music, art, dance) all use the mind's existing resources to promote physical well-being. Meditation originated in religious contexts, but subsequently assumed a variety of secular forms. Both qi gong and Reiki have a meditative component. With the ability to measure the benefits and physical changes caused by a meditative practice, scientists have found a number of measureable changes. Studies have found that meditation may reduce blood pressure, ease menopausal symptoms, and even help relieve cancer symptoms and their treatment's side effects.

Ayurveda

The Indian system of traditional medicine, called Ayurvedic medicine, is a series of medicinal preparations, and surgical procedures used to improve overall health. Ayurvedic medicine is highly integrated into the healthcare system in India, and relies on the fundamental aspect of considering a holistic approach during diagnosis and therapy. Multiple state-run hospitals exclusively practicing Ayurveda exist throughout India despite there being no scientific evidence for its effectiveness.

Ayurvedic medicine was developed in India between 2000 and 1000 BCE.The term is derived from the Sanskrit words *ayur* (life), and *veda* (knowledge). Ayurvedic treatments include the prescription of herbal or proprietary compounds, dietary recommendations, physical activity, massage techniques, and other lifestyle changes. Originally documented in the Rigveda (2000 BCE) and the Atharvaveda (1500–1000 BCE), healing compounds

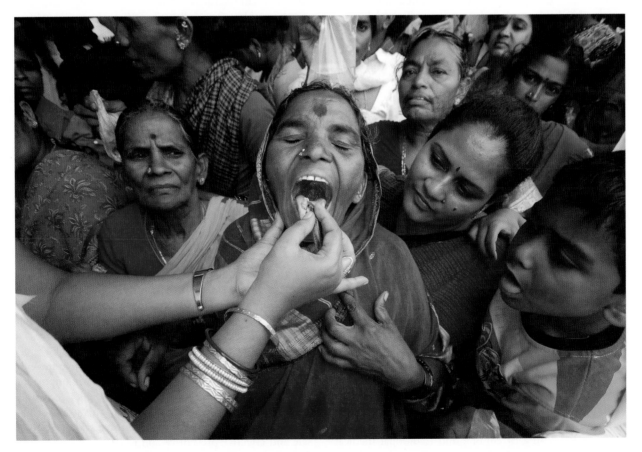

A member of the Bathini family, only hands seen, administers "fish medicine" to an asthma patient in Hyderabad, India. Started by the Bathini Goud family, the therapy is a secret formula of herbs, handed down by generations only to family members. The herbs are inserted in the mouth of a live sardine or murrel fish and slipped into a patient's throat. © *Mahesh Kumar A/AP Images.*

were derived from plant sources and regularly used in early Indian medicine. In 1000 BCE, respected scholars from the schools of medicine and surgery passed on their knowledge in two central texts, the *Charaka Samhita* and *Sushruta Samhita.*

An underlying theory of Ayurveda is that the human body and universe are linked, and the same principles govern both. Health is seen as an equilibrium maintained between three life forces referred to as Doshas: Vata, Pitta, and Kapha. Vata governs the nervous system, Pitta regulates the endocrine and glandular activities, and Kapha controls the musculoskeletal and anabolic systems. Illnesses and diseases are the result of imbalances between Doshas, hence treatments are designed specifically for each individual with the intention of regaining a natural state of balance, termed agni.

Pharmacological treatments and compounds are made of plants (e.g., roots, leaves, and berries), animal substances (e.g., milk, fats, and oils), and minerals (e.g., lead, copper sulfate, and gold). In the United States deep concerns have been raised about the products promoted as being related to Ayurvedic medicine, and researchers found that many of the Indian-manufactured products contained harmful amounts of toxic substances such as lead, mercury, and arsenic, as noted in the 2008 article "Lead, Mercury, and Arsenic in US- and Indian-Manufactured Medicines Sold via the Internet" by Robert Saper and others, published in *JAMA*. It is vital for those who consider Ayurvedic medicine as a complementary or alternative option to be made aware of the inherent risks associated with the treatment and acknowledge that unscrupulous providers take advantage of the association with Ayurvedic's cultural history.

Faith Healing

Faith healing varies across cultures and religious ideologies, but generally involves calling upon divine powers to alleviate disease, sickness, or injury. The patient's belief is used in combination with the faith healer's ability to channel the patient's faith into curing the illness or disease. Faith healing traditions exist in most of the major religions in the world, including Christianity, Islam, and Hinduism.

Safety and Oversight

In 2006, the WHO established the International Regulatory Cooperation for Herbal Medicines (IRCH) to monitor and regulate herbal compounds. Since its establishment, the IRCH's primary activities have been fostering collaboration and facilitating dialogue among national drug regulatory authorities. The WHO recommends national health authorities address the regulation and licensing of cultural and traditional medical techniques being practiced in their countries. In order to ensure patient safety, the WHO also advises that its member states establish criteria for recognizing professional

conduct and quality standards. Whereas some countries have the infrastructure to require university-level training for practicing cultural and traditional medicine, in less developed countries this knowledge is transferred orally across generations. In some circumstances, drastic differences and the lack of an agreed-upon threshold for expertise can make it difficult for consumers to identify a knowledgeable provider. In such cases, the WHO advises local health authorities to register or regulate practices.

In the United States, the Food and Drug Administration (FDA) has issued warnings on fraudulent claims made by medical products claiming to be "traditional" and implying effectiveness. One warning is in regard to products manufactured by Washington Homeopathic Products Inc., in 2009. The FDA issued multiple letters to the manufacturer regarding concerns surrounding broken glass found their products, cross-contamination risks, and inadequate microbial testing techniques. Another letter was issued to the Guilin Hospital of Sino-western Medicine regarding the false claims and sales of treatments used for the H1N1 flu virus. The company's website contained multiple statements claiming Chinese herbal teas and formulas could be used to cure the flu virus, such as "Traditional Chinese Medicine should be chosen to cut the throat of swine flu." Although the FDA regulates cultural remedies, the agency does not evaluate these products for safety or effectiveness.

⊕ Future Implications

In 2003, the WHO issued a resolution encouraging its member states to support the development of policies and regulations regarding the use of alternative and cultural medical practices. The WHO also recommended that member states begin integrating alternative and cultural medicines into their existing health systems wherever possible.

The WHO predicts that the increased use of alternative and cultural medicine by consumers and practitioners will lessen the global disease burden. The WHO's updated "Traditional Medicine Strategy: 2014–2023" declared its two key goals are: to support Member States in harnessing the potential contribution of T&CM to health, wellness and people-centred health care and to promote the safe and effective use of T&CM through the regulation of products, practices and practitioners.

As countries gradually shift toward providing individuals with universal health coverage, alternative and cultural medical therapies will continue to play an important role in providing consumers with affordable, accessible treatment options. Also included in this transformation is the ability for consumers to use a wide variety of safe and effective preventive and rehabilitative remedies. The director-general of the WHO, Dr. Margaret Chan (1947–) stated in a 2008 address at the WHO Congress on Traditional Medicine: "The two systems of traditional and Western medicine need not clash. Within the context of primary health care, they can blend together in a beneficial harmony, using the best features of each system, and compensating for certain weaknesses in each."

PRIMARY SOURCE

Folk Remedy–Associated Lead Poisoning in Hmong Children—Minnesota

SOURCE *"Folk Remedy–Associated Lead Poisoning in Hmong Children—Minnesota," from* Morbidity and Mortality Weekly Report (MMWR) *32, no. 42, (October 28, 1983): 555–556. Centers for Disease Control and Prevention (CDC). http://www. cdc.gov/mmwr/preview/mmwrhtml/00000165. htm (accessed January 25, 2015).*

INTRODUCTION *This primary source is the full text of an article in the* Morbidity and Mortality Weekly Report (MMWR), *a weekly epidemiological journal of the U.S. Centers for Disease Control and Prevention (CDC). According to the CDC website, the* MMWR *"contains data on specific diseases as reported by state and territorial health departments and reports on infectious and chronic diseases, environmental hazards, natural or human-generated disasters, occupational diseases and injuries, and intentional and unintentional injuries." The* MMWR *article addresses lead poisoning in children that was related to folk remedies among Hmong children in Minnesota in 1983. Though the case mentioned in the* MMWR *is from more than 20 years ago, such folk treatments continue to be of concern to the CDC, as noted on its website (http://www.cdc.gov/nceh/lead/tips/ folkmedicine.htm [accessed April 8, 2015]): "Lead has been found in some traditional (folk) medicines used by East Indian, Indian, Middle Eastern, West Asian, and Hispanic cultures…. Lead has been found in powders and tablets given for arthritis, infertility, upset stomach, menstrual cramps, colic and other illnesses." The CDC warns that "Consuming even small amounts of lead can be harmful. There is no safe blood lead level. Lead poisoning from folk medicines can cause illness and even death."*

Folk Remedy–Associated Lead Poisoning in Hmong Children—Minnesota

Between January 1, and June 30, 1983, 35 children with lead toxicity were identified through routine screening by the St. Paul, Minnesota, Division of Public Health. Of these, 24 (69 percent) were Hmong refugees from Northern Laos. This represents a twofold to threefold increase in the number of Hmong children found to have lead toxicity in St. Paul compared with previous years. One source of lead poisoning appears to be a Hmong folk remedy used for treating infants and children with fevers. A case report follows:

On May 3, 1983, a 6-month-old Hmong girl was found to have lead poisoning (blood lead (BL) 60 ug/dl [micrograms per deciliter], erythrocyte protoporphyrin 263 ug/dl, hematocrit 38 percent) during screening for well-baby care. She was asymptomatic at the time. Her physical examination was unremarkable. X-ray films of the wrists and knees revealed dense provisional zones of calcification suggestive of lead deposits. No environmental sources of lead, such as paint, could be identified after a thorough investigation of the family's home. After detailed questioning by the child's pediatrician, the parents admitted giving red and orange powders to the baby as a cure for high fever. Laboratory analysis of the red powder showed a lead concentration of 8 percent. The infant was given ethylene diamine tetraacetic acid (EDTA) chelation therapy as an outpatient.

Officials have been unable to obtain samples of the folk remedy from the parents of other Hmong children with lead poisoning. The remedy, generally referred to as "pay-loo-ah," consists of red and orange powders, the composition and source of which often vary; therefore, a more exact description of the material remains difficult. Believed to have originated in China or Southeast Asia, pay-loo-ah is fed to children as a cure for fever or rash. Samples of folk remedies were obtained from several Hmong households in the community, and the U.S. Food and Drug Administration confirmed that two contained lead (1% and 90%). Arsenic was found in three samples at concentrations of 70%–80%. These folk remedies were in wide use and were easily available through local Asian food stores or Hmong peddlers. To date, no cases of arsenic poisoning in the Hmong children have been reported. Reported by C Levitt, MD, Children's Hospital, St. Paul, D Paulson, MD, K Duvall, MPH, J Godes, MPH, St. Paul Div of Public Health, AG Dean, MD, State Epidemiologist, Minnesota State Dept of Health; J Roberts, J Egenberger, Minneapolis District, US Food and Drug Administration; Special Studies Br, Chronic Diseases Div, Center for Environmental Health, CDC.

Editorial Note

Editorial Note: Folk remedies have been known to cause lead poisoning. A Mexican folk medicine, azarcon, has been reported to cause lead poisoning in Mexican children in a number of southwestern states (1,2). Hmong refugees, who have emigrated from North Laos, have an estimated total population over 50,000 and live in many parts of the United States, with the largest concentrations in Fresno, Stockton, and San Diego, California, in addition to St. Paul.

Health-care providers for Hmong and Southeast Asians should be aware of this unusual lead source. Screening for elevated blood lead levels is necessary to identify additional cases, because symptoms of lead toxicity generally have not been reported by the Hmong. Reporting of cases to local or state health departments is recommended. Appropriate health education will be necessary to inform the Hmong of the health consequences associated with this folk remedy.

Lead poisoning resulting from folk remedies exemplifies the need to continue screening young children for lead toxicity. CDC recommends routine screening of EP [erythrocyte protoporphyrin] of all children between 6 months and 5 years of age. An EP level of over the CDC recommendation of 50 ug/dl indicates either iron deficiency anemia or lead toxicity (3). Lead toxicity should then be confirmed by a blood lead level.

SEE ALSO *Complementary and Alternative Medicine; Health as a Human Right and Health-Care Access; Health-Related Education and Information Access; Pharmaceutical Research, Testing, and Access; Universal Health Coverage; World Health Organization: Organization, Funding, and Enforcement Powers*

BIBLIOGRAPHY

Books

Balch, Phyllis, and Stacey J. Bell. *Prescription for Herbal Healing*, 2nd ed. New York: Avery, 2012.

Baran, George R., Mohammad F. Kiani, and Solomon P. Samuel. "Science, Pseudoscience, and Not Science: How Do They Differ?" In *Healthcare and Biomedical Technology in the 21st Century: An Introduction for Non-science Majors*, 19–58. New York: Springer, 2013.

Bauer, Brent, et al. *Mayo Clinic Book of Alternative Medicine*, 2nd ed. New York: Time Inc. Home Entertainment Books, 2010.

Beinfield, Harriet, and Efrem Korngold. *Between Heaven and Earth: A Guide to Chinese Medicine*. New York: Ballantine Books, 1991.

Cotter, Ann C., Samuel C. Shiflett, and David Kuo. "Complementary and Alternative Medicine." In *Physical Medicine & Rehabilitation: Principles and Practice*, Vol. 1, 4th ed., Joel L. DeLisa and Bruce M. Gans, eds. Philadelphia: Lippincott Williams & Wilkins, 2005.

Dikötter, Frank *The Cambridge History of Science*, Vol. 4: *18th Century Science*. New York: Cambridge University Press, 2008.

Haehl, Richard. *Samuel Hahnemann: His Life and Work: Based on Recently Discovered State Papers, Documents, Letters, &c.* New Delhi: B. Jain, 1922; reprint 1995.

Horstmanshoff, H. F. J., Martin Stol, and C. R. van Tilburg. *Magic and Rationality in Ancient Near Eastern and Graeco-Roman Medicine*. Leiden, Netherlands: Brill, 2004.

Leach, Robert. *The Chiropractic Theories: A Textbook of Scientific Research*, 4th ed. Philadelphia: Lippincott, Williams and Wilkins, 2004.

O'Reilly, Wenda, ed. *The Organon of the Healing Art by Dr. Samuel Hahnemann*, 6th ed. Redmond, WA: Birdcage Press, 2010.

Schultz, Andrea M., Samantha M. Chao, and J. Michael McGinnis. *Integrative Medicine and the Health of the Public: A Summary of the February 2009 Summit*. Washington, DC: National Academies Press, 2009.

Sointu, Eeva. *Theorizing Complementary and Alternative Medicines: Wellbeing, Self, Gender, Class*. New York: Palgrave Macmillan, 2012.

Stux, Gabriel, Brian Berman, and Bruce Pomeranz. *Basics of Acupuncture*, 5th ed. New York: Springer, 2003.

Yang, Yifan. *Chinese Herbal Medicines: Comparisons and Characteristics*, 2nd ed. New York: Elsevier, 2010.

Periodicals

Ernst, Edzard. "The Public's Enthusiasm for Complementary and Alternative Medicine Amounts to a Critique of Mainstream Medicine." *International Journal of Clinical Practice* 64, no. 11 (October 2010): 1472–1474.

Gorski, David H., and Steven P. Novella. "Clinical Trials of Integrative Medicine: Testing Whether Magic Works?" *Trends in Molecular Medicine* 20, no. 9 (September 2014): 473–476.

Juckett, Gregory. "Cross-Cultural Medicine." *American Family Physician*, 72, no. 11 (December 1, 2006): 2267–2274. Available online at http://www.aafp.org (accessed January 18, 2015).

Kupferschmidt, Kai. "Scourge of Snake Oil Salesmen Bids an Early Farewell." *Science* 333, no. 6043 (August 5, 2011): 687.

Lee, Myeong Soo, M. H. Pittler, and Edzard Ernst. "Effects of Reiki in Clinical Practice: A Systematic Review of Randomized Clinical Trials." *International Journal of Clinical Practice* 62, no. 6 (June 2008): 947–954.

Linde, Klaus, Michael M. Berner, and Levente Kriston. "St John's Wort for Major Depression." *Cochrane Database of Systematic Reviews* 4, no. CD000448 (October 8, 2008). Available online at http://summaries.cochrane.org/CD000448/DEPRESSN_st.-johns-wort-for-treating-depression (accessed January 18, 2015).

Marcus, Donald M., and Arthur P. Grollman. "Science and Government: Review for NCCAM Is Overdue." *Science* 313, no. 5785 (July 21, 2006): 301–302.

Oumeish, Oumeish Youssef. "The Philosophical, Cultural, and Historical Aspects of Complementary, Alternative, Unconventional, and Integrative Medicine in the Old World." *Archives of Dermatology* 134, no. 11 (November 1998): 1373–1386.

Saper, Robert B., et al. "Lead, Mercury, and Arsenic in US- and Indian-Manufactured Medicines Sold via the Internet." *JAMA* 300, no. 8 (August 2008): 915–923.

Servick, Kelly. "Outsmarting the Placebo Effect." *Science* 345, no. 6203 (September 19, 2014) 1446–1447.

Wieland, L. Susan, Eric Manheimer, and Brian M. Berman. "Development and Classification of an Operational Definition of Complementary and Alternative Medicine for the Cochrane Collaboration." *Alternative Therapies in Health and Medicine* 17, no. 2 (March/April 2011): 50–59.

Websites

"Acupuncture: Definition." *Mayo Clinic*. http://www.mayoclinic.org/tests-procedures/acupuncture/basics/definition/prc-20020778 (accessed January 20, 2015).

"Benchmarks for Training in Ayurveda." *World Health Organization (WHO)*, 2010. http://apps.who.int/medicinedocs/en/m/abstract/Js17552en/ (accessed January 20, 2015).

"Benchmarks for Training in Naturopathy." *World Health Organization (WHO)*, 2010. http://apps.who.int/medicinedocs/en/m/abstract/Js17553en/ (accessed January 20, 2015).

"Benchmarks for Training in Traditional Chinese Medicine." *World Health Organization (WHO)*, 2010. http://apps.who.int/medicinedocs/en/m/abstract/Js17556en/ (accessed January 20, 2015).

Brown, David. "Critics Object to 'Pseudoscience' Center." *Washington Post*, March 17, 2009. http://www.washingtonpost.com/wp-dyn/content/article/2009/03/16/AR2009031602139.html (accessed January 18, 2015).

Chan, Margaret. "Address at the WHO Congress on Traditional Medicine." *World Health Organization (WHO)*, November 7, 2008. http://www.who.int/dg/speeches/2008/20081107/en/ (accessed May 27, 2015).

"Chinese Herbal Medicine." *American Cancer Society*. http://www.cancer.org/treatment/treatmentsandsideeffects/complementaryandalternativemedicine/herbsvitaminsandminerals/chinese-herbal-medicine (accessed January 20, 2015).

Cochrane Collaboration. http://www.cochrane.org/ (accessed January 20, 2015).

"Complementary, Alternative, or Integrative Health: What's in a Name?" *National Center for Complementary and Integrative Health.* http://nccih.nih.gov/health/integrative-health (accessed January 20, 2015).

"Funding Strategy." *National Center for Complementary and Integrative Health.* http://nccih.nih.gov/grants/strategy (accessed January 21, 2015).

"NCCIH Facts-at-a-Glance and Mission." *National Center for Complementary and Integrative Health.* http://nccih.nih.gov/about/ataglance (accessed January 21, 2015).

"Quality Control Methods for Herbal Materials." *World Health Organization (WHO).* http://apps.who.int/medicinedocs/en/m/abstract/Jh1791e/ (accessed November 15, 2014).

"Research Funding Priorities." *National Center for Complementary and Integrative Health.* http://nccih.nih.gov/grants/priorities (accessed January 21, 2015).

"Safety Issues in the Preparation of Homeopathic Medicines." *World Health Organization (WHO)*, 2010. http://apps.who.int/medicinedocs/en/m/abstract/Js16769e/ (accessed January 21, 2015).

"Traditional and Complementary Medicine Policy. (MDS-3: Managing Access to Medicines and Health Technologies, Chapter 5)." *World Health Organization (WHO)*, 2012. http://apps.who.int/medicinedocs/en/m/abstract/Js19582en/ (accessed January 21, 2015).

"Traditional Medicines: Definitions." *World Health Organization (WHO)*, 2000. http://www.who.int/medicines/areas/traditional/definitions/en/ (accessed December 17, 2014).

Weil, Andrew. "Meet Dr. Weil." *DrWeil.com.* http://www.drweil.com/drw/u/ART03076/A-Health-Care-Call-to-Action-by-Andrew-Weil-MD.html (accessed May 27, 2015).

"WHO Guidelines on Basic Training and Safety in Chiropractic." *World Health Organization (WHO)*, 2005. http://apps.who.int/medicinedocs/en/m/abstract/Js14076e/ (accessed January 21, 2015).

"WHO Traditional Medicine Strategy: 2014–2023." *World Health Organization (WHO)*, 2013. http://apps.who.int/medicinedocs/en/m/abstract/Js21201en/ (accessed January 21, 2015).

Margaret Loraine Scott
Martin Frigaard

Dengue

⊕ Introduction

Dengue is a mosquito-borne viral infection afflicting tropical and subtropical regions of the world. Symptoms of the disease include high fever, severe headache, joint and muscle pain, and rash, among other flu like symptoms. Dengue hemorrhagic fever and dengue shock syndrome are more severe forms of dengue fever and can be fatal if not properly treated. There is no specific treatment or approved vaccine for dengue fever.

More than one-third of the world lives in areas at risk of dengue. The World Health Organization (WHO) estimates that between 50 million and 100 million people are infected with dengue every year. Worldwide, there are approximately 500,000 cases of dengue hemorrhagic fever annually. More than 20,000 people die of dengue every year, primarily children. It is one of the most important mosquito-transmitted diseases in the world along with malaria and yellow fever.

With the geographic spread of mosquitoes that carry the disease, the number of cases of dengue fever has reached epidemic proportions. Before 1970, only nine countries had severe dengue epidemics. Dengue was endemic in 2014, meaning it occurs naturally every year, in more than 100 countries in the Americas, Asia, Africa, and Oceania. Between 2004 and 2010, Brazil was the most highly endemic country in the world for dengue, followed by Indonesia, Vietnam, and Mexico, according to the WHO.

Dengue is a virus spread primarily by the bite of female mosquitoes of the species *Aedes aegypti*, also known as the yellow fever mosquito, although there are additional species capable of serving as the vector for dengue. Humans represent the reservoir of the virus. There are four known closely related subtypes of the dengue virus, dubbed serotypes: *DENV 1, DENV 2, DENV 3,* and *DENV 4*. A fifth serotype, *DENV 5*, was discovered in Malaysia in 2007, although it does not seem to be sustained in human populations. Once infected, a person becomes immune to that particular dengue serotype.

Subsequent infections by a different serotype are generally more severe and can result in the development of a more serious condition resulting in dengue hemorrhagic fever or dengue shock syndrome.

⊕ Historical Background

The first record of a disease with symptoms resembling those of dengue fever was in the Chinese *Encyclopedia of Disease Symptoms and Remedies* published during the Jin dynasty between 265 and 420 CE. Outbreaks of illnesses that matched the symptoms of dengue fever were recorded on the Caribbean islands of Martinique and Guadeloupe in 1635 and in Panama in 1699. "Thus, a dengue-like illness had a wide geographic distribution before the 18th century," writes Duane J. Gulder in *New Treatment Strategies for Dengue and Other Flaviviral Diseases,* published by the Novartis Foundation.

The disease most likely gets its name from the Swahili phrase *Ki-Dinga pepo,* used during dengue like epidemics in Zanzibar and the coast of East Africa in 1823 and 1870. The West-Indian Spanish word *dengue* means careful or fastidious, which could also describe the care used in walking or moving by people afflicted with the bone pain of dengue.

During an epidemic in Cuba in 1828, the illness was called *dunga,* though later accounts used the word *dengue*. Medical historians have pointed out that in many cases dengue may have been confused with chikungunya, and vice versa, due to similar fever like symptoms and bone pain. Observations from past outbreaks pinpoint dengue as the probable cause of illnesses in the 18th and 19th centuries in colonists in tropical Asia, Australia, the Caribbean, and the Mississippi basin of the United States.

Molecular evidence shows that modern dengue probably evolved approximately 1,000 years ago. It most likely moved from a monkey-mosquito cycle to a human-mosquito cycle between 125 and 320 years ago, concludes the University of Oxford's S. Susanna Twiddy and

Global Dengue Risk, 2012

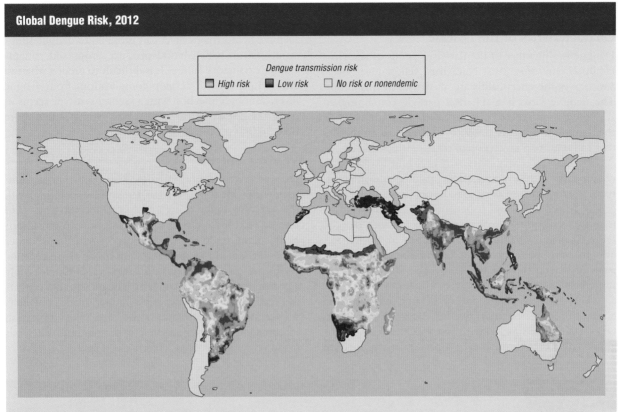

Dengue transmission risk

☐ High risk   ■ Low risk   ☐ No risk or nonendemic

SOURCE: Adapted from "Figure 2. Distribution of global dengue risk (determination of risk status based on combined reports from WHO, the United States Centers for Disease Control and Prevention, Gideon online, ProMED, DengueMap, Eurosurveillance and published literature (Simmons CP et al, 2012)," in *Global Strategy for Dengue Prevention and Control 2012–2020*, World Health Organization (WHO), 2012, p. 2, http://apps.who.int/iris/bitstream/10665/75303/1/9789241504034_eng.pdf (accessed January 15, 2015).

The risk of dengue fever is highest in tropical and subtropical regions of the world due to it being a mosquito-borne viral infection.

colleagues in their article "Inferring the Rate and Time-Scale of Dengue Virus Evolution" in the journal *Molecular Biology and Evolution*. The dengue virus transmits between mosquitoes and nonhuman primates in jungle environments, the so-called sylvatic cycle. "Evidence suggests that the human dengue virus evolved as a parasite of subhuman primates," states Scott Halstead in his book *Dengue*. He continues, "The probable spread from Africa during historical times of *Aedes aegypti* throughout the world created an ecological niche permitting an urban transmission cycle."

Historians recorded the first outbreaks of severe dengue (dengue complicated by hemorrhage) from 1897 to 1902 in Australia, in 1928 in Greece, and in 1931 in Taiwan. Subsequent outbreaks during the 1950s represented a resurgence of dengue. In the 1950s, dengue hemorrhagic fever outbreaks occurred in the Philippines and Thailand. Sporadic reports of dengue hemorrhagic fever originated from Curaçao, Honduras, Jamaica, and Puerto Rico in the late 1960s and 1970s. During the 1980s and 1990s there was a marked geographic spread of the disease in South America, infecting people from Venezuela, Peru, Brazil, and as far south as Argentina. A Cuban outbreak of dengue hemorrhagic fever that

began in 1981 marked the start of severe dengue in the Americas that continued into the 2010s.

Dengue was isolated first in August 1942 during a Japanese outbreak. Tens of thousands of soldiers fighting in the Pacific during World War II (1939–1945) came down with dengue fever. Scientists injected blood taken from infected patients into the brains of mice, causing debility, tremors, and limb paralysis. Further characterization allowed researchers to name the Southeast Asian dengue serotype *DENV 1* and the serotype circulating in the Americas *DENV 2*, though *DENV 2* initially was found in New Guinea in 1944. In 1956 an outbreak of dengue hemorrhagic fever led to the discovery of two new serotypes of dengue, *DENV 3* and *DENV 4*, isolated from children in the Philippines.

The first decade of the 2000s saw an outbreak of dengue cases around the world. In 2010 Brazil reported more than 1.2 million cases of dengue. In 2011 Lahore, Pakistan, had an outbreak that killed more than 300 people. Dengue is regarded as endemic to 100 countries worldwide. Severe dengue is endemic in most countries in Southeast Asia. Latin America is contending with an ongoing regional pandemic of dengue.

⊕ Impacts and Issues

Characteristics of the Disease

Dengue is a member of the flavivirus genus of the virus family *Flaviviridae*. West Nile virus, yellow fever virus, and tick-borne encephalitis are all viruses in this genus. The dengue virus is a spherical particle containing an RNA genome. Infected persons develop immunity when their immune systems produce neutralizing antibodies that can bind to a glycoprotein on the virus surface.

Dengue fever manifests as a high, flu like fever in conjunction with severe headache, pain behind the eyes, nausea, vomiting, swollen glands, and rash. If dengue is recognized early and a patient's body fluid volume is maintained, mortality is rare in patients with dengue fever. As many as half of all dengue cases are asymptomatic, meaning patients do not exhibit clinical characteristics of having the disease. This makes disease control more challenging.

The main complications of dengue include fluid accumulation, respiratory distress, organ impairment, or excessive bleeding. There is no specific treatment or approved vaccine for dengue. Proper supportive medical care including maintaining body fluid balance is critical to keeping patients with complications of dengue alive. Dengue hemorrhagic fever can progress to dengue shock syndrome, in which blood pressure drops and patients exhibit circulatory failure. It is difficult to predict when an affected person will develop complications from dengue fever, although infection with a second serotype seems to make the disease worse. The WHO estimates that more than 20,000 people die of severe dengue per year.

Vector Control

Dengue fever is found in tropical and subtropical countries worldwide. The spread of dengue fever coincides with the widening range of two mosquito species. The *Aedes aegypti* and *Aedes albopictus* mosquitoes have spread primarily along trade routes. The two types of mosquitoes are well adapted to urban and semi-urban environments. As disease-carrying insects, this makes them increasingly a primary public health concern. The mosquitoes primarily breed in standing water left in human-made containers such as discarded tires and bottle caps. This disposition for breeding in any container with standing water has made vector control particularly challenging.

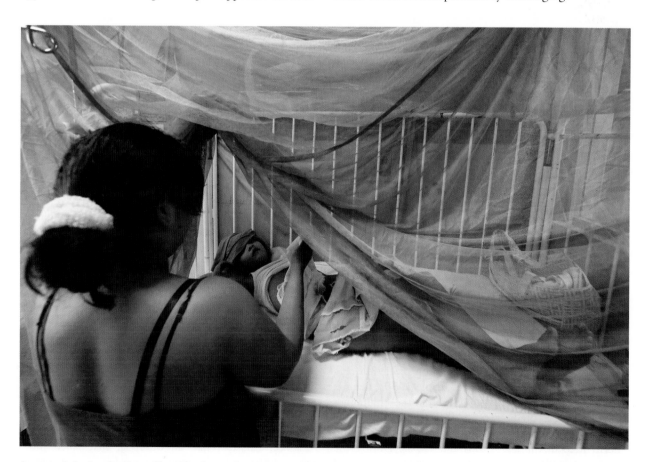

A woman helps her daughter affected by dengue fever in a room at La Mascota hospital in Managua, Nicaragua. The Nicaraguan government issued a health red alert as a dengue fever epidemic spread in 2013. Dengue, transmitted by the *Aedes aegypti* mosquito, occurs in Central America mostly during its rainy season from May to November. The disease causes fever, muscle and joint ache, as well as potentially fatal dengue hemorrhagic fever and dengue shock syndrome. © *Inti Ocon/AFP/Getty Images.*

Public health officials rely on a multipronged approach to control dengue-carrying mosquitoes. One tactic is educating the public on mosquito behavior, habitat, and breeding sites. Access to egg-laying habitats to remove water or kill mosquito eggs and larvae is a constant challenge around the world. Education is key in informing the public about the need to cover or clean domestic water storage containers and minimize mosquito breeding habitats.

Another strategy for vector control is surveillance. Public health authorities constantly monitor regional mosquito activity to best tackle an outbreak when it occurs. Funding, resources, and human action are limiting factors to proper surveillance. Integrated surveillance between the local and international level is needed, WHO officials note. "A harmonized effort across national dengue surveillance systems is needed to obtain the critical data of the disease's burden necessary to assess progress in reaching mortality and morbidity reduction goals," says a WHO report titled *Global Strategy for Dengue Prevention and Control 2012–2020*. An additional strategy to controlling dengue-carrying mosquitoes is fumigation with insecticides and larvicides. However, gaining access to housing in at-risk neighborhoods has been challenging. Many residents are reluctant to allow authorities entrance to their homes to spray chemicals. Education programs are therefore paramount.

The female *Aedes aegypti* mosquito is well adapted to carrying and transmitting the dengue virus. The mosquito acquires the virus by feeding off the blood of an infected human. The virus infects the mosquito's mid-gut and spreads to the salivary glands over a period of 8 to 12 days. This incubation period can fluctuate depending on ambient temperatures.

Aedes aegypti is the quintessential urban mosquito. Its domestication alongside humans has allowed it to adapt keenly to urban and semi-urban conditions. Female *Aedes aegypti* mosquitoes are daytime biters, striking most often in the early morning and just before dusk. The mosquitoes can breed in almost any human-made container that holds standing water.

Eradication efforts following World War II saw the heavy use of the synthetic insecticide DDT, also known as dichlorodiphenyltrichloroethane. The widespread spraying of DDT virtually eradicated *Aedes aegypti* from the Western Hemisphere before the 1970s. But reinfestation of the mosquito occurred as DDT control programs were scaled back due to

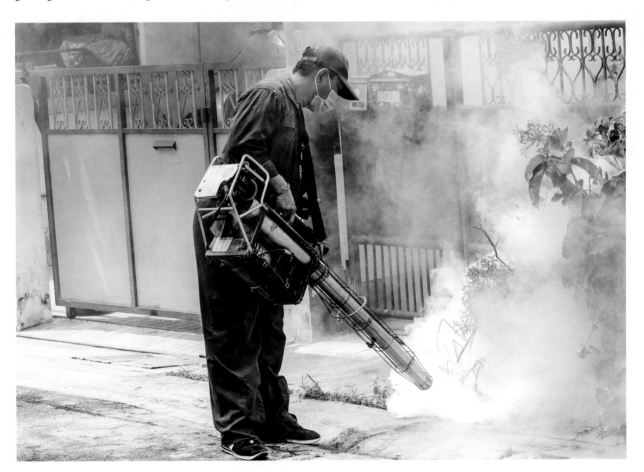

A worker sprays an insecticide meant to kill mosquitoes to stop an outbreak of dengue fever in March 2014 in Laksi, Bangkok, Thailand. © *Cbenjasuwan/Shutterstock.com.*

THE MOSQUITO VECTOR

The *Aedes aegypti* mosquito is the principal vector of dengue. *Aedes aegypti* has been living alongside humans since the drying of the Sahara Desert in Africa between 4,000 and 6,000 years ago. A northern *Aedes aegypti* species thus was separated from mosquitoes to the south, which remained in more wooded, or sylvan, conditions. In the absence of natural water sources, *Aedes aegypti* mosquitoes were left to breed in virtually any human-generated container with standing water such as tires, fountains, and flower pots. The mosquito is associated closely with humans and the urban environment and as such is referred to as domesticated.

Aedes aegypti left Africa aboard slave ships and first was introduced into the Americas following colonization by Europeans. An outbreak of yellow fever on Mexico's Yucatan Peninsula in 1648 was proof of the arrival of the *Aedes aegypti* mosquito, though yellow fever had been noted in Haiti as early as 1495. Historians suspect that an outbreak of dengue fever occurred in 1635 in the Caribbean islands of Martinique and Guadeloupe, but without more detailed records, this dengue outbreak is only a theory, according to the Pan American Health Organization.

Trade ships allowed for the globalization of the *Aedes aegypti* mosquito. The passage from Africa to the New World lasted four to six weeks. "The casks used for shipboard storage of water must have been prolific breeding sites for the mosquito, and the slaves were an abundant source of blood," writes Paul Reiter of the Pasteur Institute in France in his *Eurosurveillance* article "Yellow Fever and Dengue: A Threat to Europe?"

Throughout colonial times and into the 18th century, mosquito-borne disease outbreaks were common in port cities in the Americas, Africa, Asia, and Oceania. People in areas where the *Aedes aegypti* mosquito could breed were at risk of mosquito-borne diseases such as dengue, yellow fever, and malaria. Improved transportation facilitated the movement of people and goods around the world and also exacerbated the global dissemination of *Aedes aegypti*.

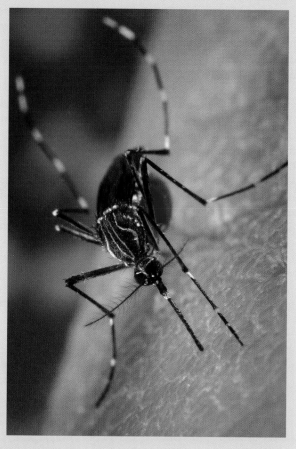

Dengue is transmitted principally by the *Aedes aegypti* mosquito, a species found living in close association with humans in most tropical urban areas. Mosquito biting activity is greatest in the morning for several hours after daybreak and in the late afternoon for several hours before dark. *James Gathany/U.S. Centers for Disease Control and Prevention.*

environmental concerns after it was linked to reduced populations of birds. "The deterioration of the control programs during the 1960s led to the reintroduction and expanding geographic distribution of the mosquito, and subsequent outbreaks caused by different dengue serotypes in several countries," writes the Pan American Health Organization's Olivia Brathwaite Dick and colleagues in their article "The History of Dengue Outbreaks in the Americas" published in the *American Journal of Tropical Medicine and Hygiene*. By 1980 more than 700,000 cases of dengue were reported in the Americas. *Aedes aegypti* has reinfested tropical and subtropical regions globally.

Another mosquito capable of transmitting dengue has been spreading throughout tropical and subtropical regions of the world. *Aedes albopictus*, also known as the Asian tiger mosquito, has been one of the fastest-spreading animal species over the past two decades, according to scientists from the Centers for Disease Control and Prevention (CDC) writing in a 2007 study titled "Spread of the Tiger: Global Risk of Invasion by the Mosquito *Aedes albopictus*." Its expansion along trade routes follows the pattern of the spread of *Aedes aegypti*, except that it originated in Asia.

Aedes albopictus is also a more competent vector of viral disease. The Asian tiger mosquito has the capacity of overwintering in climates where *Aedes aegypti* would not survive the lower temperatures. This means *Aedes albopictus* has penetrated farther into subtropical and even temperate regions. It has invaded Europe, the Mediterranean, South Africa, and North America. In concert, the two mosquitoes represent a serious public health risk.

Whereas *Aedes aegypti* can tolerate humidity and high temperatures, *Aedes albopictus* can overwinter in regions with temperature drops. Both are highly adapted to the urban environment.

Climate Change

The *Aedes* mosquitoes that carry dengue are highly sensitive to environmental conditions. The expansion of the range of *Aedes aegypti* and *Aedes albopictus* has coincided with a warming climate. Wetter conditions and increased precipitation also seem to affect the abundance of *Aedes* mosquitoes.

Global warming is not the only factor resulting in the increase of dengue cases worldwide. "Although climate may play a role in changing dengue incidence and distribution, it is one of many factors," according to the website of the CDC. Population growth, urbanization, and increased globalization are other factors that affect the spread of dengue and its mosquito hosts.

⊕ Future Implications

Dengue represents a global pandemic threat, according to the WHO. Around 2.5 billion people live in the 100 countries where the dengue virus can be transmitted. Since the early 1960s, the incidence of dengue has increased 30-fold, and the full global burden of the disease is uncertain. The economic impact of the disease on health systems is substantial yet difficult to calculate precisely.

The geographic spread of the *Aedes* mosquitoes that carry the dengue virus has been exacerbated by warming temperatures, globalization, and increased urbanization. Eradication of the mosquitoes is not financially viable. The absence of an insecticide that is devoid of side effects or environmental impacts makes impossible the global eradication of dengue-carrying mosquitoes. Thus, education and vector control measures represent the arsenal of tools for the fight against dengue.

Vaccine Development

Researchers are developing vaccines for dengue fever. As of mid-2014 no vaccine has been approved for the disease. In 2014 the French pharmaceutical company Sanofi Pasteur was in the late stages of development of a dengue vaccine in partnership with several Asian countries. The Brazilian government is working closely with its Butantan Institute to develop a dengue vaccine as well. There are several challenges to developing a vaccine, however. As it is a human disease, animal models such as mice do not reproduce dengue fever reliably. Tests on nonhuman primates are expensive. Vaccines must also protect against all four serotypes of dengue. The global dissemination of a fifth dengue serotype would be a significant setback to dengue vaccine development.

As of August 2014, the most advanced vaccine candidate was a live-attenuated chimeric yellow fever–dengue virus. Chimeric means it is composed of pieces of the yellow fever and dengue viruses. Live-attenuated means the vaccine contains a weakened, but still viable, version of the virus. Phase III clinical trials were ongoing, meaning it was being administered to large groups of volunteers to test efficacy and monitor side effects.

Genetically Modified Mosquitoes

Scientists have come up with an innovative vector control tool to contain the spread of *Aedes* mosquitoes. In developing genetically modified mosquitoes, researchers hope to stymie the spread of dengue-carrying *Aedes* mosquitoes. Public health officials in the Cayman Islands, Malaysia, and Brazil already have authorized the release of modified mosquitoes into the wild. These efforts have been met with success, albeit limited, due to the size of the trials.

In the laboratory, male mosquitoes are modified genetically to carry a lethal gene they can pass onto their offspring. The hope is that once released into the wild, these males will breed with wild female mosquitoes. The genetic trait passed on causes the offspring to die before reaching adulthood, thereby hopefully stemming future dengue outbreaks.

Some critics worry that scientists do not yet fully understand the ramifications of releasing millions of genetically modified mosquitoes into the wild. What is certain is that the cost of doing so may end up limiting the efficacy of this vector control tool. Estimates range in the millions of dollars for each release of genetically modified mosquitoes. These expensive measures would have to be repeated seasonally. They may also divert resources that otherwise could be used for surveillance, education, or alternate forms of vector control.

PRIMARY SOURCE

Epidemiology, Burden of Disease and Transmission

SOURCE *"Epidemiology, Burden of Disease and Transmission" in* Dengue: Guidelines for Diagnosis, Treatment, Prevention and Control *(New Edition, 2009). Geneva: World Health Organization (WHO) and the Special Programme for Research and Training in Tropical Diseases (TDR), 2009, 3–7. http://whqlibdoc. who.int/publications/2009/9789241547871_ eng.pdf?ua=1 (accessed January 25, 2015).*

INTRODUCTION *This primary source is from a joint publication of the World Health Organization and the Special Programme for Research and Training in Tropical Diseases. Dengue is*

Dengue

a major arthropod-borne virus, and a serious public health threat. Presented here are sections of the guidelines that describe the disease and its implications for global health, including transmission via global travel.

CHAPTER 1. EPIDEMIOLOGY, BURDEN OF DISEASE AND TRANSMISSION

1.1 DENGUE EPIDEMIOLOGY

Dengue is the most rapidly spreading mosquito-borne viral disease in the world. In the last 50 years, incidence has increased 30-fold with increasing geographic expansion to new countries and, in the present decade, from urban to rural settings. An estimated 50 million dengue infections occur annually and approximately 2.5 billion people live in dengue endemic countries. The 2002 World Health Assembly resolution WHA55.17 urged greater commitment to dengue by WHO and its Member States. Of particular significance is the 2005 World Health Assembly resolution WHA58.3 on the revision of the International Health Regulations (IHR), which includes dengue as an example of a disease that may constitute a public health emergency of international concern with implications for health security due to disruption and rapid epidemic spread beyond national borders.

1.1.6 Dengue case classification

Dengue has a wide spectrum of clinical presentations, often with unpredictable clinical evolution and outcome. While most patients recover following a self-limiting non-severe clinical course, a small proportion progress to severe disease, mostly characterized by plasma leakage with or without haemorrhage. Intravenous rehydration is the therapy of choice; this intervention can reduce the case fatality rate to less than 1% of severe cases. The group progressing from non-severe to severe disease is difficult to define, but this is an important concern since appropriate treatment may prevent these patients from developing more severe clinical conditions....

1.2 BURDEN OF DISEASE

Dengue inflicts a significant health, economic and social burden on the populations of endemic areas. Globally the estimated number of disability-adjusted life years (DALYs) lost to dengue in 2001 was 528....

The number of cases reported annually to WHO ranged from 0.4 to 1.3 million in the decade 1996—2005. As an infectious disease, the number of cases varies substantially from year to year. Underreporting and misdiagnoses are major obstacles to understanding the full burden of dengue....

Dengue afflicts all levels of society but the burden may be higher among the poorest who grow up in communities with inadequate water supply and solid waste infrastructure, and where conditions are most favourable for multiplication of the main vector, *Ae. Aegypti*.

1.3 DENGUE IN INTERNATIONAL TRAVEL

Travellers play an essential role in the global epidemiology of dengue infections, as viraemic travellers carry various dengue serotypes and strains into areas with mosquitoes that can transmit infection. Furthermore, travellers perform another essential service in providing early alerts to events in other parts of the world. Travellers often transport the dengue virus from areas in tropical developing countries, where limited laboratory facilities exist, to developed countries with laboratories that can identify virus serotypes. Access to research facilities makes it possible to obtain more detailed information about a virus, including serotype and even sequencing, when that information would be valuable. Systematic collection of clinical specimens and banking of serum or isolates may have future benefits as new technologies become available....

SEE ALSO *Insect-Borne Diseases; Neglected Tropical Diseases; Viral Diseases*

BIBLIOGRAPHY

Books

Barrett, Alan D. T., and Lawrence R. Stanberry. *Vaccines for Biodefense and Emerging and Neglected Diseases.* Amsterdam: Academic Press, 2009.

Bock, Gregory, and Jamie Goode, eds. *New Treatment Strategies for Dengue and Other Flaviviral Diseases.* Chichester, UK: Wiley, 2006.

Christophers, S. Rickard. *Aëdes aegypti the Yellow Fever Mosquito: Its Life History, Bionomics and Structure.* Cambridge, UK: Cambridge University Press, 2009.

Halstead, Scott B. *Dengue.* London: Imperial College Press, 2008.

Juang, Richard M., and Noelle Morrissette, eds. *Africa and the Americas: Culture, Politics and History.* Santa Barbara, CA: ABC-CLIO, 2008.

Lloyd, Linda S. *Mejores prácticas para la prevención y el control del dengue en las Américas.* Washington, DC: Environmental Health Project: Oficina para Programas Mundiales, Apoyo de Campo e Investigación, Oficina de Salud y Nutrición, Agencia para el Desarrollo Internacional de los Estados Unidos, 2003. Available online at http://pdf.usaid.gov/pdf_docs/PNACS816.pdf (accessed August 26, 2014).

Pan American Health Organization. *Dengue and Dengue Hemorrhagic Fever in the Americas: Guidelines for Prevention and Control.* Washington, DC: PAHO Scientific Publication, 1997.

Terrero, Clemente. *Dengue: diagnóstico, manejo y control.* Santo Domingo: Editora Universitaria, UASD, 2000.

Dengue

Periodicals

Benedict, Mark, et al. "Spread of the Tiger: Global Risk of Invasion by the Mosquito *Aedes albopictus.*" *Vector-Borne and Zoonotic Diseases* 7, no. 1 (Spring 2007): 122–129.

Brathwaite Dick, Olivia, et al. "The History of Dengue Outbreaks in the Americas." *American Journal of Tropical Medicine and Hygiene* 87, no. 4 (October 2012): 584–593. Available online at http://www.ajtmh.org/content/87/4/584.full (accessed March 31, 2015).

Powell, J. R., and Walter J. Tabachnick. "History of Domestication and Spread of *Aedes aegypti*—A Review." *Memorias Instituto Oswaldo Cruz* 108, Suppl. 1 (December 2013): 11–17.

Reiter, Paul. "Yellow Fever and Dengue: A Threat to Europe?" *Eurosurveillance* 15, no. 10 (March 2, 2010): 19509.

Twiddy, S. Susanna, et al. "Inferring the Rate and Time-Scale of Dengue Virus Evolution." *Molecular Biology and Evolution* 20, no. 1 (January 2003): 122–129.

Websites

"Dengue and Climate." *U.S. Centers for Disease Control and Prevention (CDC).* http://www.cdc.gov/Dengue/entomologyEcology/climate.html (accessed August 26, 2014).

"Dengue/Dengue Hemorrhagic Fever." *World Health Organization (WHO).* http://www.who.int/csr/disease/dengue/en/ (accessed August 27, 2014).

"Dengue Hemorrhagic Fever: Diagnosis, Treatment, Prevention and Control." *World Health Organization (WHO).* http://www.who.int/csr/resources/publications/dengue/Denguepublication/en/ (accessed August 27, 2014).

Normile, Dennis. "Surprising New Dengue Virus Throws a Spanner in Disease Control Efforts." *Science Magazine,* October 25, 2013. http://www.sciencemag.org/content/342/6157/415.summary (accessed August 26, 2014).

Aleszu Bajak

Diabetes

⊕ Introduction

Diabetes is a group of diseases resulting from impairments in insulin production, insulin action, or both. These impairments lead to chronic high blood glucose levels. According to the first edition of the International Diabetes Federation's *Diabetes Atlas*, in 2000, an estimated 151 million people worldwide had diabetes. By the publication of the sixth edition in 2013, that number had more than doubled, to more than 382 million people, 80 percent of whom lived in a low- or middle-income country. Indeed, 43 percent of people with diabetes in the world live in just two Asian countries: 98.4 million in China and 65.1 million in India.

Given the debilitating complications of untreated diabetes, including possible blindness, limb amputations, and kidney failure, and the increasingly young age of onset, the impact of this disease on productivity and economic development can be substantial. Furthermore, the mortality (death) burden from diabetes is great: in 2013, according to the *Diabetes Atlas*, diabetes accounted for 8.4 percent of global all-cause mortality in people aged 20 to 79 years. In absolute terms, 5.1 million people died annually as a direct result of diabetes, a number that likely is significantly underestimated because diabetes often is not included on death certificates as the cause of death.

The vast majority of diabetes cases (90–95 percent) are classified as type 2 diabetes, and therefore this is the primary focus of this article. Type 2 diabetes often is associated with obesity, and results from a combination of insulin resistance and inability to produce enough compensatory insulin. Most of the remaining cases of diabetes (5–10 percent) are classified as "type 1 diabetes," which results from the autoimmune destruction of insulin-producing cells (beta cells) in the pancreas. In low- and middle-income countries, access to insulin, which is essential for the survival of patients with type 1 diabetes, has been the focus of research and humanitarian efforts. As life expectancy for these persons improves

with increased access to insulin, greater attention will need to be given to treating the co-morbidities of type 1 diabetes (conditions that often accompany diabetes, including high blood pressure and high cholesterol) and to preventing long-term complications such as cardiovascular disease and kidney disease.

Although scientists do not understand fully the causes of the diabetes epidemic, industrialization, urbanization, and globalization, and the closely related demographic and nutrition transitions, are key culprits. In particular, the transition from traditional, plant-based diets to more energy-dense, animal-based diets high in fat, saturated fat, refined carbohydrates, and added sugar (Western diets), has been implicated in the global rise of obesity and diabetes. As such, prevention efforts have focused on lifestyle interventions involving dietary modifications and increased physical activity with subsequent weight loss.

⊕ Historical Background

Until 1979, physicians classified diabetes cases largely according to age at onset, with what is now considered type 1 diabetes classified as "juvenile onset diabetes" and type 2 diabetes as "adult onset diabetes." In 1979, a new classification scheme endorsed by the American Diabetes Association (ADA) and the Expert Committee on Diabetes of the World Health Organization (WHO) recognized that both subclasses of diabetes can occur at any age, thus they changed the classification to "insulin-dependent diabetes" and "non-insulin-dependent diabetes." Eighteen years later, in 1997, the ADA developed the classification scheme that continues in use in the 2010s, moving away from categories based on pharmacological treatment to categories based on etiology.

These distinctions in classification underscore the changing nature of the diabetes epidemic over time and the understanding of diabetes etiology. Three scientific observations are noteworthy in this regard. First is the

Prevalence of Diabetes by Country, 2014

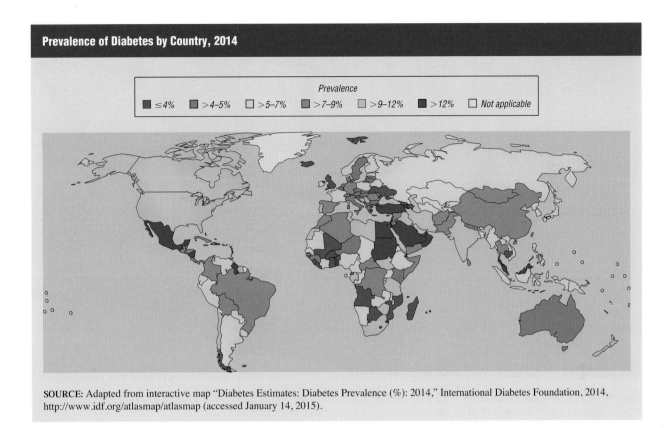

SOURCE: Adapted from interactive map "Diabetes Estimates: Diabetes Prevalence (%): 2014," International Diabetes Foundation, 2014, http://www.idf.org/atlasmap/atlasmap (accessed January 14, 2015).

observation that type 1 diabetes is not solely a disease of childhood and adolescence, but can occur at any point across the life span. Surveillance of type 1 diabetes around the world, including the seminal WHO's Multinational Project for Childhood Diabetes (DIAMOND) conducted in 57 countries between 1990 and 1999, has focused on children up to 14 years old, and a peak age of onset of 10–14 years has been reported. However, a life-table analysis by T. Lorenzen and others, published in the journal *Diabetologia* in 1994, estimated that the cumulative risk of type 1 diabetes in siblings of individuals with type 1 diabetes up to 18 years of age is 2.5 percent, up to 30 years is 6.4 percent, and up to 60 years is 9.6 percent. Furthermore, epidemiological studies from Africa, and subsequently China, have reported much later peak onset ages (early to mid-20s). Clearly, this is not just a juvenile disease.

Similarly, type 2 diabetes is not only an adult disease. Indeed, in Japan, Teruo Kitagawa and colleagues reported in the journal *Diabetes Research and Clinical Practice* (1994) that in the early 1980s, type 2 diabetes was already more common than type 1 diabetes in children less than 15 years old. In the United States, Dana Dabelea and others reported in *JAMA* (2014) on behalf of the SEARCH for Diabetes in Youth Study, a 30.5 percent overall increase in type 2 diabetes between 2001 and 2009 among youth aged 10 to 19 years. The prevalence of type 2 diabetes was highest among minority youth, particularly Native Americans (1.2 cases per 1,000 youth)

and African Americans (1.06 cases per 1,000 youth). In response to these epidemiological observations, the ADA recommends testing for type 2 diabetes in children 18 years or younger who are overweight and have at least two other risk factors.

Finally, the critical importance of beta cell dysfunction and impaired insulin production in the development of type 2 diabetes has become well recognized, and as the disease progresses, insulin therapy eventually is recommended for most persons with type 2 diabetes. Thus, the previous classification according to pharmacological treatment no longer holds. Related to this, evidence suggests that there may be substantial heterogeneity (diversity) within the category of "type 2 diabetes," because individuals of Asian ethnicity tend to develop type 2 diabetes at a lower body mass index (BMI) and beta cell dysfunction tends to occur at an earlier stage in disease progression when compared to Caucasians. Further research is needed to understand the underlying factors contributing to this heterogeneity and the implications for treatment.

⊕ Impacts and Issues

Screening

According to the *Diabetes Atlas* (2014), on average worldwide, nearly half (46 percent) of people with diabetes are undiagnosed, though the proportion is much

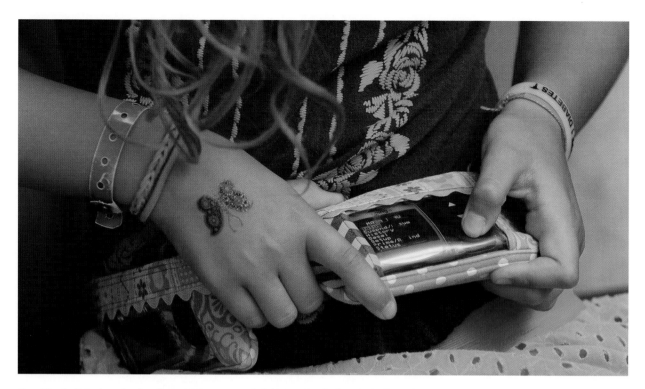

Zara Cheek, 7, looks at her insulin pump in a custom belt her mother had made for her. Cheek, who has type 1 diabetes, was entered in a "bionic pancreas" study in Boston in 2014. © *Lloyd Fox/Sun Photographer/MCT via Getty Images.*

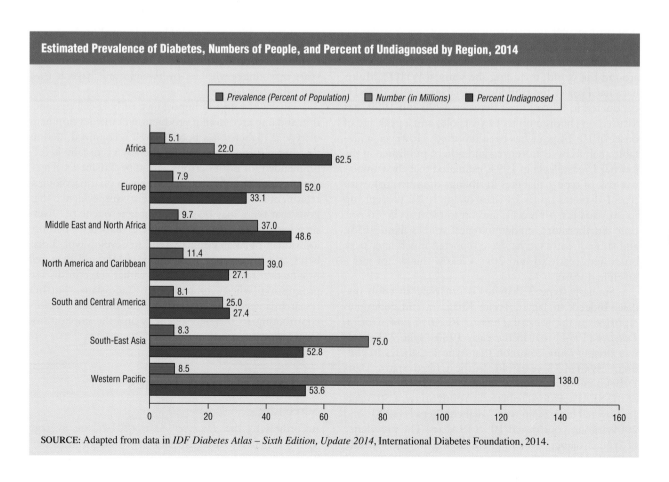

Estimated Prevalence of Diabetes, Numbers of People, and Percent of Undiagnosed by Region, 2014

Legend:
- ■ Prevalence (Percent of Population)
- ■ Number (in Millions)
- ■ Percent Undiagnosed

Region	Prevalence (Percent of Population)	Number (in Millions)	Percent Undiagnosed
Africa	5.1	22.0	62.5
Europe	7.9	52.0	33.1
Middle East and North Africa	9.7	37.0	48.6
North America and Caribbean	11.4	39.0	27.1
South and Central America	8.1	25.0	27.4
South-East Asia	8.3	75.0	52.8
Western Pacific	8.5	138.0	53.6

SOURCE: Adapted from data in *IDF Diabetes Atlas – Sixth Edition, Update 2014*, International Diabetes Foundation, 2014.

higher in low-income countries, especially in Africa (62.5 percent for the region; 75 percent in low-income countries) and the Western Pacific (53.6 overall; 63 percent in low-income countries). This relatively low rate of diagnosis stems from the fact that after onset, type 2 diabetes is asymptomatic (causes no symptoms) for many years. The scientific evidence supporting screening for undiagnosed diabetes is mixed, and the debate is ongoing as to the utility and cost-effectiveness of early diagnosis in screening-detected diabetes. Even if clear benefits are observed, challenges still remain in identifying who to screen and how often, and how to ensure adherence to protocols for screening in primary care settings.

As such, universal screening for undiagnosed diabetes is not recommended in the International Diabetes Federation's *Global Guidelines for Type 2 Diabetes* (2012). Rather, a two-step approach is used: First, high-risk individuals are identified using a questionnaire and then, in high-risk individuals, fasting blood glucose is tested via the glycated hemoglobin A1c (HbA1c) test, or an oral glucose tolerance test (OGTT) is performed. "High-risk" here and elsewhere typically refers to adults who are overweight (BMI equal to or more than 25) and have additional risk factors including physical inactivity, family history of diabetes, high-risk race/ethnicity (e.g. Asian and indigenous populations), women who had gestational diabetes, people with hypertension, low high-density lipoprotein (HDL) levels, women with polycystic ovarian syndrome, and a history of cardiovascular disease. Results (published in *The Lancet* in 2011) from an Anglo-Danish-Dutch study indicated that screening for early detection and treatment could reduce cardiovascular disease risk factors (HbA1c, cholesterol, and blood pressure) significantly when diabetes is identified. However, effects on mortality, published in *The Lancet* in 2012, were nonsignificant, suggesting that the benefits of screening may be smaller than expected.

Primary Prevention

The goal of primary prevention is to prevent or delay the onset of disease in individuals without diabetes. Given the high cost of treating diabetes—worldwide, US$548 billion in 2013 according to the *Diabetes Atlas*—primary prevention has been the focus of global health efforts to address the diabetes epidemic. Primary prevention can involve population-based policies aimed at improving healthy behaviors or targeted interventions in high-risk individuals. Both of these approaches are discussed in more detail in the sections that follow.

Population-Based Primary Prevention

It is difficult to obtain strong scientific evidence to support population-based strategies to prevent type 2 diabetes because these strategies typically are aimed

---

HIGH BLOOD GLUCOSE IN PREGNANCY

According to the *Diabetes Atlas*, published in 2013, an estimated 21.4 million live births (16.8 percent of live births worldwide) are affected by high blood glucose (hyperglycemia) during pregnancy, a condition often referred to as "gestational diabetes mellitus" or GDM. Gestational diabetes, typically with an onset mid-pregnancy (24–28 weeks), is the result of impaired insulin action, potentially arising from the effects of hormones released by the placenta. Following delivery of the child, the high blood glucose in the mother resolves.

Due to the increased prevalence of undiagnosed type 2 diabetes globally, the American Diabetes Association recommends that women with risk factors for type 2 diabetes be screened at their initial prenatal visit and that women diagnosed with diabetes in their first trimester be diagnosed with overt diabetes, not gestational diabetes. Scientific evidence supports that left untreated, high blood glucose during pregnancy can lead to a large-for-gestational-age baby, which in turn increases the risk for obstructed labor in the mother, injury and breathing problems in the baby, and cesarean section delivery. High blood glucose during pregnancy also increases the mother's risk of preeclampsia, a life-threatening complication of pregnancy stemming from sudden high blood pressure in the mother. Finally, and importantly, high blood glucose during pregnancy increases the risk of future type 2 diabetes in both the mother and child. The mechanism underlying this long-term increased risk in the child has been termed "developmental origins of adult disease," and is a key area of primary prevention research.

---

at improving the environment, and appropriate controls often are not available for comparison. Furthermore, most of these strategies are targeted at obesity, an important risk factor for diabetes, rather than diabetes itself, because following up participants over long periods until they develop diabetes is difficult and expensive. Given that many of the risk factors for diabetes, such as unhealthy diets and physical inactivity, are also risk factors for other noncommunicable diseases, policies aimed at reducing these risk factors may have beneficial effects not only on patients with diabetes but also on those with hypertension, cardiovascular disease, and some cancers. What is clear from current evidence is that information alone is inadequate and that the environment will also have to be modified to support healthful decisions. Furthermore, this broad, population-based approach requires strong collaborations across multiple sectors including the government, food industry—marketing and product formulation—health-care systems, schools, and the workplace. Several examples of population-based approaches are noted here.

The Change4Life program in the United Kingdom is an example of a national campaign to improve the nutrition and physical activity of citizens by increasing awareness of healthy lifestyles through the media and improving retail access to fresh fruits and vegetables. The HEALTHY Study in the United States was a multicomponent, school-based intervention to address risk factors for type 2 diabetes in children with the primary outcome being overweight and obesity. After following students from sixth to eighth grade, results (published in the *New England Journal of Medicine* in 2010) indicated that the proportion of participants who were overweight or obese in both the intervention and control schools decreased, with no significant difference between treatment groups. However, analysis of secondary outcomes indicated that the intervention schools had significantly greater reductions in other markers of adiposity (excess fat), for example, BMI z-score and waist circumference, and fasting insulin, supporting some positive effect on type 2 diabetes risk reduction.

Targeted Primary Prevention

Numerous trials have demonstrated that lifestyle interventions can prevent or delay the onset of type 2 diabetes in high-risk individuals. Most notably, these include the 2006 Finnish Diabetes Prevention Study, the Da Qing Diabetes Prevention Study in China published in *The Lancet* in 2008, and the 2009 Diabetes Prevention Program in the United States. One 2007 meta-analysis published by Clare L. Gillies and colleagues in the *British Medical Journal* evaluated 17 such trials and found that individuals with impaired glucose tolerance (known as prediabetes) who received a lifestyle intervention had half the risk of developing diabetes compared to those who received standard advice. A 30 percent reduction in risk was also observed in individuals who received oral diabetes drugs when compared to those who received standard advice. In regard to specific prevention program goals, the ADA recommends a weight loss of 7 percent of initial body weight for overweight individuals, along with increasing physical activity to at least 150 minutes per week.

These results demonstrate that type 2 diabetes can be prevented. The key challenge is translating expensive clinical trials with limited reach to real-world settings, especially to socially and economically disadvantaged groups. Preliminary results from a 2011 statewide diabetes prevention program in Australia ("Life!") and a first-ever nationwide diabetes prevention program in Finland, are especially promising. Also of note is the DE-PLAN study, which is being implemented across Europe with the aim of preventing type 2 diabetes in community-based settings. It is clear from this literature that the development and evaluation of such trials will need to be setting-specific, particularly in regard to recruitment and retention strategies (follow-up counseling is important

for success), frequency and duration of sessions, culturally appropriate content, and who is delivering the sessions.

Secondary Prevention

The goal of secondary prevention is to prevent or delay the onset of complications in individuals with diabetes. Cardiovascular disease is the leading cause of death among people with diabetes, and therefore, treating risk factors of cardiovascular disease such as high blood pressure and high cholesterol are key aspects of treatment.

Studies have previously shown that intensive control of blood glucose levels in persons with type 2 diabetes can help reduce the development of complications such nephropathy (kidney disease) and retinopathy (damage to the retina of the eye). However, along with lower blood glucose targets comes an increased risk of low blood glucose, an acute complication of diabetes that can interfere with quality of life, and in serious cases can be life threatening. One randomized controlled trial, Action to Control Cardiovascular Risk in Diabetes, also found increased mortality among patients in the intensive control group, further contributing to the complexity surrounding treatment for type 2 diabetes.

The effects of intensive treatment for blood glucose control in persons with diabetes on other complications, particularly cardiovascular disease, are mixed. Recent evidence has not shown a significant reduction in cardiovascular disease with intensive blood glucose control in patients with long-standing type 2 diabetes. Given these unexpected results, the ADA, in collaboration with the American College of Cardiology Foundation and the American Heart Association, published a position statement in 2009 in the journal *Diabetes Care* regarding the implications for treatment of type 2 diabetes. They concluded that the additive benefits on cardiovascular disease of intensive glycemic control in patients with long-standing type 2 diabetes (and therefore in those who likely already have established atherosclerosis—fatty deposits in the arteries) are likely modest compared to other treatments such as statin therapy to lower cholesterol, aspirin, and blood pressure treatment.

Increased Risk of Tuberculosis among Individuals with Diabetes

A systematic review of 13 studies conducted in 2008 concluded that people with type 2 diabetes are three times as likely to contract tuberculosis compared to people without diabetes. People with type 2 diabetes are also nearly twice as likely to die from tuberculosis. Diabetes-associated tuberculosis is therefore an important consideration in the context of global diabetes, especially in low- and middle-income countries such as China and India, which have the highest prevalence of both type 2 diabetes and tuberculosis.

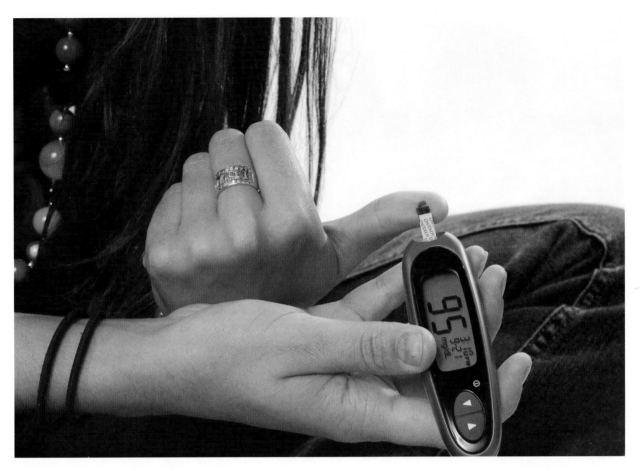

A young diabetic girl carries out a blood glucose test. After a finger stick that releases a blood droplet, she tests the blood glucose level by bringing the drop into contact with a monitoring device. Keeping one's glucose level close to normal helps prevent, or delay, some diabetes problems, such as eye disease, kidney disease, and nerve damage. *Amanda Mills/U.S. Centers for Disease Control.*

Experimental studies in mice support the biological plausibility of this association, providing evidence that the underlying mechanism involves direct impairment of the immune response by high blood glucose. Key players in this immune impairment include interferon-gamma and T-helper cells, which play a role in adaptive immunity and countering the proliferation of tuberculosis. There is clearly a need for coordinated health-care delivery between global communicable and noncommunicable disease programs. Tuberculosis control programs are beginning to target patients with type 2 diabetes, and screening, diagnosis, and treatment of type 2 diabetes may in turn have a positive impact on tuberculosis control. The dual treatment of tuberculosis and type 2 diabetes is challenging, particularly because the drugs used to treat tuberculosis can worsen blood glucose control. In the mid-2010s, there is limited evidence to inform clinical practice guidelines, and this is an important issue that will need to be addressed in future studies.

Pollution as a Risk Factor for Diabetes

While largely banned in most parts of the world, persistent organic pollutants such as DDT continue to be used in some low- and middle-income countries, especially India, for malaria control. Given that these countries also are experiencing unprecedented increases in diabetes, and the observation that symptoms of acute poisoning from these pollutants include high blood glucose, researchers have suspected for several years a link between pollutants and diabetes. A U.S. National Toxicology Program Workshop published in the journal *Environmental Health Perspectives* in 2013 concluded that evidence is sufficient to support an association of some persistent organic pollutants, particularly *trans*-Nonachlor, DDE (a metabolite of DDT), polychlorinated biphenyls (PCBs), and dioxins, with type 2 diabetes. Experimental studies in mice and rats tend to support that chronic exposure to low doses of persistent organic pollutants impairs insulin regulation in muscle and fat tissues.

In addition to persistent organic pollutants, other environmental pollutants also have been linked to type 2 diabetes. Air pollution in particular has risen in the scientific literature as a possible contributor to insulin resistance. Prospective studies in Denmark, Canada, the United States, and elsewhere have demonstrated associations between traffic-related air pollution and incident

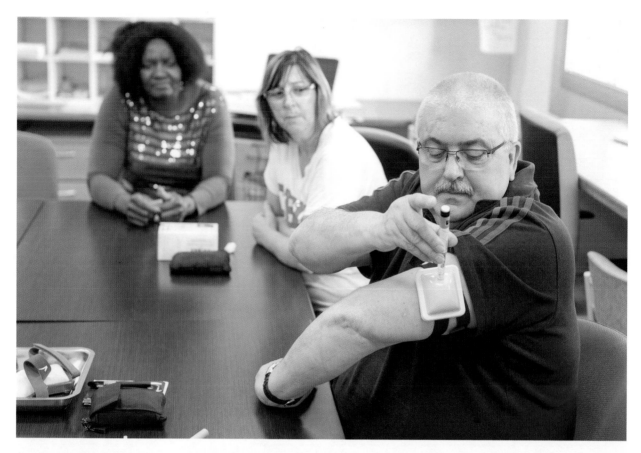

A man practices giving himself an insulin shot at an education program for diabetic patients in France.   © *Phanie / Alamy.*

diabetes. Pollution abatement policies may therefore have the added benefit of preventing diabetes.

⊕ Future Implications

In September 2011, the first United Nations high-level meeting on noncommunicable diseases was held in New York. One of the outcomes of this meeting was the development and adoption of a Global Monitoring Framework including 9 global targets and 25 indicators by the World Health Assembly in May 2013 (commonly referred to as "25 by 25"). One of the nine targets is to halt the rise in diabetes and obesity, with the diabetes-specific indicator being the age-standardized prevalence of high blood glucose in adults 18 years and older. Several other targets and indicators also are related to the prevention of diabetes, including a target to reduce the prevalence of insufficient physical activity by 10 percent and indicators relating to fruit and vegetable intake.

Given the large body of scientific evidence summarized previously, the global health community and large governmental organizations such as the U.S. National Institutes of Health are focusing on late-stage translational research, taking science from clinical practice to "real-world" settings. While diabetes is a key target of

these efforts, emphasis on strengthening health systems and integrated health-care delivery ensure that all noncommunicable diseases are addressed. Key constraints include funding, infrastructure, trained personnel, institutional support, and national policy frameworks. Nonetheless, diabetes increasingly is becoming an important aspect of global and national health agendas, and addressing the epidemic of this disease undoubtedly will require multidisciplinary and multi-sector collaborations to successfully implement evidence-based practices and policies.

PRIMARY SOURCE

Diabetes Fact Sheet

SOURCE *"Diabetes,"* Fact Sheet *No. 312. World Health Organization (WHO), January 2015. http://www.who.int/mediacentre/factsheets/fs312/en/ (accessed February 6, 2015).*

INTRODUCTION *This primary source contains information from a fact sheet from the World Health Organization (WHO) on the topic of diabetes, a noncommunicable disease that has emerged as a major cause of death globally. Along with key facts, the sheet describes the disease and methods of prevention and treatment. The fact sheet is updated periodically by the WHO.*

DIABETES

Fact sheet N°312
Updated January 2015

Key facts

- In 2014 the global prevalence of diabetes * was estimated to be 9% among adults aged 18+ years.

- In 2012, an estimated 1.5 million deaths were directly caused by diabetes.

- More than 80% of diabetes deaths occur in low- and middle-income countries.

- WHO projects that diabetes will be the 7th leading cause of death in 2030.

- Healthy diet, regular physical activity, maintaining a normal body weight and avoiding tobacco use can prevent or delay the onset of type 2 diabetes.

What is diabetes?

Diabetes is a chronic disease that occurs either when the pancreas does not produce enough insulin or when the body cannot effectively use the insulin it produces. Insulin is a hormone that regulates blood sugar. Hyperglycaemia, or raised blood sugar, is a common effect of uncontrolled diabetes and over time leads to serious damage to many of the body's systems, especially the nerves and blood vessels....

What are common consequences of diabetes?

Over time, diabetes can damage the heart, blood vessels, eyes, kidneys, and nerves.

- Diabetes increases the risk of heart disease and stroke. In a multinational study, 50% of people with diabetes die of cardiovascular disease (primarily heart disease and stroke).

- Combined with reduced blood flow, neuropathy (nerve damage) in the feet increases the chance of foot ulcers, infection and eventual need for limb amputation.

- Diabetic retinopathy is an important cause of blindness, and occurs as a result of long-term accumulated damage to the small blood vessels in the retina. One percent of global blindness can be attributed to diabetes.

- Diabetes is among the leading causes of kidney failure.

- The overall risk of dying among people with diabetes is at least double the risk of their peers without diabetes.

How can the burden of diabetes be reduced?

Prevention

Simple lifestyle measures have been shown to be effective in preventing or delaying the onset of type 2 diabetes. To help prevent type 2 diabetes and its complications, people should:

- achieve and maintain healthy body weight;

- be physically active—at least 30 minutes of regular, moderate-intensity activity on most days. More activity is required for weight control;

- eat a healthy diet of between three and five servings of fruit and vegetables a day and reduce sugar and saturated fats intake;

- avoid tobacco use—smoking increases the risk of cardiovascular diseases.

Diagnosis and treatment

Early diagnosis can be accomplished through relatively inexpensive blood testing.

Treatment of diabetes involves lowering blood glucose and the levels of other known risk factors that damage blood vessels. Tobacco use cessation is also important to avoid complications.

Interventions that are both cost saving and feasible in developing countries include:

- moderate blood glucose control. People with type 1 diabetes require insulin; people with type 2 diabetes can be treated with oral medication, but may also require insulin;

- blood pressure control;

- foot care.

---

* Defined as fasting blood glucose >= 7 mmol/l or on medication for raised blood glucose or with a history of diagnosis of diabetes.

SEE ALSO *Cardiovascular Diseases; High Blood Pressure; Noncommunicable Diseases (Lifestyle Diseases); Nutrition; Obesity; Tuberculosis (TB)*

BIBLIOGRAPHY

Books

Bergman, Michael. *Global Health Perspectives in Prediabetes and Diabetes Prevention.* Singapore: World Scientific, 2014.

Guariguata, Leonor, et al. *IDF Diabetes Atlas*, 6th ed. Brussels: International Diabetes Federation, 2013.

International Diabetes Federation. *Diabetes Atlas.* Brussels: International Diabetes Federation, 2000.

International Diabetes Federation, Clinical Guidelines Task Force. *Global Guidelines for Type 2 Diabetes.* Brussels: International Diabetes Federation, 2012.

Narayan, K. M. Venkat, et al., eds. *Diabetes Public Health: From Data to Policy.* New York: Oxford University Press, 2011.

World Health Organization. *Diagnostic Criteria and Classification of Hyperglycaemia First Detected in Pregnancy.* Geneva: World Health Organization, 2013.

World Health Organization. *Global Action Plan for the Prevention and Control of Noncommunicable Diseases, 2013–2020.* Geneva: World Health Organization, 2013.

Periodicals

American Diabetes Association. "Report of the Expert Committee on the Diagnosis and Classification of Diabetes Mellitus." *Diabetes Care* 20, no. 7 (July 1997): 1183–1197.

American Diabetes Association. "Standards of Medical Care in Diabetes–2014." *Diabetes Care* 37, Supplement 1 (January 2014): S14–S80.

American Diabetes Association, American College of Cardiology Foundation, and American Heart Association. "Intensive Glycemic Control and the Prevention of Cardiovascular Events: Implications of the ACCORD, ADVANCE, and VA Diabetes Trials: A Position Statement of the American Diabetes Association and a Scientific Statement of the American College of Cardiology Foundation and the American Heart Association." *Diabetes Care* 32, no. 1 (January 2009): 187–192.

Baker, Meghan A., et al. "The Impact of Diabetes on Tuberculosis Treatment Outcomes: A Systematic Review." *BioMed Central Medicine* 9 (July 2011): 81–96.

Dabelea, Dana, et al. "Prevalence of Type 1 and Type 2 Diabetes among Children and Adolescents from 2001 to 2009." *JAMA* 311, no. 17 (May 7, 2014): 1778–1786.

Diabetes Prevention Program Research Group. "10-Year Follow-Up of Diabetes Incidence and Weight Loss in the Diabetes Prevention Program Outcomes Study." *The Lancet* 374, no. 9702 (November 14, 2009): 1677–1686.

DIAMOND Project Group. "Incidence and Trends of Childhood Type 1 Diabetes Worldwide 1990–1999." *Diabetic Medicine* 23, no. 8 (August 2006): 857–866.

Gillies, Clare L., et al. "Pharmacological and Lifestyle Interventions to Prevent or Delay Type 2 Diabetes in People with Impaired Glucose Tolerance: Systematic Review and Meta-Analysis." *British Medical Journal* 334, no. 7588 (February 10, 2007): 299–308.

Griffin, Simon J., et al. "Effect of Early Intensive Multifactorial Therapy on 5-Year Cardiovascular Outcomes in Individuals with Type 2 Diabetes Detected by Screening (ADDITION-Europe): A Cluster-Randomised Trial." *The Lancet* 378, no. 9786 (July 9, 2011): 156–167.

HEALTHY Study Group. "A School-Based Intervention for Diabetes Risk Reduction." *New England Journal of Medicine* 363, no. 5 (July 2010): 443–453.

Hectors, Tine L. M., et al. "Environmental Pollutants and Type 2 Diabetes: A Review of Mechanisms That Can Disrupt Beta Cell Function." *Diabetologia* 54, no. 6 (June 2011): 1273–1290.

International Association of Diabetes and Pregnancy Study Groups Consensus Panel. "International Association of Diabetes and Pregnancy Study Groups Recommendations on the Diagnosis and Classification of Hyperglycemia in Pregnancy." *Diabetes Care* 33, no. 3 (March 2010): 676–682.

Jeon, Christie Y., and Megan B. Murray. "Diabetes Mellitus Increases the Risk of Active Tuberculosis: A Systematic Review of 13 Observational Studies." *PLoS Medicine* 5, no. 7 (July 2008): e152.

Kitagawa, Teruo, Misao Owada, Tatsuhiko Urakami, and Naoko Tajima. "Epidemiology of Type 1 (Insulin-dependent) and Type 2 (Non-Insulin-Dependent) Diabetes Mellitus in Japanese Children." *Diabetes Research and Clinical Practice* 24, Supplement (October 1994): S7–S13.

Li, Guangwei, et al. "The Long-Term Effect of Lifestyle Interventions to Prevent Diabetes in the China Da Qing Diabetes Prevention Study: A 20-Year Follow-Up Study." *The Lancet* 371, no. 9626 (May 24, 2008): 1783–1789.

Lindström, Jaana, et al. "Sustained Reduction in the Incidence of Type 2 Diabetes by Lifestyle Intervention: Follow-Up of the Finnish Diabetes Prevention Study." *The Lancet* 368, no. 9548 (November 11, 2006): 1673–1679.

Liu, Cuiqing, et al. "Epidemiological and Experimental Links between Air Pollution and Type 2 Diabetes." *Toxicologic Pathology* 41, no. 2 (February 2013): 361–373.

Lorenzen, T., F. Pociot, P. Hougaard, and J. Nerup. "Long-Term Risk of IDDM in First-Degree Relatives of Patients with IDDM." *Diabetologia* 37, no. 3 (March 1994): 321–327.

National Diabetes Data Group. "Classification and Diagnosis of Diabetes Mellitus and Other Categories of Glucose Intolerance." *Diabetes* 28, no. 12 (December 1979): 1039–1057.

Ohkubo, Yasuo, et al. "Intensive Insulin Therapy Prevents the Progression of Diabetic Microvascular Complications in Japanese Patients with Non-Insulin-Dependent Diabetes Mellitus: A Randomized Prospective 6-Year Study." *Diabetes Research and Clinical Practice* 28, no. 2 (May 1995): 103–117.

Simmons, Rebecca K., et al. "Screening for Type 2 Diabetes and Population Mortality over 10 Years (ADDITION-Cambridge): A Cluster-Randomised Controlled Trial." *The Lancet* 380, no. 9855 (November 17, 2012): 1741–1748.

Stevenson, Catherine R., et al. "Diabetes and Tuberculosis: The Impact of the Diabetes Epidemic on Tuberculosis Incidence." *BioMed Central Public Health* 7 (2007): 234–242.

Taylor, Kyla W., et al. "Evaluation of the Association between Persistent Organic Pollutants (POPs) and Diabetes in Epidemiological Studies: A National Toxicology Program Workshop Review." *Environmental Health Perspectives* 121, no. 7 (July 2013): 774–783.

UK Prospective Diabetes Study Group. "Intensive Blood-Glucose Control with Sulphonylureas or Insulin Compared with Conventional Treatment and Risk of Complications in Patients with Type 2 Diabetes (UKPDS 33)." *The Lancet* 352, no. 9131 (September 12, 1998): 837–853.

Whittemore, Robin. "A Systematic Review of the Translational Research on the Diabetes Prevention Program." *Translational Behavioral Medicine* 1, no. 3 (September 2011): 480–491.

Websites

"Diabetes Basics." *American Diabetes Association.* http://www.diabetes.org/diabetes-basics/?loc=db-slabnav (accessed January 6, 2015).

"Facts and Figures about Diabetes." *World Health Organization (WHO).* http://www.who.int/diabetes/facts/en/ (accessed January 6, 2015).

"Gestational Diabetes and Pregnancy." *U.S. Centers for Disease Control and Prevention (CDC).* http://www.cdc.gov/pregnancy/diabetes-gestational.html (accessed January 6, 2015).

Lindsay M. Jaacks

Drug/Substance Abuse

⊕ Introduction

Illegal drug and substance use and abuse is a global concern. Although primary drugs of abuse vary between and within regions and countries, the four main drugs of abuse worldwide are opiates (heroin is the most widely known), cocaine, cannabis (marijuana is the most well-known), and the amphetamine-type drugs (not including Ecstasy). In nearly every country, whether developed, wealthy, developing, middle income, undeveloped, or impoverished, drug manufacture, possession, and distribution or trafficking are illegal. Some countries have well-articulated policies, procedures, and laws regarding consequences for drug-related crime, others do not. Among those with criminal laws related to drugs, their enforcement varies from place to place.

The United Nations' 2012 *World Drug Report* states that roughly 5 percent of the global population, or more than 230 million people, self-reported use of illicit drugs during 2010. About 27 million people worldwide are believed to have significant issues with drug and substance abuse and addiction. Although global drug use is believed to be neither increasing not decreasing, disproportionate increases in numbers among people living in some of the developing countries are reported. About 200,000 individuals die annually as a result of drug use, with the highest overall mortality rate among heroin and cocaine users. Drug and substance use is closely associated with the spread of some communicable diseases, particularly HIV/AIDS. Drug and substance use negatively impact productivity, work and school performance, economic and social stability and growth, and significantly contribute to crime, particularly crimes of a violent nature.

In 2011, roughly 7,000 tons of opium were produced worldwide, with the largest amount produced in Afghanistan. Coca production has been steadily decreasing since 2000, with total cultivation area down by more than 33 percent since the start of the 21st century.

Although there has been some measurable success in decreasing the production of plant-based drugs, there has been a burgeoning industry devoted to the production of synthetic drugs. Synthetic drugs have not yet come under international control.

The primary goals of the United Nations' approach to the management of all aspects of illicit substance use are to develop an integrated, interagency, global approach to target prevention, to promote effective and safe treatment, to encourage the development of alternative crops for those cultivating plants used for illegal drugs, and to protect and promote basic human rights.

⊕ Historical Background

Using a variety of substances to enhance and alter mood is a practice as old as humanity. Drugs have been used for medical purposes; consciousness-altering and hallucinogenic substances have been incorporated into religious practice; and a variety of substances have been used recreationally since very early history. A Sumerian pictogram illustrates the recreational use of opium as early as 5000 BCE. Manual laborers have chewed coca leaves for thousands of years. In 3500 BCE, the ancient Egyptians created instructions, on papyrus scrolls, for the production of alcoholic beverages. Swiss lake dwellers, around 2500 BCE, were reported to eat poppy seeds for their euphoric and hallucinogenic effects. Concern for negative effects associated with the use of alcohol and drugs began as early as 2000 BCE in Egypt, where students were warned to avoid local taverns because the mood-altering substances they encountered there caused them to make poor choices.

During the 9th century CE, it was reported that opium was in wide recreational use throughout much of Asia. At the end of the 15th century (c. 1493), Christopher Columbus brought dried tobacco leaves back from his journeys and introduced the concept of smoking tobacco to the European populace. By the early 1600s,

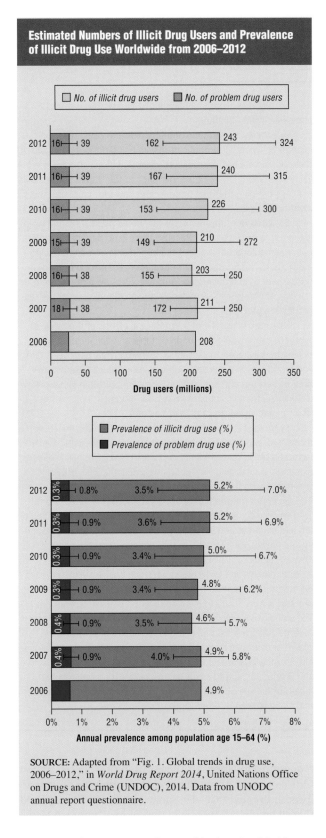

Estimated Numbers of Illicit Drug Users and Prevalence of Illicit Drug Use Worldwide from 2006–2012

□ No. of illicit drug users   ▨ No. of problem drug users

Year			
2012	16	39	162	243	324
2011	16	39	167	240	315
2010	16	39	153	226	300
2009	15	39	149	210	272
2008	16	38	155	203	250
2007	18	38	172	211	250
2006			208		

Drug users (millions)

▨ Prevalence of illicit drug use (%)
■ Prevalence of problem drug use (%)

Year			
2012	0.3%	0.8%	3.5%	5.2%	7.0%
2011	0.3%	0.9%	3.6%	5.2%	6.9%
2010	0.3%	0.9%	3.4%	5.0%	6.7%
2009	0.3%	0.9%	3.4%	4.8%	6.2%
2008	0.4%	0.9%	3.5%	4.6%	5.7%
2007	0.4%	0.9%	4.0%	4.9%	5.8%
2006			4.9%		

Annual prevalence among population age 15–64 (%)

SOURCE: Adapted from "Fig. 1. Global trends in drug use, 2006–2012," in *World Drug Report 2014*, United Nations Office on Drugs and Crime (UNDOC), 2014. Data from UNODC annual report questionnaire.

was subject to criminal penalties; users were sometimes severely punished.

In the early 1500s, an opium derivative called laudanum was incorporated into medical practice as a pain reliever and cough suppressant. It was extremely potent, and contained many of the opium alkaloids, including morphine (pain reliever) and codeine (both a pain reliever and a cough suppressant). Dover's powder, an opium-based preparation touted as a cure for gout, was extremely popular for about 150 years. In 1805, German chemist Friedrich W. A. Sertürner (1783–1841) isolated and described the drug morphine. Laudanum, morphine, and other opium derivatives were sold commercially until the early 20th century, when opium's addictive properties were recognized and its use became controlled.

Around 1800, Napoleon's army brought cannabis from Egypt into France, primarily in the form of hashish. Its popularity quickly spread, particularly among artists, writers, and musicians. In 1841, French psychiatrist Jacques-Joseph Moreau (1804–1884), used hashish to treat mental illness in patients at the Bicêtre Hospital, located in the southern portion of Paris. Cocaine was chemically isolated for the first time in the mid-1800s.

In 1852, the American Pharmaceutical Association was founded. One of its stated goals was to restrict the dispensing and sale of prescribed medications to properly educated apothecaries and druggists.

In Ghent, Belgium, in 1864, German chemist Johann Friedrich Wilhelm Adolf von Baeyer (1835–1917) synthesized the first barbiturate, barbituric acid. In the late 1800s, Austrian psychiatrist and neurologist Sigmund Freud (1856–1939), now known as the founder of psychoanalysis, reported his use of cocaine for the treatment of depression. In 1874, heroin was first synthesized from morphine. It was produced commercially by the Bayer Pharmaceutical Company in 1898. The original intent was to use heroin in place of the widely abused morphine, as it was not initially believed to be addictive. It quickly became apparent that heroin was highly addictive, and its use was restricted. Heroin was made illegal in most places around the globe.

In 1914, the Harrison Narcotic Act was passed by the U.S. Congress as a means of regulating and taxing the importation, production, and distribution of opiates and coca products. The legal interpretation of this law was that physicians could judiciously prescribe these classes of narcotic to their patients, but they were not to be used to treat addictions. In 1924, heroin production in the United States was made illegal. The Marihuana Tax Act of 1937 imposed a tax on the sale of all forms of cannabis in the United States.

In the late 1950s and early 1960s, the World Health Organization (WHO) began to look at the most effective

American tobacco growers began shipping the dried leaves to Europe. Tobacco was considered an addictive and dangerous drug in many countries, and its possession or use

WHAT EXACTLY ARE SYNTHETIC DRUGS AND WHAT DO THEY DO?

Synthetic drugs are manufactured, rather than grown or cultivated. They are often targeted and marketed to children and youth, who are given the impression that these substances, which are often sold commercially and are therefore readily accessible to young populations, particularly in the developed or more affluent countries, are harmless. However, they actually are reported to be harmful, and sometimes deadly.

Synthetic drugs are increasing in production and availability worldwide. The most commonly sold are synthetic cannabinoids designed to mimic the experience and effects of marijuana, colloquially referred to as "K-2" or "spice." They are most often marketed commercially as forms of incense, although they are typically smoked or ingested. Because they are often marketed with labels indicating that they are not suitable for consumption by humans, they are not subject to any form of regulatory oversight or quality control. However, in 2011, the U.S. Drug Enforcement Administration (DEA) began to regulate possession and sale of some of the chemicals used, and in 2012, additional chemicals were added to the list of those banned. However, development and production of new synthetic cannabinoids is reported to be significantly increasing, with 51 new types identified in 2012, up from just 2 in 2009. Manufacturers continue to try to use new formulations to work around the DEA bans.

Synthetic cannabinoids are often touted as a legal way to achieve an altered state of consciousness (colloquially, to get "high"). They are eaten, smoked, sprayed onto the skin or into the mouth or applied to incense, which is then burned and inhaled. Sometimes, the drug is sprayed onto potpourri, which is then heated and the vapor inhaled.

According to data published in the United States in an annual survey conducted by the National Institute on Drug Abuse at the National Institutes of Health, called "Monitoring the Future," synthetic cannabinoids were the second-most-popular drug of abuse in the United States, after marijuana, in 2012. Of the 12th-grade students surveyed, 36.4 percent reported use of marijuana within the previous calendar year, and 11.3 percent reported use of synthetic cannabinoids. In the 2013 survey, the percent of marijuana use remained the same, though synthetic marijuana use dropped to 7.9 percent.

Synthetic cathinones are a human-made substance similar in effect to amphetamine. They are often referred to as "bath salts" or "jewelry cleaner." Their development and production is on the rise, with 31 new types identified in the United States in 2012, compared with 4 in 2009.

In addition to synthetic cannabinoids and cathinones, an increasing variety of synthetic drugs are being developed, manufactured, distributed, and consumed worldwide, with a reported 76 new and different varieties identified in the United States alone in 2012, bringing the total there to 158 new synthetic substances identified.

So, what does this mean for the global population and what is the risk to public health? Because there is no national or international regulation of many of the ingredients or manufacturing methods, as the products are not categorized as food or medications, there is no regulation or quality control. As a result, there is a lack of consistency in materials or ingredients used, as well as production processes.

Reported physical and psychological effects of the range of synthetic cannabinoids are unpredictable and can include: agitation, extreme anxiety, hallucinations, sharp increases in heart rate and blood pressure, nausea, tremors, vomiting leading to dehydration, seizures and severe headache, unpredictable behaviors including extreme risk taking, very poor judgment and choice-making, and suicidal thoughts or gestures.

Synthetic cathinones' effects are reported to be similar to those associated with significant amphetamine use: significantly increased blood pressure and heart rate, chest pain, hallucinations, extreme paranoid thinking, delusions, and behavior sufficiently violent to cause threat or physical harm to self or others.

Synthetic drugs are developed, produced, marketed and utilized worldwide. While they are especially prevalent in developed or affluent countries and in urban area of city centers, their accessibility and prevalence is steadily increasing regardless of demographics. They are readily available both in commercial establishments such as local markets and convenience stores as well as via the Internet. Because they are constantly shifting ingredients and manufacturing processes, it is difficult to regulate or legislate these compounds. The world community is attempting to categorize synthetic drugs as illegal or illicit substances based on overall similarity of the grown or cultivated drugs they are synthesized to mimic. There are efforts underway to impose criminal penalties on their manufacture and distribution and to create safety standards around them as a means of harm reduction while the global community scrambles to find effective means of reducing supply and demand.

---

ways to treat drug addiction. At that time, it was believed that inpatient stays in institutional settings were probably the most effective. In 1961, the United Nations' "Single Convention on Narcotic Drugs of 10 March 1961" also suggested that drug addicts without criminal convictions should be institutionalized for treatment. In 1971, U.S. President Richard Nixon (1913–1994) stated that drug abuse was the most severe problem in the country and requested legislation for the creation of a Special Action Office of Drug Abuse Prevention. During the same year, Turkish President Cevdet Sunay (1899–1982) mandated that all opium production in the country be ended by the end of the following year.

Beginning in the early 1970s, vehicles moving between Mexico and the United States were searched for illicit drugs and, by the 1980s, drug traffic, particularly involving cannabis, was believed to be steadily increasing. During the late 1980s, Boris Yeltsin (1931–2007), then the Communist Party leader of the Soviet Union and later the first president of the Russian Federation, declared that drug addiction was becoming an epidemic among the youth of Russia.

By the early years of the 21st century, it was widely recognized that drug and substance use were very significant global issues. Rather than continuing to simply attempt to eradicate drug production, trafficking, and use, which had not proven an effective means of decreasing addiction or of eliminating drugs and illegal substances, there was a burgeoning movement toward harm reduction. This is a process in which there is acceptance that drug abuse exists and must be treated as a serious issue without necessarily being able to completely eradicate it. Some of the ways in which harm reduction is implemented include enacting legal protections that increase safety for users and decrease the spread of communicable diseases related to substance use by creating needle exchange programs. Other important methods of the harm reduction movement include providing oversight of habitual users and those with addictions to help ensure their safety and health, as well as aiding in their ability to remain functional members of society.

⊕ Impacts and Issues

The global disease burden of drug and substance abuse remains significant despite ebb and flow in types of substances and means of administration. The WHO and the United Nations Office on Drugs and Crime (UNDOC) estimate that between 3.4 and 6.6 percent of individuals between the ages of 1 and 64 report illegal drug or substance use. Of those, between 10 and 13 percent of users have significant issues related to dependence or addiction. Roughly one-fifth of injectable drug or illicit substance users are HIV positive or diagnosed with AIDS. About 47 percent of those users have hepatitis C, and nearly 15 percent have been diagnosed with hepatitis B. Approximately 1 percent of adult deaths are directly attributable to causes related to drug or illicit substance use or to overdose.

According to UNODC data, the drugs and illicit substances that pose the greatest global concerns are cannabis, opioids, opiates, cocaine, amphetamine and

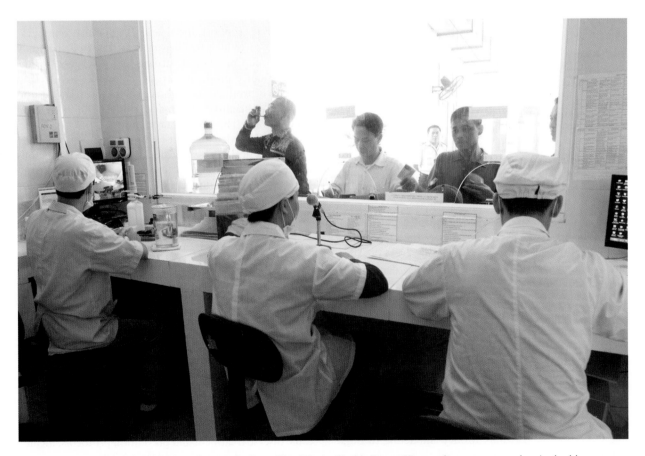

Drug addicts get their daily methadone doses at the Long Bien District Health Center. Vietnam has many comprehensive health programs aimed at the prevention of HIV and to help drug addicts. At this health center, there are comprehensive HIV services, including HIV testing, antiretroviral treatment, distribution of clean needles and condoms, and methadone maintenance therapy for drug addicts.
© Chau Doan/LightRocket via Getty Images.

amphetamine-like stimulants, and Ecstasy. By prevalence percentages and numbers of self-reported users, cannabis is the most prevalent, followed by amphetamine-type stimulants and opioids.

Drugs and other illicit substances move within regions and countries as well as between regions, countries, and continents. An understanding of the patterns of production, movement, trafficking and use increases the effectiveness of interventions developed. The WHO and the United Nations utilize trend analysis as an integral part of their research and data collection methods, which enables pattern analysis, with a goal of decreasing both demand and supply of illegal drugs and other substances. Closely aligned with the research and trending processes are interagency partnerships.

In order to be most effective at both interdiction and prosecution of those involved in drug trade, it is imperative to have international cooperation. UNODC has made inroads on the creation of regional and cross regional infrastructures aimed at sharing information both inside and across borders, allowing for cooperation with international and cross-regional initiatives. Involving multiple jurisdictions and existing law enforcement agencies increases continuity and assures consistent protocols throughout the supply and trafficking chain, which has been shown to be an effective deterrent for those involved in the drug and illegal substance trades.

UNODC has adopted a broad approach to interrupting international drug and substance movement by sea and air called the Container Control Programme, as large shipping containers filled with legitimate goods are often used to transport illicit substances in southern and western areas of Asia as well as to move heroin along the Balkan route to southeastern Europe. They have developed a regional/international hub to interrupt ground and air-based substance movement in the Caribbean and Central America. The hub is located in Panama and works closely with strengthened and increasingly trained law enforcement agencies in Mexico and the Dominican Republic. A parallel part of the effort involves education and programming aimed at reducing the demand for drugs and other illegal substances.

Globally, centers of excellence are being established to reduce demand. Evidence-based best practices are employed in interruption of material flow, demand reduction, prosecution and law enforcement, and education concerning the negative aspects of drug and substance use.

Two issues intimately involved in the drug and substance trade that make it difficult to permanently reduce or eliminate production and flow are money laundering and economic hardship. Money laundering through regional and international organized crime syndicates is an integral part of the drug trade. The economic base of many areas is supported by income from drug and substance production and distribution. Developing alternative means of income by substituting different cash-producing crops and providing financial and other incentives (housing, education, etc.) aids in the development of sustainable economic security and contributes to increasing cooperation by producers. UNODC's overarching goal is to clearly show, and support, the lasting benefits of decreasing supply and demand, as well as to illustrate the long-term benefits of cooperation between and among law enforcement agencies as a means of taking power away from organized crime syndicates. By interrupting drug and substance flow (decreasing supply) while working to decrease demand, the financial base for production and trafficking will be greatly reduced or eliminated.

Research and best-practice methodology have shown that criminal prosecution and punishment or incarceration is significantly less effective globally and longitudinally than shifting incentives, shoring up economies, creating new means of livelihood, and developing quality rehabilitation and harm reduction programs. The processes must be viewed as synergistic: reducing demand and supply must be coupled with increasing programming to develop alternative livelihoods, rehabilitation, and resocialization. Methods must be effective and provide lasting support in order to support social and community reintegration and to reduce recidivism. It is reported that only around one-fourth of all farmers and growers of drug- and substance-producing crops historically involved in substance production have access to the training and economic incentives necessary to create shifts in crop production. This percentage must be dramatically increased in order to effect lasting change.

It is critical to provide education and other programming in order to interrupt progression while simultaneously working to reduce demand, particularly in countries where drug and substance use is on the increase. Central and Western African countries have reported increasing use of cocaine; heroin and opium use have been rising in Afghanistan and the Islamic Republic of Iran.

⊕ Future Implications

Reducing drug and substance supply and demand involves much more than just the redirection of a worldwide and very lucrative industry; there is an extremely critical parallel process involving human rights, physical health, and mental health. Drug and substance use are accompanied by a host of addiction, treatment, and rehabilitation concerns; overdose, morbidity, and mortality issues; and physical health and infectious and communicable disease treatment and prevention protocols, including widespread hepatitis and HIV/AIDS.

Drug and illegal substance production and trafficking are often accompanied by several different types of violent crime: murder is not uncommon, particularly

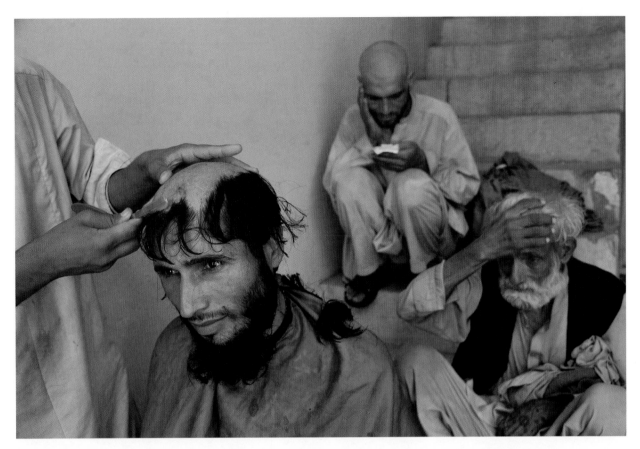

A barber shaves the head of an Afghan drug addict entering rehabilitation at a drug treatment center in Jalalabad, Afghanistan. In 2014, Afghanistan was the source of over 90 percent of the illicit opium in the world. In addition to the illicit cultivation, manufacture, and export of heroin around the world, the country faces the problem of rising domestic drug abuse with at least a million people addicted to heroin, according to research by the International Narcotics Control Board. © *Noorullah Shirzada/AFP/Getty Images.*

among lower-level traffickers and recruiters for local drug and substance distribution. Kidnapping and human trafficking are common, presenting very serious human rights violation concerns. The sex trades exist symbiotically with the worldwide drug and illicit substance mega-industries.

Overall, global drug and illicit substance production and use have remained relatively consistent with the exception of a significant increase in opium production in Afghanistan after a sharp decrease due to crop failure in 2010; this does not reflect a true rise, but represents a return to previous crop levels. Although overall data remains mostly consistent, there is considerable ebb and flow by type of drug within and across regions and nations. With ever-increasing attention to programming with the stated goals of reduction of demand and supply, the maintenance of the status quo is actually very concerning, as it means that current efforts are not effective. There is very significant ability on the part of those involved in the illicit drug trade to recover and shift priorities in order to maintain levels. Put more succinctly, when one type of drug or route of trafficking/production is squeezed shut, another venue is found and opened.

Traditionally, drug and substance use monitoring, programming, interdiction and other concerns have been focused on the more developed and economically stable countries. Over time, the pattern has shifted, and more of the developing and lower-income countries are struggling with the myriad issues related to drugs. Because they have less infrastructure and stability, they are not as well equipped to manage and mitigate, and their stressors are relatively greater as a result. Demographics suggest that population shifts are rapidly occurring toward developing countries, with a steep rise in younger populations that are historically most vulnerable to engagement with illegal drugs and other substances. While males have been reported as generally the most likely to utilize drugs and other illegal substances, the gender gap is diminishing. This is due in part to the improving socioeconomic status of females in many countries around the globe as well as to decreasing sociocultural barriers that previously prevented many females from engaging with the world outside their immediate families or within their small communities. Rural populations are shrinking, and urban growth is exponential, increasing access to the global community.

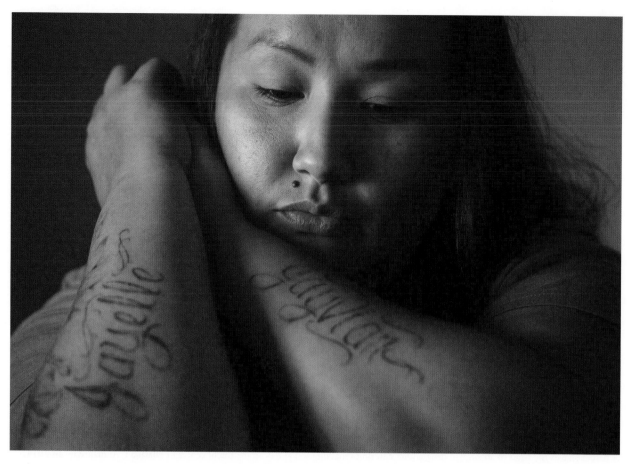

Native American Rachelle Baker has tattoos on her arms to cover up needle scars from being addicted to heroin and methamphetamine on the Fort Berthold Indian Reservation in New Town, North Dakota. In 2014 Fort Berthold was the epicenter of the fracking and oil boom where many tribal members financially benefited from fracking leases and oil royalties. With the money also came a dramatic increase in crime in the form of methamphetamines and heroin use and trafficking, drunk driving, assaults, and domestic violence. Baker is looking at a 56-month jail term for using and selling drugs. She believes the reservation could benefit from a methadone clinic and a narcotics anonymous group. *© Linda Davidson/The Washington Post/Getty Images.*

As global population growth, socioeconomic development and migration trends experience shifts, drug and illicit substance demands are likely to change, perhaps in unexpected ways. As females make inroads in the efforts to achieve equality of social status, education and earning power, trends in type and nature of substance and drug use will change. Decreasing rural populations with rapid growth of city centers significantly impacts supply, demand, and substance use choices. More youthful populations are more likely to move toward synthetic drugs and away from some of the more traditional drugs of abuse such as heroin, opioids and opiates. Increasingly complex social, educational, and occupational demands are often accompanied by a rise in the use of amphetamine-type substances. As countries develop and populations become more affluent, more expensive drug and illegal substance demand and use rises accordingly. In developing or undeveloped countries, where money is more scarce and the ability to obtain and maintain gainful employment is sharply limited, the demand for less-expensive drugs and other illicit substances tends to increase. Any time there is a change in the prevailing moral code, value system, age or gender balance, or level of poverty or affluence, the demand for, and use of, drugs and illegal substances is likely to rise.

Predictive statistics suggest that the use and desirability of heroin, injectable drugs, and cocaine will progressively decrease. Cannabis is predicted to remain stable as the most popular and prevalent illicit drug. Many regions are decriminalizing it, which is likely to impact law enforcement protocols and programming. Distribution and production will likely become more globally standardized over the next several decades. The creation, development and distribution of a wide variety of illegal synthetic drugs are expected to continually increase.

SEE ALSO *Alcohol Use and Abuse; HIV/AIDS; Mental Health Treatment Access; Viral Hepatitis; Vulnerable Populations*

BIBLIOGRAPHY

Books

Ghodse, Hamid, et al., eds. *Substance Abuse Disorders: Evidence and Experience.* Chichester, UK: Wiley-Blackwell, 2011.

Kuhar, Michael J. *The Addicted Brain: Why We Abuse Drugs, Alcohol, and Nicotine.* Upper Saddle River, NJ: FT Press, 2012.

Lawson, Gary, and Ann W. Lawson, eds. *Alcoholism and Substance Abuse in Diverse Populations*, 2nd ed. Austin, TX: PRO-ED, 2011.

Mills, China. *Decolonizing Global Mental Health: The Psychiatrization of the Majority World.* New York: Routledge, Taylor & Francis, 2014.

Montvilo, Robin Kamienny, ed. *Addictions & Substance Abuse.* Ipswich, MA: Salem Press, 2013.

Murati, Kristina A., and Allison G. Fischer, eds. *Substance Abuse, Assessment, and Addiction.* New York: Nova Science, 2011.

Nutt, David J., and Liam Nestor. *Substance Abuse.* Oxford: Oxford University Press, 2013.

Ruiz, Pedro, and Eric C. Strain. *The Substance Abuse Handbook*, 2nd ed. Philadelphia: Wolters Kluwer Health, 2014.

Walters, Scott T., and Frederick Rotgers, eds. *Treating Substance Abuse: Theory and Technique*, 3rd ed. New York: Guilford Press, 2012.

Periodicals

Hammer, Rachel, et al. "The Experience of Addiction as Told by the Addicted: Incorporating Biological Understandings into Self-Story." *Culture, Medicine and Psychiatry* 36, no. 4 (2012): 712–734.

Kaye, Kerwin. "Rehabilitating the 'Drugs Lifestyle' Criminal Justice, Social Control, and the Cultivation of Agency." *Ethnography* 14, no. 2 (2013): 207–232.

Lisi, Donna M. "Designer Drugs: Patients May Be Using Synthetic Cannabinoids More Than You Think." *Jems* 39, no. 9 (2014): 14.

Serec, Masa, et al. "Health-Related Lifestyle, Physical and Mental Health in Children of Alcoholic Parents." *Drug and Alcohol Review* 31, no. 7 (2012): 861–870.

Wechsberg, Wendee M., et al. "Substance Use, Gender Inequity, Violence and Sexual Risk among Couples in Cape Town." *Culture, Health & Sexuality* 15, no. 9–10 (2013): 1221–1236.

Websites

"Drug Addiction." *Mayo Clinic.* http://www.mayoclinic.com/health/drug-addiction/DS00183 (accessed March 2, 2015).

"Global Strategy to Reduce Harmful Use of Alcohol." *World Health Organization (WHO).* http://www.who.int/substance_abuse/activities/gsrhua/en/ (accessed March 1, 2015).

"Persons Who Use Drugs (PWUD)." *U.S. Centers for Disease Control and Prevention (CDC).* http://www.cdc.gov/pwud/default.html (accessed March 2, 2015).

"Substance Abuse." *World Health Organization (WHO).* http://www.who.int/topics/substance_abuse/en/ (accessed March 2, 2015).

"Substance Abuse and Mental Health Services Administration (SAMHSA)." *U.S. Department of Health and Human Services.* http://www.samhsa.gov/ (accessed March 2, 2015).

Pamela V. Michaels

Ebola Virus Disease

⊕ Introduction

Ebola virus disease (EVD) is a highly deadly viral disease that is hemorrhagic; that is, it involves the destruction of blood cells. As the disease progresses, the walls of blood vessels break down and blood gushes from every tissue and organ. The disease is caused by the Ebola virus, named after the river in Zaire (now the Democratic Republic of the Congo) where the first known outbreak occurred in 1976.

The disease is extremely contagious and exceptionally lethal. Whereas a 10 percent mortality rate is considered high for most infectious diseases, Ebola can kill up to 90 percent of its victims, usually within only a few days after exposure. Direct contact with contaminated blood or bodily fluids seems to transmit the disease. Health personnel and caregivers are often the most likely to be infected. Even after a patient has died, preparing the body for a funeral can be deadly for family members.

In March 2014 Guinea officials notified the World Health Organization (WHO) about possible cases of EVD. Subsequent lab tests confirmed the presence of Ebola. The disease spread quickly across the nearby borders with Liberia and Sierra Leone to become the largest and most deadly outbreak of Ebola in history.

More than a year after the first cases were reported, the worst EVD outbreak in history continued to claim lives in the West African countries of Guinea, Liberia, and Sierra Leone. By March 18, 2015, the outbreak had resulted in more than 24,701 cases of EVD, including 10,194 deaths, and the outbreak continued. For multiple reasons, including reporting methods and cultural taboos, experts estimate the actual numbers for both cases and deaths related to EVD are substantially higher.

⊕ Historical Background

After the first outbreak of EVD in 1976, subsequent EVD epidemics occurred periodically, usually in remote villages in Central Africa. Prior to the 2014 outbreak in West Africa, the outbreaks resulted in no more than a few hundred deaths before the epidemic's dying out. (See table.) The high lethality of the disease, the quickness with which it kills, actually worked against the spread of disease outbreaks in remote areas.

Before the 2014 West Africa outbreak, the two worst documented EVD outbreaks occurred in 1976 and 1995 in the Democratic Republic of the Congo, killing an estimated 280 and 254 people, respectively, according to the WHO. In the 1995 EVD outbreak, as in many others, some of the first victims were health workers. Doctors and nurses performed exploratory surgery on a lab technician who became ill with unexplained symptoms. The lab worker who was the patient and the surgery team all died of the disease.

Over the years, prior to the 2014 outbreak in West Africa, health officials had confirmed Ebola cases only in Sudan, the Democratic Republic of the Congo, Gabon, Uganda, the Ivory Coast (Côte d'Ivoire), Guinea, Liberia, Sierra Leone, and Nigeria. During the 2014 outbreak in West Africa, cases were exported to multiple countries, including the United States. All cases outside of Africa were individuals who had recently lived, visited, or worked in the 2104 West Africa outbreak zone, or were traced to contact with such individuals (e.g., Ebola infection acquired by medical personnel treating infected patients).

EVD typically kills between 50 to 90 percent of those who fall ill with the virus. It is most contagious in victims with high viral loads of the disease, usually those at the height of illness or recently deceased. Ebola is not transmitted prior to the development of symptoms. Ebola's incubation period, from exposure to onset of illness, ranges from 2 to 21 days. After the incubation period, symptoms develop and progress very rapidly. The disease spreads by direct contact with contaminated blood or bodily fluids.

Initially, EVD causes humans to experience a high fever, headache, muscle aches, abdominal pain, tiredness, and diarrhea. Some people also will display bloody diarrhea and vomit blood. As the disease progresses, the

Ebola Virus Disease Outbreaks from 1976–2012

Year	Country	Cases	Deaths	Case fatality
2012	Democratic Republic of Congo	57	29	51%
2012	Uganda	7	4	57%
2012	Uganda	24	17	71%
2011	Uganda	1	1	100%
2008	Democratic Republic of Congo	32	14	44%
2007	Uganda	149	37	25%
2007	Democratic Republic of Congo	264	187	71%
2005	Congo	12	10	83%
2004	Sudan	17	7	41%
2003 (Nov–Dec)	Congo	35	29	83%
2003 (Jan–Apr)	Congo	143	128	90%
2001–2002	Congo	59	44	75%
2001–2002	Gabon	65	53	82%
2000	Uganda	425	224	53%
1996	South Africa (ex-Gabon)	1	1	100%
1996 (Jul–Dec)	Gabon	60	45	75%
1996 (Jan–Apr)	Gabon	31	21	68%
1995	Democratic Republic of Congo	315	254	81%
1994	Cote d'Ivoire	1	0	0%
1994	Gabon	52	31	60%
1979	Sudan	34	22	65%
1977	Democratic Republic of Congo	1	1	100%
1976	Sudan	284	151	53%
1976	Democratic Republic of Congo	318	280	88%

SOURCE: Adapted from "Table: Chronology of previous Ebola virus disease outbreaks," in *Ebola Virus Disease, Fact sheet N°103*, World Health Organization (WHO), updated September 2014.

walls of blood vessels break down, causing internal and external bleeding, followed by shock and death. EVD in its initial stages presents symptoms similar to many tropical diseases, including malaria and typhoid fever. Physicians usually detect the presence of Ebola when patients present advanced symptoms such as internal and external bleeding, internal tissue necrosis, and organ failure, or through laboratory testing.

The Ebola virus is one of two members of a family of RNA viruses called the *Filoviridae*. The other Filovirus causes Marburg hemorrhagic fever, named after the German town where it was contracted first, by laboratory workers handling imported primates infected with the virus. Researchers have identified five species within the genus *Ebolavirus*, based on differences in their genetic sequences. Three of the species regularly cause disease in humans: Zaire ebolavirus (isolated in 1976), Sudan ebolavirus (isolated in 1976), and Bundibugyo ebolavirus (isolated in 2008). The fourth species, called Ebola-Reston, causes disease in primates and is capable of infecting humans but so far has not resulted in disease in humans. Ebola-Reston is named

for the U.S. military primate research facility where scientists isolated the virus during a 1989 outbreak of the disease caused by infected monkeys that had been imported from the Philippines for research. Taï Forest ebolavirus (TFEV) was identified in 1995 and initially was known as Côte d'Ivoire ebolavirus. The only human case of TFEV occurred in a researcher who was performing necropsies on primates who had died of the virus.

Ebola-Reston inspired public awareness of hemorrhagic diseases. At that time, there was fear that Ebola-Reston could spread to neighboring Washington, D.C. Study of the cause of this outbreak determined that these particular Ebola viruses could remain infectious after becoming dispersed in the air. Four researchers at the facility tested positive for Ebola-Reston antibodies but showed no signs of illness. Later it was determined that Ebola-Reston, unlike other forms of Ebola, does not cause disease in humans.

Although genetic testing dates Ebola to the earliest parts of the 20th century, scientists do not yet understand fully the history of Ebola and its evolution to causing infections in humans. The current evidence suggests fruit bats (*Pteropodidae*) are the likely natural host (a natural reservoir) for the virus. Monkeys and other primates are thought to have played a significant role in the early transmission of EVDs to humans. Accordingly, health officials discourage the killing and eating of bats, primates, and other bushmeat to reduce human contact with disease reservoirs.

The 2014 West African Outbreak

In August 2014, an international group of experts on the Ebola virus and EVD subsequently assembled by the WHO unanimously concluded that the ongoing EVD outbreak in the East African countries of Guinea, Liberia, Nigeria (Africa's most populous country), and Sierra Leone met criteria specified in the governing International Health Regulations (IHR) to warrant declaration of a public health emergency of international concern. The committee concluded that the EVD outbreak in West Africa was an "extraordinary event" and that the consequences of further international spread of the disease mandated a coordinated international response. Announcing its decision in a press release, committee members cited the virulence of the virus, the patterns of transmission—especially in health facilities and among health-care workers—and the weak health-care systems in the region of the outbreak.

The WHO initially estimated mortality from the West Africa EVD outbreak at just over 50 percent. However, updated figures suggest that as many as 70 percent of those infected in the West Africa outbreak died of the disease. As medical infrastructure developed and supportive care increased, the death rate declined.

The outbreak remained most virulent and centered in Guinea, Liberia, and Sierra Leone, with related and quickly contained cases spread by travelers to Nigeria. Senegal officials also reported a case of EVD in a traveler. After 42 days (double the normal incubation time) with no reports of new Ebola cases, on October 17 and 20, 2014, respectively, the WHO declared outbreaks of EVD in Senegal and Nigeria to be over.

However, the disease had begun to appear outside of Africa. In early October 2014, a nursing assistant in Spain was diagnosed with EVD. She had been part of the medical team that treated two Spanish priests who contracted the Ebola virus in West Africa, were transported to Spain for medical care, and later died. The nursing assistant later recovered and was released from the hospital in November 2014.

Though transmission to humans has never been documented, and according to the CDC, there is limited evidence that dogs can become infected with carriers of the Ebola virus, the Spanish government ordered

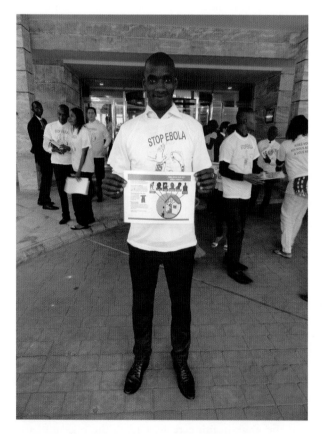

An employee of a hotel located in the West African city of Conakry, Guinea, wears a "STOP EBOLA" T-shirt depicting two hands stopping the Ebola virus and dialing the Guinea Ebola Hotline number 115 on a cell phone. He also holds a handout received during a training seminar he and his colleagues attended inside educating them as to the proper methods and protocols to be implemented when dealing with Ebola hemorrhagic fever. *Sally Ezra/U.S. Centers for Disease Control and Prevention.*

that the dog belonging to the nursing assistant be euthanized. The World Small Animal Veterinary Association subsequently called for the quarantine of dogs exposed to the EVD instead of automatic euthanasia.

In late September 2014, a traveler from Liberia carried the Ebola virus to the United States. The patient, the first person to be diagnosed with and die of EVD in the United States, had close contact with Ebola-infected people while in Liberia. Fears for his immediate family and contacts in the United States eased as no new cases among them were reported during their 21-day quarantine. However, the traveler, who eventually died of EVD, infected health-care workers at the hospital in Dallas, Texas, where he sought treatment.

CDC officials confirmed in October that there were two cases of transmission to nurses who cared for the patient in Dallas. The nurses were sent to special facilities near Washington, D.C., and Atlanta, Georgia, for treatment. Both nurses responded to supportive care and experimental treatments, including plasma from patients who previously recovered from EVD. Both were eventually declared free of the Ebola virus. Physicians at Emory Hospital in Atlanta had previous success treating health-care workers infected in Africa who were repatriated to the United States. Although there is still no definitive cure for EVD, physicians said that early supportive care, including aggressive hydration and treatment with experimental drugs, holds promise to reduce the lethality of the disease where such care is available.

Subsequent to the Ebola death in Dallas and the confirmed transmission to health-care workers, U.S. President Barack Obama (1961–) convened a special cabinet meeting centered on coordinating the U.S. response to the Ebola virus. Prior to the meeting, the United States committed troops to help build clinics and other health-care infrastructure in the outbreak areas in Africa. The CDC activated its Emergency Operations Center and announced it would work with the Customs and Border Protection agency to begin fever screening measures for travelers from West Africa arriving at selected U.S. airports with a high number of travelers from Guinea, Liberia, and Sierra Leone.

Following the infection of health-care workers in the United States, the CDC reviewed and tightened treatment protocols, including new guidelines for the use of personal protective equipment (PPE). Ebola is transmitted by contact with bodily fluids, and the new guidelines reduce the potential for transmission to health-care workers by eliminating any exposure of skin. Because many infections occur during the removal of PPE, the CDC also recommended more intensive training in the donning and removal of disposable gowns, masks, face shields, hoods, shoe covers, and so forth. Although Ebola is not an airborne virus, the virus can be transmitted in droplets of fluid exuded by patients, especially in close quarters where

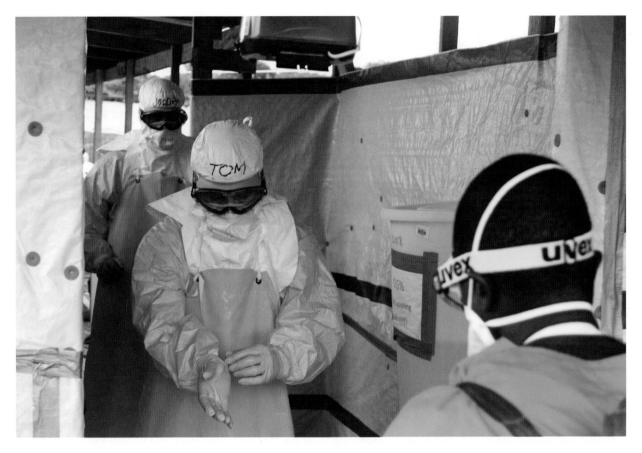

Dr. Tom Frieden, director of the U.S. Centers for Disease Control and Prevention (CDC), who is dressed in his personal protective equipment, undergoes a protocol-required decontamination procedure as he prepares to exit the Ebola treatment unit (ETU), known as ELWA 3, which opened on August 17, 2014, in Monrovia, Liberia. Staff members of Médecins Sans Frontières, or Doctors Without Borders, who operate the ELWA 3 ETU, were conducting this decontamination process. *Sally Ezra/U.S. Centers for Disease Control and Prevention.*

contamination by droplets produced by sneezing, vomiting, and diarrhea is possible. Accordingly, akin to protocols used in specialized biocontainment units, the new CDC guidelines also require a higher protective level of breathing masks (e.g., N95 respirators or other air-purifying respirators).

In late October 2014, the New York City Department of Health and Mental Hygiene confirmed that a physician returning from treating EVD patients in Guinea tested positive for the Ebola virus. New York and other states quickly introduced controversial policies requiring mandatory quarantines of health-care workers returning from treating patients in Guinea, Liberia, and Sierra Leone. The patient recovered. In November 2014 a surgeon who contracted Ebola while working in Sierra Leone was returned to the United States to receive treatment at the Nebraska Medical Center biocontainment unit. The surgeon arrived in extremely critical condition and died soon after his arrival.

In November 2014, Mali reported its first Ebola reported deaths, joining Nigeria, Spain, Senegal, and the United States as countries outside the core outbreak area in Guinea, Liberia, and Sierra Leone to report

deaths from Ebola. Mali eventually reported eight cases, including six deaths. The WHO declared Mali Ebola free on January 18, 2015, after 42 days without any additional cases.

While the Ebola outbreak in West Africa continued to expand, in September 2014, the WHO announced an unrelated EVD outbreak in the Democratic Republic of the Congo. As of October, the outbreak had infected at least 60 people, resulting in 49 deaths. WHO officials announced that laboratory testing confirmed that the Congo outbreak is of a different zoonotic origin than the strain responsible for the EVD outbreak originating in West Africa.

⊕ Impacts and Issues

Since the mid-1970s, disease researchers, physicians, and health workers from organizations that include the WHO, CDC, and Médecins Sans Frontières (MSF, or Doctors Without Borders) have responded to EVD outbreaks by providing research assistance, frontline medical care, and quarantine facilities. Organizations such as

COLLEGES ENHANCE MONITORING FOR EBOLA VIRAL DISEASE (EVD)

The declaration by the World Health Organization that the 2014 Ebola outbreak constituted a public health emergency of international concern caught college administrators in the United States off guard. With just weeks or days before faculty and students would start to return from EVD outbreak regions, schools faced tough decisions regarding isolation and quarantine measures.

Harvard University, with a reputation for a globally diverse faculty and student body, required faculty, staff, and students returning from outbreak areas be screened by Harvard University Health Services before returning to campus.

Harvard University Health Services published the following recommendation to prevent EVD transmission:

- Maintain good personal and environmental hygiene; frequently wash hands with soap and water;
- Ensure thorough cooking of food before consumption;
- Avoid close contact with ill persons and avoid contact with blood and body fluids of infected people, including items that may have come in contact with an infected person's blood or body fluids;
- Avoid contact with animals;
- After returning from travel in an affected area, travelers should observe closely their health condition for 21 days.
- Seek medical advice promptly if a fever develops greater than 100.4 degrees Fahrenheit (38 degrees Celsius), or if diarrhea, vomiting, rash, or bleeding occurs.

Though the guidelines were developed for the students at Harvard, they are useful for anyone who is concerned that he or she could have been exposed to EVD.

the International Committee of the Red Cross also have helped local governments and health officials conduct critical public information campaigns to educate people on how to identify symptoms and prevent the spread of the disease.

Ebola affects people in the most basic way. It strikes with little warning and can sweep through a village in a short time. In the rural settings where the disease usually occurs, medical care is minimal, and health-care providers are stretched to their limits to contain the infection and provide basic comforts to those who are ill.

Part of the reason for the ferocity of an Ebola outbreak is a lack of understanding of the disease among those who are most affected by it. More education targeting those who are at risk of acquiring the infection is still needed. For example, burial customs in many African cultures include an open viewing of the deceased, which potentially exposes the mourners to the virus. This

practice can amplify the spread of the virus—that is, the virus can affect more people than it otherwise would. Amplification is an important means by which a variety of viral and bacterial diseases can spread. In the case of Ebola and mourning customs, learning to pay respect to the deceased person without touching or even seeing them would help reduce the spread of Ebola.

During some initial outbreaks, well-meaning medical personnel helped spread the virus. The infection of health-care workers is, unfortunately, a common aspect of Ebola outbreaks. The use of protective measures, such as masks and gloves, lessens the risk of passing the infection to caregivers. In some rural clinics, however, such measures—commonplace in medical clinics in developed countries—are a luxury.

Aggressive Vaccine Development and Distribution

In August 2014, three internationally respected and influential viral disease specialists signed a joint statement asking that WHO allow experimental drugs and vaccines used on American aid workers who contracted Ebola be produced and distributed more broadly to alleviate suffering and stop the outbreak in Africa. Peter Piot (1949–), director of the London School of Hygiene and Tropical Medicine (and codiscoverer of ebolavirus in 1976); David Heymann (1946–), director of the Chatham House Centre on Global Health Security; and Jeremy Farrar (1961–) of the Wellcome Trust argued that others working in the infected zone areas be given an equal chance at experimental treatments. The statement said that the WHO was "the only body with the necessary international authority to allow such treatments" as part of a "more robust international response" to the outbreak.

The length and extent of the West Africa Ebola virus outbreak mobilized the international public health community on a scale unprecedented for any previous Ebola outbreak. The severity of the outbreak also pushed the development of new Ebola virus drugs and vaccines. Although limited amounts of experimental drugs used during the 2014 outbreak proved potentially effective, there remained no definitive and tested vaccine, antiviral drug, or cure for EVD during the outbreak.

Advances in Research

Working at a pace quickened by the 2014 EVD outbreak in Africa, in August 2014, Harvard University researchers and researchers from the Broad Institute and other research facilities—in turn, working in cooperation with government and public health officials in Africa—sequenced and analyzed Ebola virus genomes. The breakthroughs offered hope for development of more sensitive and rapid field diagnostic tests for the presence of Ebola virus and EVD.

While evolutionary change in viral genomes is normal, researchers concluded that genetic changes observed in the Ebola strains contributing to the 2014 EVD outbreak were occurring faster and more frequently than genetic changes observed in previous outbreaks.

Public Health Response

In accord with existing IHRs, WHO officials recommended that in countries with EVD outbreaks, governments declare a state of national emergency and activate their emergency management response systems. WHO officials also urged governments to use whatever means necessary to ensure that medical supplies, including PPE, were consistently and reliably available to health-care providers. In areas of intense transmission, the WHO recommended that "extraordinary supplemental measures such as quarantine should be used as considered necessary" and that countries affected should conduct exit screening of "all persons at international airports, seaports and major land crossings."

In order to minimize the risk of international spread of EVD, the committee recommended "probable and suspect cases should immediately be isolated and their travel should be restricted." In addition, mass gatherings should be postponed. Although the WHO did not impose a general ban on international travel or trade, individual airlines and other companies began to impose targeted bans on travel and trade, raising fears of damage to the economies in outbreak areas.

The OPEC Fund for International Development approved an emergency assistance grant of US$500,000 to support WHO in its attempts to stop the international spread of EVD. The World Bank offered to provide up to $200 million to countries in the outbreak region.

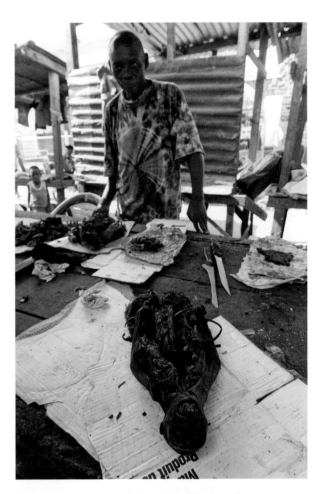

Bushmeat, including smoked monkeys like those shown, is a common food staple in many countries, especially during times of conflict or other disruptions. However, the consumption of bushmeat increases the chances of zoonotic hemorrhagic diseases such as that caused by the Ebola virus. © *Sergey Uryadnikov/ Shutterstock.com.*

⊕ Future Implications

Factors critical to a country's ability to deal with health-care emergencies include (1) the robustness or fragility of component health-care systems (e.g., whether they have significant deficits in personnel, financial, and material resources); (2) experience with a particular disease; perceptions or misperceptions about the disease (including critical factors such as how the disease is transmitted, incubation periods, susceptibility of the population, etc.); and an ability to track and control movements of the population across regions or borders.

On a broader scale, Ebola is a striking example of how human encroachment on regions that were previously uninhabited can bring people into contact with microorganisms to which they had not been previously exposed.

In the case of Ebola, human encroachment on previously uninhabited areas includes increased contact with the natural host of the disease. The blurring of the boundaries between the human and the natural worlds has brought people into closer contact with primates, who are either the natural reservoir of the virus or who acquire the infection from the natural reservoir, possibly a fruit bat. The virus can spread to humans who kill and eat apes or chimpanzees. Bushmeat, including the meat of primates, has long been eaten by rural Africans, and its sale is still an important part of the rural economy.

The link between the consumption of bushmeat and the spread of Ebola has spurred efforts to restrict poaching. A 2005 meeting involving 23 African nations and representatives of the United Nations addressed the problem of the declining great ape population and urged stricter controls on poaching and deforestation (which increases the access of people to ape territory). While admirable, the effectiveness of the campaign is debatable. Ape meat is still available for sale in many local markets in regions of Africa and is sought by buyers in Western countries.

PRIMARY SOURCE

Ebola and Marburg Virus Disease Epidemics: Preparedness, Alert, Control, and Evaluation

SOURCE *"Introduction,"* in Ebola Strategy: Ebola and Marburg Virus Disease Epidemics: Preparedness, Alert, Control, and Evaluation. *Geneva: World Health Organization (WHO), August 2014, 9–15. http://apps.who.int/iris/bitstream/10665/130160/1/WHO_HSE_PED_CED_2014.05_eng.pdf?ua=1 (accessed January 25, 2015).*

INTRODUCTION *This primary source is taken from the introduction of a 2014 report prepared by the World Health Organization on the Ebola and Marburg virus epidemics. The selected text gives an overview of the transmission of the diseases.*

TRANSMISSION

In Africa, fruit bats of the family *Pteropodidae* are considered natural hosts of filoviruses—the viruses that cause Marburg and Ebola viruses. Fruit bats belonging to the genus *Rousettus* are considered potential hosts of the Marburg virus, and bats belonging to the genera *Hypsignathus, Epomops*, and *Myonycteris* are considered possible hosts of the Ebola virus. However, Ebola and Marburg have also been found in other bat species. The geographic distribution of Ebola and Marburg viruses probably corresponds to that of fruit bats of the family *Pteropodidae*. Consequently, Ebola and Marburg viruses are considered endemic throughout Sub-Saharan Africa.

In Africa, the infection of human cases with Ebola virus disease has occurred through the handling of infected chimpanzees, gorillas, monkeys, bats of the species *Hypsignathus* and *Epomops*, forest antelopes, and porcupines. Most primary (index) cases (cases) of Marburg infection occurred following an extended stay in or near mines or caves inhabited by bats of the *Rousettus* species.

Person-to-person transmission of Ebola and Marburg virus occurs through direct contact with the blood, secretions, organs, or other body fluids of infected persons, putting health-care workers and the community at risk. Burial ceremonies in which relatives and friends have direct contact with the body of the deceased person also play a significant role in the transmission of the virus. Health-care workers have been infected while treating Ebola and Marburg patients, through close contact without correct infection control precautions and inadequate barrier nursing procedures. To date, approximately 9% of Ebola or Marburg victims have been health-care workers. During EVD and MVD outbreaks, only strict compliance with biosafety guidelines (i.e. appropriate laboratory practices, infection control precautions, barrier nursing procedures, use of personal protective equipment by health-care workers handling patients, disinfection of contaminated objects and areas, safe burials, etc.) can prevent the epidemic from spreading and reduce the number of victims.

In order to control outbreaks effectively, it is important to develop comprehensive social mobilization campaigns that include feasible, culturally-appropriate, and technically sound interventions for the affected populations. These sensitive and essential measures identify behaviours that may put people at risk and are crucial in supporting the adoption of practices that can help prevent infection or reduce transmission within the community. During outbreaks, social mobilization programmes help affected populations understand and comply with control measures, which may seem to patients and family members to be austere, such as isolating sick people.

Severely ill patients must be given symptomatic treatment and intensive care. There is no specific treatment or vaccine for either Ebola or Marburg. Several candidate vaccines are being developed, but it will be several years until they are available for utilization by outbreak response teams working in the field. Similarly, several candidate drugs show promise but their safety and efficacy in humans is not yet known.

PRIMARY SOURCE

Public Health Matters Blog

SOURCE *Esapa, Lisa. "On the Ground in Nigeria: Ebola Response,"* Public Health Matters Blog, U.S. Centers for Disease Control and Prevention (CDC), August 29, 2014. http://blogs.cdc.gov/publichealthmatters/2014/08/on-the-ground-in-nigeria-ebola-response/ (accessed January 25, 2015).

INTRODUCTION *This primary source is a blog written by Lisa Esapa, a public health adviser for the U.S. Centers for Disease Control and Prevention (CDC). The author works in Lagos, Nigeria, for the Global Immunization Division of the CDC, and this blog briefly describes a typical workday for her team.*

On the Ground in Nigeria: Ebola Response

By Lisa Esapa, CDC-Nigeria

For the last few months, there has been a constant buzz about Ebola among my friends and colleagues in Abuja, the capital of Nigeria. Everyone had a theory about if, when, or how Ebola would come to Nigeria. When we heard about a probable case in Lagos, my heart sank. Lagos is one of the most densely populated cities in the world, with a population of 15 to 20 million people.

Lagos is crowded and loud, with sprawling slum areas that occupy the spaces between the river banks, markets, and developed areas. The stakes for stopping this outbreak from spreading are incredibly high.

For the past 17 months, I've been stationed in Abuja, Nigeria, with the Global Immunization Division, working on polio eradication and routine immunizations as part of CDC's emergency response efforts. I was deployed from Abuja to Lagos just over a week ago to work on setting up Nigeria's own Emergency Operations Center (EOC) for Ebola. I'm a public health advisor, which I have learned in my 6 years at CDC means I have to be a jack-of-all-trades. This is certainly true for this response. Nine CDC staff in Lagos are working with Nigeria and non-governmental organizations (NGOs) on infection control, airport screening, contact tracing, epidemiology and surveillance, communications, and management. I fit into the last category, but really my job is to be sure that all the different pieces are coming together and working. Our days start around 7:30 am with discussions over breakfast at the hotel. We then move to the Ebola EOC, temporarily located in a psychiatric hospital.

The drive to the EOC is the first adventure of the day. Traffic in Lagos can be quite challenging; lanes are congested with cars, while street venders move between the lanes of traffic at intersections selling daily papers—Ebola is the headline in 80 point font in all of them.

Talking to people, you can tell they are nervous and scared. Part of the work of the EOC is to put out accurate messages on prevention and counter the misinformation about Ebola that circulates. For example, the current rumor is that drinking salt water can prevent Ebola. There is a lot of stigma around Ebola and anyone associated with the disease. Many of the people who had contact with Ebola patients have been shunned by their communities. We are working with UNICEF and the U.S. Consulate to determine ways to support this group of people.

During the course of the day, some team members go to an isolation ward (which houses the current patients), the airport, the lab, or the U.S. Consulate. In a "typical" day, I may work on a number of varying tasks, such as finalizing guidance documents that can be shared with states or healthcare workers, meeting with teams leads and partners, drafting a budget for specific activities, and explaining Nigerian culture to the team members. Luckily, this is part of my toolkit—being able to work in a different culture and help ensure my team doesn't run into problems. Even a job like coordinating the motor pool is no small task, since security is always a concern in Nigeria and we have to travel in armored vehicles around the city. Connectivity has also been a major challenge this week. Sometimes the simplest tasks, like sending an email, can be the hardest to achieve!

The days are long; the team arrives back at the hotel between 9pm–10pm each night. As we eat dinner, we discuss the events of the day and plan for the next day. The pace is extremely hectic, but, we all understand the urgency of the situation. We are all tired and at times frustrated when things don't happen as quickly as we might like. In this type of environment, patience can sometimes wear thin.

Yesterday, we got word from the hospital that another one of the patients with Ebola had died. This was the fourth death from Ebola in Nigeria. I might not have known the patient personally, but I'm still deeply saddened by the news. We're all a part of the response and working as hard as we can to ensure that no one else will become infected. With the bad news, there was also good news from the hospital that other patients are recovering and may be ready for discharge in the coming days. Compared to other countries in the West Africa Ebola outbreak, case numbers in Nigeria are low and we're all holding our breath hoping that we've done enough to prevent any further spread of the disease.

SEE ALSO *Epidemiology: Surveillance for Emerging Infectious Diseases; Health-Care Worker Safety and Shortages; Hemorrhagic Diseases; Isolation and Quarantine; Médicins Sans Frontières; NGOs and Health Care: Deliverance or Dependence; Viral Diseases; Zoonotic (Animal-Borne) Diseases*

BIBLIOGRAPHY

Books

Acton, Q. Ashton, ed. *Ebola Virus: New Insights for the Healthcare Professional.* Atlanta: Scholarly Editions, 2012.

Alton, Joseph. *The Ebola Survival Handbook: An MD Tells You What You Need to Know Now to Stay Safe.* New York: Skyhorse, 2014.

Calisher, Charles H. *Lifting the Impenetrable Veil: From Yellow Fever to Ebola Hemorrhagic Fever and SARS.* Red Feather Lakes, CO: Rockpile Press, 2013.

Centers for Disease Control and Prevention (U.S.). *West Africa Ebola Outbreak.* Atlanta: U.S. Department of Health and Human Services, 2014.

Evans, David. *The Economic Impact of the 2014 Ebola Epidemic: Short- and Medium-Term Estimates for West Africa.* Washington, DC: World Bank Group, 2014.

Garrett, Laurie. *Ebola: Story of an Outbreak.* New York: Hachette Books, 2014.

Quammen, David. *Ebola: The Natural and Human History of a Deadly Virus.* New York: Norton, 2014.

Troh, Louise. *My Spirit Took You In.* Boston: Weinstein Books, 2015.

Valle, Carmen. *Psychological First Aid: During Ebola Virus Disease Outbreaks.* Geneva: World Health Organization, 2014.

Periodicals

Farmer, Paul. "Ebola Diary." *London Review of Books* 36, no. 20 (2014): 38–39.

Feldmann H., and T. W. Geisbert. "Ebola Hemorrhagic Fever." *The Lancet* 377, no. 9768 (2011): 849–862.

Sharts-Hopko, N. "Ebola." *American Journal of Nursing* 115, no. 3 (2015): 13.

Wilkinson, Annie, and Melissa Leach. "Briefing: Ebola-Myths, Realities, and Structural Violence." *African Affairs: The Journal of the Royal African Society* 114, no. 454 (2015): 136–148.

Websites

"Ebola." *Doctors Without Borders.* http://www.doctorswithoutborders.org/our-work/medical-issues/ebola (accessed March 18, 2015).

"Ebola (Ebola Virus Disease)." *U.S. Centers for Disease Control and Prevention (CDC).* http://www.cdc.gov/vhf/ebola/index.html (accessed March 18, 2015).

"Ebola Outbreak." *BBC News.* http://www.bbc.com/news/world-africa-28754546 (accessed March 18, 2015).

"Ebola Virus Disease." *World Health Organization (WHO).* http://www.who.int/csr/disease/ebola/en/ (accessed March 18, 2015).

"Global Ebola Response." *United Nations.* http://ebolaresponse.un.org (accessed March 18, 2015).

Preston, Richard. "The Ebola Wars." *New Yorker,* October 27, 2014. http://www.newyorker.com/magazine/2014/10/27/ebola-wars (accessed March 18, 2015).

K. Lee Lerner

Epidemiology: Surveillance for Emerging Infectious Diseases

⊕ Introduction

Epidemiology is an investigative and analytical field of study concerned with the sources, causes, and distribution of disease in populations and the distinction between correlation and causation in matters of public health. Epidemiology is a deeply mathematical science, relying on statistical analysis as well as laboratory data. Epidemiologists are inherently concerned with detecting trends related to health issues, predicting the course of disease outbreaks, and maintaining surveillance for emerging infectious diseases and other threats to public health. Ongoing surveillance enables timely development of effective therapies to treat emerging diseases and vaccines to prevent additional cases.

Epidemiologists seek to determine the origin and risk factors for emerging diseases, defined by the World Health Organization (WHO) as diseases that appear in vulnerable populations for the first time, or diseases that may have existed previously but which begin to increase rapidly in occurrence or spread geographically into new areas with vulnerable populations. The term generally is applied to infectious diseases such as influenza (flu), drug-resistant infections, Ebola, HIV/AIDS, and measles. Emerging diseases can be previously unrecognized, such as HIV/AIDS was in the 1980s, or be reemergent. Diseases like tuberculosis and measles were once well controlled in developed nations, but both have again become public health problems in areas where outbreaks were rare.

Pathogens (bacteria, viruses, or other microorganisms that can cause disease) are constantly evolving. Genetic changes can increase a pathogen's virulence (capacity to cause disease) or transmissibility (ability to spread within a population). Mutations can make microbes more capable of infection or survival in the environment, resistant to antibiotics, and so forth. Disease also can exist at low levels and in places where it can remain undetected in a population until an outbreak occurs. For example, Ebola existed in its natural

reservoir before emerging in outbreaks that took place in remote villages in Central Africa in the 1970s and, more recently, in the outbreak that began in West Africa in 2014. Populations can also allow diseases such as measles to reemerge (become emergent again in a vulnerable population) by failing to maintain sufficient levels of immunization (i.e., herd immunity) within the population.

Epidemiologists evaluate factors such as disease transmissibility from an infected person to a susceptible individual (a factor specific to each disease), the number of average contacts an infected person has within a susceptible population, and the length of exposure to determine whether a disease outbreak has the potential to spread or become an epidemic or pandemic.

One technique of epidemiology, contact tracing, identifies people who have been in direct contact with someone who is sick or contagious. The tracing helps track down not only the source of disease but also identifies those potentially infected so that they can receive treatment immediately, which in turn can slow the spread of disease. The accompanying table prepared by the U.S. Centers for Disease Control and Prevention (CDC) shows how contact tracing works and how it is used to reduce the impact of an emerging disease such as Ebola.

The epidemiologist is concerned with the interactions of organisms and their environments. Environmental factors related to disease may include geographical features, climate, the concentration of pathogens in soil and water, or other factors. Epidemiologists determine the numbers of individuals affected by a disease, the environmental contributions to disease, the causative agent or agents of disease, and the transmission patterns and lethality of disease.

Using statistical analysis, case study investigations, and laboratory data, epidemiologists can, for example, determine if the geographic locations of children born with birth defects correlates strongly enough to their

What is contact tracing?
Contact tracing can stop the Ebola outbreak in its tracks

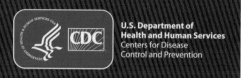

U.S. Department of Health and Human Services
Centers for Disease Control and Prevention

Contact tracing is finding everyone who comes in direct contact with a sick Ebola patient. Contacts are watched for signs of illness for 21 days from the last day they came in contact with the Ebola patient. If the contact develops a fever or other Ebola symptoms, they are immediately isolated, tested, provided care, and the cycle starts again—all of the new patient's contacts are found and watched for 21 days. **Even one missed contact can keep the outbreak going.**

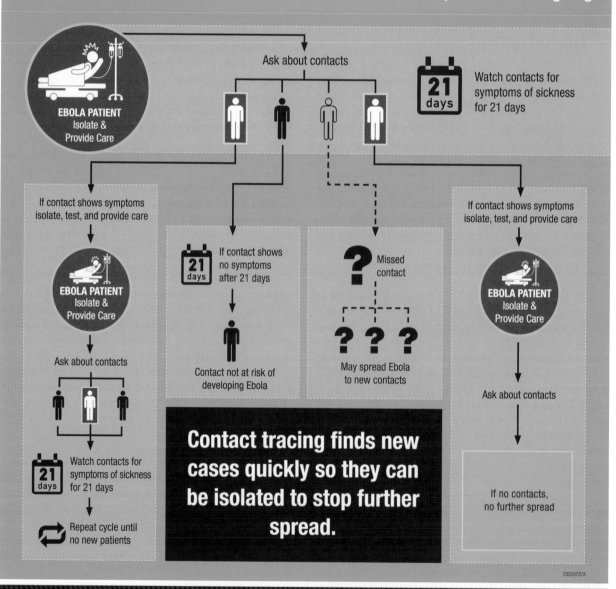

This infographic created by the U.S. CDC provides the viewer with a basic understanding of the steps involved in the process known as contact tracing, a tool implemented by epidemiologists during an outbreak investigation that will help lead investigators to the source of a responsible pathogen, or to whom the pathogenic organism might have been spread.   *Caitlin Shockey/U.S. Centers for Disease Control and Prevention.*

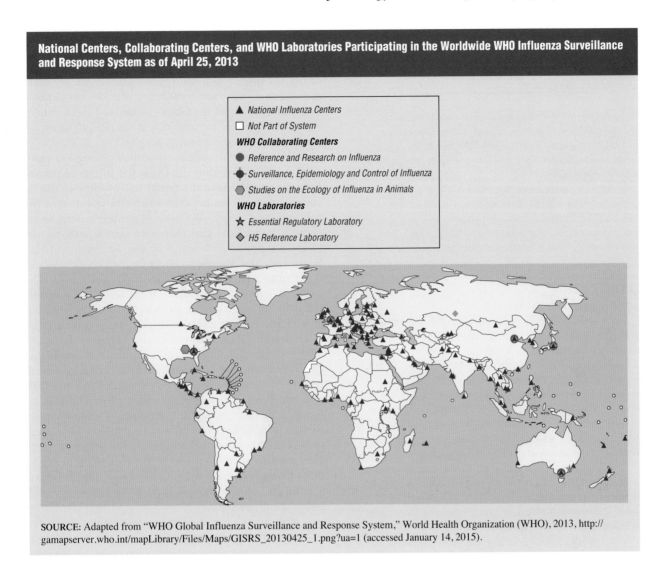

National Centers, Collaborating Centers, and WHO Laboratories Participating in the Worldwide WHO Influenza Surveillance and Response System as of April 25, 2013

▲ National Influenza Centers

☐ Not Part of System

WHO Collaborating Centers

● Reference and Research on Influenza

◆ Surveillance, Epidemiology and Control of Influenza

⬡ Studies on the Ecology of Influenza in Animals

WHO Laboratories

☆ Essential Regulatory Laboratory

◇ H5 Reference Laboratory

SOURCE: Adapted from "WHO Global Influenza Surveillance and Response System," World Health Organization (WHO), 2013, http://gamapserver.who.int/mapLibrary/Files/Maps/GISRS_20130425_1.png?ua=1 (accessed January 14, 2015).

proximity to hazardous waste sites to warrant action to remove or mitigate the threat. This can occur even in the absence of definitive articulation of the physiological or molecular mechanisms of causation.

Using both field observational data and reports from public health agencies, epidemiologists can track the spread of influenza throughout the world and, using statistical methods, can predict case load or the extinction of an outbreak. As shown in the accompanying map illustration, epidemiologists rely on data from a WHO Global Influenza Surveillance and Response System to help characterize influenza outbreaks.

Epidemiology is commonly thought to be limited to the study of infectious diseases, but that is only one aspect of the medical specialty. More recently, scientists have broadened the worldwide scope of epidemiology to a variety of health-related fields, including studies of violence, heart disease due to lifestyle choices, and the spread of disease due to environmental degradation.

🌐 Historical Background

The first physician known to consider the fundamental concepts of disease causation was the ancient Greek Hippocrates (c. 460–c. 377 BCE), when he wrote that medical thinkers should consider the climate and seasons; the air; the water that people use; the soil; and people's eating, drinking, and exercise habits in a region. Subsequently and until recent times, these causes of diseases were often considered but not quantitatively measured. In 1662, John Graunt (1620–1674), a London haberdasher (clothing dealer), published an analysis of the weekly reports of births and deaths in London, the first statistical description of population disease patterns. Among his findings, he noted a higher death rate for men than women, a high infant mortality rate, and seasonal variations in mortality. Graunt's study, with its meticulous counting and disease pattern description, set the foundation for modern public health practice.

JOHN SNOW, CHOLERA DETECTIVE

Although reports of cholera-like diseases date to antiquity, the first pandemic of modern cholera reached Great Britain in 1831. At the time, cholera claimed the lives of around half those who acquired it. The cause was unknown, though there were several theories.

Some doctors assumed that miasmata (bad air) or toxins in the air spread disease. Others believed the disease spread only via direct contagion from one person to another but did not understand the mechanism for how this occurred. The germ theory of disease, which holds that pathogens, such as viruses and bacteria, are the causative infectious agents of diseases such as yellow fever, smallpox, typhoid, cholera, and others, was still developing, and it would not be widely accepted for another generation.

When the 1831 outbreak in Great Britain began, John Snow (1813–1858) was a doctor's apprentice gaining his first experience with the disease, noting its symptoms of diarrhea and extreme dehydration. Snow first began a serious scientific investigation of cholera transmission during the 1848 London epidemic. In his classic essay, *On the Mode of Communication of Cholera,* published on August 29, 1849, he postulated that polluted water was a source of cholera—especially water contaminated by the waste of an infected person, a not-uncommon occurrence at the time. When an outbreak erupted in central London at the end of August 1854, close to where Snow himself lived, he resumed his research. Snow constructed a map of cases and published it in 1855. Snow linked the local cases, shown as dark blocks, to a commonly used water pump in Broad Street. (See primary source.)

It is partially thanks to John Snow's work in the Broad Street area that Britain suffered fewer major outbreaks of cholera after this time. An influential figure in medical circles, he was elected president of the Medical Society of London in 1855. Fortunately for British public health, the successful proof of his theory on the transmission of cholera—from person to person via contaminated water—took hold, and the "bad air" theory eventually died away. Although the actual causative agent, the bacterium *Vibrio cholerae,* would not be identified until 1883, Snow's preventive methods worked. Indeed, they are still effective today, for despite the advent of vaccination and antibiotics, hand washing and the avoidance of contaminated food and water are still fundamental ways of preventing infection.

Graunt's data collection and analytical methodology was furthered by the physician William Farr, who assumed responsibility for medical statistics for England and Wales in 1839 and set up a system for the routine collection of the numbers and causes of deaths. In analyzing statistical relationships between disease and such circumstances as marital status, occupations such as mining and working with earthenware, elevation above sea level and imprisonment, he addressed many of the basic methodological issues that contemporary epidemiologists study. These issues include defining populations at risk for disease and the relative disease risk between population groups, and considering whether associations between disease and the factors mentioned above might be caused by other factors, such as age, length of exposure to a condition, or overall health.

The advent of modern epidemiology began a generation later in London. In 1854, the British physician John Snow (1813–1858) tested the hypothesis that a cholera epidemic in London was being transmitted by contaminated water. By examining death rates from cholera, he realized that they were significantly higher in areas supplied with water by the Lambeth and the Southwark and Vauxhall companies, which drew their water from a part of the Thames River that was grossly polluted with sewage. When the Lambeth Company changed the location of its water source to another part of the river that was relatively less polluted, rates of cholera in the areas served by that company declined, while no change occurred among the areas served by the Southwark and Vauxhall. Areas of London served by both companies experienced a cholera death rate that was intermediate between the death rates in the areas supplied by just one of the companies. The geographic pattern of infections was carefully recorded and plotted on a map of London. In recognizing the grand but simple natural experiment posed by the change in the Lambeth Company water source, Snow was able to make a uniquely valuable contribution to epidemiology and public health practice.

After Snow's seminal work, investigations by epidemiologists have come to include many chronic diseases with complex and often still unknown causal agents, and the methods of epidemiology have become similarly complex. Today, researchers use genetics, molecular biology, and microbiology as investigative tools, and the methods used to establish relative disease risk make use of the most advanced statistical techniques available. Yet reliance on meticulous counting and categorizing of cases and the imperative to think logically to avoid the pitfalls in mathematical relationships in medical data remain at the heart of all of the research used to show elevated disease risk in population subgroups and to prove that medical treatments are safe and effective.

Today, epidemiologists study not only infectious diseases, such as cholera and malaria, but also noninfectious diseases, such as lung cancer and certain heart disorders.

Epidemiological Practice

The primary focus of epidemiology is groups of persons, rather than individuals. The primary effort of epidemiologists is in determining the etiology (cause) of the disease and identifying measures to stop or slow its spread. This information, in turn, can be used to create strategies by which the efforts of health-care workers and facilities in communities can be most efficiently allocated for this purpose.

In tracking a disease outbreak, epidemiologists may use any or all of three types of investigation: descriptive epidemiology, analytical epidemiology, and experimental epidemiology.

Descriptive epidemiology is the collection of all data describing the occurrence of the disease, and usually includes information about individuals infected, and the place and period during which it occurred. Such a study is usually retrospective; that is, it is a study of an outbreak after it has occurred.

Analytical epidemiology attempts to determine the cause of an outbreak. Using the case control method, the epidemiologist can look for factors that might have preceded the disease. Often, this entails comparing a group of people who have the disease with a group that is similar in age, sex, socioeconomic status, and other variables but does not have the disease. In this way, other possible factors, for example, genetic or environmental, might be identified as factors related to the outbreak.

Using the cohort method of analytical epidemiology, the investigator studies two populations, one who has had contact with the disease-causing agent and another that has not. For example, the comparison of a group that received blood transfusions with a group that has not might disclose an association between blood transfusions and the incidence of a blood-borne disease, such as hepatitis B.

Experimental epidemiology tests a hypothesis about a disease or disease treatment in a group of people. This strategy might be used to test whether or not a particular antibiotic is effective against a particular disease-causing organism. One group of infected individuals is divided randomly so that some receive the antibiotic and others receive a placebo—an inactive drug that is not known to have any medical effect. In this case, the antibiotic is the variable, that is, the experimental factor being tested to see if it makes a difference between the two otherwise similar groups. If people in the group receiving the antibiotic recover more rapidly than those in the other group, it may logically be concluded that the variable—antibiotic treatment—made the difference. Thus, the antibiotic is effective.

Basic Concepts

The most basic concepts in epidemiology are the measures used to discover whether a statistical association exists between various factors and disease. These measures include various kinds of rates, proportions, and ratios. Mortality (death) and morbidity (disease) rates are the raw material that researchers use in establishing disease causation. Morbidity rates are most usefully expressed in terms of disease incidence (the rate with which members of a population or research sample contract a disease) and prevalence (the proportion of the group that has a disease over a given period of time).

The most important task in epidemiology is the assessment or measurement of disease risk. The population at risk is the group of people that could potentially contract a disease, which can range from the entire world population (e.g., at risk for the flu) to a small group of people within a remote and isolated community (e.g., at risk for contracting a particular, ecologically restricted parasite). The most basic measure of a population group's risk for a disease is relative risk—the ratio of the prevalence of a disease in one group with particular biological, demographic, or behavioral characteristics to the prevalence in another group with different characteristics.

The simplest measure of relative risk is the odds ratio, which is the ratio of the odds that a person in one group has a disease to the odds that a person in a second, comparator group has the disease. The odds for contracting a disease are the ratio between the proportion of people in a population group that share particular characteristics that put them at risk for a disease to the proportion of people in a reference or control population (often the general population in a certain region or jurisdiction).

The mortality rate is the ratio of the number of deaths in a population, either in total or disease-specific, to the total number of members of that population, and is usually given in terms of a large population denominator, so that the numerator can be expressed as a whole number.

Assessing disease frequency is more complex because of the factors of time and disease duration. For example, disease prevalence can be assessed at a point in time (point prevalence) or over a period of time, usually a year (period prevalence, annual prevalence). This is the prevalence that is usually measured in illness surveys that are reported to the public in the news. Researchers can also measure prevalence over an indefinite time period, as in the case of lifetime prevalence, which is the prevalence of a disease over the course of the entire lives of the people in the population under study up to the point in time when the researchers make the assessment. Researchers calculate this by determining for every person in the study sample whether or not he or she has ever had the disease, or by checking lifetime health records for everybody in the population for the occurrence of the disease, counting the occurrences, and then dividing by the number of people in the population.

The other basic measure of disease frequency is incidence, the number of cases of a disease that occur in a given period of time. Incidence is a critical statistic in describing the course of a fast-moving epidemic, in which medical decision makers must know how quickly a disease is spreading. The incidence rate is the key to public health planning because it enables officials to understand what the prevalence of a disease is likely to be in the future. Prevalence is mathematically related to the cumulative incidence of a disease over a period of time as well as the expected duration of a disease, which can be a week in the case of the flu or a lifetime in the case of juvenile onset diabetes. Therefore, incidence not only indicates the rate of new disease cases, but is the basis of the rate of change of disease prevalence.

Epidemiologists use statistical analysis to discover associations between death and disease in populations and various factors—including environmental (e.g., pollution), demographic (e.g., age and gender), biological (e.g., body mass index or "BMI" and genetics), social (e.g., educational level), and behavioral (e.g., tobacco smoking, diet or type of medical treatment)—that could be implicated in causing disease.

By identifying specific factors and how they are ultimately related to the disease, it is sometimes possible to determine which preventive actions can be taken to reduce the occurrence of the disease. In the case of myocardial infarction, for example, these preventive actions might include a change in diet, treatment for hypertension, eliminating smoking, and beginning a regular schedule of exercise.

Emergent Diseases

All diseases were once emergent. Smallpox, formerly the scourge of populations in Europe and Asia for hundreds of years, has been eradicated, which means it has been eliminated from every country in the world. Poliomyelitis (polio), another age-old infection, was common around the world until vaccines for it were developed in the 1950s and 1960s. By 2014 polio was under control in all but three countries where it remained endemic (naturally occurring)—Pakistan, Nigeria, and Afghanistan. The ability to control such diseases was in part due large-scale immunization programs that were directed by epidemiological research and methods.

About 75 percent of emerging infections are zoonotic (transmitted from animals to humans). Human encroachment into wild habitats brings people into contact with animal hosts of pathogens that can cause disease in humans. An example of a zoonotic disease in the northeast United States is Lyme disease, which is caused by tick bites from ticks that have been infected with the disease by wild deer and rodents.

In the 1980s, classic epidemiology discovered that a puzzling array of illnesses was linked, and it came to be known as acquired immune deficiency syndrome (AIDS). Epidemiologists traced the disease to sexual contact, then to contaminated blood supplies, then proved the virus that caused AIDS, human immunodeficiency virus (HIV), could cross the placental barrier, infecting babies born

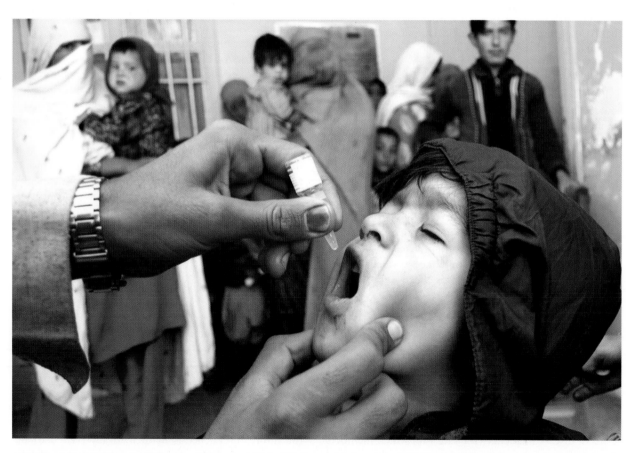

A health worker administers polio vaccine drops to a child during three days of an anti-polio campaign at the Pakistan-Afghanistan border in January 2014 in Chaman, Afghanistan. Success in combating diseases such as smallpox and polio is reliant on epidemiological methods of surveillance and study of the sources, causes, and effective methods of treatment. *© Asianet-Pakistan/Shutterstock.com.*

to HIV-infected mothers. Since the identification of the virus responsible for AIDS, multiple genetic studies have established that HIV passed into humans in Central Africa from a mutation in the simian immunodeficiency virus (SIV) in chimpanzees that were probably butchered for meat around sometime before World War I (1914–1918). The disease then migrated to Leopoldville in the Belgian Congo (now known as Kinshasa in the Democratic Republic of the Congo), where the disease mutated repeatedly before becoming HIV, subgroup M—the strain of the disease that has infected millions around the world. Haitians working in the Congo in the 1960s became infected and carried the disease to Haiti and then to the United States.

Before being identified in the United States in the early 1980s, what eventually became known as AIDS was effectively hidden because it existed in people living in remote areas and occurred at low population levels. What is now known as AIDS was previously misdiagnosed as other diseases. For example, doctors in Africa often listed leukemia as the cause of death for persons who had AIDS.

Epidemiologists at the Epidemic Intelligence Service (EIS) of the CDC have played important roles in other landmark epidemiologic investigations. Those include an investigation of the definitive epidemic of Legionnaires' disease in 1976 and identification of tampons as a risk factor for toxic-shock syndrome. EIS officers are increasingly involved in the investigation of noninfectious disease problems, including the risk of injury associated with all-terrain vehicles, cell phone use, and cluster illness and deaths related to contaminated food.

Epidemiologists are often integrated into the public health structure of a local community, and work closely with public health officials to track and manage local outbreaks of disease. Other times, epidemiologists are part of larger national or international health organizations, and work to identify and track the emergence of new diseases worldwide. In either case, epidemiologists rely on observations and data collected at the source of an outbreak, and rapid dissemination of the data among colleagues.

For example, when a dangerous pneumonia surfaced in February 2003 in China, Chinese authorities were at first hesitant to implement isolation procedures and investigate the outbreak. Within a month, the disease spread to a hospital in Vietnam, where Carlo Urbani, an Italian medical epidemiologist working with the WHO in Hanoi, recognized the influenza-like disease as unusual. Urbani worked at the hospital, collecting samples for testing, compiling data, instituting isolation and other infection control measures, and notifying health authorities worldwide. The disease was SARS (severe acute respiratory syndrome), and Urbani is credited with identifying and containing the epidemic. In mid-March 2003, Urbani traveled to Thailand to present data to CDC officials. Feeling ill upon landing at the airport, Urbani again insisted upon isolating himself and for protective equipment for those coming in contact with him. He died of SARS two weeks later.

⊕ Impacts and Issues

Another way epidemiologists may view etiology of disease is as a "web of causation." This web represents all known predisposing factors and their relations with each other and with the disease. For example, a web of causation for myocardial infarction (heart attack) can include diet, hereditary factors, cigarette smoking, lack of exercise, susceptibility to myocardial infarction, and hypertension. Each factor influences and is influenced by a variety of other factors.

Among the important environmental factors that affect an epidemic of infectious diseases are poverty, overcrowding, lack of sanitation, and such uncontrollable factors as the season and climate.

Diseases can also reemerge when vulnerable populations such as unvaccinated people are exposed to the disease. According to the CDC, before the availability of the measles vaccine in 1963, practically all children had measles by the time they were teenagers. In the United States, several million people were infected each year and between 400 and 500 deaths, 48,000 hospitalizations, and 4,000 cases of encephalitis (swelling of the brain) were attributable to measles. Although measles was eliminated in the United States in 2000 (elimination is defined as no continuous transmission of disease for 12 months or longer in a specific geographic area), the United States had outbreaks of measles cases in 2013, 2014, and 2015. The majority of outbreaks occurred in unvaccinated communities, underscoring the importance of vaccination. The December 2014 to February 2015 multistate outbreak likely started when a traveler infected with measles visited a California amusement park. The CDC reports that the U.S. outbreak was the same strain of measles responsible for 21,420 cases and 110 deaths in the Philippines during 2014. The WHO has committed to eliminating measles by 2020.

The emergence and reemergence of infectious diseases is influenced by a number of factors such as economic development, availability of health care and vaccination programs, and the overall health and nutritional status of citizens. In developing countries, poor conditions in any of these areas can increase susceptibility to infectious diseases. Of the nearly 40 million people worldwide living with AIDS, two-thirds live in sub-Saharan Africa. Epidemiologists are well poised to articulate the factors for appropriate action. Epidemiology is also essential to monitoring progress toward remediation of hazards and disease.

In some cases, surveillance and advanced medical research is able to restrict emerging infection outbreaks to relatively small geographic areas and short periods. Outbreaks are part of a greater web of natural and social factors, and understanding how changes in these factors can heighten the risk of the emergence of infectious diseases helps to strengthen efforts to prevent these threats to public health.

Screening

Screening a community using relatively simple diagnostic tests is one of the most powerful tools that healthcare professionals and public health authorities have in preventing or combating disease. Familiar examples of screening include HIV testing to help prevent AIDS, tuberculin testing to screen for tuberculosis, and hepatitis C testing by insurers to detect subclinical infection that could result in liver cirrhosis over the long term. In undertaking a screening program, authorities must always judge whether the benefits of preventing the illness in question outweigh the costs and the number of cases that have been mistakenly identified, called false positives.

The ability of the test to identify true positives (sensitivity) and true negatives (specificity) makes screening a valuable prevention tool. However, the usefulness of the screening test is proportional to the disease prevalence in the population at risk. If the disease prevalence is very low, there are likely to be more false positives than true positives, which would cast doubt on the usefulness

and the cost-effectiveness of the test. For example, if the prevalence of a disease in the population is only 2 percent and a test with a false positive rate of 4 percent is given to everyone (normally a good rate for a screening test), then individuals falsely identified as having the disease would be twice as frequent as individuals accurately identified with the disease. This would render the test results virtually useless. Public health officials deal with this situation by screening only population subgroups that have a high risk of contracting the disease. In infectious disease, screening tests are valuable for infections with a long latency period, which is the period during which an infected individual does not show disease symptoms, or which have a lengthy and ambiguous symptomatic period.

Changes in environment or social infrastructure can also fuel epidemics. For example, a breakdown in sanitation frequently offers conditions favorable to the spread of disease. An epidemic can result from an alteration in the environment that normally acts to limit disease. In

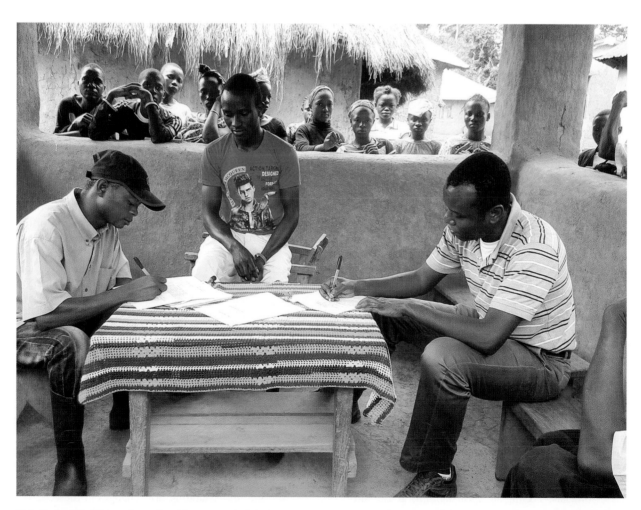

U.S. Centers for Disease Control and Prevention (CDC) Epidemic Intelligence Service (EIS) officer, Dr. Djawe, seated on the right, completes his daily tally sheets from his contact tracing visit in the city of Kamian, Guinea. Contact tracing is one of the tools implemented in an epidemiologic investigation in order to contain the spread of a pathogen, in this case, the Ebola virus. *U.S. Centers for Disease Control.*

other cases, ecological imbalances can also increase the spread of disease. For example, an increase in mosquitoes, vectors for a number of diseases, can offer continuing challenges to public health officials. In addition to tracking the origins of disease, epidemiologists may investigate the factors causing the increase in vector populations.

Despite improvements in global surveillance and the international response to the 2014 Ebola epidemic in West Africa that was centered in Liberia, Guinea, and Sierra Leone, the epidemic claimed thousands of lives.

🌐 Future Implications

The control of infectious disease is an urgent mission for epidemiologists employed in various state and federal public health agencies and their partners in private industry and research foundations.

Infectious disease epidemiology requires accurate and timely incidence and prevalence data such as is provided with comprehensive disease surveillance of usual and emerging diseases. Although the development of an organized surveillance system is critical to the provision of these data, the system's effectiveness depends on the willingness and ability of health-care providers to detect, diagnose, and report the incidence of cases that the system is supposed to track. A reporting system functions at four levels: (1) the basic data are collected in the local community where the disease occurs; (2) the data are assembled at the district, state, or provincial levels; (3) information is aggregated under national auspices (e.g., the CDC in the United States); and (4) for certain prescribed diseases, the national health authority reports the disease information to the WHO.

The reporting of cases at the local level is mandated for notifiable illnesses that come to the attention of health-care providers. Case reports provide patient information, suspect organisms, and dates of onset with basis for diagnosis, consistent with patient privacy rights. Collective case reports are compiled at the district level by diagnosis, stipulating the number of cases occurring within a prescribed time. Any unusual or group expression of illness that may be of public concern should be reported as an epidemic, whether the illness is included in the list of notifiable diseases and whether it is a well-known identified disease or an unknown clinical entity.

Because of the emergence or reemergence of HIV/AIDS and resistant strains of tuberculosis, malaria, gonorrhea, and *Escherichia coli*, among others, infectious disease epidemiology, once thought to be waning in importance due to significant advances in public sanitation and immunization programs, has reemerged as an urgent challenge. Air travel has created a situation in which travelers can return home from areas where particular pathogens are endemic, which can potentially precipitate an epidemic. Infectious diseases pose a threat to social order in some developing nations and pose extremely difficult public health problems even in the wealthiest societies. Lifestyle disease epidemics like obesity create a serious economic and medical resource burden on even the most advanced societies.

In order to prepare for a pandemic, or respond to any other threat to public health, health officials need to share information quickly and accurately. Early warning and adequate response to a health crisis often relies on both surveillance and epidemiological modeling. The official reporting agency for the WHO is the Global Outbreak Alert and Response Network (GOARN), a consortium of independent laboratories and reporting networks. GOARN works with public health authorities worldwide to rapidly identify and respond to disease outbreaks. Other internationally important resources include the Global Public Health Intelligence Network (GPHIN), developed by the Public Health Agency of Canada. GPHIN is one of several organizations that provide real-time global coverage of public health news. The Program for Monitoring Emerging Diseases, also known as ProMED-mail, is an Internet-based global reporting system for the exchange of news reports, field notes, and epidemiological analysis about infectious diseases. ProMED first reported an outbreak of unusual pneumonia in China in 2003 that was subsequently known as SARS. Both ProMED and GPHIN collect and report information about disease outbreaks from countries around the world.

PRIMARY SOURCE

John Snow's Map of the Broad Street Pump Outbreak, 1854

SOURCE *Snow, John.* On the Mode of Communication: Cholera. *London: John Churchill, 1855, 45. Copyright © 1855 John Churchill.*

INTRODUCTION *This primary source is a detail from a map drawn in 1854 by Dr. John Snow, showing the locations of London cholera cases, which are marked by bars perpendicular to the streets. The map shows the most dense cluster, surrounding a water pump on Broad Street. Snow then took samples of the water and studied them under a microscope, discovering a new bacterium in the water pumped from the Broad Street pump. The cholera outbreak abated when the handle of the pump was removed. Snow's map is a famous early example of epidemiology, which enabled identification of the epidemic's source.*

SEE ALSO *Centers for Disease Control and Prevention (CDC); Health-Related Education and Information Access; International Health Regulation,*

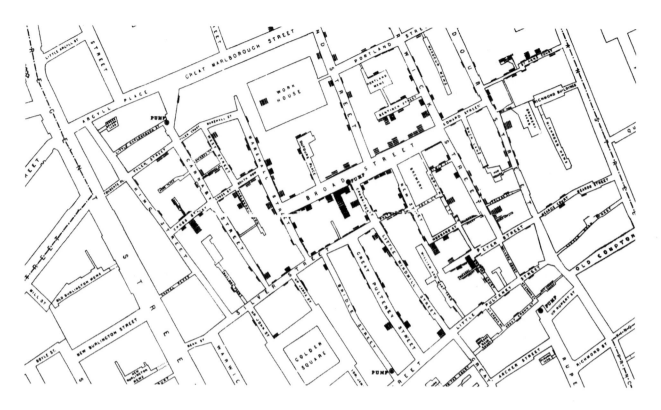

Surveillance, and Enforcement; Pan American Health Organization (PAHO); Population Issues; World Health Organization: Organization, Funding, and Enforcement Powers

BIBLIOGRAPHY

Books

Ahrens, Wolfgang, and Iris Pigeot, eds. *Handbook of Epidemiology*, 2nd ed. New York: Springer, 2014.

Broadbent, Alex. *Philosophy of Epidemiology*. New York: Palgrave Macmillan, 2013.

Büttner, Petra, and Reinhold Muller. *Epidemiology*. South Melbourne, Australia: Oxford University Press, 2011.

Koehler, Steven A., and Peggy A. Brown. *Forensic Epidemiology*. Boca Raton, FL: CRC Press, 2010.

Krieger, Nancy. *Epidemiology and the People's Health: Theory and Context*. New York: Oxford University Press, 2011.

Law, Graham R., and Shane W. Pascoe. *Statistical Epidemiology*. Wallingford, UK: CABI, 2013.

Merrill, Ray M. *Introduction to Epidemiology*, 6th ed. Sudbury, MA: Jones and Bartlett, 2010.

Tu, Yu-Kang, and Darren C. Greenwood, eds. *Modern Methods for Epidemiology*. New York: Springer, 2012.

Periodicals

Faria, Nuno R., et al. "HIV Epidemiology. The Early Spread and Epidemic Ignition of HIV-1 in Human Populations." *Science* 346, no. 6205 (October 2014): 56–61.

Valdiserri, Ronald O. "Commentary: Thirty Years of AIDS in America: A Story of Infinite Hope." *AIDS Education and Prevention* 23, no. 6 (December 2011): 479–494.

Websites

"Emerging Infectious Diseases." *U.S. Centers for Disease Control and Prevention (CDC)*. http://wwwnc.cdc .gov/eid/ (accessed April 1, 2015).

"Emerging Infectious Diseases/Pathogens." *U.S. National Institute of Allergy and Infectious Diseases (NIAID)*. http://www.niaid.nih.gov/topics/emerging/Pages/ Default.aspx (accessed April 1, 2015).

"Frequently Asked Questions about Measles in the U.S." *U.S. Centers for Disease Control and Prevention (CDC)*. http://www.cdc.gov/measles/about/faqs .html#measles-elimination (accessed March 5, 2015).

"Global Tuberculosis Report 2014." *World Health Organization (WHO)*. http://apps.who.int/iris/bitstr eam/10665/137094/1/9789241564809_eng .pdf?ua=1 (accessed April 1, 2015).

"Measles History." *U.S. Centers for Disease Control and Prevention (CDC)*. http://www.cdc.gov/measles/ about/history.html (accessed April 1, 2015).

"Measles in the Philippines." *U.S. Centers for Disease Control and Prevention (CDC)*. http://wwwnc .cdc.gov/travel/notices/watch/measles-philippines (accessed April 1, 2015).

K. Lee Lerner

Family Planning

⊕ Introduction

Family planning is the practice of controlling the number of children a woman has and the intervals between their births, by means of contraception or fertility treatment. The promotion of family planning is important in improving the health and independence of women around the world and in supporting the health and development of their children, communities, and wider societies. According to the World Health Organization (WHO), there are an estimated 222 million women in developing countries who would like either to delay or stop childbearing, but are not using an effective method of family planning. At the same time, there are around 50 million couples worldwide who would like to start or add to a family but are affected by infertility and find themselves unable to conceive.

Many would agree that people have a right to determine the number and spacing of their children. Family planning helps them to do this, through a combination of education and technologies, such as the contraceptive pill and, where infertility is the issue, in vitro fertilization. Reducing the overall number of pregnancies a woman has, and increasing the intervals between them, has many benefits for not only her own health but that of her children. For younger women, early childbearing before the body is fully developed can be dangerous, and pregnancy also may be risky in older women. Closely spaced and multiple pregnancies contribute to higher rates of infant mortality. Access to effective contraception reduces the need for unsafe abortion. Having smaller families means that more can be invested in each child, improving their chances in life. Family planning empowers women by enabling them to make informed choices and leaves them more time to invest in education. It also slows down unsustainable population growth, thereby alleviating otherwise negative impacts on the economy, environment, and national development efforts. There is a wide and effective range of both contraceptive methods and fertility treatments available. The challenge is to make these more readily available to those who wish to use them around the world.

⊕ Historical Background

The origins of modern family planning lie in the late 18th-century writings of economist Thomas Malthus (1766–1834), who attributed society's problems to population expansion. He advocated sexual abstinence as a method of limiting family size. In the early 20th century, socialists and feminists began to call for birth control as a way of women achieving their independence. Their work was taken up by pioneers such as Margaret Sanger (1879–1966) and Marie Stopes (1880–1958), but efforts were diverted toward poor, black families and immigrants in an attempt to counter falling birth-rates among native-born whites. Indeed, the early campaigners for birth control often openly advocated eugenics as a policy.

There was huge population growth in the countries of the Southern Hemisphere following World War II (1939–1945). This led to family planning efforts being targeted toward the so-called Third World, based upon the neo-Malthusian belief that the "population explosion" was responsible for poverty, political instability, and environmental degradation. With the advent of modern contraceptives such as the contraceptive pill, there was a massive international expansion in family planning programs. In 1979, China introduced its one child policy in an attempt to reduce the country's population. Those adhering to it were rewarded with higher wages and various forms of preferential treatment. Though the government allowed exceptions, those breaking the rule were punished with fines and loss of employment. The International Conference on Population and Development in 1994 marked a turning point, however, with a new emphasis on women's reproductive health and human rights and a shift away from the previous numerical population goals.

⊕ Impacts and Issues

There have been many years of international agreements, with participation of a wide range of governmental and nongovernmental organizations, aimed at improving the health of women and children. Despite these efforts, rates of mortality and poor health among women and newborns in developing countries both remain unacceptably high. Sociologists see family planning as vital to these goals because of its many potential benefits.

There is evidence that investing in the reproductive health of women is worthwhile on many levels. It means fewer unintended pregnancies and fewer maternal and newborn deaths. Family planning also has the potential to improve women's health, status, and rights. Healthier mothers and children mean more productive families who have better prospects for education and work. This in turn strengthens local and national economies as well as reducing pressure on natural resources. Family planning therefore has an important role to play in helping countries reach the United Nations Millennium Development Goals (MDGs). Indeed, improving maternal health is named as MDG 5, and there is an international

consensus that a comprehensive health package for all people should include sexual and reproductive health services.

In most developing regions, the use of family planning has increased since the late 20th century, although it remains very low in Africa. The level of contraceptive use also varies significantly around the world. It has increased in many regions since the 1990s, including in Asia and Latin America, but remains particularly low in sub-Saharan Africa. Between 1990 and 2003, the percentage of married women aged 15 to 49 using modern contraception grew from 47 to 56 worldwide, with regional variations. For example, in Asia the increase was from 52 to 62 percent, in Latin America and the Caribbean from 53 to 65 percent, but in Africa only from 13 to 21 percent. By 2011, according to the United Nations *World Contraceptive Patterns 2013*, the estimated use of any contraception (including traditional methods) among women worldwide in marriages or unions was 63 percent. The percentage of those using modern contraceptive methods was 57 percent, with percentages ranging from almost 70 percent in North America to less than 10 percent in some countries in Africa. In Latin America and the Caribbean

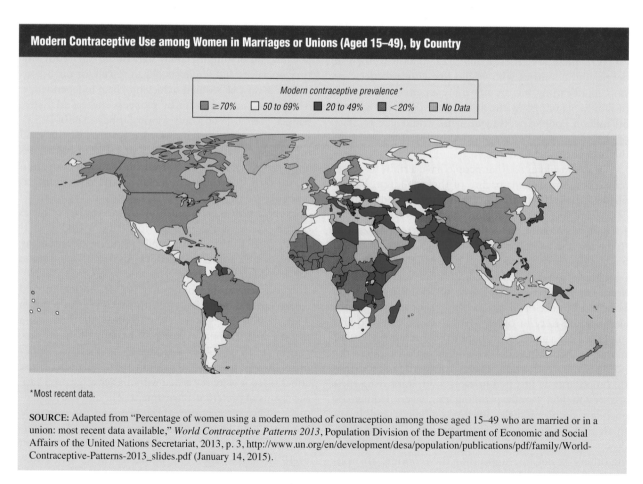

Modern Contraceptive Use among Women in Marriages or Unions (Aged 15–49), by Country

Modern contraceptive prevalence*

■ ≥70%   □ 50 to 69%   ■ 20 to 49%   ■ <20%   □ No Data

*Most recent data.

SOURCE: Adapted from "Percentage of women using a modern method of contraception among those aged 15–49 who are married or in a union: most recent data available," *World Contraceptive Patterns 2013*, Population Division of the Department of Economic and Social Affairs of the United Nations Secretariat, 2013, p. 3, http://www.un.org/en/development/desa/population/publications/pdf/family/World-Contraceptive-Patterns-2013_slides.pdf (January 14, 2015).

Sub-Saharan Africa remains an area where use of modern family planning methods are used the least. Approximately 45 million women in the region use traditional family planning methods or no methods at all.

CONTRACEPTION METHODS

Contraception, also known as birth control, is a way of avoiding becoming pregnant by interfering with the natural processes of ovulation, fertilization, or implantation. There are several contraceptive methods available, divided into broad groups according to how they work. Traditional methods are widely used, as they are without cost and require no medical intervention, however, they are not as effective as modern contraceptive methods. In the case of modern contraception, there are barrier methods, such as the condom, and hormonal methods, such as the contraceptive pill. These methods are reversible when a couple wants another child. Male and female sterilization are modern contraceptive methods that are permanent.

Traditional Methods

The withdrawal method, also known as coitus interruptus, involves a man withdrawing his penis from the vagina before ejaculation, in an attempt to avoid sperm entering the woman's body. This is one of the least effective methods of contraception because it is hard to time the moment of withdrawal. If it is done even seconds too late, then it is likely that sperm will enter the vagina.

The other traditional method of contraception is the rhythm method, also known as fertility awareness. The woman monitors her menstrual cycle, and intercourse is avoided during the fertile days around ovulation. The method can also be used in reverse when a woman wishes to become pregnant and has intercourse on the fertile days. The cycle is monitored by noting changes in cervical mucus thickness and temperature. Traditional methods do not have any side effects and may be preferred for religious reasons. However, they require commitment and motivation if they are to be effective in avoiding pregnancy.

Hormonal Contraception and Interuterine Devices

Combined oral contraceptives generally contain two hormones, estrogen and progestogen, which work to prevent ovulation. Used properly and consistently, they have greater than 99 percent effectiveness in preventing pregnancy. A progestogen-only pill, sometimes called the mini-pill, is slightly less effective and works by thickening cervical mucus, to prevent sperm and egg from meeting. Hormonal methods are available in pill, implant, and injectable forms. There is also emergency contraception in the form of a pill containing the hormone levonorgestrel, which is used to prevent implantation after unprotected intercourse.

The intrauterine device (IUD) is a small flexible plastic device that contains copper wire. It is inserted into the uterus where it has a long-term action. The copper in the device damages sperm and so prevents fertilization from occurring. There is also an IUD that that releases the hormone levonorgestrel and works by suppressing the growth of the uterine lining. Both these methods are more than 99 percent effective, if correctly used.

Barrier Methods

Male condoms are one of the oldest methods of contraception. A condom is a thin plastic sheath that fits over the penis, trapping sperm on ejaculation so they do not enter the woman's body. There are also female condoms that are fitted into the vagina. The diaphragm, or cap, is a shallow, silicone cap that is inserted into the vagina so as to cover the cervix and prevent the entry of sperm. It usually is used with a spermicide, which is a chemical gel or cream that kills sperm.

Barrier methods are slightly less effective than hormonal methods in preventing pregnancy. For instance, when the diaphragm is used correctly, 6 women out of 100 will get pregnant each year, rising to 12 in 100 if it is not used correctly or consistently. Condoms have the advantage of affording some protection against sexually transmitted infections, including HIV.

Sterilization

Male sterilization, or vasectomy, involves cutting through the vas deferens, which are the tubes that carry sperm from the testicles. This keeps sperm out of the ejaculated semen, so it does not enter the woman's body. Female sterilization, known as tubal ligation, blocks or cuts the Fallopian tubes, which carry eggs from the ovaries. Both male and female sterilization can be considered as being permanent methods of contraception, although there are instances in which they are not 100 percent effective. For this reason, voluntary and informed choice are essential, as the man or woman concerned is effectively losing fertility. If an individual is certain that he or she does not want children, or any more children, then sterilization is a common solution, as there will be no further need to practice contraception.

about 66.6 percent of women used modern contraception; in Asia it was 61.2 percent; and in Africa it was 26 percent, with substantial differences in rates depending on the region, for example in southern African countries the rate was around 61.7 percent on average, while in middle African countries it averaged only 8.8 percent.

The overall increase in family planning use has contributed to a general decline in fertility rates and in maternal and infant death rates. However, rates of unintended pregnancy, maternal and infant death, and unsafe abortion remain unacceptably high. There is still far from universal access to effective family planning, largely due to funding shortfalls and lack of infrastructure. MDG 5 calls for a reduction in maternal mortality by 75 percent between 1990 and 2015, but progress has been slow and the goal clearly will not be met.

According to the WHO, in 2008 modern contraceptive use avoided 188 million unintended pregnancies, 1.2 million newborn deaths, and 230,000 maternal deaths and other negative health outcomes for women. Savings in health-care costs also resulted from the avoidance of unsafe abortion and complications of childbirth.

Pregnancy, Childbirth, and Women's Health

There was a decline in the rate of unintended pregnancies of 20 percent in developing countries between 1995 and 2008, which has been attributed to an increase in contraceptive use. However, the rate of unintended pregnancy remains high in Africa, at 86 per 1,000 women aged between 15 and 44. Given the low rate of contraceptive use in the region, this is not surprising. What is less expected, however, is the relatively high rates of unintended pregnancy in Latin America and the Caribbean, at 72 per 1,000, which has been linked to high rates of discontinuation of contraceptive use and incorrect and inconsistent use. In Asia, the rate of unintended pregnancy is lower, 49 per 1,000, probably because of the widespread use of long-acting contraceptives and sterilization, and lower levels of sexual activity among unmarried women.

For women in developing countries, pregnancy and childbirth are a major source of ill health. Around 99 percent of all maternal deaths occur in the developing world, more than half of them in sub-Saharan Africa. One in 22 women in this region die during pregnancy or childbirth, compared with 1 in nearly 6,000 in more developed regions. Although the rate of maternal mortality has decreased somewhat, the total number of deaths remains around the same, because of an increase in the global population.

Unmet Need for Family Planning

According to the WHO, an unmet need for family planning occurs in those women who are fertile and sexually active, and therefore likely to become pregnant, and who have expressed a desire either to not have more children or to delay their next child. It describes the gap between what women's reproductive intentions are and their actual contraceptive behavior. For monitoring, unmet need is expressed as a percentage based on women who are married or in a consensual relationship. Unmet need is particularly high among adolescents, migrants, urban slum dwellers, refugees, and women immediately after childbirth. Two-thirds of women who want to avoid pregnancy want no more children, and the rest want to delay their next pregnancy. There is therefore a difference in their contraceptive needs.

The underlying reasons for unmet family planning need vary by country. Sometimes it is a case of lack of resources and health-care infrastructure, which means that women who want contraceptives cannot access them. However, in many cases women do not want to use certain family planning methods for a variety of other reasons:

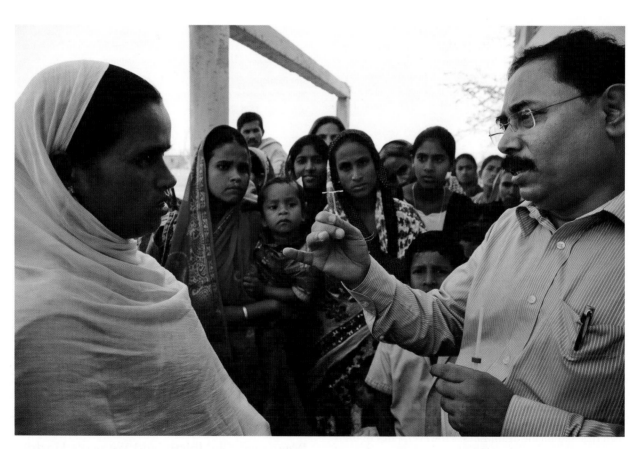

Dr. Ilias Ali, head of India's family planning program in Assam, displays a Copper T, an intrauterine contraceptive device (IUD), to a migrant Muslim woman during an awareness and service camp for the National Rural Health Mission in February 2014 at a very remote Baralakhaiti village on the sandbars of River Brahmaputra, about 43 miles (70 kilometers) north of Gauhati, India. Ali blends religious scriptures with science to popularize birth control as he explained the use of Copper T to migrant Muslims living in remote areas.
© Anupam Nath/AP Images.

there may be concern over side effects, objection from the woman's partner, lack of knowledge or understanding, or cultural or religious objections to contraceptive use.

In sub-Saharan Africa, concern over the health effects of contraceptives and opposition to family planning by the woman and her partner are the main reasons for unmet need. In south-central Asia, one in three cited religious or cultural opposition as their reason, whereas in Southeast Asia, two out of five women were worried about side effects of contraceptives. Across these three regions, lack of access to, and cost of, family planning was not the most significant reason for unmet need. In some instances, of course, women and partners actually desire to have a large family and do not require family planning. In this situation, there would be a low unmet need for contraception.

Countries Compared A comparison of unmet need for family planning in Niger, Uganda, Nepal, and Colombia shows how availability of family planning and fertility expectations interact and differ by region. In Niger, large families are the cultural norm and contraceptive use is low, at 5 percent, and unmet need also is low. In Uganda, again contraceptive use is relatively low, at 18 percent, but women there want to have fewer children, so unmet need is higher. In Nepal, there is a higher use of contraceptives, at 43 percent, but unmet need is high because young women increasingly want to postpone pregnancy yet fear that contraceptives will make them infertile. Finally, in Colombia, family planning programs are well established and the cultural norm is for small families. Contraceptive use here is very high, at 73 percent, and unmet need is low.

Unmet Need in Africa Unmet need for family planning is highest in sub-Saharan Africa. Approximately 49 million women in the region, which is around a quarter of the childbearing population, either use traditional family planning or no method at all, yet wish to avoid pregnancy. The emphasis is upon spacing births, rather than limiting the number. Within the region, there are still significant country-by-country variations. In Zimbabwe, unmet need is as low as 13 percent, where 58 percent of married women use modern contraceptives, while it is as high as 41 percent in Togo, with only 12 percent of women using a modern method.

Use of contraception tends to be higher among wealthier women. In Ethiopia, unmet need is 32 percent among poorer women, compared with 15 percent among wealthier women. However, the picture is complex, with unmet need being similar between wealthier and poorer women in both the Democratic Republic of the Congo and Liberia.

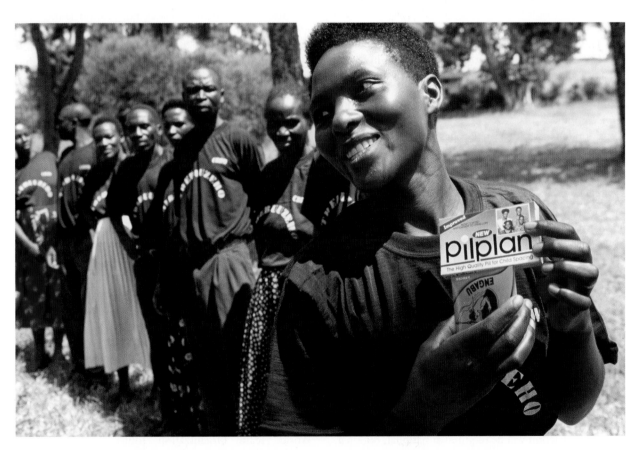

Community reproductive health worker volunteers educate villagers on the use of contraceptives in Uganda. © *Alan Gignoux / Alamy.*

Meeting Family Planning Needs

To meet family planning needs, first of all, more resources should be mobilized. Health planners and policy makers also need to look at a wide range of implementation challenges, such as training more health-care workers and putting an effective infrastructure in place, as well as addressing some of the cultural barriers to family planning. It is difficult to give exact figures for how much a family planning service costs, but one WHO estimate puts this at $3.1 billion for current use of family planning service, going up to $6.7 billion, if unmet need were to be addressed totally. This investment would bring sterilization, long-acting contraceptives, oral contraceptives, and condoms to millions more women and men. If the unmet need were fulfilled, the WHO believes, 53 million unwanted pregnancies, 640,000 newborn deaths, and 150,000 maternal deaths would be averted each year.

Nongovernmental Organizations Many nongovernmental organizations (NGOs) are involved in family planning. For some, such as the WHO, it is just one element of their work in health, education, and development. Others have family planning, including contraception, as their main focus. NGOs can offer funding, expertise, education, and other resources. They can point to many improvements and success stories, but their success ultimately depends on how well they can work with governments, other NGOs, health-care providers, and additional stakeholders.

The International Planned Parenthood Federation (IPPF) was founded in the early 1950s. It works in maternal and child health, reproductive rights, contraception, and abortion, making services available to women in 172 countries around the world. IPPF currently has 65,000 service points.

Founded in 1976, Marie Stopes International (MSI) also works with women and families on all aspects of family planning. It measures its outcomes by a measure called couple years of protection, which is the number of years of protection from unintended pregnancy given to a sexually active couple by use of family planning. In 2013, MSI gave 24.5 million couple years of protection around the world through its work. This avoided 368,000 maternal deaths and 6.2 million unintended pregnancies. MSI's goal is to double the number of women it serves from 10 million to 20 million by 2020.

⊕ Future Implications

Much more funding, from national governments and the international community, is required to fulfill the universal right to modern family planning. Investment in the mid-2010s is both insufficient and unpredictable. Much stronger political commitment to previous agreements is needed, and action will be required at national, regional, and international levels.

Weaknesses in health systems that need to be addressed include poor supply systems, a lack of trained health-care professionals, and insufficient physical capacity. There are also societal, cultural, and religious barriers against a woman's right to safe and effective family planning, such as stigma against unmarried women who are sexually active. All of this will need effective leadership, which could come from many organizations, such as the WHO, NGOs, the private sector, charities, health-care providers, and governments at all levels.

To achieve the goals of MDG 5, it is necessary to expand and improve family planning for women around the world. Investment in family planning already has been shown to yield significant health and economic benefits. Further investment is justified because it would lead to big gains in health and productivity, would save millions of lives, and have broad and multiple benefits for both women and society at large. Family planning efforts in the mid-2010s are not keeping pace with growing demand, and there are still unacceptably high levels of unintended pregnancies, particularly in developing countries. Family planning is a wise investment, the benefits of which would continue to flow for many years into the future.

There have been many milestones along the family planning road. One of these was the 2012 London Summit on Family Planning, at which the UK government and the Bill & Melinda Gates Foundation launched a new effort to make contraceptives, services, and information available to an additional 120 million women and girls around the world by 2020. This would have a big impact, not least on infant mortality, with 3 million fewer babies dying in the first year of life. Whether the pledge will prove more successful than MDG 5 depends upon the commitment of the many stakeholders involved.

SEE ALSO *Gender and Health; Maternal and Infant Health; Pregnancy Termination*

BIBLIOGRAPHY

Books

McVeigh, Enda, Roy Homburg, and John Guillebaud. *Oxford Handbook of Reproductive Medicine and Family Planning*, 2nd ed. Oxford: Oxford University Press, 2013.

Parry, Manon. *Broadcasting Birth Control: Mass Media and Family Planning.* New Brunswick, NJ: Rutgers University Press, 2013.

United Nations, Department of Economic and Social Affairs, Population Division. *World Contraceptive Patterns 2013*, October 2013. Available online at http://www.un.org/en/development/desa/population/publications/family/contraceptive-wallchart-2013.shtml (accessed February 18, 2015).

World Health Organization, Johns Hopkins Bloomberg School of Public Health, and USAID. *Family*

Planning: A Global Handbook for Providers. Baltimore: Johns Hopkins Bloomberg School of Public Health, 2011. Available online at http://whqlibdoc.who .int/publications/2011/9780978856373_eng. pdf?ua=1 (accessed May 20, 2015).

Periodicals

Carr, Bob, Melinda Gates, Andrew Mitchell, and Rajiv Shah. "Giving Women the Power to Plan Their Families." *The Lancet* 380, no. 9837 (July 14, 2012): 80–82.

van Braeckel, Dirk, Marleen Temmerman, Kristien Roelens, and Olivier Degomme. "Slowing Population Growth for Wellbeing and Development." *The Lancet* 380, no. 9837 (July 14, 2012): 84–85.

Websites

"Family Planning." *World Health Organization (WHO).* http://www.who.int/topics/family_planning/en/ (accessed February 18, 2015).

"Our Work." *International Planned Parenthood Federation.* http://www.ippf.org/our-work (accessed February 18, 2015).

Provost, Claire. "Teenage Pregnancy and Access to Contraception under the Spotlight at Global Summit." *Guardian*, November 12, 2013. http:// www.theguardian.com/global-development/2013/ nov/12/teenage-pregnancies-contraception-global-summit (accessed February 18, 2015).

United Nations Population Fund (UNFPA) and the Guttmacher Institute. "Adding It Up: Costs and Benefits of Investing in Family Planning and Maternal and Newborn Health." *UNFPA.org.* http:// www.unfpa.org/public/publications/pid/4461 (accessed February 18, 2015).

"What We Do." *Marie Stopes International.* http:// mariestopes.org/what-we-do (November 18, 2014)

Susan Aldridge

Food Safety and Food Preparation

🌐 Introduction

Food safety is the discipline of preparing, handling, and storing food in a way that prevents food-borne illness. There are more than 250 food-borne illnesses, many of which are caused by ingesting raw or processed foods that have been contaminated by pathogens (disease-causing organisms) such as microbial pathogens, zoonotic diseases, parasites, mycotoxins (toxins produced by fungi), antibiotic drug residues, and pesticide residues. Most food-borne illnesses cause abdominal cramps, diarrhea, nausea, and vomiting, and in the most severe cases, organ failure and death. Chemical contamination of food tends to cause chronic illnesses such as cancer.

Contamination of a food source can happen anywhere along the food chain: in primary production, improper handling and storage, and improper preparation and cooking in the home or in other places where food is consumed. Food-borne illness is entirely preventable. There are international rules and guidelines—and in many countries laws—in place to try to control contamination on the production end. Consumers can prevent food-borne illnesses by keeping cooking surfaces clean; washing their hands; separating raw meat, poultry, and seafood from other foods; cooking foods thoroughly; keeping food at safe temperatures; and using safe water and raw materials to make the food.

And yet, the World Health Organization (WHO) estimates that at least 2 billion people per year contract a food-borne illness, and about 2.2 million people, many of whom are children, die from those illnesses. Those who do not die can face other serious consequences including kidney and liver failure, brain and neural disorders, and reactive arthritis.

Food safety is a critical, international public health concern. Since the mid-20th century, the food chain from production to consumption has become more global. While this globalization has many health, economic, and social benefits, it also means that what once might have been a small outbreak of a food-borne illness somewhere in the world has the potential to become an international incident. Further, new technologies in food production and processing, changes in animal husbandry, antimicrobial resistance in food-borne pathogens, and the emergence of new pathogenic microorganisms and chemical substances in the food supply can make keeping food safe a challenge.

🌐 Historical Background

From the misadventures of opportunistic eaters in the Stone Age, to lead contamination in the Roman Era, to widespread mold poisonings of the Renaissance, food-borne illness has been an unwelcome visitor since the dawn of humankind. Over the ages, it has killed composers such as Franz Schubert (1797–1828), kings such as Henry I of England (1068–1135), inventors such as Wilbur Wright (1867–1912), and even a U.S. president, Zachary Taylor (1784–1850). The impact of food-borne illness on human history has been profound, as Morton Satin, an American molecular biologist, wrote in an entry in the *Encyclopedia of Food Safety*, "Who knows how different the world would have turned out had lead poisoning not reduced the intellectual capacities of some of the great Greek and Roman leaders? Empires may have been won or lost over a few unsuspected molecules."

It was not until the end of the 19th century that scientists started to grasp fully the nature of food spoilage and disease, due primarily to the work of French chemist and biologist Louis Pasteur (1822–1895). This knowledge led to new technologies in food processing and production. Better preservation of food around this time also bolstered food exportation around the world and the need for regulating food crossing borders.

The dawn of the 20th century saw several nations creating government agencies and laws designed to ensure food safety. In 1945, the Food and Agriculture Organization of the United Nations (FAO) was founded. Three years later, the WHO followed. At a joint committee meeting of the FAO and the WHO in 1950, members

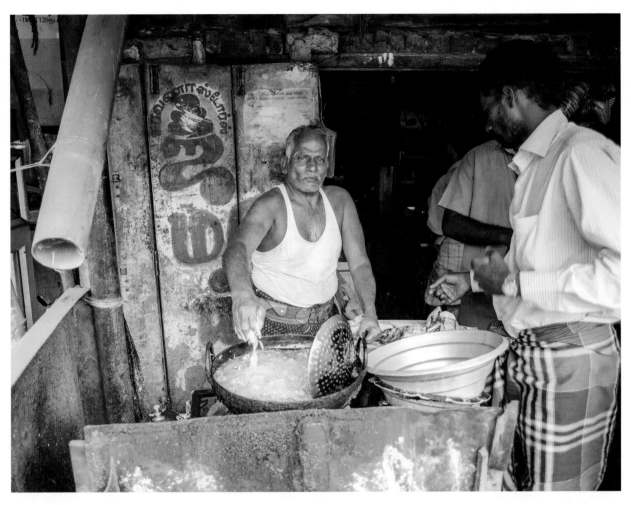

A street food vendor uses his hands to drop food into a vat of frying oil. The Indian government has been trying to educate street food vendors and the public about precautions to prevent food-related illness. *© Ailisa/Shutterstock.com.*

of the two entities agreed there needed to be a uniform set of standards governing food regulations. Work to that end began in 1951.

Ten years later, the FAO and the WHO established the *Codex Alimentarius*. Latin for "Book of Food," the *Codex* is a set of internationally recognized standards, recommendations, and guidelines for food regulation and safety. In 1963, the Codex Alimentarius Commission was formed to oversee the Codex program.

In the 2010s, the *Codex* is still the international standard for food safety best-practice recommendations. As for the commission, its role has evolved to include ensuring fair-trade practices in the food trade, as well as promoting coordination of all food standards work undertaken by international governmental and nongovernmental organizations.

In addition to international bodies overseeing food safety, several nations have their own regulatory agencies. Those nations include Australia, China, France, Germany, Hong Kong, India, New Zealand, Pakistan, South Korea, the United Kingdom, and the United States.

⊕ Impacts and Issues

Food-borne illnesses enter the body through food or water that contains contaminants such as microbial pathogens, zoonotic diseases, parasites, mycotoxins, antibiotic drug residues, or pesticide residues. Genetically modified foods also can contain allergens or toxins. Uncooked meat, poultry, or fish, fruits and vegetables contaminated with feces, and seafood infected with marine biotoxins are just a few of the ways that food can be unsafe and cause disease. The pathogens that infect these foods can lead to illnesses that range from severe diarrhea to debilitating infections to disability and death. Vulnerable populations such as infants, children, pregnant women, people with underlying health conditions, and the elderly are often the hardest hit.

Common Food-Borne Illnesses

There are hundreds of known food-borne illnesses, and new ones are emerging all the time. According to the WHO, food-borne illnesses usually are "caused by bacteria, viruses, parasites, or chemical substances entering

Food-Borne Illness-Causing Organisms in the United States

Organism	Common Name of Illness	Onset Time After Ingesting	Signs & Symptoms	Duration	Food Sources
Bacillus cereus	*B. cereus* food poisoning	10–16 hrs	Abdominal cramps, watery diarrhea, nausea	24–48 hours	Meats, stews, gravies, vanilla sauce
Campylobacter jejuni	Campylobacteriosis	2–5 days	Diarrhea (possibly bloody), cramps, fever, and vomiting	2–10 days	Raw/undercooked poultry, unpasteurized milk, contaminated water
Clostridium botulinum	Botulism	12–72 hours	Vomiting, diarrhea, blurred or double vision, difficulty swallowing, muscle weakness. Possible respiratory failure/death	Variable	Improperly canned foods, especially home-canned vegetables, fermented fish, baked potatoes in aluminum foil
Clostridium perfringens	Perfringens food poisoning	8–16 hours	Intense abdominal cramps, watery diarrhea	Usually 24 hours	Meats, poultry, gravy, dried or precooked foods
Cryptosporidium	Intestinal cryptosporidiosis	2–10 days	Diarrhea (usually watery), stomach cramps, upset stomach, slight fever	May be remitting and relapsing over weeks to months	Uncooked food/food contaminated by an ill food handler, contaminated water
Cyclospora cayetanensis	Cyclosporiasis	1–14 days, usually at least 1 week	Diarrhea (usually watery), loss of appetite and/or weight, stomach cramps, nausea, vomiting, fatigue	May be remitting and relapsing over weeks to months	Various types of fresh produce
E. coli (Escherichia coli) producing toxin	*E. coli* infection, or "travelers' diarrhea"	1–3 days	Watery diarrhea, abdominal cramps, some vomiting	3–7 or more days	Water or food contaminated with human feces
E. coli O157:H7	Hemorrhagic colitis or *E. coli* O157:H7 infection	1–8 days	Severe (often bloody) diarrhea, abdominal pain and vomiting. Can lead to kidney failure	5–10 days	Undercooked beef (especially hamburger), unpasteurized milk/juice, raw fruits/vegetables, and contaminated water
Hepatitis A	Hepatitis	28 days average (15–50 days)	Diarrhea, dark urine, jaundice and flu-like symptoms, i.e., fever, headache, nausea, and abdominal pain	Variable, 2 weeks–3 months	Raw produce, contaminated water, uncooked foods and cooked foods contaminated by an ill food handler; contaminated shellfish
Listeria monocytogenes	Listeriosis	9–48 hrs for gastrointestinal symptoms, 2–6 weeks for invasive disease	Fever, muscle aches, and nausea or diarrhea. Infection in pregnant women can lead to premature delivery or stillbirth. Elderly or immuno-compromised patients may develop bacteremia or meningitis	Variable	Unpasteurized milk, soft cheeses made with unpasteurized milk, ready-to-eat deli meats
Noroviruses	Viral or acute nonbacterial gastroenteritis, winter diarrhea, food poisoning or infection	12–48 hrs	Nausea, vomiting, abdominal cramping, diarrhea, fever, headache. Diarrhea is more prevalent in adults, vomiting more common in children	12–60 hrs	Raw produce, contaminated water, uncooked foods or cooked foods contaminated by an ill food handler; contaminated shellfish
Salmonella	Salmonellosis	6–48 hours	Diarrhea, fever, abdominal cramps, vomiting	4–7 days	Eggs, poultry, meat, unpasteurized milk/juice, cheese, contaminated raw fruits/vegetables
Shigella	Shigellosis or Bacillary dysentery	4–7 days	Abdominal cramps, fever, and diarrhea. Stools may contain blood and mucus	24–48 hrs	Raw produce, contaminated water, uncooked foods or cooked foods contaminated by an ill food handler
Staphylococcus aureus	Staphylococcal food poisoning	1–6 hours	Sudden onset of severe nausea and vomiting. Abdominal cramps. Diarrhea and fever may be present	24–48 hours	Unrefrigerated or improperly refrigerated meats, potato and egg salads, cream pastries
Vibrio parahaemolyticus	*V. parahaemolyticus* infection	4–96 hours	Watery (occasionally bloody) diarrhea, abdominal cramps, nausea, vomiting, fever	2–5 days	Undercooked or raw seafood, such as shellfish
Vibrio vulnificus	*V. vulnificus* infection	1–7 days	Vomiting, diarrhea, abdominal pain, blood-borne infection, fever, bleeding under the skin, ulcers. Can be fatal to the immuno-compromised or with liver disease.	2–8 days	Undercooked or raw seafood, such as shellfish (especially oysters)

SOURCE: U.S. Food and Drug Administration Center for Food Safety and Applied Nutrition, 2014.

the body through contaminated food or water." These illnesses provoke a host of maladies from severe diarrhea to longer-term, more debilitating illnesses such as meningitis and cancer and can be found in numerous sources including raw animal meats, fruits and vegetables contaminated with feces, and raw shellfish containing marine biotoxins.

Though there are many food-borne illnesses, the WHO has identified some as the most common. When it comes to bacteria, *Salmonella*, *Campylobacter*, and *Escherichia coli* are major concerns, affecting millions of people annually. Symptoms are fever, headache, nausea, vomiting, abdominal pain, and diarrhea. *Salmonella* causes salmonellosis, which usually lasts four to seven days and typically does not require medical treatment. It usually is transmitted via eggs, poultry, and other meats. *Campylobacter* causes campylobacteriosis, which usually lasts about a week and is transmitted through raw milk, raw or undercooked poultry, and contaminated drinking water.

Escherichia coli, the third-most-common bacteria to cause a food-borne illness, can be very serious. Whereas most *E. coli* infections clear up within a week, some can lead to hemolytic uremic syndrome (HUS). According to the CDC, this can lead to kidney failure and often requires dialysis and transfusions. Some people develop chronic kidney failure or neurologic impairment. About 3 to 5 percent of those afflicted with HUS die. The major source of transmission is ground beef, but other sources include unpasteurized milk and juice, sprouts, lettuce, and salami, and contact with cattle. The CDC states that "waterborne transmission occurs through swimming in contaminated lakes or pools or drinking inadequately chlorinated water."

Another serious bacterial infection can be caused by *Listeria*. The infection can lead to spontaneous abortions in pregnant women and death in newborn babies. *Listeria* is found in unpasteurized dairy products and ready-to-eat foods and can grow at refrigeration temperatures. *Vibrio cholerae* causes cholera, which people can get from eating contaminated food—rice, vegetables, millet gruel, and various types of seafood have all been linked to outbreaks—or contaminated water. The WHO notes

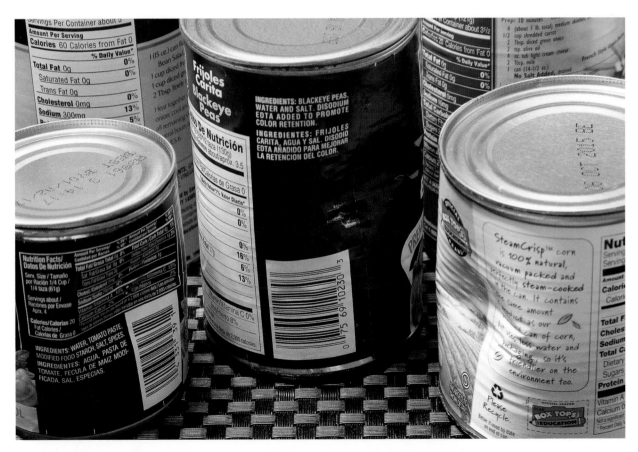

According to the U.S. Centers for Disease Control and Prevention (CDC), each of the dented cans of foods portrayed should raise concern for consumers as to the safety of the contents. The CDC recommends always checking to be sure a package or can is intact before purchasing and keeping an eye out for "leaking, bulging, rusting, or badly dented cans; cracked jars; jars with loose or bulging lids; canned food with a foul odor; or any container that spurts liquid when opening." This caution should be taken because these signs can mean that the food contains a toxin produced by the bacteria *Clostridium botulinum*. Botulism can be a deadly danger even in small amounts. *Debora Cartagena/U.S. Centers for Disease Control and Prevention.*

OUTBREAKS IMPACT WORLD TRADE

There are many challenges to keeping global food supplies safe. Transporting food around the globe has increased dramatically since the 1960s. This shift in the food supply from local to global fundamentally changed the way consumers eat and how countries produce goods. As a result, rural areas urbanized, agriculture has become more industrialized to keep up with demand from growing populations, people are traveling and eating out more, and consumers are demanding more exotic and out-of-season foods, all of which serve to elongate and complicate the food chain from producer to consumer.

A product can be grown in one country, processed in another, and consumed in yet another, and vulnerabilities can develop anywhere along that food chain. When those vulnerabilities lead to an outbreak of a food-borne illness, it can affect numerous markets around the world. Localized incidents of food-borne disease have the potential to spread globally. Furthermore, governments of some countries may not trust the practices employed by another country. That mistrust can lead to trade restrictions and losses for everyone in the chain.

Every continent has had a serious food-borne disease outbreak since 2005, many made worse by global trade. Examples cited by the WHO include infant formula contaminated with melamine in 2008 that affected 300,000 infants and young children and caused six deaths in China alone. In Germany in 2011, an *Escherichia coli* (*E. coli*) outbreak linked to contaminated fenugreek sprouts spread to eight countries in Europe and North America. This *E. coli* outbreak led to 53 deaths, US$1.3 billion in losses for farmers and industries, and US$236 million in emergency aid payments to 22 European Union member states, according to the WHO.

that symptoms may include "abdominal pain, vomiting, and profuse watery diarrhea, which may lead to severe dehydration and possibly death."

Viruses also can be sources for food-borne illness. Norovirus infections are among the most common viral food-borne illness. Characterized by nausea, vomiting, watery diarrhea, and abdominal pain, norovirus infections can be contracted by coming into contact with feces or vomit from an infected person. This can happen as a result of touching an infected surface, or eating foods contaminated by the virus due to poor hygiene.

Hepatitis A is a virus that affects the liver and can be transmitted through food, objects, or drinks contaminated with the feces, even in microscopic amounts, of an infected person or from contact with an infected person. The disease course ranges from mild and lasting only a few weeks to severe and lasting several months.

Parasites can wreak havoc when it comes to food safety. For example, fish-borne trematodes, which are flatworms, are transmitted only through food. Other parasites, however, can be transmitted through food or direct contact with animals. For example, *Echinococcus* species, also known as small tapeworms, usually are transmitted by dogs. A dog typically becomes infected by eating organs of animals that have hydatid cysts (cysts containing the larval parasites). These tapeworms grow inside the dog. The tapeworm eggs then are released from the dog through the animal's fecal matter. People can get infected by accidentally eating soil, water, or food that has been contaminated by the fecal matter of an infected dog. Persons with cystic echinococcosis usually do not show symptoms until hydatid cysts grow large enough to cause discomfort, pain, nausea, and vomiting. This can take several years. The cysts can grow in the liver, lungs, spleen, kidneys, heart, bone, central nervous system, brain, and eyes. Some cysts go away on their own, whereas others need to be removed surgically. Other parasites, such as *Entamoeba histolytica*, and *Giardia*, have been known to enter the food chain via water, soil, or fresh produce.

Naturally occurring toxins and environmental pollutants can cause a host of food safety issues. According to the WHO, such toxins include mycotoxins, marine biotoxins, cyanogenic glycosides, and toxins occurring in poisonous mushrooms. Foods with high levels of mycotoxins such as aflatoxin and ochratoxin can include corn or cereals. Long-term exposure to these toxins can affect the immune system, development, or cause cancer.

Compounds that accumulate in the environment and the body are called persistent organic pollutants. Examples of these include dioxins and polychlorinated biphenyls, which are by-products of industrial processes and waste incineration. They tend to accumulate in animal food chains. The WHO warns that "dioxins are highly toxic and can cause reproductive and developmental problems, damage the immune system, interfere with hormones, and cause cancer."

Environmental contamination with heavy metals, which include lead, cadmium, and mercury, also can contaminate both the land-based and oceanic elements of the food chain. Ingestion of these contaminated food sources by humans can cause neurological and kidney damage. Heavy metals usually enter the animal and human food chain through pollution of air, water, and soil.

Keeping Global Food Supplies Safe

Food safety is a critical factor in food security. When food is scarce, the population will consume whatever is available, even food that is unsafe or contaminated, leading to an increase in food-borne illnesses. And when there is a food safety scare in a country where food is scarce, it typically causes a disruption in the existing food supply, waste of the contaminated (or suspect) food, and thus even less available food. Furthermore, efforts to increase food production significantly in these countries can mean an increase in the use of fertilizers, pesticides, and veterinary medicines that can add potential risks.

Safe Minimum Cooking Temperatures and Rest Times for Meat, Poultry, Seafood, and Other Foods

Category	Food	Temperature (°F/°C)	Rest Time
Ground Meat & Meat Mixtures	Beef, Pork, Veal, Lamb	160/71	None
	Turkey, Chicken	165/74	None
Fresh Beef, Veal, Lamb	Steaks, roasts, chops	145/63	3 minutes
Poultry	Chicken & Turkey, whole	165/74	None
	Poultry breasts, roasts	165/74	None
	Poultry thighs, legs, wings	165/74	None
	Duck & Goose	165/74	None
	Stuffing (cooked alone or in bird)	165/74	None
Pork and Ham	Fresh pork	145/63	3 minutes
	Fresh ham (raw)	145/63	3 minutes
	Precooked ham (to reheat)	140/60	None
Eggs & Egg Dishes	Eggs	Cook until yolk and white are firm.	None
	Egg dishes	160/71	None
Leftovers & Casseroles	Leftovers	165/74	None
	Casseroles	165/74	None
Seafood	Fin Fish	145/63 or cook until flesh is opaque and separates easily with a fork.	None
	Shrimp, lobster, and crabs	Cook until flesh is pearly and opaque.	None
	Clams, oysters, and mussels	Cook until shells open during cooking.	None
	Scallops	Cook until flesh is milky white or opaque and firm.	None

SOURCE: Foodsafety.gov, U.S. Department of Health and Human Services, 2014.

Proper food handling and cooking can prevent food-borne illness from occurring.

Additionally, food safety has tremendous impacts on national economies, trade, and tourism and is key to sustainable development. The magnitude of risk of an outbreak to public health and its effect on the economy varies. Sometimes, the mere perception of a food safety breakdown is enough to cause governments and consumers to lose confidence in a product. This can result in long-term impacts for the economy, sustainability of the food supply, and ultimately human development in the affected countries.

Because a food-borne illness event can have such tremendous consequences, international agencies such as the WHO and the FAO have been urging governments around the world to make food safety a priority and harmonize regional safety regulations with internationally agreed upon standards as much as possible. By doing this, governments can ensure that food producers and suppliers are following best practice guidelines and responsibly supplying safe food to consumers. However, some countries, particularly developing ones, find some food safety trade regulations are too demanding. And although officials of these countries agree food should be safe, some of the regulations do not take into account the financial burden it poses to smaller economies and ultimately can lead to trade barriers.

Closer to home, many food-borne diseases arise simply from foods improperly prepared or mishandled in the kitchen, in food service establishments, by street vendors, or in markets. To avoid this, food handlers and consumers can follow procedures that keep contamination to a minimum. When preparing food at home, it is important to wash hands with soap and water before preparing the food. Next wash all produce and cutting boards and continue to do so throughout the preparation process. Hands, utensils, and cutting boards should all be cleaned again, any time they have been in contact with raw meat or poultry and before touching another food. It is also important use a food thermometer to cook meat and poultry to proper temperatures and refrigerate food within two hours of serving. Refrigerated foods needs to be kept at 40 degrees Fahrenheit (4.4 degrees Celsius) or cooler. Bacteria grows rapidly in what is often referred to as the "Danger Zone," which is 40 to 140 degrees Fahrenheit (4.4 to 60 degrees Celsius).

⊕ Future Implications

Even as more countries modernize and improve food safety standards, new challenges to the health of the global food supply are emerging constantly. Among them is the occurrence of new pathogens in food. For example, there have been multiple outbreaks of bovine spongiform encephalopathy (BSE), also known as mad cow disease, in cattle. The human form of the disease, variant Creutzfeldt-Jakob disease, is contracted by eating beef from an infected cow. Another emergent pathogen is H5N1 influenza, which can be transmitted by handling a contaminated bird or eating raw or undercooked contaminated poultry.

In addition, there has been a surge in the number of antibiotic resistant pathogens in food animals. As farms have become more industrial, the use of antibiotics to keep animals healthy has increased. Likewise, humans have increased their use of antibiotics. In both instances, this has resulted in drug-resistant pathogens.

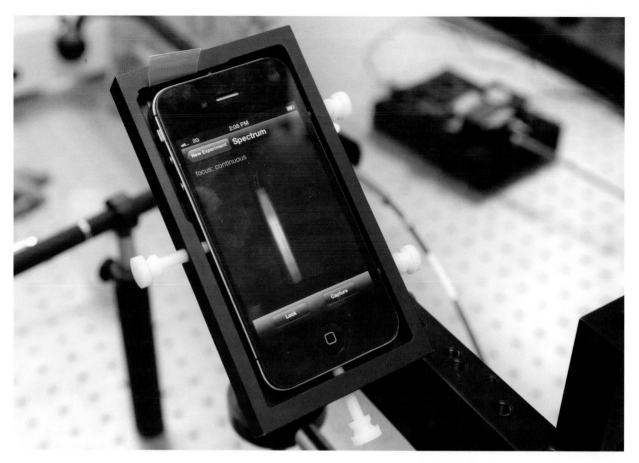

A handheld biosensor developed by researchers at the University of Illinois, Urbana-Champaign, is shown. An app can turn a smartphone into a handheld biosensor, promising the ability to run on-the-spot tests for food safety, environmental toxins, medical diagnostics, and more.   © *Michael Conroy/AP Images.*

The overuse, and sometimes misuse, has been connected to the emergence and proliferation of antibiotic-resistant bacteria. The concern is that these pathogens may get passed on to the food supply. However, the extent of this problem is contested, and generally it is agreed that more study is needed to understand the full impact of antibiotic-resistant pathogens.

New technologies at times have been a boon to food safety, such as those that can detect and analyze various pathogens and toxins in foods. Scientists state that these technologies will aid in early warning of food-borne pathogens. However, the downside of new technology means growing concerns over the safety of processed food additives and novel food ingredients, biotechnology, and irradiation.

Some studies also show that climate change will have an effect on food safety moving into the future. One challenge is that people may change what they eat due to increasing costs of food resulting from climate change. For example, consumers may switch from fresh to frozen poultry. This can increase the likelihood of people ingesting *Salmonella*, but lowers the possibility of ingesting *Campylobacter*.

Another challenge to food safety when it comes to climate change is that food will be produced in altered ecosystems. Climate change may alter the patterns of pests and diseases, causing an increase in the use of herbicides, fungicides, and antibiotics for animals in food production. All of these can increase the risk to the food supply.

PRIMARY SOURCE

Notes from the Field: Multistate Outbreak of Listeriosis Linked to Soft-Ripened Cheese

SOURCE *Choi, Mary J., et al. "Notes from the Field: Multistate Outbreak of Listeriosis Linked to Soft-Ripened Cheese—United States, 2013," from* Morbidity and Mortality Weekly Report *63, no. 13 (April 4, 2014): 294–295. Centers for Disease Control and Prevention (CDC). http://www.cdc.gov/ mmwr/preview/mmwrhtml/mm6313a5.htm?s_ cid=mm6313a5_w (accessed January 25, 2015).*

INTRODUCTION *This primary source is from a weekly publication of the U.S. Centers for Disease Control and Prevention (CDC). The issue presented here describes the CDC's investigation of a multistate outbreak of listeriosis, which was traced to one cheese producer and brought under control.*

Notes from the Field: Multistate Outbreak of Listeriosis Linked to Soft-Ripened Cheese—United States, 2013

Weekly
April 4, 2014 / 63(13);294–295

On June 27, 2013, the Minnesota Department of Health notified CDC of two patients with invasive *Listeria monocytogenes* infections (listeriosis) whose clinical isolates had indistinguishable pulsed-field gel electrophoresis (PFGE) patterns. A query of PulseNet, the national molecular subtyping network for foodborne disease surveillance, identified clinical and environmental isolates from other states. On June 28, CDC learned from the Food and Drug Administration's Coordinated Outbreak Response and Evaluation Network that environmental isolates indistinguishable from those of the two patients had been collected from Crave Brothers Farmstead Cheese during 2010–2011. An outbreak-related case was defined as isolation of *L. monocytogenes* with the outbreak PFGE pattern from an anatomic site that is normally sterile (e.g., blood or cerebrospinal fluid), or from a product of conception, with an isolate upload date during May 20–June 28, 2013. As of June 28, five cases were identified in four states (Minnesota, two cases; Illinois, Indiana, and Ohio, one each). Median age of the five patients was 58 years (range: 31–67 years). Four patients were female, including one who was pregnant at the time of infection. All five were hospitalized. One death and one miscarriage were reported.

Case—case analysis of *Listeria* Initiative data was conducted, comparing food exposure frequencies among the five outbreak-related cases identified by June 28 with food exposure frequencies in 1,735 sporadic listeriosis cases reported to CDC during 2004–2013. The analysis indicated that any soft cheese consumption during the month before illness onset was associated with outbreak-related listeriosis: five of five (100%) in the outbreak-related cases versus 569 of 1,735 (33%) in the sporadic cases (odds ratio = 10.8; 95% confidence interval = 1.8–∞).

The five patients were reinterviewed to assess their cheese exposures. All five patients had definitely or probably eaten one of three varieties of Crave Brothers soft-ripened cheese (Les Frères, Petit Frère, or Petit Frère with truffles). Three patients had purchased the cheese at three different restaurants, and two had purchased the cheese at two different grocery stores. The cheeses were shipped as intact wheels to the three restaurants and two grocery stores, where they had been cut and served or repackaged and sold to customers.

Testing at the Minnesota Department of Agriculture identified the outbreak pattern of *L. monocytogenes* in two cheese wedges (Les Frères and Petit Frère with truffles) collected from two different grocery stores in Minnesota. Inspection of the cheese-making facility revealed that substantial sanitation deficiencies during the cheese-making process itself, after the milk was pasteurized, likely led to contamination. On July 1, Crave Brothers halted production of Les Frères, Petit Frère, and Petit Frère with truffles. On July 3, Crave Brothers issued a voluntary recall of these products with a production date of July 1, 2013, or earlier. On July 11, the company voluntarily halted production of all cheese products manufactured at the facility. After product recall, one additional case was identified in Texas through whole genome sequencing, bringing the total case count for the outbreak to six.

This outbreak was linked to soft cheeses that were likely contaminated during the cheese-making process. Pasteurization eliminates *Listeria* in milk. However, contamination can occur after pasteurization. Cheese-making facilities should use strict sanitation and microbiologic monitoring, regardless of whether they use pasteurized milk.

Persons at greater risk for listeriosis, including older adults, pregnant women, and those with immunocompromising conditions, should be aware that certain soft cheeses made with unpasteurized milk, or made under unsanitary conditions, regardless of whether the milk was pasteurized, have been shown to cause severe illness. These soft cheeses include fresh (unripened) cheeses, such as queso fresco, and soft-ripened cheeses, such as the cheeses implicated in this outbreak.

SEE ALSO *Antibiotic/Antimicrobial Resistance; Avian (Bird) and Swine Influenzas; Bacterial Diseases; Cholera and Dysentery; Climate Change: Health Impacts; Dengue; Ebola Virus Disease; Epidemiology: Surveillance for Emerging Infectious Diseases; Food Security and Hunger; Hemorrhagic Diseases; Marine Toxins and Pollution; Neglected Tropical Diseases; Parasitic Diseases; Prion Diseases; Sanitation and Hygiene; Viral Diseases; Vulnerable Populations; Water Supplies and Access to Clean Water; Waterborne Diseases; Zoonotic (Animal-Borne) Diseases*

BIBLIOGRAPHY

Books

Booth, Michael, and Jennifer Brown. *Eating Dangerously: Why the Government Can't Keep Your Food Safe—and How You Can.* Lanham, MD: Rowman and Littlefield, 2014.

Motarjemi, Yasmine, Gerald Moy, and E. C. D. Todd, eds. *Encyclopedia of Food Safety.* Boston: Academic Press, 2014.

Perrett, Heli. *The Safe Food Handbook: How to Make Smart Choices about Risky Food.* New York: Experiment, 2011.

Periodicals

Mitka, Mike. "Food Safety." *JAMA* 305, no. 18 (May 11, 2011): 1850.

Sun, Juanjuan. "The Evolving Appreciation of Food Safety." *European Food and Feed Law Review.* 7, no. 2 (2012): 84–90.

Websites

Anderson, Ross. "Bugs through the Ages: The Foodborne Illness Fight." *FoodSafetyNews.com*, January 3, 2011. http://www.foodsafetynews.com/2011/01/fbi-through-the-ages/#.VJJPWHuYTXQ (accessed January 7, 2015).

"Campylobacter: General Information." *U.S. Centers for Disease Control and Prevention (CDC).* http://www.cdc.gov/nczved/divisions/dfbmd/diseases/campylobacter/ (accessed January 7, 2015).

"Enterohemorrhagic *Escherichia coli.*" *U.S. Centers for Disease Control and Prevention (CDC).* http://www.cdc.gov/ncidod/dbmd/diseaseinfo/enterohemecoli_t.htm (accessed January 7, 2015).

"Food Safety." *U.S. Centers for Disease Control and Prevention (CDC).* http://www.cdc.gov/foodsafety/ (accessed January 7, 2015).

"Food Safety," Fact Sheet No. 399. *World Health Organization (WHO)*, November 2014. http://www.who.int/mediacentre/factsheets/fs399/en/ (accessed January 7, 2015).

"Foodborne Illness, Foodborne Disease (Sometimes Called 'Food Poisoning')." *U.S. Centers for Disease Control and Prevention (CDC).* http://www.cdc.gov/foodsafety/facts.html (accessed January 7, 2015).

"Hepatitis A FAQs for the Public." *U.S. Centers for Disease Control and Prevention (CDC).* http://www.cdc.gov/hepatitis/A/aFAQ.htm (accessed January 7, 2015).

"Norovirus." *U.S. Centers for Disease Control and Prevention (CDC).* http://www.cdc.gov/norovirus/index.html (accessed January 7, 2015).

"Parasites—Echinococcosis." *U.S. Centers for Disease Control and Prevention (CDC).* http://www.cdc.gov/parasites/echinococcosis/index.html (accessed January 7, 2015).

"Prion Diseases." *U.S. Centers for Disease Control and Prevention (CDC).* http://www.cdc.gov/ncidod/dvrd/prions/ (accessed January 7, 2015).

"What Is Salmonellosis?" *U.S. Centers for Disease Control and Prevention (CDC).* http://www.cdc.gov/salmonella/general/ (accessed January 7, 2015).

Melanie R. Plenda

Food Security and Hunger

⊕ Introduction

A key target of the eight United Nations (UN) Millennium Development Goals (MDGs) agreed to in 2000 was to halve, from 1990 to 2015, the proportion of people who suffer from hunger. In 2014, one year away from the target, the UN Food and Agriculture Organization (FAO) published updated estimates of the number of hungry people in the world in *The State of Food Insecurity in the World 2014: Strengthening the Enabling Environment for Food Security and Nutrition*. At least 805 million people (one in nine) worldwide were chronically undernourished in 2012–2014, and the vast majority (791 million people, or 98 percent) lived in low- and middle-income countries. However, trends in global hunger reduction are promising: the proportion of undernourished people dropped from 18.7 percent in 1990–1992 to 11.3 percent in 2012–2014; thus, the hunger target of MDG 1 is within reach.

There is substantial regional variability in the proportion of people who suffer from hunger. Worldwide, according to the FAO report, the greatest progress in reducing hunger over the 25 years covered in the report has been in Latin America, where the prevalence of undernourishment dropped from 14.4 percent in 1990–1992 to just 5.1 percent in 2012–2014. The governments in this region are now committed to reaching 0 percent by 2025, as declared in the Hunger-Free Latin America and the Caribbean Initiative. Over that same period, southern Asia and sub-Saharan Africa reduced the proportion of hungry people in those regions, from 33.3 percent to 23.8 percent and from 24.0 percent to 15.8 percent, respectively, but the reductions have been inadequate so far for reaching the MDG 1.

In addition to the UN MDG to halve the proportion of people who suffer from hunger, the World Food Summit set a goal in 1996 to halve the number of people who suffer from hunger, a much more difficult target. While 63 low- and middle-income countries had already achieved the MDG in 2014, only 25 had achieved the World Food Summit goal. Of those 25 countries, most were in Latin America and the Caribbean (Cuba, Saint Vincent and the Grenadines, Brazil, Chile, Guyana, Nicaragua, Peru, Uruguay, and Venezuela), though a few sub-Saharan Africa countries (Cameroon, Djibouti, Ghana, Mali, and São Tomé and Principe) and several Asian countries (Myanmar, Thailand, and Vietnam) also achieved the World Food Summit goal.

The World Food Summit of 1996 also led to the international adoption of a uniform definition for food security; "food security exists when all people, at all times, have physical and economic access to sufficient, safe and nutritious food that meets their dietary needs and food preferences for an active and healthy life." This definition includes four key dimensions: availability, access, utilization, and stability. It therefore recognizes that food security does not simply involve having sufficient quantities of food, but also the quality and diversity of food, being able to acquire food in a socially and legally acceptable way, food safety, and not being at risk to lose access to food. Because of this expanded definition, the FAO now collects data on multiple indicators of food security, not just the number of people who suffer from hunger (e.g. "undernourishment," which is based on national annual per capita calorie consumption). These FAO indicators include, for example, the share of calories derived from cereals, roots and tubers, the average supply of animal-source proteins, domestic food price index and volatility, fluctuations in domestic food supply, access to water and sanitation, and the prevalence of anemia.

While the measurement and ongoing surveillance of food security and hunger is important for targeting policies to improve global health, understanding the root causes of food insecurity is essential for informing the content of such interventions. It is now widely accepted that both nature- and human-based factors lead to hunger. Drought, natural diasters, wars and civil strife, and the AIDS epidemic are just a few of the underlying causes of food insecurity around the world. Therefore, continued progress in alleviating hunger will require that not only agricultural practices and food storage and distribution infrastructure be addressed, as discussed in detail in the sections that follow, but also political and economic

Percent of the World Population Who is Undernourished, by Country, 2012–2014

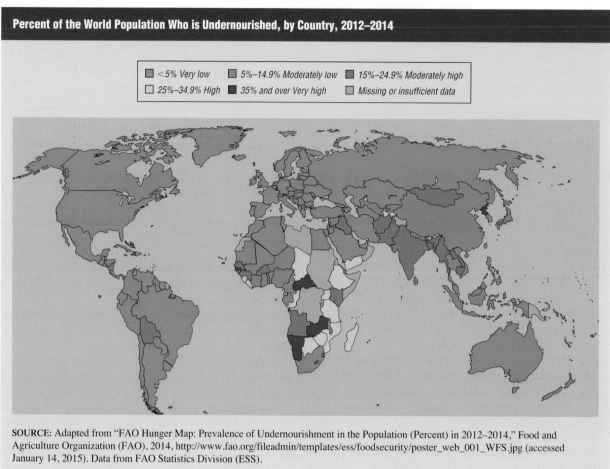

☐ <5% Very low   ☐ 5%–14.9% Moderately low   ☐ 15%–24.9% Moderately high

☐ 25%–34.9% High   ■ 35% and over Very high   ☐ Missing or insufficient data

SOURCE: Adapted from "FAO Hunger Map: Prevalence of Undernourishment in the Population (Percent) in 2012–2014," Food and Agriculture Organization (FAO), 2014, http://www.fao.org/fileadmin/templates/ess/foodsecurity/poster_web_001_WFS.jpg (accessed January 14, 2015). Data from FAO Statistics Division (ESS).

Between 2012 and 2014 at least one in nine people worldwide was undernourished. The majority of undernourished live in low- and middle-income countries.

stability. As with many aspects of global health, improving food security necessitates close collaborations across multiple disciplines and sectors.

⊕ Historical Background

In 1798, Thomas Malthus (1766–1834) predicted in his essay *On the Principle of Population* that human population growth would soon outpace food production, and any gains in living standards would be lost. The Industrial and Agricultural Revolutions of the 19th century and the Green Revolution of the 20th century proved that farmers' ability to increase food production, particularly of maize, wheat, rice, oats, and barley, could be improved substantially with technology. According to Nikos Alexandratos and Jelle Bruinsma of the FAO, from 2005 to 2007, world average per capita food availability was 2,770 calories per person per day after accounting for food waste, animal feed, and nonfood uses. This is much higher than the caloric intake recommended for sedentary, adult (31–50 years old) men (2,200 to

2,400 calories per day) and women (1,800 calories per day) by the U.S. Departments of Agriculture and Health and Human Services in the 2010 *Dietary Guidelines for Americans*. In light of the persistence of hunger around the world, this also highlights important disparities in the distribution of food between and within countries.

Two modern-day global food crises are worth noting here, the 1972–1974 crisis and the 2007–2008 crisis. In 1971, the United States liberalized exports of grains, particularly wheat, to the Union of Soviet Socialist Republics (USSR), Eastern Europe, and China. Then, in 1972, after a relatively long period of grain surpluses and stable food prices (related to the large grain reserves, which could be used to buffer price fluctuations), cereal production worldwide dropped by 3 percent as a result of climatic conditions (harsh winters, droughts, and tropical cyclones). Around the same time, the Organization of the Petroleum Exporting Countries (OPEC) dramatically increased the price of petroleum, which in turn increased the price of fertilizers and transportation. Consequently, food prices increased, and food aid to developing countries dropped, resulting in a global food crisis.

From their peak in the mid-1970s, food prices steadily decreased until early in the first decade of the 21st century. Then, beginning in 2006 and lasting until mid-2008, food prices surged. Derek Headey and Shenggen Fan of the International Food Policy Research Institute stated in a 2010 report that the relative contribution of various factors to the 2007–2008 crisis is still uncertain, but possible causes include increasing energy prices and demand for biofuels. Experts predict that the 2007–2008 food crisis marks the beginning of a period of high and volatile food prices, and indeed, according to the FAO's 2014 Report, the number of food emergencies has risen since the mid-1990s, particularly in Africa, where the number has tripled. Shifts in the way crops are grown and livestock is raised are needed in order to reverse this alarming trend.

⊕ Impacts and Issues

A 2010 review published by H. Charles J. Godfray and colleagues in the journal *Science* highlighted five strategies for achieving food security in a sustainable manner: (1) closing the yield gap (e.g., the difference between what is actually produced and what could be produced using current technologies), (2) increasing production limits, (3) reducing waste, (4) changing diets, and (5) expanding aquaculture (farmed fish). A key limitation of these strategies is that they largely focus on the first dimension of food security—availability—while overlooking the remaining dimensions of access, utilization, and stability.

Strategies (1) and (2): Sustainable Intensification Strategies one and two, closing the yield gap and increasing production limits, relate to increasing crop productivity and the availability of food. According to a 2011 review by Jonathan A. Foley and colleagues published in the journal *Nature*, average global crop yields increased by about 20 percent between 1985 and 2005, down from a 56 percent increase calculated between 1965 and 1985. This 20 percent increase was above and beyond a 7 percent increase in harvested cropland area owing to fewer crop failures, less fallow land (e.g., land left unseeded), and increased multiple cropping (e.g., growing at least two crops on the same area during a single season). This is important because methods used in the past to increase food productivity, such as increasing cultivated land area and exploiting new fisheries, are no longer viable options. Foley and colleagues state: "agriculture has already cleared or converted 70 percent of the grassland, 50 percent of the savanna, 45 percent of the temperate deciduous forest, and 27 percent of the tropical forest biome."

Thus, farmers will need to produce more food with the same amount (or less) land while reducing the negative environmental impacts of agriculture, a concept known as "sustainable intensification." Negative environmental impacts include nutrient runoff from fertilizers, overextraction of water, soil degradation, release of greenhouse gases, and decreased biodiversity. It is also increasingly clear that this shift toward sustainability will need to occur rapidly in order to achieve global food security.

Sustainable intensification is particularly difficult to implement in low-income countries, where food production is still dominated by smallholder farmers and land rights are not secure. This results in a disincentive to invest in, for example, closing the yield gap, because inputs (e.g., irrigation systems, fertilizer, improved crop and livestock varieties, machinery, and storage infrastructure) can be expensive and the immediate payoffs can be low. Nonetheless, several cost-effective and environmentally friendly strategies are available to farmers to increase yields, including minimum tillage to conserve soils and precision farming (e.g., applying expensive inputs such as pesticides and fertilizers only to those areas that need it).

Adoption of crop varieties that have been bred for improved characteristics can also increase yields. However, this practice inevitably leads to lower genetic diversity among crop varieties compared to wild varieties. With the introduction of improved varieties in low-income countries, it is important to ensure that genetic adaptations to local environments are not lost. Retaining genetic diversity is also important for adaptation to changing environments resulting from climate change.

Strategy (3): Reducing Waste According to the aforementioned review in the journal *Science* by Godfray and colleagues, approximately 30–40 percent of food is lost to waste. In developed countries such as the United States and the United Kingdom, most food is lost at home, while in developing countries, the majority of food is lost on-farm or in transport and processing. For example, according to Christian Nellemann of the UN Environment Programme (2009), 35–40 percent of fresh produce is lost in India because wholesale and retail outlets do not have cold storage. Thus, building and strengthening food chain infrastructure in low- and middle-income countries will be a key component of reducing food waste and improving the sustainability of the global food system.

In high-income countries, most of the food waste arises at the home stage of consumption, perhaps because food is relatively cheap and therefore consumers are not incentivized to reduce waste. Furthermore, "sell by" and "use by" dates with very wide safety margins often lead to the disposal of food that is suitable for consumption. Because these are individual-level behaviors, tackling food waste in high-income countries will be difficult and require legislation, possibly relating to composting of food waste and reform of the sell by and use by dates.

Strategy (4): Changing Diets According to the 2012 FAO report *World Agriculture towards 2030/2050*, approximately one-third of cereals produced worldwide

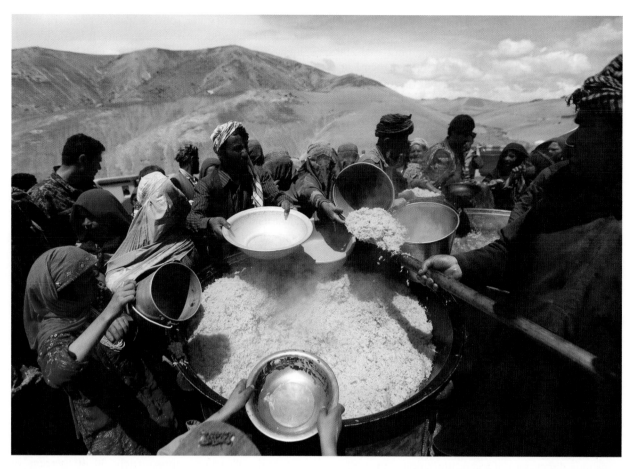

Villagers displaced by a deadly landslide receive lunch in the Argo district of Badakhshan Province, Afghanistan, on May 7, 2014. Between 500 and 2,700 people were estimated dead, and aid agencies rushed supplies to more than 4,000 displaced by the landslide. It is believed that climate change will precipitate an increase in natural disasters such as floods and landslides, which may lead to periodic decreases in food security in some of the poorest countries of the world. © *Mohammad Ismail/Reuters.*

goes into animal feed. Given that the plant-to-animal conversion efficiency is only about 10 percent, many people now accept that significant shifts in dietary patterns will need to occur if an increasing number of people on a decreasing amount of land are to be supported. However, it is also accepted that not all livestock production is equal in its externalities. For example, grass-fed livestock are often fed on land that could not be cultivated without great environmental costs, and manure can be used as a natural fertilizer. Furthermore, livestock can be an important source of income and nutrients for poorer communities. More research is needed to understand the impacts of decreasing animal products in the human diet.

Strategy (5): Expanding Aquaculture Aquaculture, or fish-farming, provides the world's human population with about 7 percent of the protein it consumes. Both in developing countries and in areas where the local wild-caught fish are no longer in abundance due to overfishing, aquaculture practices are increasing to meet a growing demand for dietary protein. Currently, Asia leads the world in aquaculture, with China alone

accounting for over more than 50 percent of global aquaculture production. Current challenges for increasing global protein supply via aquaculture include building inland aquaculture infrastructure in rainy subtropical areas of Africa and ensuring sustainable environmental practices.

Climate Change

Climate change is thought to contribute to the increased frequency of food emergencies since the mid-1990s and represents a threat to the progress of reducing hunger, particularly in the poorer parts of the world. In particular, the Intergovernmental Panel on Climate Change's Fifth Assessment Report published in 2013 predicts that climate change has and will continue to result in increased global temperatures and increased frequency and duration of heat waves, droughts, heavy precipitation, tropical cyclones, and extremely high sea levels. In general, the report predicts that rainfall during summer monsoons in Asia will increase, while parts of northern and southern Africa will become drier. Emissions of

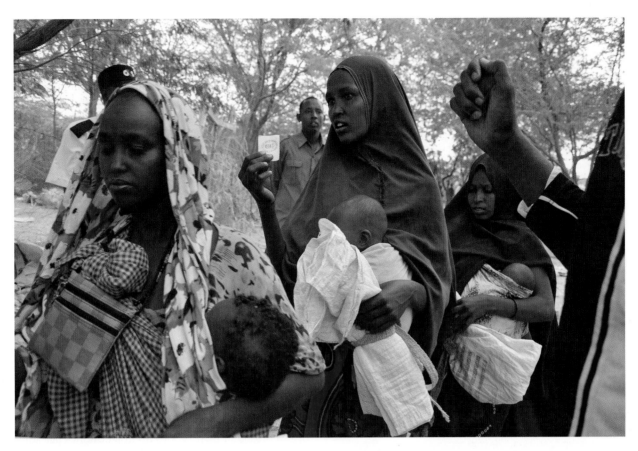

Somalis at one of the Dadaab refugee camps run by the office of the United Nations High Commissioner for Refugees wait in line for food aid in Dadaab, Kenya. In 2010 and 2011, drought and food insecurity in the Horn of Africa and war in Somalia led to over 485,000 displaced people becoming refugees in Dadaab. By January 2015, though drought conditions had ended, 353,590 refugees still remained. © *hikrcn/Shutterstock.com.*

greenhouse gases will also impact crop production, as demonstrated by a World Bank analysis published as part of their *Development Report* in 2010.

A recent meta-analysis by Jerry Knox and colleagues published in the journal *Environmental Research Letters* in 2012 found that crop yields will decline, on average, by 7.7 percent by the 2050s in Africa and South Asia, two regions that already have the highest proportion of people who suffer from hunger. They found that the scientific evidence for climate change impacts on crop productivity in this region are most robust for the staples, wheat (average decline of 12.1 percent), maize (average decline of 7.2 percent), sorghum (average decline of 13 percent), and millet (average decline of 8.8 percent), and less robust for rice, cassava, sugarcane, yams, pulses (legumes), vegetables, and grasslands for livestock as these crops are less studied. Downstream of crop productivity, a 2009 report by Gerald C. Nelson and colleagues at the International Food Policy Research Institute found that climate change will lead to increases in the price of staple crops including wheat, maize, soybeans, and rice, and that food energy availability in 2050 will be lower than that in 2000, thus eliminating progress made to date on alleviating hunger.

Genetically Modified Crops

Genetically modified (GM) crops have been an area of lively debate since they were first commercialized in 1996. According to a 2013 International Service for the Acquisition of Agri-biotech Applications (ISAAA) report, while only 27 countries currently plant GM crops, the number of hectares of GM crops has increased by over 100-fold worldwide since their introduction into global markets: from 1.7 million hectares in 1996 to 175 million hectares in 2013. The top countries in terms of hectares of GM crops are the United States (173.2 million acres [70.1 million hectares]), Brazil (100 million acres [40.3 million hectares]), Argentina (60.3 million acres [24.4 million hectares]), India (27.2 million acres [11 million hectares]), and Canada (26.7 million acres [10.8 million hectares]). China, Paraguay, South Africa, Pakistan, Uruguay, and Bolivia also plant 2.5 million acres (1 or more million hectares) of GM crops annually.

The most common applications of GM technology include tolerance to broad-spectrum herbicides and resistance to insects via insertion of a gene for a toxin, specifically in maize, cotton, soybeans, and oilseeds. According to Godfray and colleagues, researchers are also looking into the use of GM technology to improve

FOOD SECURITY AND NUTRITION

Food security and nutrition are intricately related, with food security being necessary, though not sufficient, for achieving good nutrition. This topic is especially important for mothers, infants, and children who are particularly vulnerable to malnutrition due to their increased nutrient requirements. Most estimates of hunger focus on undernourishment, which is an undersupply of calories. However, micronutrient deficiencies, particularly iron, zinc, vitamin A, and folate, may still persist, leading to what some public health researchers refer to as "hidden hunger." Thus, food security efforts are now focused not only on supplying appropriate calories through macronutrients (carbohydrates, fat, and protein) but also micronutrients.

One approach that has been explored is the nutritional biofortification of staple crops, most notably, golden rice. An analysis by Hans De Steur and colleagues published in the journal *New Biotechnology* in 2012 found that introducing multi-biofortified rice (rice enhanced with vitamin A, zinc, iron, and folate) could lower the disability-adjusted life year (DALY) burden by up to 46 percent at a cost of less than US$10 per DALY. However, public concern over the safety of genetically modified crops and political debates over international intellectual property rights continue to pose significant barriers to wide implementation of such interventions.

Other approaches include crop and livestock diversification and nutrition education through school and workplace gardens. Marie Ruel and colleagues of the International Food Policy Research Institute emphasize in the book *The Road to Good Nutrition*, published in 2013, the importance of food safety and access to clean water and sanitation in achieving both food and nutrient security. As an example, Ruel and colleagues say that young children must be free of recurrent infections and diarrhea in order for the nutrients in foods to be absorbed and utilized effectively by the body for growth. Poverty, inequality, cultural beliefs and practices, and the status of women all influence food and nutrition security; thus, more holistic approaches to prevention are needed.

drought, salinity (high salt levels in soil), and high-temperature tolerance, as well as to increase nitrogen-use and photosynthetic efficiency. Indeed, according to the 2013 ISAAA report, two new drought-tolerant crops have been introduced: maize in the United States and sugarcane in Indonesia. The ultimate goal of these technologies is to reduce the inputs (e.g., water and fertilizer) needed to produce the same output level and to adapt to climate change (e.g., desertification and increased frequency of droughts).

In stark contrast to these positive views of the role of GM crops in the reduction of hunger, others have argued that this technology will worsen global food insecurity. Uncertainties over environmental and human health effects, the role of GM crops in industrial agriculture, negative impacts on traditional agricultural practices, excessive corporate dominance, and intellectual property rights are the key issues brought up by those opposed to this technology. While these concerns undoubtedly need to be addressed, the evidence supporting the use of GM crops to increase crop productivity is relatively strong. A review of 49 peer-reviewed publications of farmer surveys published in the journal *Nature Biotechnology* in 2010 found that 73.8 percent of reported results found higher yields in adopters compared to non-adopters, 19 percent found no difference in yields, and 7.7 percent found lower yields in adopters compared to non-adopters.

In addition to the potential direct effects of increasing crop productivity and thus the availability of food worldwide, GM crops may also indirectly increase food availability through improving the economic situation of smallholder farmers. According to the 2008 *World Bank Development Report*, which focused on agriculture, half of undernourished people are smallholder farmers in low- and middle-income countries. In one of the first studies to analyze the effects of adopting Bt cotton (insecticide-producing cotton) on food security in India, published in the journal, *PLOS ONE*, in 2013, Matin Qaim and Shahzad Kouser found that if all non-adopters switched to Bt cotton, the proportion of food-insecure households would decrease by 20.3 percent. Per hectare of Bt cotton, an increase of 73.7 total calories per adult equivalent per day was observed and an increase of 23.2 calories from nutritious foods (pulses, fruits, vegetables, and animal products) per adult equivalent per day was also observed, suggesting potential positive impacts on both quantity and quality of food.

⊕ Future Implications

According to the 2012 UN world population projections (published in 2013), the world population will increase to 9.6 billion by 2050, representing a deceleration in population growth compared to the 20th century. Nonetheless, combined with the increasing impacts of climate change, this population increase of about 2.4 billion over the next 35 years will require drastic changes at all levels of the food system.

In addition to a higher demand for total calories to prevent undernourishment, with economic development in low- and middle-income countries will come a higher demand for processed foods, meat, dairy, and fish. The world's food system will need to adapt to these demands in an environmentally and socially sustainable way. In addition to total calories, the nutritional quality of crop commodities will need to be considered. Researchers, farmers, manufacturers, retailers, legislators, and consumers must work together to carry out the discussed strategies and create a radically different food system capable of providing healthful diets for future generations.

PRIMARY SOURCE

Codex Alimentarius Ad Hoc Intergovernmental Task Force on Foods Derived from Biotechnology

SOURCE *Food and Agriculture Organization of the United Nations, 2000, "FAO Statement on Biotechnology" from Codex Alimentarius Ad Hoc Intergovernmental Task Force on Foods Derived from Biotechnology. http://www.fao.org/biotech/ fao-statement-on-biotechnology/en/ (accessed January 25, 2015).*

INTRODUCTION *This primary source is a statement released at the time of the 2000 conference of the Food and Agriculture Organization (FAO) of the United Nations. It broadly covers the range of the FAO's concerns at that time regarding modern technology in the production of food worldwide, a discussion that is still ongoing. It recognizes the benefits associated with the application of biotechnology, such as the genetic engineering of plants and animals, to raise production for food security in impoverished nations, while also noting possible risks.*

FAO Statement on Biotechnology

The statement was published in March 2000 on the occasion of the "Codex Alimentarius Ad Hoc Intergovernmental Task Force on Foods Derived from Biotechnology" meeting in Japan.

Biotechnology provides powerful tools for the sustainable development of agriculture, fisheries and forestry, as well as the food industry. When appropriately integrated with other technologies for the production of food, agricultural products and services, biotechnology can be of significant assistance in meeting the needs of an expanding and increasingly urbanized population in the next millennium.

There is a wide array of "biotechnologies" with different techniques and applications. The Convention on Biological Diversity (CBD) defines biotechnology as: *"any technological application that uses biological systems, living organisms, or derivatives thereof, to make or modify products or processes for specific use."*

Interpreted in this broad sense, the definition of biotechnology covers many of the tools and techniques that are commonplace in agriculture and food production. Interpreted in a narrow sense, which considers only the new DNA techniques, molecular biology and reproductive technological applications, the definition covers a range of different technologies such as gene manipulation and gene transfer, DNA typing and cloning of plants and animals.

While there is little controversy about many aspects of biotechnology and its application, genetically modified organisms (GMOs) have become the target of a very intensive and, at times, emotionally charged debate. FAO recognizes that genetic engineering has the potential to help increase production and productivity in agriculture, forestry and fisheries. It could lead to higher yields on marginal lands in countries that today cannot grow enough food to feed their people. There are already examples where genetic engineering is helping to reduce the transmission of human and animal diseases through new vaccines. Rice has been genetically engineered to contain pro-vitamin A (beta carotene) and iron, which could improve the health of many low-income communities.

Other biotechnological methods have led to organisms that improve food quality and consistency, or that clean up oil spills and heavy metals in fragile ecosystems. Tissue culture has produced plants that are increasing crop yields by providing farmers with healthier planting material. Marker-assisted selection and DNA fingerprinting allow a faster and much more targeted development of improved genotypes for all living species. They also provide new research methods which can assist in the conservation and characterization of biodiversity. The new techniques will enable scientists to recognize and target quantitative trait loci and thus increase the efficiency of breeding for some traditionally intractable agronomic problems such as drought resistance and improved root systems.

However, FAO is also aware of the concern about the potential risks posed by certain aspects of biotechnology. These risks fall into two basic categories: the effects on human and animal health and the environmental consequences. Caution must be exercised in order to reduce the risks of transferring toxins from one life form to another, of creating new toxins or of transferring allergenic compounds from one species to another, which could result in unexpected allergic reactions. Risks to the environment include the possibility of outcrossing, which could lead, for example, to the development of more aggressive weeds or wild relatives with increased resistance to diseases or environmental stresses, upsetting the ecosystem balance. Biodiversity may also be lost, as a result of the displacement of traditional cultivars by a small number of genetically modified cultivars, for example.

FAO supports a science-based evaluation system that would objectively determine the benefits and risks of each individual GMO. This calls for a cautious case-by-case approach to address legitimate concerns for the biosafety of each product or process prior to its release. The possible effects on biodiversity, the environment and food safety need to be evaluated, and the extent to which the benefits of the product or process outweigh its risks assessed. The evaluation process should also take into consideration experience gained by national regulatory authorities in clearing such products. Careful monitoring of the post-release effects of these products and processes is also essential to ensure their continued safety to human beings, animals and the environment.

Current investment in biotechnological research tends to be concentrated in the private sector and oriented towards agriculture in higher-income countries where there is purchasing power for its products. In view of the potential contribution of biotechnologies for increasing food supply and overcoming food insecurity and vulnerability, FAO considers that efforts should be made to ensure that developing countries, in general, and resource-poor farmers, in particular, benefit more from biotechnological research, while continuing to have access to a diversity of sources of genetic material. FAO proposes that this need be addressed through increased public funding and dialogue between the public and private sectors.

FAO continues to assist its member countries, particularly developing countries, to reap the benefits derived from the application of biotechnologies in agriculture, forestry and fisheries—through, for example, the network on plant biotechnology for Latin America and the Caribbean (REDBIO), which involves 33 countries. The Organization also assists developing countries to participate more effectively and equitably in international commodities and food trade. FAO provides technical information and assistance, as well as socio-economic and environmental analyses, on major global issues related to new technological developments. Whenever the need arises, FAO acts as an "honest broker" by providing a forum for discussion.

For instance, together with the World Health Organization, FAO provides the secretariat to the Codex Alimentarius Commission which has just established an ad hoc Intergovernmental Task Force on Foods Derived from Biotechnologies, in which government-designated experts will develop standards, guidelines or recommendations, as appropriate, for foods derived from biotechnologies or traits introduced into foods by biotechnological methods. The Codex Alimentarius Commission is also considering the labelling of foods derived from biotechnologies to allow the consumer to make an informed choice.

Another example is the FAO Commission on Genetic Resources for Food and Agriculture, a permanent intergovernmental forum where countries are developing a Code of Conduct on Biotechnology aimed at maximizing the benefits of modern biotechnologies and minimizing the risks. The Code will be based on scientific considerations and will take into account the environmental, socio-economic and ethical implications of biotechnology. As in applications in medicine, these ethical aspects warrant responsible consideration. Therefore the Organization is working towards the establishment of an international expert committee on ethics in food and agriculture.

FAO is constantly striving to determine the potential benefits and possible risks associated with the application of modern technologies to increase plant and animal productivity and production. However, the responsibility for formulating policies towards these technologies rests with the Member Governments themselves.

SEE ALSO   *Child Health; Climate Change: Health Impacts; Malnutrition; Maternal and Infant Health; Nutrition; Population Issues; Water Supplies and Access to Clean Water*

BIBLIOGRAPHY

Books

Alexandratos, Nikos, and Jelle Bruinsma. *World Agriculture towards 2030/2050: The 2012 Revisions.* Rome: Food and Agriculture Organization, 2012. ESA Working Paper No. 12-03.

Food and Agriculture Organization. *The State of World Aquaculture.* Rome: Food and Agriculture Organization, 2006.

Food and Agriculture Organization, International Fund for Agricultural Development, and World Food Programme. *The State of Food Insecurity in the World 2014: Strengthening the Enabling Environment for Food Security and Nutrition.* Rome: Food and Agriculture Organization, 2014. Available online at http://www.fao.org/3/a-i4030e.pdf (accessed February 11, 2015).

Headey, Derek, and Shenggen Fan. *Reflections on the Global Food Crisis: How Did It Happen? How Has It Hurt? And How Can We Prevent the Next One?* Washington, DC: International Food Policy Research Institute, 2010.

Intergovernmental Panel on Climate Change. *Climate Change 2013: The Physical Science Basis.* Cambridge, UK: Cambridge University Press, 2013.

International Service for the Acquisition of Agri-biotech Applications (ISAAA). *Global Status of Commercialized Biotech/GM Crops: 2013.* Ithaca, NY: ISAAA, 2014.

Nellemann, Christian, et al., eds. *The Environmental Food Crisis: The Environment's Role in Averting Future Food Crises.* Arendal, Norway: UNEP, 2009.

Nelson, Gerald C., et al. *Climate Change: Impact on Agriculture and Costs of Adaptation.* Washington, DC: International Food Policy Research Institute, 2009.

Ruel, Marie, et al., eds. *The Road to Good Nutrition.* New York: Karger, 2013.

United Nations. *World Population Prospects: The 2012 Revision.* New York: United Nations, 2013. Available online at http://esa.un.org/unpd/wpp/Documentation/pdf/WPP2012_%20KEY%20FINDINGS.pdf (accessed February 10, 2015).

U.S. Department of Agriculture, U.S. Department of Health and Human Services. *Dietary Guidelines for Americans, 2010*, 7th ed. Washington, DC: U.S. Government Printing Office, 2010.

World Bank. *World Bank Development Report 2008: Agriculture for Development.* Washington, DC: World Bank, 2008.

World Bank. *World Bank Development Report 2010: Development and Climate Change.* Washington, DC: World Bank, 2010.

Periodicals

Carpenter, Janet E. "Peer-Reviewed Surveys Indicate Positive Impact of Commercialized GM Crops." *Nature Biotechnology* 28, no. 4 (April 2010): 319–321.

De Steur, Hans, et al. "Potential Impact and Cost-Effectiveness of Multi-biofortified Rice in China." *New Biotechnology* 29, no. 3 (February 2012): 432–442.

Foley, Jonathan A., et al. "Solutions for a Cultivated Planet." *Nature* 478 (October 2011): 337–342.

Godfray, H. Charles J., et al. "Food Security: The Challenge of Feeding 9 Billion People." *Science* 327 (February 2010): 812–818.

Knox, Jerry, Tim Hess, Andre Daccache, and Tim Wheeler. "Climate Change Impacts on Crop Productivity in Africa and South Asia." *Environmental Research Letters* 7 (September 2012): 1–8.

Qaim, Matin, and Shahzad Kouser. "Genetically Modified Crops and Food Security." *PLOS ONE* 8, no. 6 (June 2013): e64879.

Websites

"Climate Change: How Climate Change Affects Hunger." *World Food Programme.* http://www.wfp.org/climate-change (accessed February 11, 2015).

"Food Security." *CARE International.* http://www.care-international.org/what-we-do/food-security.aspx (accessed February 11, 2015).

"Food Security." *World Health Organization (WHO).* http://www.who.int/trade/glossary/story028/en/ (accessed February 11, 2015).

"Global Food Security." *United Nations (UN).* http://www.un-foodsecurity.org/ (accessed February 11, 2015).

"Hunger." *World Food Programme.* http://www.wfp.org/hunger (accessed February 11, 2015).

Lindsay M. Jaacks

Fungal Diseases

⊕ Introduction

The fungi are a diverse group of organisms, ranging from microscopic molds and yeasts to mushrooms with more complex structures. They are not plants, because they lack chlorophyll, nor are they bacteria, because their cells have nuclei. Microscopic fungi are everywhere in the environment and, like bacteria and viruses, may cause disease if they get onto the skin or inside the body.

Fungal diseases, also known as mycoses, can affect anyone. Most fungal diseases do not make people ill but tend to have irritating symptoms, such as itching or discharge. However, when fungi enter the body, they can cause life-threatening disease, usually among people who are already ill.

Those with weakened immunity are more at risk of serious fungal disease. This means that fungal disease is a particular problem for those with HIV/AIDS (human immunodeficiency virus/acquired immune deficiency syndrome). Many of those with, or at risk of, fungal disease live in places affected by poverty and weak health systems. Therefore diagnosis and treatment can be difficult, which is why the U.S. Centers for Disease Control and Prevention (CDC) states that fungal diseases are a global health problem. The CDC and partners such as the World Health Organization (WHO) are working to bring both antifungal diagnostics and antifungal medications to those who need them.

There are more than 100,000 fungi, many of which are still to be studied and classified. Most are harmless, and some are even used in the manufacture of medicines, foods, and beverages. Fungi derive their nutrients from their surroundings; when these happen to be human, animal, or plant tissue, then disease may result.

A fungal infection may be either local or systemic, with the latter tending to be more serious. Local fungal infections occur on the skin, mouth, and vagina. Common examples of local fungal infections are athlete's foot, where the fungus *Tinea pedis* affects the skin on the feet and between the toes, and oropharyngeal and genital or vulvovaginal candidiasis (generally called thrush when it involves infection of the mouth and "yeast infection" in the vagina) by fungus in the genus *Candida*, usually *Candida albicans*. *Candida* fungus normally live on human skin and in the mucus membranes without causing problems, however, in certain conditions the overgrowth of the fungus can cause problems. Nonsystemic mycoses also can be classified according to how far they penetrate the body's tissues. Superficial mycoses remain on the skin or hair. Cutaneous mycoses include athlete's foot or ringworm, where the superficial layer of skin, nails, or hair are involved. The subcutaneous mycoses penetrate below the skin and involve subcutaneous, connective, and even bone tissue.

In a systemic fungal infection, the fungus usually is inhaled and enters the bloodstream, where it may start to attack internal organs. Examples of systemic fungal infections include aspergillosis and cryptoccosis, caused by inhalation of *Aspergillus* and *Cryptococcus* fungi, respectively. Meanwhile, the *Candida* species, though it normally lives inside the body, may cause a systemic infection called invasive candidiasis, in which the fungus enters the bloodstream and other parts of the body in which it does not normally live; this type of infection can be serious.

Fungal diseases, or infections, are either opportunistic or primary. Most fungi are not actually pathogenic, save in a human host that has reduced immunity. In these circumstances, an opportunistic infection may occur that would not in a healthy person. Important causes of compromised immunity include HIV/AIDS, diabetes, leukemia, and other cancers of the blood. Treatment with steroids, cancer chemotherapy, immunosuppressants after an organ transplant, and spending time in the intensive care unit also tend to undermine the immune system, putting the patient at risk of opportunistic fungal disease. Infections that occur as a result of medical treatment in the hospital setting are known as nosocomial, or hospital-acquired, infections. They can be caused by either fungi or bacteria and may be very difficult to treat.

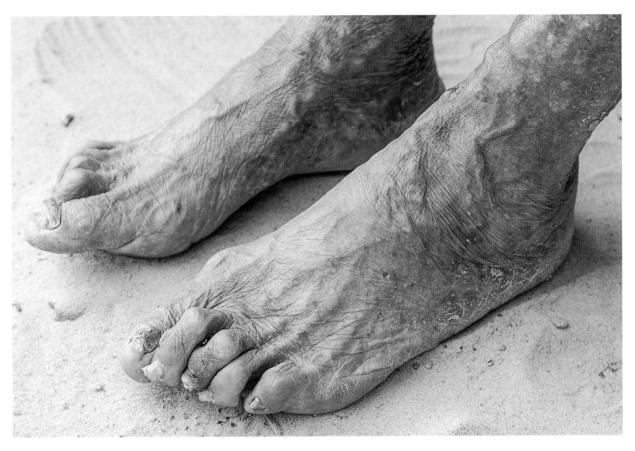

Onychomycosis (also called tinea unguium) is a fungal infection caused by several types of fungus that affect the nails. Fungal infections are also the cause of yeast infections, ringworm, and jock itch. © *ra3rn/Shutterstock.com.*

Typical systemic opportunistic fungal infections include candidiasis and aspergillosis. If a patient has severely compromised immunity, the infection may be acute and life threatening, with progressive pneumonia, dissemination of infection throughout the body, or fungemia, the presence of fungi in the blood, which can lead to multiple organ failure. Primary fungal infections affect healthy people and tend to be chronic rather than acute. Indeed, months often pass before the person seeks a diagnosis.

If a patient is suspected of having a systemic fungal disease, the doctor should take a travel history in case he or she has been exposed to a fungus endemic in another location. Samples of sputum may be needed for lab culture if the lungs are affected. There are many antifungal drugs and, in the case of local infections such as athlete's foot, treatment usually is straightforward.

⊕ Historical Background

The ancient Greek physician Hippocrates (c. 460–c. 377 BCE) wrote of aphthae, or sores in the mouth, which would now be recognized as oral thrush. Fungi are one of the earliest-known infections of humans, other animals, and plants. It was Hungarian physician David Gruby (1810–1898) who first wrote in detail about fungi as a cause of human disease in the mid-19th century.

Around this time, fungal infections of the skin, such as ringworm, were well known. Gruby was able to link specific fungi to infections of the scalp. Soon, fungi became part of the germ theory of disease. By the 20th century, researchers recognized three types of human disease that could be caused by fungi. There were infections affecting the skin, nails, hair, blood, and internal organs. Then there was fungal disease caused by fungal toxins. Finally, there were allergic reactions to fungi. In the 1980s a fourth, and somewhat controversial, category was added, which was the idea of the fungal overgrowth. According to William G. Crook (1917–2002) in his book *The Yeast Connection* (1986), this phenomenon could be responsible for a number of chronic conditions, such as inflammatory bowel disease and chronic fatigue syndrome.

Modern Trends in Fungal Disease

Medical and social advances have brought about changes in the type of fungal disease most commonly seen. Mass schooling provided ideal conditions for the spread of ringworm of the scalp among children. The rise of college sport with communal changing rooms drove the increase in the incidence of athlete's foot.

More serious yeast infections began to emerge with the development of medical treatments. For instance, antibiotic treatments alter the gut flora, which allows opportunistic yeast infections with fungus such as *Candida* to take hold. Cancer chemotherapy and steroid treatment following organ transplantation lowered immunity, which also opened the door to opportunistic yeast infection, including candidiasis and aspergillosis. Previously, these opportunistic yeast infections had been rare, and they were regarded as diseases of people who are already ill.

⊕ Impacts and Issues

Candidiasis

The *Candida* species are the most common cause of human fungal infections, from local skin and mucous membrane infections to invasive infections of the blood and body organs. There are more than 150 species of *Candida*, of which 9 are human pathogens. *Candida* species live inside the human body, rather than in the environment, and are the most common fungal component of normal human gut flora. They become the cause of opportunistic infections only when the human host has compromised immunity or if there are changes in the host's normal flora, usually caused by the use of broad-spectrum antibiotics.

Candida albicans is the most common cause of human yeast infections, from the trivial to the deadly serious. However, other *Candida* species are emerging as significant causes of disease. These include *C. glabrata*, *C. krusei*, *C. parapsilosis*, and *C. tropicalis*. Mortality from blood infections from these *Candida* species is similar to that found with *Candida albicans*.

Local *Candida* infection commonly involves the skin, mouth, esophagus, and vagina. Candidiasis involving the folds of the skin is known as intertrigo. In babies, it is one of the causes of diaper rash. *Candida* infection may also affect the fingernails and toenails. Oral candidiasis, or thrush, is particularly common among people with HIV/AIDS who are not on antiretroviral drugs. It also occurs in babies, those on inhaled drugs for asthma, those having radiotherapy for head and neck cancer, and in leukemia and transplant patients. Esophageal candidiasis affects around 3 million, which is around 20 percent of patients with HIV/AIDS who are not on antiretroviral therapy. Vulvovaginal candidiasis is a common infection among women of childbearing age. Repeated attacks affect at least 80 million women each year and can have a significant impact on quality of life.

Because *Candida* normally live inside the gut, any breach in the body's normal defenses will allow these normally harmless organisms to turn opportunistic. Examples include HIV/AIDS, low white blood cell counts induced by cancer chemotherapy, and stem cell or solid organ transplantation. Other risk factors for systemic candidiasis include diabetes, use of antibiotics, extreme age, and the use of intravenous or urinary catheters.

There are around 400,000 invasive candidiasis (candidemia) infections worldwide each year. *Candida* species are the fourth-most-common cause of nosocomial (health-care acquired) infections in the United States, and such infections have a mortality rate of 30 to 61 percent. Nosocomial candidiasis also is associated with increased hospital stays and health-care costs. One reason for this high mortality rate is that *Candida* species are capable of forming a hard-to-remove biofilm on medical devices such as catheters. All patients with candidemia need intensive treatment with antifungal drugs if they are to survive, along with removal of all catheters.

Meanwhile, *Candida* peritonitis (inflammation of the peritoneum or tissue that lines the abdomen) may develop in patients who are on peritoneal dialysis, after gastrointestinal surgery or as a complication of candidemia. Research suggests that there are around 60,000 to 100,000 cases per year, with a mortality rate of 38 percent.

Aspergillosis

Aspergillosis is an opportunistic infection that is caused by the inhalation of the spores of the mold *Aspergillus*, which is ubiquitous in the environment. There are several *Aspergillus* species, among which *A. fumigatus* is the most common cause of invasive pulmonary disease. *Aspergillus* tends to infect open cavities in the body such as cavities in the lungs caused by previous lung disorders, such as tuberculosis (TB). The ear canals or the sinuses may also be affected. A movable fungus ball within a cavitary lesion is a common finding. Such infections tend to be locally invasive, but systemic spread may occur in persons with reduced immunity.

Around 10 percent of all new leukemia patients and 10 percent of those having a stem cell transplant will go on to develop invasive aspergillosis. In chronic obstructive pulmonary disease, around 1 to 2 percent will become infected. However, aspergillosis is unusual in those with HIV/AIDS. Invasive aspergillosis is very serious, with a mortality rate of around 50 percent, even with treatment. Acute invasive pulmonary aspergillosis causes cough, with blood, chest pain, and breathlessness. If untreated, it can progress to fatal respiratory failure.

Meanwhile, allergic bronchopulmonary aspergillosis (ABPA) tends to affect those with asthma or bronchiectasis. Around 5 million people, out of 193 million people worldwide with asthma, will develop ABPA. Around 15 people of people with cystic fibrosis develop ABPA.

Histoplasmosis

The mold *Histoplasma capsulatum* is found in soil, where its growth is supported by the nitrogen present in bird and bat droppings. It occurs all around the world. In the United States, *H. capsulatum* is endemic in the Ohio-Mississippi River valleys, parts of Florida, and along the St. Lawrence River and the Rio Grande. When soil is disturbed, the mold becomes airborne, and its spores can be inhaled and invade the tissue of the lung from where they can spread rapidly throughout the body. As it infects the lung, it changes into yeast form.

Most histoplasmosis infections are self-limiting and asymptomatic. However, in the immunosuppressed patient, or in the very old, dissemination of histoplasmosis becomes progressive. This form of the disease has a poor prognosis without treatment, with mortality rates of more than 90 percent. Fever and weight loss are the most common symptoms. Progressive disseminated histoplasmosis is one of the most common opportunistic infections in those with HIV/AIDS. Sometimes the HIV/AIDS patient's state may worsen without obvious explanation. There are also an increasing number of patients at risk of histoplasmosis following the use of newer immune-modulating agents, such as tumor necrosis factor, following organ transplantation and for other conditions.

Cryptococcal Meningitis

Cryptococcal meningitis is a deadly brain infection that is caused by the soil yeast *Cryptococcus neoformans*. It is the most common infection arising from this organism. The yeast is present all around the world and is found in soil that is contaminated with droppings, particularly those of pigeons. It is inhaled, and it disseminates rapidly, particularly to the brain and meninges. Most cases occur in people with compromised immunity, and the infection only came to the fore from the 1980s.

Originally, cryptococcal meningitis was found mainly in people with lymphoma or in those on steroid therapy. In the 2010s the disease was found mainly among those with advanced HIV/AIDS, particularly those with a low CD4 cell count, in whom it is a major cause of morbidity and mortality. At the peak of the HIV/AIDS epidemic in the United States during the mid-1990s, between 5 and 10 percent of those with the disease had cryptococcal meningitis.

With the advent of antiretroviral therapy, incidence has declined, but it is still important in resource-poor settings. According to the CDC, more than 1 million people with AIDS develop cryptococcal meningitis each year, resulting in around 625,000 deaths, of which around 70 percent are in sub-Saharan Africa. In some countries with a high prevalence of HIV/AIDS, cyptococcal meningitis may cause more deaths than TB. Patients with HIV/AIDS may also develop a disseminated form of crypococcal infection.

There is a simple blood test, based on the presence of a chemical marker for *Cryptococcus*, which can detect early cryptococcal infection in HIV-infected patients before it develops into meningitis. This is particularly useful for people with advanced HIV infection, for research has shown deaths from cryptococcal meningitis can be prevented if antifungal medication is taken to fight the early stage of the infection when the patient starts anti-HIV medication.

The diagnostic test is inexpensive and accurate for detecting both early and late stage cryptococcal infection more than 95 percent of the time. The CDC is working in several countries to stop deaths from cryptococcal meningitis by developing screening programs and building laboratory capacity to support this, as well as improving access to treatment.

Other Fungal Infections

Coccidiomycosis, or valley fever, is infection with the soil fungus *Coccidiomycosis immitis*, which produces symptoms similar to tuberculosis. The fungus occurs in desert soils, and infection tends to affect travelers, oil and construction workers, and the military. The fungus is endemic to southern and central California, southern Arizona, and New Mexico, as well as parts of Central and South America, including Honduras, Guatemala, Colombia, and Venezuela. There are around 25,000 cases in the United States each year, and many more in Central and South America.

Sporotrichosis is a chronic fungal infection caused by exposure to the mold *Sporothrix schenckii*, which affects the skin and lymph glands. The fungus is distributed widely on plant debris in soil and on the bark of trees, shrubs, and garden plants. It is particularly common in tropical and temperate zones. Activities most closely linked to sporotrichosis include gardening, farming, carpentry, and horticulture. Patients with HIV/AIDS are more susceptible to more severe forms of sporotrichosis.

The mold normally enters the body through small cuts and abrasions, rather than by inhalation. Skin nodules in sporotrichosis may spread through the lymphatic system and produce abscesses and ulcers. This is a chronic and mild form of the disease, although occasionally it may spread to joints and organs. There also is a pulmonary form of the disease, in which the mold is inhaled.

The fungus *Exserohilum rostratum* came to public attention during a multistate fungal meningitis outbreak investigation in 2012. During the outbreak, the CDC and U.S. Food and Drug Administration determined that medication vials of the steroid methylprednisolone acetate, which is used in epidural spinal injections given to patients for pain management, were contaminated at a compounding pharmacy with the mold *Exserohilum rostratum*. *Exserohilum* is commonly

ANTIFUNGAL DRUGS

There are many different antifungal drugs available. They range from creams and suppositories to treat vaginal candidiasis, to powders for athlete's foot, to injectable medications for systemic candidiasis and aspergillosis. There is an ongoing need for access to affordable antifungal drugs in many resource-poor parts of the world. At present, antifungal drugs are largely unavailable in sub-Saharan Africa and Asia. Furthermore, researchers need to continue to develop new antifungal drugs, as fungi continue to develop resistance to existing medications.

Nystatin

The first widely used antifungal drug was nystatin, originally known as fungicidin, which was discovered by Elizabeth Lee Hazen (1885–1975) and Rachel Fuller Brown (1898–1980) in 1950 at the New York State Department of Health. In fact, the name *nystatin* comes from the name of these labs. Nystatin works by binding to ergosterol, which is a component of the fungal cell membrane. This action kills the fungus by creating pores in the membrane. Ergosterol does not occur in either animal or plant cell membranes, so the action of nystatin on fungi is specific.

Nystatin is active against many molds and fungi, including *Candida* species. It continues to be widely used and is regarded as an essential drug in places with just basic health systems. Nystatin is available only in oral and topical forms, so other drugs are needed for systemic fungal infections.

Amphotericin B

Amphotericin B has long been the drug of choice for the treatment of serious systemic fungal infection. Its mode of action is similar to that of nystatin. However, although effective, amphotericin B also is relatively toxic and is being superseded as first-line therapy by drugs in the azole class.

Amphotericin B, although it does not have good penetration into the cerebrospinal fluid, still is effective for cryptococcal meningitis. The drug has to be given by infusion, and it produces various symptoms such as chills, nausea, and headache during, and for several hours after, the infusion. These can be alleviated by giving the amphotericin in a lipid formulation, which also makes the drug less toxic to the kidneys.

Other Antifungals

Azole antifungals block the synthesis of ergosterol, rather than binding to it. They are oral drugs, so do not have to be given by infusion. The first azole to be used in the treatment of fungal infection was ketoconazole. These have been supplanted by more effective and less toxic drugs, namely fluconazole (introduced in 1990), itraconazole, bifonazole, posaconazole, and voriconazole.

The echinocandins are water-soluble compounds that inhibit the enzyme glucan synthase, thereby destroying the fungal cell wall. These drugs must be administered by intravenous injection rather than orally. They are very effective against clinically important *Candida* species, but less so against *Aspergillus*.

Flucytosine is a nucleic acid analog, which works by interfering with the DNA and RNA synthesis of the fungus. Usually it is given alongside another antifungal drug and mainly is used to treat cryptococcosis, but also is useful for candidiasis and severe invasive aspergillosis.

Resistance to Antifungal Drugs

As with antibiotics and antiviral drugs, resistance to antifungal drugs is growing. This is occurring in a situation where both invasive fungal infections are becoming more common and more antifungal drugs are being introduced to combat them. This means that susceptibility testing in the lab of the fungal strains involved against antifungal agents has become an essential part of patient management.

Such testing detects the presence of antifungal drug resistance, showing which drugs will not work. It also has an important surveillance function, revealing the existence of resistance in a particular location and how it is spreading.

Resistance occurs when the fungus develops ways of interfering with the mechanism of action of the antifungal drug. A number of different mechanisms have been identified. For instance, *Candida* species can resist azoles via an efflux mechanism, which means they pump the drug molecules out of their cells.

What antifungal drug resistance means is that the minimum inhibitory concentration of the drug increases. In other words, more and more drug is needed to produce a therapeutic effect in the patient. This has been shown to be linked to a poorer clinical outcome.

found in warm, humid climates in the soil and on plants. It rarely causes infections in people, however, in this case, when injected directly into the spinal column, it was linked to fungal meningitis and persistent fungal infections in several hundred people and the deaths of dozens in more than 20 states, according to the CDC.

Finally, the burden of less serious fungal infections should not be forgotten. Skin and nail infections and athlete's foot affect around 25 percent of the world's population. Ringworm of the scalp affects around 200 million children worldwide.

⊕ Future Implications

Serious systemic fungal infections are on the increase around the world. At the same time, resistance to antifungal drugs also is rising. This means that the development of new antifungal drugs should be a priority. Equally important is to put in place, and support, the infrastructure needed to get these drugs to those who need them.

In the future, more rapid and accurate methods of diagnosing fungal infections likely will become more widely available. Antigen and DNA-based molecular

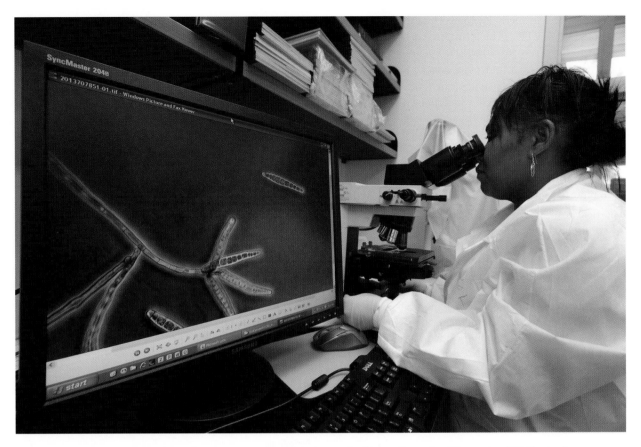

During the multistate outbreak of fungal meningitis in 2012, U.S. Centers for Disease Control and Prevention (CDC) scientist Carol Bolden examines microscopic slides on her computer screen that show *Exserohilum rostratum*. © *James Gathany/U.S. Centers for Disease Control and Prevention.*

tests will replace traditional methods that use fungal culture and radiography. The new methods already are being applied in the diagnosis of invasive aspergillosis, invasive candidiasis, and cryptococcal meningitis. This is likely to improve the outcome for the patient caught up in the growing public health issue of fungal infection, so long as these new tests are made available to all who need them.

PRIMARY SOURCE

Notes from the Field: Fatal Fungal Soft-Tissue Infections after a Tornado—Joplin, Missouri, 2011

SOURCE *"Notes from the Field: Fatal Fungal Soft-Tissue Infections after a Tornado—Joplin, Missouri, 2011," from* Morbidity and Mortality Weekly Report *60, no. 29 (July 29, 2011): 992. Centers for Disease Control and Prevention (CDC). http://www.cdc.gov/ mmwr/preview/mmwrhtml/mm6029a5.htm?s_ cid=mm6029a5_w (accessed January 25, 2015).*

INTRODUCTION *This primary source is a weekly bulletin issued by the U.S. Centers for Disease Control and Prevention. This edition reports on 18 suspected cases of fungal soft-tissue infection following a tornado in 2011.*

Notes from the Field: Fatal Fungal Soft-Tissue Infections after a Tornado—Joplin, Missouri, 2011

Weekly
July 29, 2011 / 60(29);992

On May 22, 2011, at 5:34 p.m. a tornado with winds >200 mph struck Joplin, Missouri, injuring approximately 1,000 persons and causing 159 deaths. On June 3, a local physician notified the Springfield-Greene County Health Department and the Missouri Department of Health and Senior Services (MODHSS) of two patients hospitalized with tornado injuries who had suspected necrotizing fungal soft-tissue infections. MODHSS initiated active surveillance for such infections at hospitals and laboratories serving patients injured in the tornado, and CDC began assisting MODHSS with identification of fungal isolates. By June 10, eight patients with necrotizing fungal soft-tissue wound infections caused by

Mucormycetes (formerly Zygomycetes) were identified. On June 14, a CDC field team arrived in Missouri to assist with the onsite investigation.

As of July 19, a total of 18 suspected cases of cutaneous mucormycosis had been identified, of which 13 were confirmed. A confirmed case was defined as 1) necrotizing soft-tissue infection requiring antifungal treatment or surgical debridement in a person injured in the tornado, 2) with illness onset on or after May 22, and 3) positive fungal culture or histopathology and genetic sequencing consistent with a Mucormycete. No additional cases have been reported since June 17.

The field team reviewed medical charts to describe the 13 confirmed cases. The median age of the patients was 48 years (range: 13–76 years); seven were female, and all were white. Injuries sustained during the tornado included lacerations (12 patients), fractures (11), and blunt trauma (nine). The 13 patients had an average of four wounds documented in the medical chart when they were examined at the emergency department. Post-trauma wound management included surgical debridement for all 13 patients and removal of a foreign body from six. Wooden splinters were the most common foreign body, found in the wounds of four patients. Two patients had diabetes, and none were immunocompromised. Ten patients required admission to an intensive-care unit, and five died.

CDC received 48 clinical specimens, including 32 fungal isolates and 16 tissue blocks collected from wounds for microscopic evaluation, immunohistochemical staining, and DNA sequencing; specimens from all 13 patients yielded the Mucormycete *Apophysomyces trapeziformis*. Further laboratory and epidemiologic studies are ongoing, including case-control studies to evaluate risk factors for infection.

Cutaneous mucormycosis is a rare infection caused by fungi of the order Mucorales, which typically are found in soil and decaying wood and other organic matter. Although cutaneous mucormycosis often is opportunistic, affecting patients with diabetes, hematologic malignancy or solid organ transplant, *A. trapeziformis* often is associated with immunocompetent hosts after traumatic implantation of fungal spores. The case-fatality rate for cutaneous mucormycosis has ranged from 29% to 83%, depending on severity of disease and underlying medical condition of the patient. Early diagnosis, aggressive surgical debridement, and administration of systemic antifungals have been associated with improved outcomes.

Cutaneous mucormycosis has been reported after previous natural disasters; however, this is the first known cluster occurring after a tornado. None of the infections were found in persons cleaning up debris. Healthcare providers should consider environmental fungi as potential causes of necrotizing soft-tissue infections in patients injured during tornados and initiate early treatment for suspected infections. Additional information is available at http://www.cdc.gov/mucormycosis.

SEE ALSO *Antibiotic/Antimicrobial Resistance; HIV/AIDS*

BIBLIOGRAPHY

Books

Crook, William. *The Yeast Connection.* New York: Vintage Books, 1986.

Daniel, Thomas M., and Gerald L. Baum. *Drama and Discovery: The Story of Histoplasmosis.* Westport, CT: Greenwood Press, 2002.

Homei, Aya, and Michael Worboys. *Fungal Disease in Britain and the United States 1850–2000: Mycoses and Modernity.* New York: Palgrave Macmillan, 2013.

Olsen, LeighAnne, Eileen Choffness, David Relman, and Leslie Pray. *Fungal Diseases: An Emerging Threat to Human, Animal, and Plant Health.* Washington, DC: National Academies Press, 2011.

Richardson, Malcolm D., and David W. Warnock. *Fungal Infection: Diagnosis and Management,* 4th ed. New York: Wiley-Blackwell, 2012.

Periodicals

Kousha, M., R. Tadi, and Ayman O. Soubani. "Pulmonary Aspergillosis: A Clinical Review." *European Respiratory Review* 20, no. 121 (September 2011): 156–174.

Nucci, Marcio and Kieren Marr. "Emerging Fungal Diseases." *Clinical Infectious Diseases* 41, no. 4 (August 2005): 521–526.

Websites

"Aspergillosis." *Merck Manual.* http://www.merckmanuals.com/professional/infectious_diseases/fungi/aspergillosis.html (accessed January 26, 2015).

"Fungal Diseases." *U.S. Centers for Disease Control and Prevention (CDC).* http://www.cdc.gov/fungal (accessed January 26, 2015).

Fungal Infection Trust. http://www.fungalinfectiontrust.org (accessed January 26, 2015).

"Fungal Infections." *Medline Plus.* http://www.nlm.nih.gov/medlineplus/fungalinfections.html (accessed January 26, 2015).

"Global Fungal Diseases." *U.S. Centers for Disease Control and Prevention (CDC).* http://www.cdc.gov/fungal/global/index.html (accessed January 26, 2015).

Susan Aldridge

Gender and Health

Introduction

There are many notable differences in the health outcomes and health behaviors of men and women. Many of these cannot be explained by biology alone but rather by a combination of the influence of economic, social, cultural, religious, and political factors. There is a significant health disparity between men and women across the world. Much of this is a result of gender discrimination against women; however, gender norms and values are shown to have negative effects for both men and women. Social norms may cause men to be less likely to seek medical attention, for both physical and mental health conditions.

From an early age, gender affects a child's health. The practice of son preference may begin at or even before birth in cases of female infanticide—the deliberate killing of female infants, or the selective abortion of female fetuses. Another example of son preference is related to nutrition and food allocation. Although children of both sexes require the same nutrients, in some cultures in developing countries young boys are given priority and greater access to food because they are seen as being eventual breadwinners.

Despite socioeconomic advantages, men generally have shorter life spans than women. On average, women live six to eight years longer, due to both biological factors and certain social advantages, such as lower occupational hazards and the greater tendency toward high-risk behaviors in men. However, in some regions of the world, such as in parts of Asia, gender discrimination against women overrides these advantages, resulting in a lower life expectancy for females than for than men.

Women may live longer than men on average, but women have more nonfatal illnesses throughout life, even when excluding reproductive conditions. Examples of such chronic non-life-threatening conditions include eczema, colitis, headaches, and arthritis. Although the chronic conditions that women suffer may appear minor by comparison, they play a large role in lowering women's quality of life. Men, by contrast, suffer more life-threatening chronic conditions that tend to have onset later in life, such as heart disease, kidney disease, cancer, and stroke.

Some differences in the health of men and women can be linked to the sex chromosomes. Women are born with two X chromosomes, whereas men are born with only one X, and one Y. Having only one X chromosome makes men more vulnerable to some genetic mutations of X-linked genes that cause conditions such as Hunter syndrome and hemophilia. Women may have the same mutations in one X chromosome, but because they have another "backup" copy, this usually will not result in women developing the same condition.

Historical Background

Types of gender disparities vary across cultures, but one of the most important differences in health care is in the field of reproductive health. Reproductive health has been and continues to be an important and contentious aspect of women's health. Religious and cultural norms prevent women from seeking reproductive health care, especially in developing countries where the rates of maternal mortality are highest. Access to family planning reduces the number of abortions, including unsafe illegal abortions, which are estimated by the World Health Organization (WHO) to cause 47,000 maternal deaths annually. Abortion was illegal in the United States until the U.S. Supreme Court ruling on *Roe v. Wade* in 1973, and it remains illegal or severely restricted in many countries, especially in the developing world, putting women at risk for complications or death resulting from unsafe procedures. It is estimated by the WHO that 222 million women in developing countries would like to be on some form of birth control but lack the proper access.

Inequity in biomedical and behavioral research has been a problem traditionally, as a result of the disproportionate number of male human and animal subjects used in drug trials and studies on health problems such as heart disease. This has slowed progress in the area of women's health. Recent changes to protocols put in place by the U.S. National Institutes of Health (NIH) and recommendations by the Institute of Medicine (IOM) have put a focus on correcting this inequity and focusing on women in research and clinical trials and reporting of data by sex.

A lack of education regarding women's health in medical schools has also been a problem historically. This is the result of gender bias and of curriculum design being almost exclusively in the hands of men. In recent decades, surveys of medical school curricula have shown an improvement in this area. There has also been an increase in the number of women working as health-care providers. Incorporating sex- and gender-based science in the education of health-care professionals is essential to ensure they will provide proper care to female patients.

⊕ Impacts and Issues

Men's Health

Several factors have been attributed to men's higher mortality rates. Men are more likely to engage in risk-taking behaviors such as drug and alcohol abuse, reckless driving, and using weapons. For example, in 2010, 3.14 million men died from causes related to alcohol abuse, whereas the number for women was 1.72 million. High-risk behaviors such as heavy drinking are associated with notions of masculinity in many cultures and also are related to increased risk of injury and death.

Due to the inequality of women and men in the workforce across all cultures, men are exposed disproportionately to occupational hazards such as accidents and chemical exposure in the workplace. For example, in the United States, occupations such as mining, agriculture, and commercial fishing are mostly the occupations of men and are associated with the highest rates of workplace injury and mortality.

Another factor in men's poorer health is the prevalence of social norms that lead men to be less likely to seek medical attention, and less likely to report symptoms if they do see a physician. Stereotypical notions about masculinity may lead men to feel it is a sign of weakness to seek medical attention or report symptoms of disease or illness. This is due in part to cultural beliefs that men are less vulnerable and stronger than women. Studies have shown that the more an individual subscribes to hegemonic ideals of masculinity, the less likely it is that the person will seek preventive health care such as prostate screenings, even when controlling for other socioeconomic and demographic factors.

Women's Health

During their reproductive years, women deal with challenges, disorders, or illnesses related to menstruation, such as premenstrual syndrome and premenstrual dysphoric disorder. Some health concerns occur during and as a result of menopause, such as symptoms including hot flashes, vaginal dryness, and mood changes. Women suffer more from osteoporosis than men—a result of lowered bone density after menopause due to the fact that bone density relies on estrogen production.

Some of the health challenges related to gender are shared across cultures, but many are varied depending on conditions and atmosphere of a region. There are striking differences in women's health in low-income countries compared to high-income countries. For example, 99 percent of maternal deaths annually occur in developing countries, and women in poorer countries tend to have shorter life spans than those in wealthier countries, with a majority of female deaths occurring in children, adolescent girls, and young women. Regardless of whether a country is low income or high income, socioeconomic factors affect the levels of mortality and illness. Even in developed countries, women in poorer households have higher mortality rates.

Education is one of the strongest predictors of physical health, and in many parts of the world women are denied equal access to education. Women's literacy rates are lower than men's in much of the world, and the lack of education both in schools and via participation in public life in turn hinders their ability to make informed health decisions and discuss concerns with health-care workers.

Women generally have a lower economic status than men, in part because they are paid less for doing the same jobs regardless of whether they live in a developing or an industrialized nation. This means they have fewer resources and less of an economic safety net if they become ill.

In developing countries, women are more likely than men to go to traditional healers, to self-treat, or to use alternative medicines. The reasons for this may be varied. It may be due to cost or women's inability to access clinics during business hours because of the multiple demands on them. It may also be because traditional healers provide easier and less intimidating explanations, and women may have negative experiences with non-traditional health-care workers treating them with condescension or as inferior due to their lack of education.

Religious and cultural norms in some conservative cultures have consequences for women in relation to health. For instance, in some cases women are banned from receiving medical care from a male doctor, and their movements may be restricted such that they cannot seek medical care or go to a clinic without the accompaniment and approval of a male family member. Due to these restrictions, and in some instances the indifference of male family members, women are deprived of necessary care, leading to further health problems and even premature death.

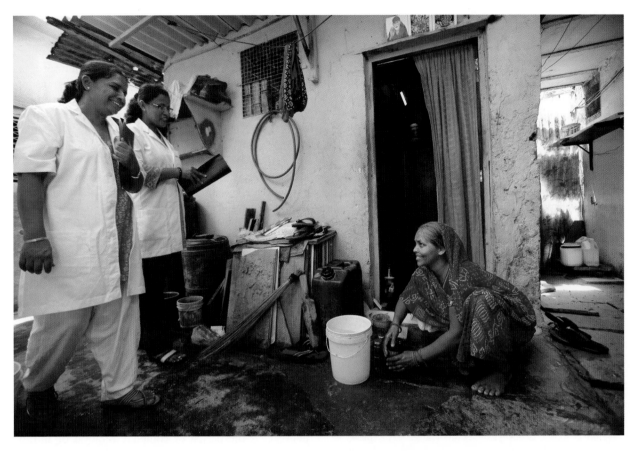

Health workers from Tata Memorial Hospital visit Usha Devi, right, who was suffering from cervical cancer, at her home in a slum in Mumbai, India. A simple vinegar test slashed cervical cancer death rates by one-third in a remarkable study of 150,000 women in the slums of India, where the disease is the top cancer killer of women. Experts called the outcome "amazing" and said this quick, cheap test could save tens of thousands of lives each year in developing countries by spotting early signs of cancer, allowing treatment before it is too late. Devi, one of the women in the study, says it saved her life. *© Rafiq Maqbool/AP Images.*

Women's Reproductive and Sexual Health

Complications due to pregnancy and childbirth (also known as maternal mortality) are the leading cause of death in women ages 15 to 19 in developing countries. Often this is the result of a woman's lack of access to family planning, or control of reproductive decisions with a male partner. According to the 2012 United Nations Summit on Family Planning, more than 220 million girls and women who would like to access contraceptives and family planning services are denied this access. There are an estimated 60 million unplanned pregnancies annually, which increases the risk of death during pregnancy or childbirth, and also increases the instances of illegal and unsafe abortions, which also can lead to injury and cause nearly 70,000 deaths each year. Although maternal mortality is rare when pregnant women have access to appropriate obstetric health care, in many developing countries with higher fertility rates, women face considerably higher risks of death during pregnancy and labor. For example, maternal mortality in Africa may be as high as 1 in 26, compared to 1 in 7,300 in high-income countries with better access to proper medical care.

Statistics surrounding the incidence of sexual violence against women vary widely across cultures. It is estimated that one in five women (18.3 percent) in the United States has been or will be a victim of sexual assault in her lifetime. According to studies conducted by the WHO, 35 percent of women worldwide reported they had experienced physical or sexual violence at the hands of a partner or sexual violence by someone else. Approximately 30 percent reported physical or sexual violence by a partner. Studies were conducted in 10 countries and reported in "WHO Multi-Country Study on Women's Health and Domestic Violence against Women," showing rates of sexual and physical violence by a partner against women aged 15–49 ranged from 15 percent of women in Japan to 71 percent of women in Ethiopia. Between 0.3 percent and 11 percent of all women reported sexual assault committed by someone other than a partner after age 15. Many women report that their first sexual experience was forced—17 percent in Tanzania, 24 percent in Peru, and 30 percent in Bangladesh. The WHO studies have concluded that as many as 38 percent of

INTERSEX HEALTH

The term intersex describes a variety of conditions in which an individual is born with sexual or reproductive organs or chromosome patterns that do not fit into the typical definition of either male or female.

According to the Intersex Society of North America (ISNA), estimates show that approximately 1 in 1,500 or 1 in 2,000 babies are born with observably atypical genitalia; however, this does not account for the many other individuals with internal intersex traits that they may not discover until later in life, or may never discover. Causes include chromosomal abnormalities in which, rather than the typical XX chromosomes for females and XY for males, an individual may have some cells with XX chromosomes and some with XY—this is known as cellular mosaicism. Other causes include but are not limited to: congenital adrenal hyperplasia, ovo-testes, aphallia, and androgen insensitivity syndrome. Some intersex infants may have ambiguous genitalia, whereas others may have male sex organs externally and female sex organs internally, or vice versa, along with many other variations.

Many health professionals have come to believe that there is valid evidence of sexual variation in human beings, and that the belief in strict sexual dimorphism is incorrect— therefore an individual being intersex is not necessarily a cause for medical intervention. There is also evidence that intersex conditions do not pose serious medical problems or threats to an individual's health (with the exception of congenital adrenal hyperplasia, which may cause salt imbalance and insufficient cortisone production).

However, since the 1950s the practice of surgical sex assignment has been standard in cases of intersex infants. The consequences of these infant surgeries are a major concern relating to intersex health. Critics of the practice say that it lacks scientific basis and long-term follow-up, and studies show that it does not lead to improved psychosocial outcomes in the patients, nor does it predict that the individual will identify with the gender assigned by the surgery. Many intersex individuals oppose the practice, believing individuals should have agency in deciding whether or not to undertake surgical genital intervention later in life.

Many individuals who had sex assignment surgery in infancy report significant trauma later in life as a result, including impaired sexual function, reproductive health issues including sterility, feelings of violation by health-care professionals, and feelings of dysphoria with regard to their bodies. An advocacy group for intersex individuals and their families, ISNA, was formed in 1993 and has the stated mission "to end shame, secrecy, and unwanted genital surgeries for people born with an anatomy that someone decided is not standard for male or female."

female murders are committed by a partner. Risks for physical and sexual violence increase in war zones and refugee camps.

Violence and sexual assault affect women disproportionately and make them vulnerable to sexually transmitted infections as well as mental health consequences such as post-traumatic stress disorder (PTSD) and depression. Due to economic hardship or domestic difficulties, women may engage in survival sex or may be forced into sex trafficking, which puts them at a higher risk of sexual assault. Many women are unable to leave their abusive partners for economic reasons, unable to work due to injuries as a result of abuse, or are unable to report abuse or harassment by an employer for fear of termination or retaliation. Although children of both genders are victims of physical abuse, evidence shows that girls are far more likely to suffer sexual abuse. In addition to immediate physical consequences of injury, disability, and death, the abuse has long-term consequences including PTSD, depression, and suicide. Survivors of rape are stigmatized and may be forced into marriages to preserve family honor in some cultures. The stigmatization of victims of sexual and physical abuse occurs across cultures and leads to victims remaining silent and not seeking out the necessary medical and psychiatric care.

The practice of female genital mutilation or cutting (FGM/C) poses serious health risks to women and girls. FGM/C is the partial or complete removal of and/or other harmful procedures to external female genitalia for nonmedical reasons. FGM generally is performed on girls between infancy and age 15, and can result in shock, severe bleeding, urinary problems, infection, cysts, infertility, and complications during childbirth. The practice of FGM takes place in nearly 60 countries, concentrated in Africa and the Middle East. It is considered a human rights abuse against women and girls by the United Nations.

Transgender Health

The term transgender includes a spectrum of gender identities in which an individual identifies as a gender other than the one correlating with the sex they were assigned at birth. Some but not all transgender people undergo hormone therapy and/or sex reassignment surgery and other surgical procedures. The percentage of transgender people in the United States is estimated to be around one percent, comparable to the number of blind people or individuals with epilepsy in the country. Repeated surveys have shown that many transgender patients have been refused care due to their transgender status. Specific needs of transgender patients include mental health care (due to increased rates of depression, anxiety, and substance abuse) as well as health care related to transitioning, such as hormone therapy and sex reassignment surgery. Transgender individuals also have specific needs in terms of reproductive health. For example, many transgender men still require pelvic exams, and transgender women may require prostate exams. Even after mastectomy, transgender men may develop breast cancer. Campaigns aiming to improve the health-care experience and create a more welcoming environment for transgender patients have emphasized implementing certain changes such as including space on intake forms for a patient's preferred name and gender pronouns.

Mental Health and Gender

Rates of depression and anxiety are higher in women, and women are more likely to seek help when dealing with these issues. However, there is evidence to suggest that men may experience depression at an equal rate to women, but because of social norms surrounding masculinity are less likely to seek professional help and more likely to remain silent about their depression, even among friends. Men and women also express feelings of depression differently. For example, crying or experiencing changes in appetite may be more common among women, whereas depression in men may manifest in the

form of drug or alcohol abuse. Alcohol abuse is linked to suicide, putting men at an increased risk for this as well. The American Foundation for Suicide Prevention states that the rate of suicide is four times higher for men, even though the number of suicide attempts by women is higher. One explanation for this is the difference in suicide methods commonly used by men and women. Men tend to use methods that are more likely to be fatal, with firearms being the most common method. Women are more likely to attempt suicide by poisoning or drowning, which increases the chances that they may be resuscitated. Nonetheless, suicide is the seventh-leading cause of death worldwide for women ages 20–59 and is even more prevalent in Western countries. Risk factors such as a history of sexual assault and domestic violence increase a woman's chances of suicide.

In industrialized countries, gender and nutrition also are linked, often in relation to the prevalence of eating disorders, which are more common in women than in men. Eating disorders, including anorexia nervosa, bulimia, and binge eating, are thought to be caused in

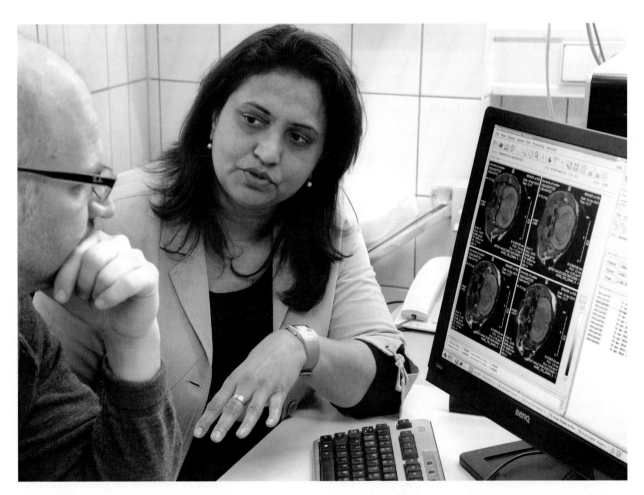

Dr. Alia Matysik discusses pictures of mouse brains on the screen with Daniel Huster, the director of the Institute for Medical Physics and Biophysics of the University in Leipzig in Germany. Matysik searches for an explanation why more women than men are affected by Alzheimer's disease. © *Waltraud Grubitzsch/picture-alliance/dpa/AP Images.*

part by biological factors such as serotonin levels in the brain, as well as cultural factors such as the perpetuation of an idealized female body image in Western media. Eating disorders do occur in men, more commonly among athletes and gay men.

Disparities in Health Research

In recent years it has come to the attention of researchers that biomedical studies and clinical trials have historically been gender biased, resulting in significant gaps in knowledge regarding women's specific health concerns. This has been the result of the overwhelming majority of male lab personnel, scientists, and both human and animal subjects. Women have not been equally represented in many clinical drug trials, with researchers traditionally using male lab animals in order to reduce variability. This has resulted in a lack of accurate data on the effects these drugs have on women. However, there is now a growing realization that women and men do not always have the same results in health testing. Recent efforts by the NIH have emerged with the aim of funding more clinical trials studying women participants and encouraging the study of sex as a biological variable in medical research. The IOM has recommended disclosure of the sex of the source of cell and tissue cultures used in research, and medical journals also recommend that reports include a breakdown of data by sex.

HIV/AIDS and Sexually Transmitted Infections (STIs)

Human immunodeficiency virus (HIV) and acquired immune deficiency syndrome (AIDS) affect both men and women, however, they present different challenges for each. The stigmatization of homosexuality makes men who have sex with men, who are at an increased risk for HIV infection, less likely to voice concerns or seek medical care, thus making their partners (both male and female) more vulnerable to transmission. According to the WHO, HIV is the leading cause of death among women of reproductive age worldwide (and the sixth-leading cause of death for females of all ages). Fear of violence at the hands of a partner may prevent women from seeking medical attention or demanding a partner use protection. Notions of masculinity may inhibit men from getting tested, coming to terms with an HIV-positive status, and taking the necessary steps to manage their disease.

Other sexually transmitted infections (STIs) have different challenges for men and women as well. Women often have more severe STIs due to the fact that some infections are more likely to be asymptomatic in women than in men. For example, chlamydia is the most common STI in women and is asymptomatic in the majority of cases. U.S. statistics for 2012 show 643.3 cases of chlamydia per 100,000 women, nearly double the figure reported for men. One of the STIs causing the greatest concern for women is human papillomavirus (HPV) because of its

relationship to cervical and other gynecological cancers. HPV infection causes nearly all cases of cervical cancer, however, there are many strains of HPV that do not cause cancer. HPV also can lead to cancers in men, with oropharyngeal (throat) cancers being the most common. For this reason, the U.S. Centers for Diseases Control and Prevention (CDC) recommends that young women between the ages of 11 and 26, young men between the ages of 11 and 21, and all men who have sex with men get vaccinated for HPV. Among men, those who have sex with men are at increased risk for STIs. In cases of syphilis infection, men who had sex with men constituted 75 percent of reported cases in 2012, according to the CDC. Many women are denied education about reproductive health and safer sex, and due to inequality are not in positions to demand or negotiate safer sex practices with a male partner.

⊕ Future Implications

Public outreach programs aimed at men's health are being established with increasing frequency. Many of these programs focus on encouraging healthy lifestyle changes such as smoking cessation and weight loss. Men who are racial minorities, men who have sex with men, and men in prison have higher rates of disease and lower life expectancy, and some campaigns have targeted these populations. There also has been an emergence of campaigns encouraging men to pursue routine preventive health-care services. Real Men Wear Gowns is a campaign started in 2008 by the Agency for Healthcare Research and Quality (part of the U.S. Department of Health and Human Services) and the Ad Council, which consists of print, radio, and television ads urging men to educate themselves about preventive health care, and get the routine tests required of them. Another public health campaign that has grown globally since it started in Australia and New Zealand in 2004 is known as "Movember." The campaign encourages men to grow mustaches during the month of November to raise awareness for issues related to men's health such as prostate cancer and to encourage men to get regular screenings and foster a dialogue surrounding men's health issues.

Additionally, global initiatives and social campaigns with the aim of changing and challenging gender norms are emerging as a response to the problem of gender disparity and its effects on women's health. Large organizations such as the WHO, the United Nations (UN), and the NIH have implemented women's health initiatives in recent years.

In 2010 the UN General Assembly created UN Women, an entity designed to accelerate the UN's goals regarding gender equality and the empowerment of women. Many of the UN Women's campaigns and initiatives are aimed at addressing issues related to women's health. Acknowledging the fact that education is one of the most important predictors of health, UN Women facilitates conferences and outreach programs to promote education and access to technology for women in developing countries. The UN observes the International Day for the Elimination of Violence against Women on November 25 each year, encouraging individuals to organize activist events around the world and interact via social media to raise awareness about the issue of violence against women. The NIH Office of Research on Women's Health monitors and reports on the efforts of the NIH to facilitate inclusion of women and women's health concerns in biomedical research in the United States.

The WHO's Gender and Women's Health Program outlines its mission as follows: "to increase health professionals' awareness of the role of gender norms, values, and inequality in perpetuating disease, disability, and death, and to promote societal change with a view to eliminating gender as a barrier to good health." In 2012 the program announced a new approach to address issues related to gender and health which they refer to as Gender Mainstreaming. The Gender Mainstreaming program aims to ensure that gender is a consideration from the start in health research, health reforms, education, outreach, and health policies, as opposed to being an afterthought or addition. The goal of Gender Mainstreaming is to educate health professionals so that they have a knowledge and awareness of the effects of gender on health and to ensure that this is a core part of their practice.

SEE ALSO *Body Image and Eating Disorders; Child Health; Family Planning; Genital Modification; Health as a Human Right and Health-Care Access; Life Expectancy and Aging Populations; Maternal and Infant Health; Social Theory and Global Health; Stigma; Vulnerable Populations; World Health Organization: Organization, Funding, and Enforcement Powers*

BIBLIOGRAPHY

Books

Bird, Chloe E., and Patricia Perri Rieker. *Gender and Health: The Effects of Constrained Choices and Social Policies.* Cambridge, UK: Cambridge University Press, 2008.

Hunt, Kate, and Ellen Annandale, eds. *Gender and Health: Major Themes in Health and Social Welfare.* Abingdon, UK: Routledge, 2012.

Pal, Manoranjan, et al., eds. *Gender and Discrimination: Health, Nutritional Status, and Role of Women in India.* New Delhi: Oxford University Press, 2009.

Pérez, Miguel A., and Raffy R. Luquis, eds. *Cultural Competence in Health Education and Health Promotion*, 2nd ed. San Francisco, CA: Jossey-Bass, 2014.

Sen, Gita, and Piroska Östlin, eds. *Gender Equity in Health: The Shifting Frontiers of Evidence and Action.* New York: Routledge, 2010.

World Health Organization. *Women and Health: Today's Evidence, Tomorrow's Agenda.* Geneva: World Health Organization, 2009. Available online at http://whqlibdoc.who.int/publications/2009/9789241563857_eng.pdf (accessed January 8, 2015).

World Health Organization. *WHO Multi-Country Study on Women's Health and Domestic Violence against Women.* Geneva: World Health Organization, 2005. Available online at http://www.who.int/reproductivehealth/publications/violence/24159358X/en/ (accessed May 28, 2015).

World Health Organization and United Nations Population Fund. *Women, Ageing, and Health: A Framework for Action: Focus on Gender.* Geneva: World Health Organization, 2007. Available online at http://www.who.int/gender/documents/ageing/9789241563529/en/ (accessed January 8, 2015).

Periodicals

Baker, Peter A., et al. "The Men's Health Gap: Men Must Be Included in the Global Health Agenda." *Bulletin of the World Health Organization* 92, no. 8 (August 1, 2014): 618–620.

Callanan, Valerie J., and Mark S. Davis. "Gender Differences in Suicide Methods." *Social Psychiatry & Psychiatric Epidemiology* 47, no. 6 (June 2012): 857–869.

Chase, Cheryl. "Rethinking Treatment for Ambiguous Genitalia." *Pediatric Nursing* 25, no. 4 (July/August 1999): 451–455.

Currin, James B., Bert Hayslip, and Jeff R. Temple. "The Relationship between Age, Gender, Historical Change, and Adults' Perceptions of Mental Health and Mental Health Services." *International Journal of Aging and Human Development* 72, no. 4 (2011): 317–341.

Huang, Audrey. "X Chromosomes Key to Sex Differences in Health." *JAMA and Archives Journals* 295 (March 22/29, 2006): 1428–1433.

Johnson, Katherine, and Browne, Kath. "Trans and Intersex Issues in Health and Care." *Diversity and Equality in Health and Care* 9, no. 4 (2012): 235–237.

Kim, Glen, Rabih Torbay, and Lynn Lawry. "Basic Health, Women's Health, and Mental Health among Internally Displaced Persons in Nyala Province, South Darfur, Sudan." *American Journal of Public Health* 97, no. 2 (February 2007): 353–361.

Powell, J. R., and Walter J. Tabachnick. "Gender Differences in Determinants and Consequences of Health and Illness." *Journal of Health, Population and Nutrition* 25, no. 1 (March 2007): 47–61.

Redfern, Jan S., and Bill Sinclair. "Improving Health Care Encounters and Communication with Transgender Patients." *Journal of Communication in Healthcare* 7, no. 1 (2014): 25–40.

Ross, Catherine E., Ryan K. Masters, and Robert A. Hummer. "Education and the Gender Gaps in Health and Mortality." *Demography* 49, no. 4 (November 2012): 1157–1183.

Springer, Kristen W., and Dawne M. Mouzon. "'Macho Men' and Preventive Health Care: Implications for Older Men in Different Social Classes." *Journal of Health and Social Behavior* 52, no. 2 (June 13, 2001): 212–227.

Websites

"About Movember: Vision, Values and Results We Seek to Achieve." *Movember.* http://us.movember.com/about/vision-goals (accessed January 8, 2015).

Clancy, Carolyn M. "Real Men Wear Gowns—and Help Their Health." *Agency for Healthcare Research and Quality,* May 6, 2008. http://www.ahrq.gov/news/columns/navigating-the-health-care-system/050608.html (accessed January 8, 2015).

"Female Genital Mutilation," Fact Sheet No. 241. *World Health Organization (WHO),* Updated February 2014. http://www.who.int/mediacentre/factsheets/fs241/en/ (accessed January 8, 2015).

"Gender and Genetics." *World Health Organization Genomic Resource Centre.* http://www.who.int/genomics/gender/en/index1.html (accessed January 8, 2015).

"How Common Is Intersex?" *Intersex Society of North America.* http://www.isna.org/faq/frequency (accessed January 8, 2015).

"LGBT Health and Well-being." *U.S. Department of Health and Human Services.* http://www.hhs.gov/lgbt/ (accessed January 8, 2015).

"Men's Health: Sexually Transmitted Diseases." *U.S. Centers for Disease Control and Prevention (CDC).* http://www.cdc.gov/men/az/std.htm (accessed January 8, 2015).

"New Study Shows HPV Vaccine Helping Lower HPV Infection Rates in Teen Girls." *U.S. Centers for Disease Control and Prevention (CDC), 2013.* http://www.cdc.gov/media/releases/2013/p0619-hpv-vaccinations.html (accessed January 8, 2015).

"Violence against Women," Fact Sheet No. 239. *World Health Organization (WHO),* Updated November 2014. http://www.who.int/mediacentre/factsheets/fs239/en/ (accessed May 28, 2015)

Hailey Wojcik

Genetic Testing and Privacy Issues

🌐 Introduction

Genetic testing refers to a form of medical screening that geneticists can use to uncover information found in human chromosomes, proteins, and genes. This information can help confirm a diagnosis, locate and inform carriers for potentially harmful copies of genes, and identify genetic markers for certain disorders and diseases. Genetic tests also may be used to detect prescription drug reactions, determine an individual's ancestry or heritage, and even establish forensic evidence in legal cases. A variety of government agencies and humans rights organizations have raised concerns about private sector biotech companies providing citizens with advanced diagnostic tools in regard to ensuring the protection of individuals against discrimination and violations of confidentiality.

Genetic screenings offer individuals unique predictive opportunities to identify their risk of a variety of inherited diseases. Screening exists for a number of diseases, including cystic fibrosis, Alzheimer's disease, and Huntington's disease. However, genetic predisposition to a certain malady or ailment does not necessitate genetic destiny. Most diseases are the result of a complicated interaction between an individual's underlying genetic makeup and environmental factors. For example, a genetic test might reveal a person has an increased risk for heart disease or obesity. This information may prompt lifestyle changes (e.g., eating a more healthful diet and getting regular exercise) to reduce the risk of developing complications later in life.

Although individual health information typically is considered to be sensitive and private, genetic tests are regarded as deserving additional safeguards due to their unique predictive capacity. The scientific and medical community is still in the process of uncovering the full prognostic value of genetic tests, and many questions remain about the benefit of genetic screening. For-profit companies also have started producing direct-to-consumer genetic tests, thus raising concerns that these results and genetic information could be obfuscated or misunderstood. As these innovative technologies continue advancing, there is an equally pressing need to provide the appropriate level of safekeeping for genetic information.

🌐 Historical Background

James Watson (1928–) and Francis Crick (1916–2004) first published their research on the double helix structure of DNA in 1953. Since this discovery, numerous diagnostic tests have built upon the unique structure and characteristics of genetic material to predict the onset of illness, develop better drugs, and create individualized treatments. Human DNA molecules consist of chains of nucleic acids that carry the cellular blueprints and serve as a mechanism of biological inheritance—the passing of genetic information between generations. The basic building blocks of DNA are four nucleotides: adenine, guanine, cytosine, and thymine. These molecules often are represented as the single letter base pairs A, C, G, and T.

The arrangement of nucleotides within the strands of DNA resembles a twisted ladder. The sides of the ladder are made of the sugar deoxyribose (the "D" in DNA). The rungs on the ladder are held together by hydrogen bonds between base pairs (adenine with thymine, and cytosine with guanine). These alternating base pairs (AT, TA, CG, and GC) make up the genetic code that contains all of the information necessary to reproduce every cell in an organism. The double helix structure is essential to how DNA transfers genetic information.

Inside the cell nucleus, enzymes separate the DNA base pairs, exposing them to free floating nucleotides. As the nucleotides attach, they form a new molecule referred to as messenger RNA (mRNA). Continuing with the ladder analogy, the mRNA now resembles a ladder with rungs that have been cut in half down the center. The new mRNA molecule duplicates the original base pair sequence with one caveat: The nucleotide uracil replaces the thymine (T becomes U). These mRNA molecules copy small sections of the original DNA sequence and pass out of the nucleus into the main body of the cell. In the cell, the mRNA connects to a second kind of RNA called transfer RNA (tRNA). The specific base pair sequence in the tRNA attaches to a unique corresponding section of mRNA. When these bases connect, the amino acids located at the opposite end of the tRNA align to form a specific protein. Through this mechanism, RNA molecules serve as intermediaries during the conversion of DNA sequences into proteins via the genetic code. Bit-by-bit, the rungs of the ladder are reconstructed. This process ensures the precise duplication of genetic code is transferred from generation to generation.

Chromosomes are structures made up of long DNA strands and proteins that carry an organism's hereditary information. Humans inherit 23 pairs of chromosomes from their parents—one pair of sex chromosomes (X and Y) and 22 autosomal, non-sex chromosomes. The term gene typically applies to a distinct segment of DNA that carries information for a particular amino acid sequence, and each gene section codes for a particular protein. Each parent passes one copy of his or her genes to his or her offspring. These slightly differing copies of similar genes are referred to as alleles. The pairs of inherited alleles located on the chromosomes combine to create a person's genotype. Although a significant portion of human genetic information is shared across populations, there are many variations in individual physical appearances and characteristics. The observable manifestation of these different traits represents a person's phenotype.

Alterations to the amino acid sequences in DNA are termed mutations. Genetic mutations can result in changes to the structure and function of the original protein. Under certain circumstances, mutations can bring about the development of genetic diseases. Single mutations that result in diseases are easier to detect and predict. For example, sickle-cell disease is caused by a mutation in the gene that codes for the hemoglobin protein, located on chromosome 11. This mutation results in a sickle shape of the red blood cell, making it less effective at transporting oxygen to internal organs and tissues. Diseases such as heart disease, cancer, and mental disorders have a combination of genetically inherited and environmental factors. Separating the influence of each component is difficult, which in turn reduces the associated predictive ability of genetic testing for these diseases.

Types of Genetic Tests

There are currently more than 100 genetic tests available, with additional tests being developed. The most commonly used genetic tests are newborn screening tests. Newborn screenings are used to find mutations in specific genes or proteins. These tests require a small sample of blood, usually taken from the newborn's heel. All infants in the United States are tested for phenylketonuria (a metabolic disorder that can cause severe mental retardation if left untreated) and congenital

hypothyroidism (a condition in which the thyroid gland fails to develop properly).

Predictive genetic testing usually is conducted later in life but before the development of major symptoms or features of the condition or disease. Common predictive genetic tests exist for breast and colon cancer, type 2 diabetes, and hemochromatosis (a condition that results in excess iron causing damage to the liver, heart, and pancreas). These tests typically require collecting a sample of cells from inside a person's cheek, referred to as the buccal swab. In some instances, predictive tests are recommended for the family members of an individual with a genetic disorder. Huntington's disease is a neurodegenerative disorder that results in progressive cognitive decline and a loss of muscle coordination. Unfortunately, there are no preventive or treatment options available for family members who possess the gene mutation that causes Huntington's; everyone who has been identified with this gene alteration gets the disease.

Diagnostic testing can confirm (or rule out) the diagnosis of a suspected genetic disorder or disease after the presentation of symptoms. Duchene muscular dystrophy is a genetic disorder that leads to muscle degeneration and eventually death. Primarily present in young males, this condition is caused by a mutation to a specific gene within muscle tissues associated with structural support. Diagnostic tests also can be used to assess if (and what type of) mutations may have affected this gene. Results from diagnostic tests can help guide treatment option decisions and the management of health conditions.

Carrier screenings identify individuals who can transfer altered genes for certain types of inherited disorders. These modified genes are found on one of the 22 non-sex chromosomes and considered to be recessive. Carriers of one recessive copy of genes do not have the disease, but they can pass the altered genes on to their offspring. If both parents happen to be carriers of an altered gene, their children can inherit both copies of the gene, causing a genetic disorder.

Prenatal genetic tests are available for women to identify fetuses that may have certain diseases or disorders throughout the course of pregnancy. Prenatal testing can be used to screen for Down syndrome and spina bifida. The test procedure usually involves taking a small sample of amniotic fluid. These tests can also determine conditions associated with certain genealogical or ancestral backgrounds. For example, Tay-Sachs is a fatal nervous system disorder that begins in early pregnancy. The mutation results in a four-base insertion of amino acids, causing the premature termination of a gene involved in the production of an enzyme called hexosaminidase-A (Hex-A). The lack of Hex-A results in a detrimental accumulation of fatty substances within nerve cells. The carrier rate for the genes associated with this condition is considerably higher among individuals of Eastern European Jewish descent (approximately 1 in every 27 people) compared to the rate in the general population (approximately 1 in

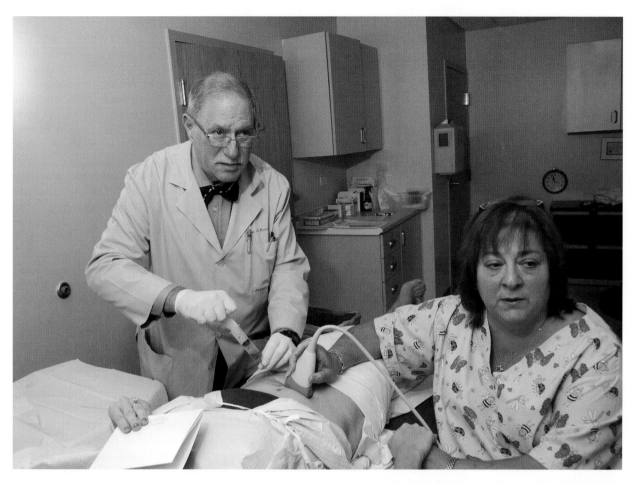

Dr. Norman Ginsberg and sonographer Sandra Concialvi draw placental tissue for prenatal genetic testing at the Reproductive Genetics Institute in Chicago, Illinois. © *Yvette Mari Dostatni/Chicago Tribune/MCT via Getty Images.*

every 250 people). For women over the age of 35, prenatal testing also can help identify chromosomal abnormalities associated with higher age pregnancies.

Pharmacogenetics, the role of a person's genetic makeup in their individual response to medicines, provides individuals with information about how certain medications and drugs are metabolized. Results from these tests can assist health-care providers in choosing treatment options that are best suited for a patient's specific genetic makeup. One illustration of how pharmacogenetic testing is used is the detection of an alteration to the gene affecting a specific liver enzyme involved in breaking down certain drugs. For example, blood clots typically are treated with the drug warfarin. If a patient suffering from a blood clot is given too little warfarin, it might not be effective in stopping the bleeding. Too much warfarin could lead to internal bleeding. Pharmacogenetic tests can guarantee that people get an ideal amount and type of medication. Particularly in human immunodeficiency virus (HIV) and cancer treatment, the use of pharmacogenetics is rapidly increasing.

Though pharmacogenetics offers physicians a means for providing customized dosages of drugs to patients,

it is also accompanied by several ethical considerations. Issues surrounding pharmacogenetics include equity in access to its benefits versus market forces, and protecting rights to know (or not know) related personal genetic information.

⊕ Impacts and Issues

Information gathered from genetic tests presents a unique set of ethical dilemmas. As with all individual health information, confidentiality remains a primary concern among stakeholders and consumers. Genetic test results have unique predictive abilities, making them particularly vulnerable to fraud and abuse. Insurance companies and employers have been known to discriminate based on genetic predispositions to certain conditions. In 2001, the Burlington Northern and Santa Fe (BNSF) Railway received an injunction from the U.S. Equal Employment Opportunities Commission (EEOC). According to multiple investigations and independent reports, BNSF had been requiring employees to undergo genetic testing after filing claims for carpal tunnel syndrome. Employees

THE U.S. FOOD AND DRUG ADMINISTRATION VS. 23ANDME

In 2008, *Time* magazine named the direct-to-consumer (DTC) DNA test the invention of the year. Created by the personal genomics company 23andMe, the at-home test kits are mailed to consumers and require only a small sample of saliva. After returning the test kit to 23andMe, the individual's genetic information is available online for that individual to access and view. In 2009, the company offered three separate types of DNA screenings: the ancestry edition, the health edition, and the complete edition. The ancestry edition enables customers to look into their genetic ancestry and determine if they have any relatives in the 23andMe database. The health edition provides consumers with screenings for many conditions and disorders, including Tay-Sachs disease, pseudocholinesterase deficiency, and Bloom's syndrome. The complete edition consists of both the ancestry and health tests, and also provides consumers with extra services via the 23andMe frequently updated online database.

The U.S. Food and Drug Administration (FDA) issued a letter to 23andMe and four other biotech companies regarding their sales of DTC genetic tests in 2010. The letter declared the companies would have to submit their products to a series of FDA tests to determine if their tests were accurate and scientifically valid. This "premarket approval" process has slowed the number of consumers purchasing DTC genetic tests considerably. The reasoning behind the FDA ruling has to do with how consumers potentially could use the information provided in the medical edition DNA test. According to the 1976 Medical Device Amendment, the FDA can review all medical devices to ensure their validity, accuracy, and safety before being sold to consumers. Initially, DTC genetic testing was not considered a medical device, making the kits exempt from premarket oversight. However, in a series of letters, the FDA concluded the products should be considered a medical device due to the possibility that DTC genetic testing "might convince consumers to make medical decisions on the basis of the genetic information provided."

Following these initial letters, communication between the FDA and 23andMe became sporadic. After finally applying for clearance on their products in 2012, 23andMe failed to cooperate with the FDA. In November 2013, after nearly four years of communication between the agency and biotech giant, the FDA issued another letter to the company. This letter described the difficulties in communication between the agency and biotech giant:

> It is now eleven months later, and you have yet to provide FDA with any new information about these tests. You have not worked with us toward de novo classification, did not provide the additional information we requested necessary to complete review of your 510(k)s, and FDA has not received any communication from 23andMe since May.

The FDA concluded that the only course of action was to demand the DTC health edition tests be removed from the company's website. As of early 2015, 23andMe offers DTC tests only for the ancestry edition. Customers could still access their raw genetic material via the company's website.

filing claims were asked to provide a blood sample to test for a gene mutation associated with chromosome 17. This altered gene allegedly was known to cause carpal tunnel syndrome. When an employee refused to participate in the screening, BNSF threatened termination. The EEOC summary indicated BNSF was in violation of the Americans with Disabilities Act and required the company to end all required genetic tests. Employees who refused the screening or cooperated during the investigation also were protected from retaliation.

Due to its ability to provide information on the health status of both individuals and family members, DNA information is both personal and ancestral. In some circumstances, the privacy considerations of an individual must be balanced against the well-being of additional family members. In the event that a genetic disorder diagnosis potentially puts additional family members (siblings, children, etc.) at risk, care must be taken to ensure that all parties receive proper ethical and medical treatment.

For example, researchers in France traced an inherited case of blindness though 30,000 descendants of a single couple who died in a small village in France in 1495. Almost half of the cases of juvenile glaucoma reported in France originated from this single couple. This gene was passed through generations with incomplete penetrance. This means not all individuals inheriting the allele become blind, but they remain carriers for the condition. Carriers of the allele unknowingly could pass the blindness onto their children. Regrettably, the symptoms of the disease are not recognizable until the individual's vision starts to deteriorate. In the late 1980s, the available treatments for this condition had to be administered before the symptoms manifested. The researchers who had identified the basis of this genetic condition wanted to share the names of individuals at risk with physicians to monitor and, if necessary, start the available treatment. Unfortunately, the existing French law prohibited the researchers from releasing the names to the doctors.

The French government decided that should the names be published, individuals carrying the alleles for the disease might suffer discrimination from insurance providers or employers. This ethical dilemma was reconciled by disseminating an educational program that encouraged concerned families to seek medical advice. However, many individuals with the potentially hazardous alleles went undetected.

Government Regulations

Although multiple countries have responded to the increased availability of genetic tests with legislation that protects the privacy of genetic information, there remains much work to be done. According to the World Health Organization (WHO) report titled "Quality & Safety in Genetic Testing: An Emerging Concern,"

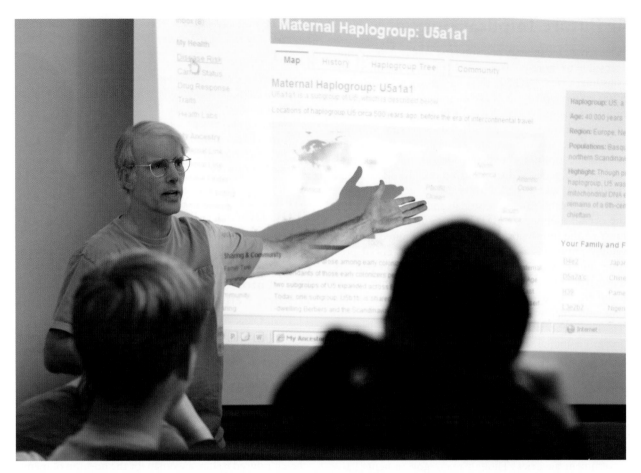

University of Iowa professor Jeff Murray talks about his genetic profile during his honors seminar on personal genetics in which students had the option of sending saliva samples so a testing company could use DNA to unlock some of their most personal health and family secrets. The class, taught at Iowa for the first time, is part of a growing movement in higher education to tackle the rapidly advancing field of personal genetics, which is revolutionizing medicine and raising difficult ethical and privacy questions. *© Brian Ray/ AP Photo.*

"Several developed countries have not yet enacted regulations based on recommendations from international, professional, and governmental sources; moreover, it is unclear how closely laboratories currently adhere to voluntary standards."

In the mid-2010s, Australia, the European Union, India, New Zealand, and the United States had policies, regulations, and protections in place for safeguarding genetic information. The WHO established the Human Genetic Programme in 1995, which focuses on advancing the technological methods involved in genetic testing; standardizing genetic testing techniques; addressing the ethical, legal, and social issues with human genetic testing; and the management of genetic approaches to the control of common diseases.

In the United States, Congress passed the Genetic Information Nondiscrimination Act (GINA) in 2008 to protect Americans from genetics-based discrimination from health insurance companies and employers. This piece of legislation took more than 13 years to become a law. Unfortunately, GINA protections do not apply to long-term-care insurance, life insurance, and disability insurance. Federal employees are awarded protection from genetic discrimination by an executive order signed in 2000 by President Bill Clinton. In 2010, the Affordable Care Act prohibited the denial of insurance coverage based on preexisting conditions, thereby reducing the ability of discrimination based on genetic factors.

Concerns over patenting issues have been raised concerning genetic material, DNA, and other forms of genetic information. In general, patents are awarded to products and processes that are new, nonobvious, and useful. Historically, patents have been designed to motivate innovation, and DNA information can be patented in certain areas under specific circumstances. In the United States, purified forms of genes and proteins can be patented. In England, naturally occurring genes cannot be patented regardless of their form, and French code on intellectual property has established that "the human body, its elements and products as well as knowledge of the partial or total structure of a human gene" is unpatentable.

⊕ Future Implications

Advances in technology continue to make genetic testing accessible to more consumers. The market for direct-to-consumer (DTC) genetic tests has grown to more than $200 billion globally as of 2014. Some of the most common reasons individuals have for purchasing DTC tests include identity-seeking genetic tests (ancestral information specific to continental, regional, and subregional geographic location); predictive/diagnostic genetic tests (for specific genes and their corresponding diseases and conditions); and basic curiosity-driven genetic testing. However, health-care professionals and physicians debate the overall usefulness of DTC genetic tests, stating that most of the information provided has "limited medical value." Physicians also have raised concerns about possible unnecessary health-care costs caused by patients misinterpreting the results of DTC tests, while others maintain that increases in health knowledge with motivate individuals to lead healthier lifestyles.

The information made available by genetic tests presents a unique set of ethical dilemmas. Progressions in genetic testing technology and increased availability must be balanced against maintaining an individual's right to personal privacy. Genetic testing or an evaluation of a family's medical history may reveal genetic information about existing or potential diseases or disorders, so individuals may choose not to seek genetic testing out of fear that the information may be disclosed to insurers, employers, or government agencies. Though many governments have adopted legislation that prohibits genetic discrimination, such discrimination still occurs, and not all countries have such laws in place. In addition, with large Internet hacking incidents occurring more frequently, including a breach that leaked the personal information of an estimated 80 million people stored by the U.S. health insurer Anthem in February 2015, people may fear that their genetic information is not secure. Although Anthem stated that the hack gained no genetic or medical data, many consumers were concerned that such information could be vulnerable to cyberattacks. Though genetic testing has the capability to treat certain conditions and potentially save many lives, people must feel that the information also cannot be used to harm them.

PRIMARY SOURCE

Fabricut to Pay $50,000 to Settle EEOC Disability and Genetic Information Discrimination Lawsuit

SOURCE *"Fabricut to Pay $50,000 to Settle EEOC Disability and Genetic Information Discrimination Lawsuit." Press Release.* U.S. Equal Employment Opportunity Commission, *May 7, 2013.*

http://www.eeoc.gov/eeoc/newsroom/release/5-7-13b.cfm (accessed February 19, 2015).

INTRODUCTION *This primary source is a press release describing the allegations and subsequent settlement agreement of a genetic discrimination lawsuit filed by the U.S. Equal Employment Opportunity Commission (EEOC). The suit is of particular interest because it was the first ever filed by the EEOC alleging genetic discrimination.*

FABRICUT TO PAY $50,000 TO SETTLE EEOC DISABILITY AND GENETIC INFORMATION DISCRIMINATION LAWSUIT

Federal Agency Files First Suit Enforcing Genetic Discrimination Law Against Fabric Distributor That Requested Family Medical History, Refused to Hire Woman

TULSA, Okla. - Fabricut, Inc., one of the world's largest distributors of decorative fabrics, will pay $50,000 and furnish other relief to settle a disability and genetic information discrimination lawsuit filed by the U.S. Equal Employment Opportunity Commission (EEOC), the agency announced today. This is the first lawsuit ever filed by the EEOC alleging genetic discrimination.

In its lawsuit, the EEOC charged that Tulsa-based Fabricut violated the Americans with Disabilities Act (ADA) when it refused to hire a woman for the position of memo clerk because it regarded her as having carpal tunnel syndrome, and violated the Genetic Information Nondiscrimination Act (GINA) when it asked for her family medical history in its post-offer medical examination.

"Employers need to be aware that GINA prohibits requesting family medical history," said David Lopez, General Counsel of the EEOC. "When illegal questions are required as part of the hiring process, the EEOC will be vigilant to ensure that no one be denied a job on a prohibited basis."

According to the EEOC's suit, Rhonda Jones, worked for Fabricut in a temporary position as a memo clerk for 90 days. When her temporary assignment was coming to an end, she applied for a permanent job in that position. Fabricut made Jones an offer of permanent employment on Aug. 9, 2011, and sent her to its contract medical examiner, Knox Laboratory, for a pre-employment drug test and physical. When Jones reported for her physical, she was required to fill out a questionnaire and disclose the existence of numerous separately listed disorders in her family medical history. The questionnaire asked about the existence of heart disease, hypertension, cancer, tuberculosis, diabetes, arthritis and "mental disorders" in her family. Jones was then subjected to medical testing, from which the examiner concluded that further evaluation was needed to determine whether Jones suffered from carpal tunnel syndrome (CTS).

Fabricut told Jones she needed to be evaluated for CTS by her personal physician and to provide the company with the results. Jones's physician gave her a battery of tests and concluded that she did not have CTS. Although Jones provided this information to Fabricut, the company rescinded its job offer because Knox Labs indicated that she did have CTS. Jones made a written request for reconsideration, emphasizing that she does not have CTS, but Fabricut ignored her plea.

Such alleged conduct violates GINA, which makes it illegal to discriminate against employees or applicants because of genetic information, which includes family medical history; and also restricts employers from requesting, requiring or purchasing such information. GINA was signed into law in 2008, and took effect the following year.

The alleged conduct also violates the ADA which prohibits discrimination against qualified individuals with disabilities, or individuals who are incorrectly regarded as having disabilities. The EEOC first attempted to settle the matter through its conciliation process.

The lawsuit and consent decree settling the case were filed at the same time on May 7, 2013, in U.S. District Court for the Northern District of Oklahoma (Civil Case No.: 13-CV-248-CVE-PJC). In addition to the $50,000 payment, Fabricut has agreed to take specified actions designed to prevent future discrimination, including the posting of an anti-discrimination notice to employees, dissemination of anti-discrimination policies to employees and providing anti-discrimination training to employees with hiring responsibilities.

One of the six national priorities identified by the EEOC's Strategic Enforcement Plan is for the agency to address emerging and developing issues in equal employment law, which includes genetic discrimination.

"We believe that when Fabricut fully understood and appreciated what happened, it took action to remedy the situation, as this quick settlement demonstrates," said EEOC Regional Attorney Barbara Seely. "Although GINA has been law since 2009, many employers still do not understand that requesting family medical history, even through a contract medical examiner, violates this law."

EEOC Senior Trial Attorney Patrick Holman added, "Fabricut has been cooperative in working with the EEOC to reach a fair and timely resolution of this case, and the company appears committed to addressing the alleged discriminatory practices at issue in order to prevent any future violations."

The EEOC enforces federal laws prohibiting employment discrimination. Further information about the agency is available on its web site at www.eeoc.gov.

SEE ALSO *Cancer; Cardiovascular Diseases; Health as a Human Right and Health-Care Access; Health-Related Education and Information Access; Mobile Health Technologies; Stigma; Vulnerable Populations*

BIBLIOGRAPHY

Books

Lackie, J. M., J. G. Coote, C. W. Lloyd, and S. E. Bradshaw, eds. *The Dictionary of Cell and Molecular Biology*, 5th ed. London: Academic Press, 2013.

Papadakis, Maxine, and Stephen McPhee. *Current Medical Diagnosis & Treatment 2013*. New York: McGraw-Hill, 2013.

Pritchard, Dorian, and Bruce Korf. *Medical Genetics at a Glance*, 3rd ed. New York: Wiley, 2013.

Periodicals

Fuller, Barbara P., et al. "Privacy in Genetics Research." *Science* 285, no. 5432 (August 27, 1999): 1359–1361.

Norrgard, Karen. "Protecting Your Genetic Identity: GINA and HIPAA." *Nature Education* 1, no. 1 (2008): 21

Peikoff, Kara. "Fearing Punishment for Bad Genes." *New York Times*, April 7, 2014.

"Stop the Genetic Dragnet." *Scientific American* 305, no. 6 (December 2011): 14.

Watson, J. D., and F. C. H. Crick. "A Structure for Deoxyribose Nucleic Acid." *Nature* 171, no. 4356 (April 25, 1953): 737–738.

Websites

"Ethical, Legal, and Social Implications (ELSI) of Human Genomics." *World Health Organization (WHO)*. http://www.who.int/genomics/elsi/en// (accessed January 9, 2015).

"Genetic Discrimination." *National Human Genome Research Institute*. http://www.genome.gov/10002077%23al-3 (accessed January 9, 2015).

"Genetic Information Nondiscrimination Act of 2008." *National Human Genome Research Institute*. http://www.genome.gov/10002328 (accessed January 9, 2015).

"Genetic Privacy." *Council for Responsible Genetics*. http://www.councilforresponsiblegenetics.org/geneticprivacy/DNA_priv.html (accessed January 9, 2015).

"Inspections, Compliance, Enforcement, and Criminal Investigations." *U.S. Food and Drug Administration*. http://www.fda.gov/ICECI/EnforcementActions/WarningLetters/2013/ucm376296.htm (accessed January 9, 2015).

"Quality & Safety in Genetic Testing: An Emerging Concern." *World Health Organization (WHO)*. http://www.who.int/genomics/policy/quality_safety/en/index1.html (accessed November 17, 2014).

Martin James Frigaard

Genital Modification

⊕ Introduction

Genital modification may be defined as any procedure in which the external genitalia are transformed, cut, stretched, repositioned or significantly altered, regardless of considerations of medical necessity and with or without informed consent. This may occur as part of a traditional societal practice, be part of a religious or cultural program, occur under the auspices of medical professionals, be considered a radical form of body art, self-expression, or sexual fetishism, or be surgically performed during the medical process of gender transition or reassignment.

There are five primary reasons for the practice of genital modification: (1) Traditional and cultural practices, as in the genital modification/mutilation/cutting (often referred to as FGM/C) of healthy, intact female external genitalia practiced primarily in the northwest regions of Africa and the Middle East (although FGM/C is practiced worldwide). Most often, this occurs between infancy and the onset of menarche, usually before the age of 15 years. By legal definition, an individual below the age of legal majority may not give fully informed consent for any medical or surgical intervention. The procedure is typically performed by a cultural practitioner or local circumciser. (2) Medically-related modification performed at birth or during early infancy as when a child is born with damaged or indeterminate external genitalia and medical staff, along with parents, opt to surgically assign a child to a specific gender. This is done without the informed consent of the child/patient. This practice has declined, and the number of individuals defined as "intersex" has risen in recent decades, particularly in the first world nations; (3) Medico-cultural and religious reasons, as in the circumcision of healthy, intact male infants for religious and cultural reasons, often in the developed world. This is often done either as a surgical procedure under sterile conditions, or by a religious or cultural leader specializing in the practice of male circumcision. (4) Genital modification may be performed as part of either a cultural practice, viewed as an art form, seen as a personal statement akin to piercing or tattooing, done for personal or sexual pleasure enhancement, or as part of an underground cultural or bondage, dominance, sadism, and masochism practice (BD/SM); and (5) Genital modification may be performed as part of the process of gender reassignment or gender transition surgery. This virtually always occurs in a hospital setting and must involve fully informed consent by the patient.

The terms genital modification and male genital mutilation may also be used to refer to the practice of involuntary male circumcision, when not performed for medically mandated reasons, or when it is performed without fully informed consent.

The traditional cultural practice of female genital modification, often referred to as female genital mutilation, is widely practiced throughout the developing, and many parts of the developed, world. In particular, it refers to the practice of making changes to the intact and healthy external female genitalia as a means of controlling sexual and social behavior or making a woman more acceptable or pleasing to a future mate. The World Health Organization (WHO) defines female genital mutilation/cutting (FGM/C) as "all procedures involving partial or total removal of the female external genitalia, or other injury to the female genital organs for non-medical reasons." Most cases of FGM/C occur in girls between infancy and age 15, according to the WHO.

Four types of FGM/C have been explicitly defined by the WHO:

1. Type I, called clitoridectomy, refers to the partial or complete removal of the external portions of the clitoris, which is a small, extremely sensitive and erectile mound of female external genital tissue, and/or the prepuce, which is the hood or covering of skin that sits over or surrounds the clitoris;

2. Type II, referred to as excision, involves the partial or total removal of the clitoris and the labia minora, the smaller segments of tissue immediately external

to the vagina with or without removal of the labia majora, which are the larger folds of skin at the outermost portion of the vaginal area (the labia are sometimes referred to as vaginal lips);

3. Type III entails the narrowing of the vaginal opening by creating a covering or seal. This is done, with or without clitoris removal, by cutting and moving either the outer or inner labia and then sewing them; and

4. Type IV encompasses all other harmful or potentially harmful procedures to the female genitalia for nonmedical purposes. Pricking, piercing, cauterization, incising, scraping, introduction of corrosive substances, and stretching all fall within this category.

⊕ Historical Background

Female Genital Modification/Mutilation

The practice of FGM/C does not seem to have a single point of cultural or traditional origin, although it is believed to date back at least 2,000 years to ancient Egypt, where it was considered a sign of upper socio-economic status. In early Arab cultures, FGM/C was thought to have been practiced as a means of controlling the behavior of female slaves. Other sources suggest that FGM/C had its origins with the inception of Islam in regions of sub-Saharan Africa. Other writers and historians suggest that some cultural and ethnic factions in sub-Saharan Africa evolved the practice as a part of adolescent and puberty rituals. It was considered a typical practice among Roman slave owners to put rings through the labia majora of female slaves as a means of prevention of pregnancy; some ancient Russian factions practiced FGM/C as a way to ensure virginity among young and adolescent females. The common theme appears to be a belief that FGM/C curtailed sexual desire, secured lasting virginity, and controlled the sexual behavior of younger females across a variety of cultures and societies.

Although it has been most prevalent in 29 African and Middle Eastern countries, FGM/C has historically been practiced throughout the world. In some areas it has been considered a ritual used to mark passage into womanhood, in others it was believed to be the way to ensure virginity until marriage. In many cultures, it was thought to be the most widely accepted means of proving eligibility for a good marriage, which has historically been a cultural and economic necessity in subsistence societies.

FGM/C was practiced in the United States and parts of Europe as a means of controlling the behavior of young females with behavioral issues or "hysteria." It has also been continued among migrants from countries in which FGM/C is culturally dominant. Sometimes, girls or young women are sent back to their countries of cultural origin in order to obtain FGM/C during school breaks or vacations and then returned home.

Male Circumcision

Although there are a number of conflicting views regarding whether male circumcision evolved as part of a religious or cultural practice, some theories suggest that it began at least 70,000 years ago, long before written history. The belief is that the ritual partial detachment of the foreskin may have heightened sexual pleasure and aided in copulation, therefore increasing birthrates, giving a selective advantage to cultures practicing the ritual. It is hypothesized to have been widely practiced before humans began the migration from Africa into other parts of the globe.

Male circumcision has been considered one of the oldest and most common surgical procedures worldwide. Male circumcision as a cultural and religious practice has occurred for more than 5,000 years in Western Africa and for more than 4,000 years in the Middle East. Ancient wall carvings and paintings, as well as sarcophagi and preserved mummies, indicate that male circumcision was practiced in Egypt at least 4,000 years ago. It is believed to have had its basis there in medical and hygienic practice, rather than religious ritual, although priests were commonly those trained to perform the procedure on young adolescent males. In desert or hot, sandy climates, circumcision was practiced as a means of preventing irritation and infections brought about by high winds and blowing sand, making it a common procedure in Mexico, the Kalahari, Egypt, Saudi Arabia, and central regions of Australia.

In Judaism and the Muslim religions, the practice was engendered by the circumcision of Abraham around 2000 BCE. Male circumcision has historically occurred primarily for cultural and religious reasons, with the highest rates globally among Muslim and Jewish males. In the United States and throughout many areas of Europe, male circumcision was popularized by the medical profession during the late 1900s. It became a routine surgery for male infants shortly after birth. It was believed that circumcision afforded a means of protection against later development of various genital cancers and syphilis. That theory came under increasing medical and public scrutiny in the 1980s, with the result that more countries began to consider male circumcision unnecessary and not beneficial, leading to reduced rates in some countries.

According to data published by the WHO and the Joint United Nations Programme on HIV/AIDS (UNAIDS), in 2007 roughly one-third of adult males worldwide were circumcised, with two-thirds of those individuals being Muslim. While medical or cultural circumcision of infant males (usually performed by a specially trained practitioner) has remained prevalent in the United States, Canada, Australia, New Zealand, Israel,

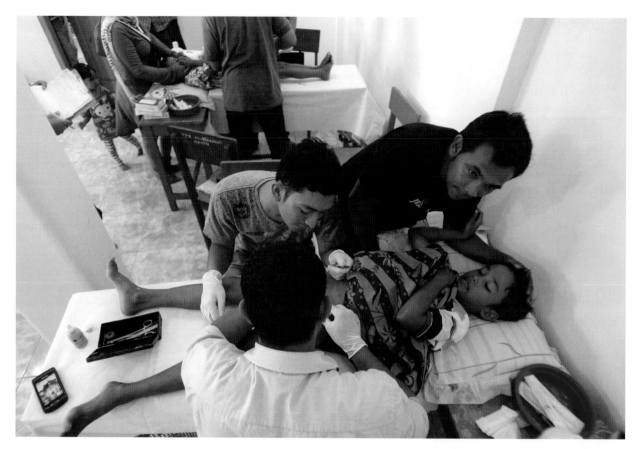

Paramedics perform circumcision on a boy during a charge-free mass circumcision in Aceh Besar, Aceh Province, Indonesia. In accordance with Islamic tradition, Indonesian Muslim boys are circumcised before they reach puberty. © *Heri Juanda/AP Images.*

many Middle Eastern, Central Asian, and West African countries, it has been relatively uncommon in southern and eastern African nations. Traditionally in those regions of Africa, male circumcision is typically part of a ritual practice occurring between middle childhood and young adulthood. However, with data showing that it may help with prevention of the spread of human immunodeficiency virus (HIV), rates in some southern and eastern African countries have been on the rise since 2008.

⊕ Impacts and Issues

Female Genital Modification/Mutilation/Cutting

The WHO, UNICEF, and many others consider nearly all forms of FGM/C "harmful traditional practices" because, although they do reflect a broad range of traditional cultural beliefs, they also cause physical harm and may cause emotional harm, and may sometimes lead to death for the girls and women who participate in them. The harm occurs during and immediately subsequent to the process of the FGM/C and may continue throughout life, particularly at the time of initial sexual experience and during pregnancy and childbirth.

FGM/C is most frequently performed by local circumcisers or tribal and cultural members who were taught by previous generations. Sterile procedure is rare, and old, used, blunt, or dirty instruments are common. There is very rarely medical supervision or oversight.

Potential medical consequences at the time of FGM/C include severe pain, heavy bleeding and sometimes hemorrhage, shock, potentially life-threatening bacterial infections, inability to urinate or to urinate fully (sometimes leading to acute or chronic urinary tract infections), sepsis resulting from open wounds, particularly in the immediate vaginal area, and injury to surrounding tissue or structures. Sometimes, the girls bleed to death as a result of the cutting; at other times the bacterial infections or sepsis that may occur result in death.

Long-term complications resulting from FGM/C include the surgical risks inherent in recutting girls or women who have experienced type III FGM/C in order to engage in sexual activity and childbirth; decreased fertility and increased rates of maternal and infant mortality; chronic or recurrent urinary tract infections, possibly leading to bladder and kidney diseases; cysts; and increased pregnancy and childbirth complications.

Most instances of FGM/C have been reported to occur in 29 countries in the Middle East and Africa, although the

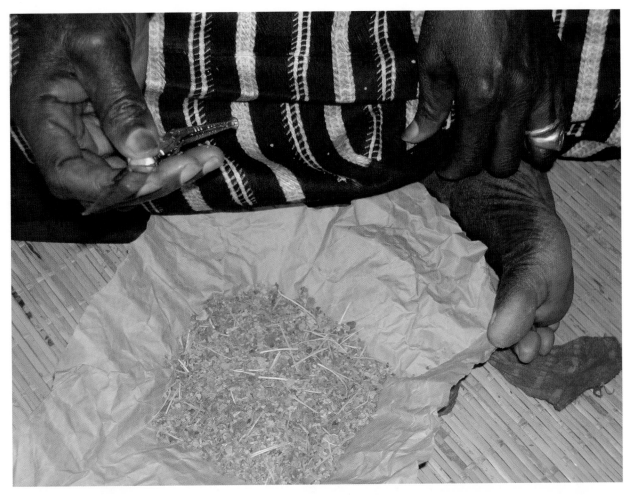

Former circumciser Mariam Coulibaly displays the tools of her trade, a knife handed down to her by her mother and herbs to heal the wounds, at her home in Salemata, southeastern Senegal. Coulibaly says that she performed circumcisions on more than 1,000 girls during her 30-year career, but gave up the practice after surrounding villages decided the practice to be dangerous. The piece of red cloth is part of one of the bright red robes she used to wear while performing the rites.   © Alexandra Zavis/AP Photo.

practice is documented in more than 60 countries in the developed million and developing world. It is estimated that between 125 million and 130 million girls and women currently alive have experienced FGM/C, with 30 million more expected to be impacted during the next decade, unless practice rates are markedly diminished, especially in those 29 countries. Many other countries either choose not to document cases of FGM/C or fail to record accurate numbers of cases. In addition, complications from FGM/C impact the global medical communities as a result of migration of affected persons, or persons supporting continuation of the practice, to other countries.

According to UNICEF statistics from 2013, the locations with the greatest number of girls and women currently living who have experienced FGM/C are as follows:

1. Egypt—27.2 million
2. Ethiopia—23.8 million
3. Nigeria—19.9 million
4. Sudan—12.1 million
5. Kenya and Burkina Faso—9.3 million
6. Mali and the United Republic of Tanzania—9 million
7. Guinea and Somalia—6.5 million
8. Ivory Coast (Cote d'Ivoire) and Yemen—5 million
9. Chad and Iraq—3.8 million
10. Eritrea and Sierra Leone—3.5 million

According to UNICEF, as of 2013 the countries with the most widely reported FGM/C practice, across more than 50 percent of the at-risk population, are: Somalia, 98 percent; Guinea, 96 percent; Djibouti, 93 percent; Egypt, 91 percent; Eritrea, 89 percent; Mali, 89 percent; Sierra Leone, 88 percent; Sudan, 88 percent; Gambia, 76 percent; Burkina Faso, 76 percent; Ethiopia,

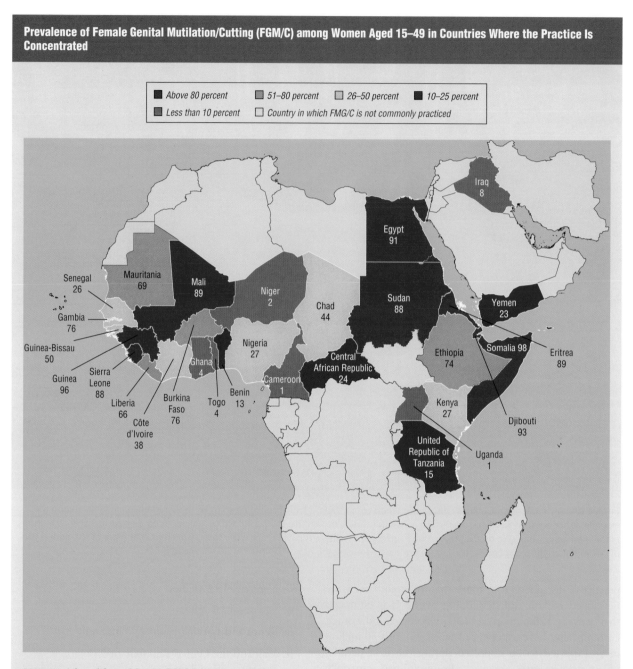

Prevalence of Female Genital Mutilation/Cutting (FGM/C) among Women Aged 15–49 in Countries Where the Practice Is Concentrated

■ *Above 80 percent*   ■ *51–80 percent*   □ *26–50 percent*   ■ *10–25 percent*

■ *Less than 10 percent*   □ *Country in which FMG/C is not commonly practiced*

Iraq 8

Egypt 91

Senegal 26

Mauritania 69

Mali 89

Niger 2

Chad 44

Sudan 88

Yemen 23

Gambia 76

Guinea-Bissau 50

Nigeria 27

Ghana 4

Central African Republic 24

Ethiopia 74

Somalia 98

Eritrea 89

Guinea 96

Sierra Leone 88

Cameroon 1

Liberia 66

Burkina Faso 76

Togo 4

Benin 13

Kenya 27

Djibouti 93

Côte d'Ivoire 38

United Republic of Tanzania 15

Uganda 1

SOURCE: Adapted from "Map 4.1 FGM/C is concentrated in a swath of countries from the Atlantic Coast to the Horn of Africa," in *Female Genital Mutilation/Cutting: A Statistical Overview and Exploration of the Dynamics of Change*, United Nations Children's Fund (UNICEF), July 2013, p. 26. Data from Demographic and Health Surveys (DHS), Multiple Indicator Cluster Surveys (MICS), and Sudan Household Health Survey (SHHS), 1997–2012.

74 percent; Mauritania, 69 percent; and Liberia, 66 percent. (See graphic.)

According to data published by UNICEF's Innocenti Research Centre in 2010, FGM/C is most frequently practiced in many countries in Africa and the Middle East, as well as a few countries in Asia and in immigrant population pockets in Europe, Australia, New Zealand, Canada, and the United States. It is important to note

that where the practice is common, it is not viewed by those involved as a human rights violation or as a dangerous activity. Rather, it is considered a cultural norm for managing and preventing premature sexual behavior in girls and young women and, more importantly, as a means of preparing them to take their place in society and to achieve a good and suitable marriage. Because familial and cultural values are at the center of the belief systems surrounding the practice, it is extremely persistent, even when outside agencies come in to provide medical and human rights education. It continues even in the face of anti-FGM/C legislation and criminal penalties for its engagement. Often, the threat of loss of social standing or ostracism by the cultural group is greater than any legal or medical sanctions against its continuing practice.

Most commonly, FGM/C is practiced with infants and minor children who are unable to give informed consent. Often, it is a cultural practice strongly encouraged across generations within families as a means of preserving virginity, encouraging chastity or fidelity, and as a means of securing a good marriage. It is considered by UNICEF, the WHO, and many other civil rights and medically related groups to be a violation of the human rights of girls and women because participants are generally believed to face substantial societal, cultural, and familial pressure to engage in a painful, harmful, and potentially lethal practice they may not desire. It is also considered a widespread means of maintaining females in roles of subjugation (unequal status and power) in comparison with males of the same culture and social standing.

The cultural practice of voluntary labial elongation engaged in by adolescent females in some countries in Africa, particularly Rwanda and Uganda, is sometimes considered an exception to the label of FGM/C, although the girls may feel substantial local cultural pressure to participate. Groups of young adolescent females who have not yet begun menstruating gather at parties and use a variety of herbs to assist them in the practice of pulling and stretching their inner labia (labia minora) as a means of enhancing sexual pleasure for both partners. The practice carries some health risks as it may cause labial irritation, tearing or infection; and the practice results in permanent stretching and tissue changes. It is engaged in as a means of enhancing sexual pleasure for both females and males, and is a highly culturally and socially valued practice.

Male Circumcision

There is substantial scientific research evidence that male medical circumcision has protective effects against a number of sexually transmitted diseases, invasive cancer of the penis, urinary tract infections, and HIV/AIDS. The data on HIV/AIDS transmission was collected during a series of randomized trials, and reduction rates in female to male transmission were shown to be as high as 50 to 60 percent. In part, this led to the articulation of Millennium Development Goal 6 (MDG 6) by the United Nations. A focus of MDG 6 involves reversing the proliferation of HIV/AIDS in areas of Africa where it has remained in epidemic proportions, with the spread of infection from females to males being particularly high. Several WHO and UNAIDS supported research projects have indicated that a very effective means of reversing infection rates involves

a large-scale increase in voluntary medical male circumcision in areas of the world where it has not been the norm.

The WHO and UNAIDS recommended that voluntary medical male circumcision (VMMC) rates be "scaled-up" in 14 highly human immunodeficiency virus/acquired immunodeficiency syndrome (HIV/AIDS)–affected eastern and southern African countries, with an overall goal of 80 percent, or 20.8 million adult males circumcised, by 2016. Those countries are Botswana, Ethiopia (focused on the Gambella Province), Kenya, Lesotho, Malawi, Mozambique, Namibia, Rwanda, South Africa, Swaziland, Tanzania, Uganda, Zambia, and Zimbabwe.

Although the pace of progress has not been as rapid as had been projected, the overall rates of VMMC have increased from a total of 21,300 in 2008 to nearly 5.9 million in 2013, according to WHO data published in July 2014. In addition to the medical benefits of VMMC regarding risk reduction for HIV, there are also considerable economic benefits: VMMC is typically a one-time procedure with few complications and little need for follow up care. By dramatically decreasing the incidence of HIV/AIDS transmission, it eliminates the lifetime economic and social burden of providing care for large numbers of individuals with new cases of HIV/AIDS. The WHO estimates that the cost of VMMC for about 20 million men would be the equivalent of US$1.5 billion, but would result in a net savings of US$16.5 billion by 2025 and would negate development of roughly 3.4 million new cases of HIV/AIDS.

It is important to note that VMMC provides only partial protection against HIV/AIDS, sexually transmitted diseases, and other diseases, and must be viewed as part of a package of programming that also includes access to HIV testing and counseling, education regarding safer sex practices—including limiting the number of sex partners (current and sequential) and avoiding penetrative sex, along with access to and teaching in the accurate use of male and female condoms, to include ongoing use of same, and treatment of existing and new sexually transmitted diseases.

⊕ Future Implications

There is a widespread belief around the globe that FGM/C is a physically and emotionally harmful and potentially lethal practice. It is considered a violation of the human rights of girls and young women, and there is considerable agreement that the practice should be ended. There are sanctions and laws condemning and criminalizing its practice, yet FGM/C still persists. Although some families and cultural groups are aware of the sanctions, the pressure to continue, coupled with the belief that their child will experience greater harm if expelled from her social group than if she is undergoes FGM/C, makes change extremely slow and difficult.

CHANGES IN SUDAN: THE SALEEMA CAMPAIGN

Historically, Sudan has had one of the highest rates of FGM/C, at more than 92 percent, with most girls being cut between the ages of 5 and 11. Women and girls who are uncut have been considered unclean, immodest, or dishonorable, and are referred to as *gulfa*, a term historically reserved for individuals of the lowest social status, often synonymous with prostitutes. Because the practice is deeply entrenched and considered an important aspect of social and kinship systems, change has been both extremely slow and difficult. The overarching belief among nongovernmental organizations (NGOs) and health policy change makers is that it is critical to shift attitudes away from support of FGM/C and toward support of human rights. In statistics published for 1989–1990, 79 percent of Sudanese girls and women between the ages of 15 and 49 believed that the practice (typically type III) of FGM/C should continue; by 2006, the percentage in favor had dropped to 51. In 1989–1990, 82 percent of married women reported that they intended to have their daughters cut, whereas only 54 percent expressed an intention to do so in 2006, according to UNICEF data published in 2010.

The United Nations Population Fund (UNFPA), in conjunction with UNICEF, supports a program created by Sudan's National Council on Child Welfare in partnership with its National Strategic Planning Centre called "The Saleema Campaign." *Saleema* is a female Arabic name meaning whole, intact, healthy in mind and body, pure, clean, perfect, and as made by God. The government worked with a variety of NGOs as well as poets and artists to design and shape the campaign. The intention is for the word saleema to replace the pejorative term *gulfa* for uncut girls and to begin the process of shifting the core beliefs away from FGM/C being the only positive indicator of social status for females and toward remaining uncut as a desirable cultural norm. The underlying strategy is not to openly discredit or speak out negatively against FGM/C, but to support a new paradigm, and to facilitate adoption of the belief that the more desirable state is to remain uncut.

The campaign began in March 2008, using colloquial (traditional) language and local culture in the form of poetry, music, dance, painting, and song to reinforce the idea of supporting children's health and well-being. It endorses the idea of close family relationships, social supports, and pride in healthy and equal, protective relationships across genders. During the induction phase of the campaign, T-shirts, shawls, and posters were widely distributed. Individuals and groups working with local communities were trained in the educational methods and communication tools to be used for effective promotion.

The core concept of The Saleema Campaign is: "Every girl is born saleema. Let her grow saleema." There are bright colors and attractive fabrics used to represent the concept of saleema, reflected in all aspects of the campaign. The goal is for the program to become progressively more explicit over time in the support of allowing girls to remain uncut and gradually supporting the notion of abandoning the practice of FGM/C.

The Saleema Campaign is now being promoted across the entirety of Sudan, with media, television, and radio support featuring progressively more songs and poems celebrating remaining saleema, while work continues in individual communities. The overarching goal is to develop collective public and specifically articulated commitments to abandon FGM/C. Because the concept of collective decision making is respected and endorsed throughout the country, public consensus is very important in order to effect lasting change.

Initially, FGM/C was not explicitly spoken about, as it was such an entrenched practice that there was concern that openly expressing negative sentiment would lead to rapid abandonment of the project and refusal by local communities to engage with the program on any level. By creating an initial approach celebrating existing social values such as pride in the family, support of beliefs around good parenting and strong communities, it was possible to create a positive groundswell before beginning to raise more the controversial subject.

In Sudan, the most extreme form of FGM/C, type III, is traditionally practiced. Although many groups have publicly declared support of abandonment, the practice declines slowly, with the most recent rate being measured at 88 percent (a decrease of 4 percent). For the first time, FGM/C is being openly discussed, and groups are reporting that they no longer view the practice as universal, leading them to consider alternatives or abandonment. Some factions have shifted to what they consider less severe forms of FGM/C, most notably clitoridectomy. In some areas, medical professionals have begun performing FGM/C rather than local practitioners, in an effort to render it safer and more hygienic. Some cultural groups have needed concrete assurances by their religious leaders that FGM/C was not mandated for spiritual practice.

One of the central takeaway messages of the Saleema Campaign's infrastructure is that change takes time. Individuals and groups require clear and repeated assurance that they are not acting alone, and that there are understandable and reasonable alternatives to entrenched cultural practices. The campaign supports the importance of the media, whether radio, television, film, or social, in promoting and supporting social change and in widely disseminating consistent messages.

FGM/C carries no health benefit, and involves the damaging, cutting, changing, or removal of healthy, intact external genital tissue or structures. According to the 2010 UNICEF Innocenti Research Centre report, "FGM/C is an infringement of the human rights of girls and women. It violates their right to health, security and physical integrity; the right to be free from torture and cruel, inhuman or degrading treatment; and the right to life when the procedure results in death. Even if it is not intended as an act of violence, the practice of FGM/C is de facto violent. It is discriminatory in nature, and assigns girls and women an inferior position in the family and society. It causes physical and psychological harm that can be extremely severe and often irreversible.

FGM/C has consequences that may affect girls and women throughout their lives."

There has been a concerted effort sponsored by UNICEF, centered in five countries, Senegal, Kenya, Egypt, Sudan, and Ethiopia, to programmatically create positive change and encourage the abandonment of the practices. Other countries have initiated education and practice leading to dramatic reductions as well, most notably Liberia and the United Republic of Tanzania. Overall, more than 30 percent fewer girls and young women experience FGM/C than did in 1985, according to UNICEF. Those positive changes notwithstanding, roughly 60 million females around the world may still be harmed by FGM/C before 2050 unless the rate of progress is significantly increased.

In order to achieve the types of lasting change that will lead to decrease in the practice, and potential elimination, of FGM/C, it is necessary for the approach to be culturally relevant and socially appropriate. A strong belief in gender inequality lies at the heart of FGM/C and associated practices such as child marriage, marriage by abduction, and forced marriage. That core belief must be changed in order for any of the social norms to shift. It is critical not only to understand the underpinnings of the belief system and how to shift those core beliefs in a culturally sensitive way, but also how to reinforce and sustain the shifts that will lead to, and then support, abandonment of a deeply ingrained, extremely long-standing tradition.

In Somalia, Ethiopia, northern portions of Sudan, and Egypt, FGM/C has been nationally widespread. In Senegal and Kenya, the practice is only common among specific groups. Efforts have been heavily concentrated since the start of the 21st century on successfully and permanently shifting cultural attitudes in an effort to bring about an end to the practices and to create a desire to abandon FGM/C and associated harmful cultural practices entirely. A first step in changing a social norm involves teaching individuals that there are alternatives. When a cultural practice is extremely widespread, there may not be awareness that it is not a global or universal practice, and that it may be possible to create new norms. FGM/C is most common in cultures where gender inequality is extreme, and females considered entirely dependent upon males for marriage, economic viability, and their own survival. They typically do not have individual rights, hold no social or political power, and have little say in matters impacting their own lives. It is least frequent in cultures in which women's rights are valued, where they hold social standing and power, and where they are imbued with the right to physical and emotional integrity and freedom from abusive, painful, or harmful practices.

In some cultures, a belief in the right of a child to protection and physical integrity, or freedom from intentional harm or pain, overrides the negative social status of females, making it easier to shift beliefs about the practice of FGM/C. By assisting the culture to adopt the belief that avoiding or ending harm and pain to children is desirable, it is possible to alter belief systems and to incorporate new norms. When groups are taught that there are other, safe and nonpainful ways of protecting their children and ensuring viable marriage and social outcomes for them, it becomes possible to contemplate abandonment of the practice of FGM/C.

The research processes carried out by UNICEF and similar groups suggest that the process of creating large cultural shifts away from ingrained and long-standing norms and practices is a gradual one. Such processes must incorporate collective work within communities and cultures in which other ways of engaging are illustrated and the communities are offered appropriate and meaningful information so that they can evaluate and reflect and make considered choices in order for the possibility of lasting change to occur. An important part of the change paradigm, in addition to public and well-communicated and considered options, is clear evidence that others of the group are willing and able to make the same changes. In other words, it is critical to believe that change can be widespread in order for it to be successful and sustained. Individuals must have agreement that there will be maintenance of social status within the new belief system.

PRIMARY SOURCE

Intensifying Global Efforts for the Elimination of Female Genital Mutilations

SOURCE Intensifying Global Efforts for the Elimination of Female Genital Mutilations. *United Nations General Assembly, Sixty-Seventh session, Agenda item 28 (a), December 20, 2012. Copyright © 2012 United Nations. http://www. un.org/en/ga/search/view_doc.asp?symbol=A/ RES/67/146&referer=http://www.un.org/en/ ga/67/resolutions.shtml&Lang=E (accessed January 25, 2015).*

INTRODUCTION *This primary source is excerpted from a resolution of the United Nations General Assembly. The resolution supports the recommendations of a committee investigating female genital mutilation practices worldwide.*

RESOLUTION ADOPTED BY THE GENERAL ASSEMBLY ON 20 DECEMBER 2012

[*on the report of the Third Committee (A/67/450 and Corr.1)*]

67/146. Intensifying global efforts for the elimination of female genital mutilations

The General Assembly,

...

Recognizing that female genital mutilations are an irreparable, irreversible abuse that impacts negatively on the human rights of women and girls, affecting about 100 million to 140 million women and girls worldwide, and that each year an estimated further 3 million girls are at risk of being subjected to the practice throughout the world,

Reaffirming that female genital mutilations are a harmful practice that constitutes a serious threat to the health of women and girls, including their psychological, sexual and reproductive health, which can increase their vulnerability to HIV and may have adverse obstetric and prenatal outcomes as well as fatal consequences for the mother and the newborn, and that the abandonment of this harmful practice can be achieved as a result of a comprehensive movement that involves all public and private stakeholders in society, including girls and boys, women and men,

Concerned about evidence of an increase in the incidence of female genital mutilations being carried out by medical personnel in all regions in which they are practised,

Recognizing that negative discriminatory stereotypical attitudes and behaviours have direct implications for the status and treatment of women and girls and that such negative stereotypes impede the implementation of legislative and normative frameworks that guarantee gender equality and prohibit discrimination on the basis of sex,

...

Deeply concerned that, despite the increase in national, regional and international efforts and the focus on the abandonment of female genital mutilations, the practice continues to exist in all regions of the world,

Deeply concerned also that a tremendous gap in resources continues to exist and that the shortfall in funding has severely limited the scope and pace of programmes and activities for the elimination of female genital mutilations,

Having considered the report of the Secretary-General on ending female genital mutilation,

1. *Stresses* that the empowerment of women and girls is key to breaking the cycle of discrimination and violence and for the promotion and protection of human rights, including the right to the highest attainable standard of mental and physical health, including sexual and reproductive health, and calls upon States parties to fulfil their obligations under the Convention on the Rights of the Child and the Convention on the Elimination of All Forms of Discrimination against Women, as well as their commitments to implement the Declaration on the Elimination of Violence against Women, the Programme of Action of the International Conference on Population and Development, the Beijing Platform for Action and the outcomes of the twenty-third special session of the General Assembly, entitled "Women 2000: gender equality, development and peace for the twenty-first century", and of the special session of the Assembly on children;

2. *Calls upon* States to enhance awareness-raising and formal, non-formal and informal education and training in order to promote the direct engagement of girls and boys, women and men and to ensure that all key actors, Government officials, including law enforcement and judicial personnel, immigration officials, health-care providers, community and religious leaders, teachers, employers, media professionals and those directly working with girls, as well as parents, families and communities, work to eliminate attitudes and harmful practices, in particular all forms of female genital mutilations, that negatively affect girls;

3. *Also calls upon* States to strengthen advocacy and awareness-raising programmes, to mobilize girls and boys to take an active part in developing preventive and elimination programmes to address harmful practices, especially female genital mutilations, and to engage community and religious leaders, educational institutions, the media and families and provide increased financial support to efforts at all levels to end those practices;

4. *Urges* States to condemn all harmful practices that affect women and girls, in particular female genital mutilations, whether committed within or outside a medical institution, and to take all necessary measures, including enacting and enforcing legislation, to prohibit female genital mutilations and to protect women and girls from this form of violence, and to end impunity;

5. *Also urges* States to complement punitive measures with awareness-raising and educational activities designed to promote a process of consensus towards the elimination of female genital mutilations, and further urges States to protect and support women and girls who have been subjected to female genital mutilations and those at risk, including by developing social and psychological support services and care, and to take measures to improve their health, including sexual and reproductive health, in order to assist women and girls who are subjected to the practice;

6. *Further urges* States to promote gender-sensitive, empowering educational processes by, as appropriate, reviewing and revising school curricula, educational materials and teacher-training programmes and elaborating policies and programmes of zero tolerance for violence against girls, including

female genital mutilations, and to further integrate a comprehensive understanding of the causes and consequences of gender-based violence and discrimination against women and girls into education and training curricula at all levels;

7. *Calls upon* States to ensure that national action plans and strategies on the elimination of female genital mutilations are comprehensive and multi-disciplinary in scope and incorporate clear targets and indicators for the effective monitoring, impact assessment and coordination of programmes among all stakeholders;

8. *Urges* States to take, within the general framework of integration policies and in consultation with affected communities, effective and specific targeted measures for refugee women and women migrants and their communities in order to protect girls from female genital mutilations, including when the practice occurs outside the country of residence;

9. *Calls upon* States to develop information and awareness-raising campaigns and programmes to systematically reach the general public, relevant professionals, families and communities, including through the media and featuring television and radio discussions, on the elimination of female genital mutilations;

10. *Urges* States to pursue a comprehensive, culturally sensitive, systematic approach that incorporates a social perspective and is based on human rights and gender-equality principles in providing education and training to families, local community leaders and members of all professions relevant to the protection and empowerment of women and girls in order to increase awareness of and commitment to the elimination of female genital mutilations;

11. *Also urges* States to ensure the national implementation of international and regional commitments and obligations undertaken as States parties to various international instruments protecting the full enjoyment of all human rights and the fundamental freedoms of women and girls;

12. *Calls upon* States to develop policies and regulations to ensure the effective implementation of national legislative frameworks on eliminating discrimination and violence against women and girls, in particular female genital mutilations, and to put in place adequate accountability mechanisms at the national and local levels to monitor adherence to and implementation of these legislative frameworks;

13. *Also calls upon* States to develop unified methods and standards for the collection of data on all forms of discrimination and violence against girls, especially forms that are underdocumented, such as female genital mutilations, and to develop

additional indicators to effectively measure progress in eliminating the practice;

14. *Urges* States to allocate sufficient resources to the implementation of policies and programmes and legislative frameworks aimed at eliminating female genital mutilations;

15. *Calls upon* States to develop, support and implement comprehensive and integrated strategies for the prevention of female genital mutilations, including the training of social workers, medical personnel, community and religious leaders and relevant professionals, and to ensure that they provide competent, supportive services and care to women and girls who are at risk of or who have undergone female genital mutilations, and encourage them to report to the appropriate authorities cases in which they believe women or girls are at risk;

16. *Also calls upon* States to support, as part of a comprehensive approach to eliminate female genital mutilations, programmes that engage local community practitioners of female genital mutilations in community-based initiatives for the abandonment of the practice, including, where relevant, the identification by communities of alternative livelihoods for them;

17. *Calls upon* the international community, the relevant United Nations entities and civil society and international financial institutions to continue to actively support, through the allocation of increased financial resources and technical assistance, targeted comprehensive programmes that address the needs and priorities of women and girls at risk of or subjected to female genital mutilations;

18. *Calls upon* the international community to strongly support, including through increased financial support, a second phase of the United Nations Population Fund-United Nations Children's Fund Joint Programme on Female Genital Mutilation/Cutting: Accelerating Change, which is currently due to end in December 2013, as well as national programmes focused on the elimination of female genital mutilations;

19. *Stresses* that some progress has been made in combating female genital mutilations in a number of countries using a common coordinated approach that promotes positive social change at the community, national, regional and international levels, and recalls the goal set out in the United Nations inter-agency statement15 that female genital mutilations be eliminated within a generation, with some of the main achievements being obtained by 2015, in line with the Millennium Development Goals;

20. *Encourages* men and boys to take positive initiatives and to work in partnership with women and girls

to combat violence and discriminatory practices against women and girls, in particular female genital mutilations, through networks, peer programmes, information campaigns and training programmes;

21. *Calls upon* States, the United Nations system, civil society and all stakeholders to continue to observe 6 February as the International Day of Zero Tolerance for Female Genital Mutilation and to use the day to enhance awareness-raising campaigns and to take concrete actions against female genital mutilations;

22. *Requests* the Secretary-General to ensure that all relevant organizations and bodies of the United Nations system, in particular the United Nations Population Fund, the United Nations Children's Fund, the United Nations Entity for Gender Equality and the Empowerment of Women (UN-Women), the World Health Organization, the United Nations Educational, Scientific and Cultural Organization, the United Nations Development Programme and the Office of the United Nations High Commissioner for Human Rights, individually and collectively, take into account the protection and promotion of the rights of women and girls against female genital mutilations in their country programmes, as appropriate and in accordance with national priorities, in order to further strengthen their efforts in this regard;

23. *Also requests* the Secretary-General to submit to the General Assembly, at its sixty-ninth session, an in-depth multidisciplinary report on the root causes of and contributing factors to the practice of female genital mutilations, its prevalence worldwide and its impact on women and girls, including evidence and data, analysis of progress made to date and action-oriented recommendations for eliminating this practice on the basis of information provided by Member States, relevant actors of the United Nations system working on the issue and other relevant stakeholders.

60th plenary meeting
20 December 2012

SEE ALSO   *Child Health; Gender and Health; Health in the WHO African Region; Maternal and Infant Health; Post-Traumatic Stress Syndrome; Stigma*

BIBLIOGRAPHY

Books

Abusharaf, Rogaia Mustafa. *Transforming Displaced Women in the Sudan: Politics and the Body in a Squatter Settlement.* Chicago: University of Chicago Press, 2009.

Denniston, George C., Frederick M. Hodges, and Marilyn Fayre Milos, eds. *Circumcision and Human Rights.* New York: Springer, 2009.

Denniston, George C., Frederick M. Hodges, and Marilyn Fayre Milos, eds. *Genital Autonomy: Protecting Personal Choice.* New York: Springer, 2010.

Jackson, J. E. "Pain and Bodies," in *A Companion to the Anthropology of the Body and Embodiment,* edited by Frances E. Mascia-Lees, 370–387. Chichester, UK: Wiley-Blackwell, 2011.

Jordan, L. *A Service Coordination Guide: Improving the Health Care of Women and Girls Affected by Female Genital Mutilation.* Victoria, BC: Family Planning Victoria, 2012.

UNICEF. *Female Genital Mutilation/Cutting: A Statistical Overview and Exploration of the Dynamics of Change.* New York: UNICEF Statistics and Monitoring Section, Division of Policy and Strategy, 2013. Available online at http://www.unicef.org/publications/index_69875.html (accessed March 3, 2015).

UNICEF Innocenti Research Centre. *Innocenti Insight: The Dynamics of Social Change. Towards the Abandonment of Female Genital Mutilation/Cutting in Five African Countries.* Florence, Italy: UNICEF Innocenti Research Centre, 2010. Available online at http://www.unicef-irc.org/publications/618 (accessed March 3, 2015).

Periodicals

Boyden, J., A. Pankhurst, and Y. Tafere, "Child Protection and Harmful Traditional Practice: Female Early Marriage and Genital Modification in Ethiopia." *Development in Practice.* Special Issue: *Child Protection in Development* 22, no. 4 (June 2012): 510–522.

Johnsdotter, S., and B. Essen. "Genitals and Ethnicity: The Politics of Genital Modifications." *Reproductive Health Matters* 18, no. 35 (May 2010): 29–37.

Kaplan-Marcusan, Adriana, et al. "Perception of Primary Health Professionals about Female Genital Mutilation: From Healthcare to Intercultural Competence." *BMC Health Service Research* 9, no. 11 (January 15, 2009): doi:10.1186/1472-6963-9-11.

Perez, Guillermo Martinez, and Harriet Namulondo. "Elongation of Labia Minora in Uganda: Including Baganda Men in a Risk Reduction Education Programme." *Health and Sexuality: An International Journal for Research, Intervention and Care* 13, no. 1 (January 2011): 45–57.

Perez, Guillermo Martinez, Harriet Namulondo, and Concepcion Tomas Aznar. "Labia Minora Elongation as Understood by Baganda Male and Female Adolescents in Uganda." *Culture, Health and Sexuality: An International Journal for Research, Intervention and Care* 15, no. 10 (2013): 1191–1205.

WORLDMARK GLOBAL HEALTH AND MEDICINE ISSUES

UNAIDS, UNICEF, and WHO. *Global AIDS Response Reporting 2014: Construction of Core Indicators for Monitoring the 2011 United Nations Political Declaration on HIV and AIDS.* Geneva: Joint United Nations Programme on HIV/AIDS (UNAIDS), January 2014.

WHO and UNAIDS. *Joint Strategic Action Framework to Accelerate the Scale-Up of Voluntary Medical Male Circumcision for HIV Prevention in Eastern and Southern Africa 2012–2016.* Geneva: Joint United Nations Programme on HIV/AIDS (UNAIDS), November 2011.

Websites

"Benefits of Infant Circumcision Outweigh Risks, Top Pediatrics Group Says." *CNN*, August 27, 2012. http://www.cnn.com/2012/08/27/health/circumcision-policy/ (accessed March 1, 2015).

Elyas, Haffiya. "A Change of Concept towards FGM in Sudan." *Sudan Vision*, August 3, 2014. http://news.sudanvisiondaily.com/details.html?rsnpid=238691 (accessed March 1, 2015).

"Female Genital Mutilation." *UNICEF.* http://www.who.int/entity/mediacentre/factsheets/fs241/en/index.html (accessed January 20, 2015).

"Female Genital Mutilation." *World Health Organization (WHO).* http://www.who.int/entity/mediacentre/factsheets/fs241/en/index.html (accessed January 20, 2015).

"Voluntary Medical Male Circumcision for HIV Prevention," Fact Sheet. *World Health Organization (WHO)*, July 2012. http://www.who.int/hiv/topics/malecircumcision/fact_sheet/en/ (accessed May 28, 2015).

"WHO Progress Brief—Voluntary Medical Male Circumcision for HIV Prevention in Priority Countries of East and Southern Africa." *World Health Organization (WHO)*, July 2014. http://www.who.int/hiv/topics/malecircumcision/male-circumcision-info-2014/en// (accessed March 3, 2015).

Pamela V. Michaels

Global Health Initiatives

🌐 Introduction

Global health initiatives (GHIs) are large-scale models of development assistance, where finance and expertise from international partnerships are brought to bear upon specific health problems affecting low- and middle-income countries.

The aim of GHIs is to reduce morbidity (illness) and mortality (deaths) from diseases such as human immuno-deficiency virus/acquired immunodeficiency syndrome (HIV/AIDS) and malaria, and to improve health systems in countries where the necessary infrastructure is lacking. GHIs involve partnerships between governments and nongovernmental organizations such as the World Health Organization (WHO) and the World Bank. Such initiatives often leverage significant amounts of money and other resources.

The WHO states that all human beings have a right to the highest possible standard of health. Advances in both medical research and public health in the 20th century provide the tools to help achieve this, yet there are still massive inequities in health around the world to be addressed. For instance, life expectancy in the 38 poorest countries in the world is only around 49 years. Although life expectancy had been on the increase in all countries around the world until about 1990, the spread of HIV/AIDS caused a sharp decrease in several sub-Saharan African countries.

GHIs are recently possible for several key reasons. In the 21st century, extensive transport and communications systems mean that there are few truly remote places on the planet. Health problems and disease do not recognize national borders, with infectious diseases such as Ebola, HIV, and severe acute respiratory syndrome (SARS) spreading far from their origins. Health issues are thus increasingly global, rather than national.

Then there is the ethical dimension. People are increasingly aware of problems such as high childhood mortality in poorer countries from diseases that are preventable and want charitable donations used wisely and effectively to alleviate this suffering. Both factors create an impetus for the creation and execution of GHIs.

Furthermore, health cannot be separated from economic and social development. High infant and maternal mortality mean fewer productive adults contributing to a country's economy, which can create political instability and a continuing need for aid from richer countries. Health, essential as it is to both the individual and society at large, does not always receive the political and financial support it should, if left to an individual government. Effective implementation of plans may only occur if organizations with a global reach become involved. These factors all justify supporting the collective effort of GHIs to improve health wherever the need for improvement is most urgent.

GHIs tend to involve many different players and each initiative may have a different array of stakeholders. A GHI always needs to work closely with the authorities in the country, or countries, affected by the health issue being targeted. In addition to governments, international organizations may be involved, some of which are public, some private. The WHO, acting as an agency of the United Nations (UN), often is involved, as is the United Nations Children's Fund (UNICEF) or the UN Program on HIV/AIDS (UNAIDS). Finance for GHIs often originates from development banks, such as the World Bank. Bilateral agencies, which are development assistance agencies in developed countries working directly with a developing nation, also play a major role in GHIs. Examples include the U.S. Agency for International Development (UNAID) and the Australian Agency for International Development. Nongovernmental foundations, such as the Rockefeller Foundation and the Bill & Melinda Gates Foundation, also may play an important role. Additionally, there are thousands of different nongovernmental organizations (NGOs) of varying sizes with the aim of improving health in the developing world, such as Save the Children and Médicins Sans

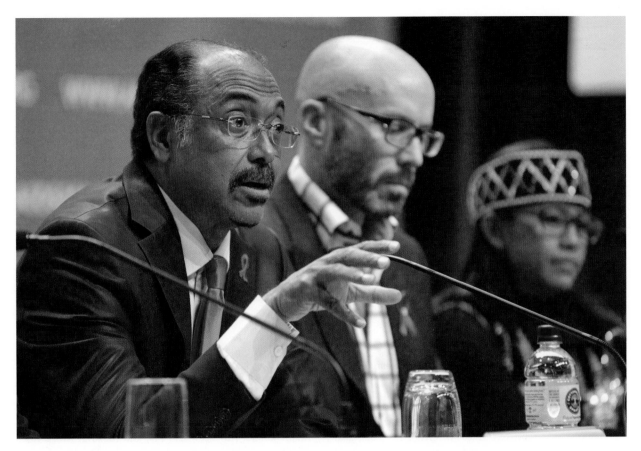

UNAIDS Executive Director Michel Sidibé from Mali speaks at a press conference during the 20th International AIDS Conference at the Melbourne Convention and Exhibition Centre in Melbourne on July 20, 2014. © *Esther Lim/Getty Images.*

Frontières (MSF, or Doctors Without Borders). There are also, increasingly, public-private partnerships that join together for cooperative work on a global health problem. Each player may take one or more roles, such as channeling finance, providing expertise, or engaging in advocacy work.

Examples of notable GHIs include the President's Emergency Plan for AIDS Relief (PEPFAR); the Global Fund to Fight AIDS, Tuberculosis and Malaria; the World Bank Multi-country AIDS Program; and the Gavi Alliance. The overall aim of these GHIs is to raise and distribute funding and coordinate action in countries where it is needed most. However, because there is no one model for how a GHI operates, their organizational structures, and the approaches they use to achieve their aims and objectives, differ widely. In the case of a GHI like PEPFAR, the U.S. government has changed its goals over time from being an agency focused on emergency response to one of promoting partnerships with countries facing HIV/AIDS epidemics. One of PEPFAR's goals has been to improve access to antiretroviral treatment (ART). The graphic shows the increasing amount of funding and number of people reached by PEPFAR from 2004 to 2012.

⊕ Historical Background

The ideal of acting globally to tackle global health problems goes back more than 150 years, with the first international conference, on cholera, taking place in 1851. Following many more such meetings, the International Office of Public Hygiene was set up in Paris in 1909, to be followed by the establishment of the League of Nations Health Office in Geneva in 1920. The focus of these early efforts on global health was giving technical advice to developing nations and setting up standards on drugs and vaccines.

WHO and UNICEF

Various agencies of the United Nations, including the WHO and UNICEF, were set up following World War II (1939–1945). During the postwar period, the focus of GHIs shifted toward helping to build health-care capacity in developing countries, particularly previous colonies that were becoming newly independent. Efforts also were directed toward reducing and even eradicating infectious disease.

In 1966, the WHO launched the most ambitious global program to date, namely the eradication

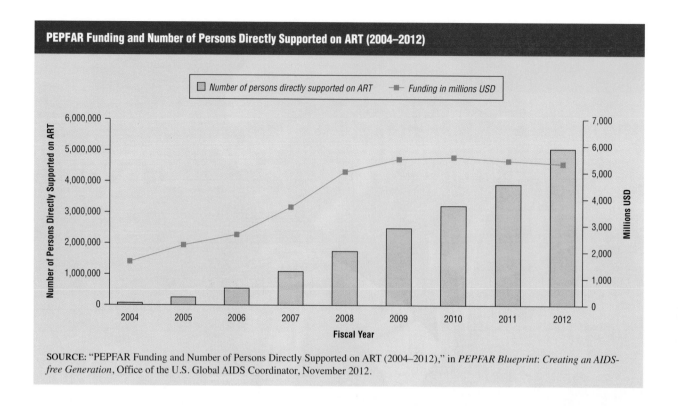

PEPFAR Funding and Number of Persons Directly Supported on ART (2004–2012)

SOURCE: "PEPFAR Funding and Number of Persons Directly Supported on ART (2004–2012)," in *PEPFAR Blueprint: Creating an AIDS-free Generation*, Office of the U.S. Global AIDS Coordinator, November 2012.

of smallpox. After several years of effort, the last case of smallpox was reported in 1978. Other projects, also led by the WHO, have focused upon the eradication of polio, lymphatic filariasis (commonly known as elephantiasis), and onchocerciasis (river blindness) and on the control of malaria and leprosy. All these diseases have a huge impact in the poorest countries in the world.

There was also a new focus upon children's health. Child survival campaigns, led by UNICEF, focused upon the so-called GOBI principles (growth monitoring, oral rehydration, breast-feeding, immunization). USAID became closely involved in the child survival agenda, as did other bilateral agencies and the World Bank.

Subsequent Developments

In the late 1980s, critics asserted that GHIs were not achieving their goals. They claimed that the GHI approach was disjointed and not grounded in a more systemic view of how to improve health services. As a result, various agencies focused on health sector reform. In 1993, the World Bank's "World Development Report" stated that the best approach to decision making on investing in health needed to be based upon cost-effectiveness analysis. This framework became the foundation for action among many of the key players in global health.

In the mid-1990s, the GHI focus was on HIV/AIDS and the devastation it was bringing to populations in sub-Saharan Africa. Many GHIs directed efforts toward making sure that antiretroviral drugs were made available by the pharmaceutical companies to those who

needed them. At the same time, GHIs targeted two other major killers, tuberculosis (TB) and malaria. More cases of TB were identified and treated by DOTS (directly observed therapy, short-course). Efforts at malaria control included provision of insecticide treated bed nets and more intensive use of effective anti-malarial drugs.

⊕ Impacts and Issues

There are many urgent health issues in the world, from HIV/AIDS and women's health to malnutrition and the possibility of emerging pandemics. Thus, there are competing, and diverse, calls on the resources of those who contribute to GHIs. There has to be some way of setting an agenda. One important approach involves the World Health Assembly, held by the WHO in Geneva each year. Here health ministers from the 194 WHO member states discuss health matters and pass resolutions to be acted upon. Such resolutions have formed the basis for important GHIs, such as smallpox eradication.

Sometimes it is a report, or a program action by the WHO, or a bilateral or multilateral development agency or health-oriented NGO that triggers GHI activity. One example was the World Bank's 1993 "World Development Report," a key document that was discussed in detail worldwide. It influenced the next generation of World Bank–funded health projects and those led by other development organizations also.

New sources of funding also can drive the GHI agenda. The Bill & Melinda Gates Foundation has provided financing to invest heavily in spreading medical technologies to developing nations to meet their health needs. In 2012, the foundation paid out nearly $4 billion on projects. The grants target four areas: infectious disease, reproductive health, vaccines, and scientific discovery. The foundation's investment in immunization and development of HIV vaccines has pushed the HIV/AIDS issue higher up the global health agenda.

In addition, there are situations where popular action, led by advocates for health, may focus attention on an issue. For instance, MSF has led the campaign for making AIDS treatment more widely available, which necessitated pressuring the pharmaceutical industry to make antiretroviral drugs more affordable. Another example is the work of Partners in Health in setting an agenda in TB and HIV. Working in Rwanda, Peru, and Haiti, researchers led by the American physician and anthropologist Paul Farmer (1959–), based at Harvard University, have championed a practical model of treating drug-resistant TB and HIV at lower cost, thereby reversing received opinion that this was not possible in resource-poor settings.

Issues of Governance

Governance is a set of rules and principles accepted by most of the key players in an organization. One criticism of GHIs is that financing and enthusiasm for projects has grown much faster than governance on a global level and that this is a significant barrier to effective collective action to improve human health. Interest in global health governance has grown since the 1990s and has been influenced by three main approaches that have led to the emergence of a number of GHIs.

The Biomedical Model Medical science has made huge strides since the 1960s, which has led to the notion that the application of science can solve the biggest global health problems such as TB, HIV/AIDS, and malaria, if only sufficient funds are invested in research. The belief in the power of science has inspired the Bill & Melinda Gates Foundation and many other global health institutions, all of which have invested large sums in research in the quest for a technical fix.

From the late 1990s, there have been a number of science-driven public-private partnership initiatives, such as the nonprofit Medicines for Malaria Venture, with its strong focus upon drug discovery. The biomedical approach to global health governance has led to the neglect of areas where complex interventions are required. Thus, vaccine development is favored over improvements in sanitation, even where the latter might bring more benefit, at least in the short term. In 2011, the Gates Foundation seemed to recognize this, when it assigned $10 million for innovative sanitation solutions in poor urban areas.

The Evidence-Based Approach Closely aligned to the biomedical model, the evidence-based approach to global health relies heavily on knowledge, procedure, and best practice. Many in the field believe that lack of accurate and complete health information in resource-poor countries is a major barrier to better health. This has led to development of evidence-based policies in some GHIs.

One example is the Global Burden of Disease Project, set up in 1998, with its focus upon health metrics, which were to be used to devise solutions to health problems. Science and evidence-based approaches to global health have been very influential in establishing health priorities. It can be argued that this stops GHIs from becoming too much driven by opinion and belief, and is therefore fairer to all concerned.

Social Determinants of Health It should not be forgotten that the greatest advances in public health in the 20th century owed as much to social reforms, such as improved nutrition, sanitation, and education, as to scientific research. In many parts of the world, living conditions are as poor as they were in Western countries before these improvements were introduced. Life expectancies in these regions reflect this.

It can therefore be argued that a broader approach to global health governance will achieve more than a narrow scientific focus. Health inequity has been the starting point for those who are seeking to reform and develop global health governance. They argue for a move away from fighting specific diseases and toward a more holistic approach to health. This would involve health policy being more closely integrated with foreign and economic policy. In short, the social determinant approach brings a political dimension to GHIs.

These are the arguments put forward by the WHO Commission on Social Determinants of Health (CSDH), which would like to see the WHO at the heart of global health governance. The WHO is the most globally representative voice, with its 194 member states, but may not be the most powerful, given the growing influence of organizations such as the World Bank. There have been calls to make the UN system more democratic, more accountable, and less influenced by the interests of richer nations.

Proliferation of GHIs There has been rapid growth in GHIs since the beginning of the 21st century, mainly driven by the three approaches to governance described above. They focus on specific diseases, technologies, health behaviors, or more specific functions such as channeling funding efforts or advocacy. Some GHIs are characterized more by who the key players are. For instance, there are the charities, the foundations, the WHO, and UNICEF, as well as the pharmaceutical and food industries. Some of these players combine in partnerships for specific purposes.

With so many different organizations and so much investment involved in global health, it has become difficult to discern what is being achieved and what governance principles these GHIs actually have in common. It is likely that there are competing and

FOCUS ON GAVI, THE VACCINE ALLIANCE

There is no typical GHI, but Gavi, the Vaccine Alliance (also known as the Global Alliance for Vaccines and Immunisation) illustrates many features of how such organizations are set up and operate. Gavi started in 2000, with a $750 million five-year pledge from the Bill & Melinda Gates Foundation. Its mission is to increase access to immunization in poor countries, thereby saving children's lives and protecting their health. This GHI works toward redressing the global inequities in access to new and underused vaccines, which is something that is taken for granted in richer nations.

Around the end of the 20th century, global immunization rates were beginning to level off, despite efforts by the Expanded Programme on Immunization (EPI), a program of the WHO that was set up in 1974 and continues as of 2015. There were still 30 million children in poor countries at risk of disease because they had not been immunized against common diseases. This was primarily because the six EPI vaccines were deemed too expensive in many countries.

Since 2000, support from Gavi's donors has allowed immunization of nearly 500 million children, which had saved an estimated 7 million lives by early 2015. Seventy-three of the world's poorest countries are covered by Gavi. The key stakeholders involved in Gavi are the WHO, UNICEF, the World Bank, the Bill & Melinda Gates Foundation, national governments, the vaccine industry, research and technical institutes, and the private sector. In early 2015, nine countries were committed to funding Gavi through yearly grants: Australia, France, Italy, the Netherlands, Norway, Spain, Sweden, South Africa, and the United Kingdom. A grant from Brazil was pending as of June 2015. Funding of $8.2 billion from 2000–2013 supported 11 vaccines, including those against rotavirus and pneumococcal disease, which are the leading preventable causes of diarrhea and pneumonia, and human papillomavirus (HPV), which causes cervical cancer.

According to Gavi's 2013 progress report, that year there were more Gavi-supported campaigns than in any single year since 2000, with 41 new projects started. In 2000, only one low-income country was routinely immunizing against *Haemophilus influenzae* type B (Hib)—the bacteria that cause meningitis and pneumonia—and hepatitis B. However, according to the report, by 2013 all low-income countries except one had introduced a pentavalent vaccine, a combination of five vaccines that protects against Hib, hepatitis B, diphtheria, tetanus, and pertussis (whooping cough). Gavi also supported six rotavirus introductions and 14 pneumococcal launches. The alliance also started to fund two vaccines that will have a significant impact on women and children's health. By the end of 2013, six countries were set to enter HPV demonstration projects, and Rwanda became the first Gavi-supported country to introduce the measles vaccine.

Child mortality fell from 78 to 73 births per 1,000 live births in countries supported by Gavi. Part of this decrease is because of the introduction of vaccines. Gavi is on track to reduce child mortality to 68 per 1,000 live births by 2015. Projections suggest that by the end of 2010, Gavi had averted 4 million deaths and another 2.2 million by the end of 2013. In 2013, around 48 million children had been immunized with Gavi-supported vaccines. The alliance is expecting to reach its target of immunizing 243 million children between 2011 and 2015 across all its vaccines programs. There is still much to do, because in 2012, 6.6 million children around the world died before the age of five and, according to the WHO, 1.5 million of these deaths would have been preventable by vaccination.

counterproductive activities, gaps, and overlaps, because there is no overall coherent view or strategy.

Some blame for the fragmentation of the GHI concept has been laid at the door of the WHO for its weak mandate, bureaucracy, lack of focus, and limited finances. There is a need for a centralized and strong leadership, which can set priorities and allocate resources accordingly. Without this, GHIs cannot reach their full potential, and the health aspirations laid out by the WHO itself cannot be fulfilled.

⊕ Future Implications

Changing Health Patterns

The players in GHIs must be flexible enough to respond quickly to changing health priorities. Smallpox has been eradicated, and polio has become rare, but infectious disease will always be an important health issue. In the 2010s, the threat comes from new and emerging infectious diseases such as Ebola, SARS, and pandemic flu. New tools may be needed to deal with these, but it is also important to build on knowledge gained from previous work on tackling infection. Preparedness for surveillance, prevention, and treatment of these new infectious diseases is vital.

Thus far, the main focus of GHIs has been on infectious disease. However, noncommunicable diseases, including diabetes, obesity, cancer, and heart disease, are becoming increasingly significant in developing countries, mainly as a result of the industrialization of these regions and the lifestyle changes it brings. The focus of GHIs to target these health conditions needs to be upon education and lifestyle change focused on nutrition and physical activity rather than on improving sanitation and access to vaccination.

Health Systems and Research

Improving global health requires far more than scientific advances, although the advent of an effective vaccine for HIV or malaria would clearly be an important step

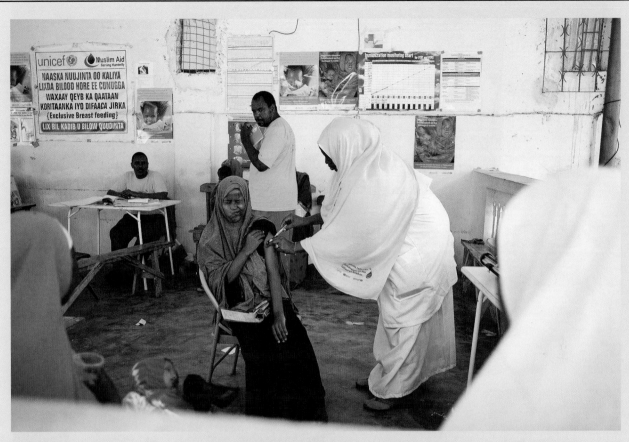

A pregnant Somali woman receives a tetanus injection at a clinic in Mogadishu, Somalia. Somali children under one year of age will now receive the pentavalent vaccine protecting against diphtheria, tetanus, pertussis, hepatitis B, and *Haemophilus influenzae* type B (Hib). The initiative was launched by Gavi, UNICEF, and the WHO. Somalia has one of the lowest immunization rates in the world.
© *Carl de Souza/Getty Images.*

forward. Development agencies need to help countries build health systems that work more effectively. Better organization and management, better training for staff and, above all, consistent financing are all essential so that countries can deliver better health care to their populations. This is perhaps a more ambitious aim than fighting a specific disease and requires strong leadership to achieve progress.

There is also a need for research efforts to fill knowledge gaps that hinder prevention and treatment of common conditions such as malaria, HIV/AIDS, and TB. Not only are products such as vaccines required, but operational aspects need to be developed to ensure that treatments get to those who need them and that they are used to maximum effectiveness.

SEE ALSO *Epidemiology: Surveillance for Emerging Infectious Diseases; Health as a Human Right and Health-Care Access; Health-Related Education and Information Access; HIV/AIDS; Maternal and Infant Health; Médicins Sans Frontières; NGOs and Health Care: Deliverance or Dependence; Pharmaceutical Research, Testing, and Access; Sanitation and Hygiene; Social Theory and Global Health; Tobacco Use; Universal Health Coverage; Vaccine-Preventable Diseases; Vaccines; World Health Organization: Organization, Funding and Enforcement Powers*

BIBLIOGRAPHY

Books

Kidder, Tracy, and Michael French. *Mountains beyond Mountains: The Quest of Dr. Paul Farmer, a Man Who Would Cure the World.* New York: Delacorte Press, 2013.

McInnes, Colin, and Kelley Lee. *Global Health and International Relations.* Cambridge, UK: Polity, 2012.

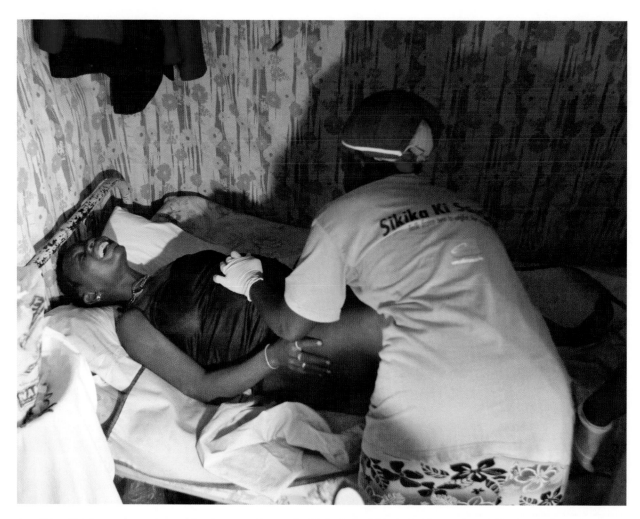

A traditional birth attendant assists a patient into a position to give birth, during labor in the Korogocho neighborhood of Nairobi, Kenya. In the first decade of the 2000s, billions of dollars were spent trying to save mothers in developing countries using strategies deemed essential by the United Nations (UN). But in two large analyses of maternal health programs—including one conducted by the UN itself— the efforts appeared almost useless, raising troubling questions about how billions of dollars are spent. Critics called for the pricey global initiatives to be significantly overhauled. © *Khalil Senosi/AP Photo.*

Skolnik, Richard L. *Essentials of Global Health.* Sudbury, MA: Jones and Bartlett, 2008.

Periodicals

Biesma, Regien, et al. "The Effects of GHIs on Country Health Systems: A Review of the Evidence from HIV/AIDS Control." *Health Policy and Planning* 24, no. 4 (December 2011): 239–252.

Marchal, Bruno, Anna Cavalli, and Guy Kegels. "Global Health Actors Claim to Support Health System Strengthening—Is This Reality or Rhetoric?" *PLoS Medicine* 6, no. 4 (April 2009): e 10000059. Available online at http://www .plosmedicine.org/article/info%3Adoi% 2F10.1371%2Fjournal.pmed.1000059 (accessed January 9, 2015).

Ravishankar, Nirmala, et al. "Tracking Development Assistance for Health from 1990–2007." *The Lancet* 373, no. 9681 (June 2009): 2113–2124.

Websites

"The GAVI Alliance 2013 Annual Progress Report." *Gavi: The Vaccine Alliance,* June 2014. http://gavipro gressreport.org/2013/ (accessed April 9, 2015).

"Global Health Initiatives." *World Health Organization.* http://www.who.int/trade/glossary/story040/ en# (accessed January 9, 2015).

"PEPFAR: A Decade of Saving Lives." *U.S. Embassy.* http://iipdigital.usembassy.gov/st/english/ pamphlet/2013/09/20130917283048. html#axzz3bTfNGJG6 (accessed May 28, 2015).

Susan Aldridge

Health as a Human Right and Health-Care Access

⊕ Introduction

The international community largely has come to recognize health care as a fundamental human right. Yet access to medical treatment varies considerably in practice depending on a country's political system and level of economic development. All wealthy industrialized nations except the United States have established universal health-care systems aiming to make medical treatment accessible to all of their population. Conversely, people inhabiting developing countries frequently have minimal or no access to health care.

Essential medicines are unavailable to a third of the world's population, approximately 2.4 billion people. Hundreds of millions of people in rural regions of developing nations will never or rarely visit a doctor in their lifetimes. Millions die annually from a host of treatable or preventable medical problems, including human immunodeficiency virus/acquired immune deficiency syndrome (HIV/AIDS), malaria, tuberculosis, tropical diseases, and malnutrition.

Although health care increasingly is identified as a legal right under international human rights law, often it is an unenforceable right because of legal or practical constraints. In light of this obstacle, health care is effectively more of an aspiration than a right for people living in countries without universal health care systems. As the World Health Organization (WHO) has observed, "there seems to be little relation between the ratification of international treaties and the existence of operational national essential medicine policies and programmes."

Universal health care has been implemented through various public policy frameworks in industrialized nations as diverse as Canada, France, Japan, and Mexico. Universal health-care systems are far from uniform, as they may give a greater or lesser role to the government and the private sector in the funding and provision of medical treatment. The case of the United States, where health care remains inaccessible to many due to its substantial cost, illustrates how realizing universal health care partly depends on regulating the price of medical insurance, drugs, and services to make them affordable to all.

⊕ Historical Background

National health-care systems already existed in certain countries prior to the rise of the modern human rights movement in the post–World War II era. The origins of national health-care systems are traceable to the emergence of the modern welfare state in the late 19th century. Otto von Bismarck (1815–1898), the influential German chancellor, was a leading figure behind this development: he backed a Sickness Insurance Law (1883) that became the world's first national health-care system. The reform created a mandatory medical insurance program jointly funded by employers and workers. Historians have suggested various reasons why Bismarck, a rather conservative aristocrat, supported the institution of a welfare state, including his effort to unify the German people, desire to placate his left-wing opposition, and the patrician principle of noblesse oblige that led certain European aristocrats to favor public assistance programs, as noted by Seymour Martin Lipset. The "Bismarck model" eventually became an example for the universal health-care systems of numerous nations worldwide.

After the landmark Universal Declaration of Human Rights of 1948, the modern human rights movement has aimed to define health care as a fundamental human right. The declaration stresses that "everyone has the right to a standard of living adequate for the health and well-being of himself and of his family, including … medical care." While the declaration is not a binding treaty, it is a statement of ideal human rights standards that has served as a stepping-stone for the modern human rights movement. Subsequent international treaties likewise have identified health care as a human right.

International Human Rights Treaties

The most significant treaty relating to health care may be the International Covenant on Economic, Social and

Cultural Rights (ICESCR), which aims to promote "the inherent dignity of the human person," as well as "freedom from fear and want." The covenant entered into force in 1976. A total of 162 countries had adhered to this treaty as of 2014.

Article 12 of the ICESCR stipulates that states adhering to its provisions "recognize the right of everyone to the enjoyment of the highest attainable standard of physical and mental health." It goes on to identify four categories of steps to be addressed by states party to the treaty: (1) reducing stillbirths, infant mortality, and problems affecting the healthy development of children; (2) improving "environmental and industrial hygiene"; (3) preventing, treating, and controlling "epidemic, endemic, occupational and other diseases"; and (4) creating "conditions which would assure to all medical service and medical attention in the event of sickness." Article 7(b) also provides a right to "safe and healthy working conditions."

In practice, however, the ICESCR is less a binding treaty than a declaration of ideal rights and aspirations, much like the Universal Declaration of Human Rights.

THE UN MILLENNIUM DEVELOPMENT GOALS

In 2000, the United Nations adopted eight major Millennium Development Goals (MDGs), ranging from halving extreme poverty to improving basic public health. In particular, the following objectives pertain to medical care:

1. Goal 4: Reduce by two-thirds the mortality rate of children under 5 years old by 2015
2. Goal 5: Improve maternal health by reducing the maternal mortality ratio by three-quarters and achieving universal access to reproductive care by 2015
3. Goal 6: Halt and reverse the spread or incidence of HIV/AIDS, malaria, and other major diseases by 2015; and achieve universal access to treatment for HIV/AIDS by 2010

Various experts such as Jeffrey D. Sachs believe that the progress made toward realizing the MDGs is encouraging even though many of the targets will not be met by the 2015 deadline. Scores of people continue to live in extreme poverty with no or minimal health care. For example, the maternal mortality rate declined from 380 deaths per 100,000 live births in 1990 to 210 deaths by 2013, still far below the target of 100 deaths by 2015. Notable improvements in the prevention and treatment of malaria have otherwise been achieved due to the provision of medicine and insecticide-treated bed nets to destitute persons in sub-Saharan Africa. Malaria nonetheless claimed 627,000 lives in 2012, 80 percent being children under five years old.

It is noteworthy that the MDGs regarding health care are not entirely the first of their kind. Another ambitious project, the Ottawa Charter for Health Promotion of 1986, illustratively aimed to achieve "health for all" by 2000.

Article 2 of the ICESCR notably indicates that a state adhering to the treaty must take steps "to the maximum of its available resources" in view of "achieving progressively the full realization of the rights recognized in the [treaty]." This clause signifies that the obligation to provide health care under the treaty is limited by a state's economic and financial capabilities. The ICESCR's impact thus seems relatively modest, as it officially has been adopted by a large number of developing countries whose population has little or no access to medical treatment.

Certain legal experts may therefore argue that the ICESCR does not technically create a human right to health care because a veritable socioeconomic right would entail a precise duty on the part of a government to provide medical treatment. A general duty to strive to offer health care without a definite timeframe to fulfill that obligation may be considered by some as too vague to constitute a genuine right.

In addition, the ICESCR provides no concrete remedy in case states fail to meet their duty to provide health care under the treaty: Article 16 merely stipulates that states must submit regular reports to the United Nations (UN) indicating the progress achieved toward meeting the treaty's objectives. The Committee on Economic, Social and Cultural Rights was created in 1985 to monitor compliance with the treaty. Nevertheless, the committee only can issue reports with recommendations and lacks the authority to bind states party to the ICESCR to provide medical treatment to their population. Accordingly, certain scholars also may deem that because the provisions of the ICESCR are unenforceable, they do not truly create a right to health care in light of the longstanding legal principle known as *ubi jus ibi remedium* (i.e., where there is a right, there is a remedy).

However, other legal experts such as Cass R. Sunstein (1954–) find it appropriate for socioeconomic rights to be prescriptive or aspirational in nature. That is arguably the dominant perspective, as suggested by the adoption of the ICESCR by numerous countries. Various other international human rights treaties or declarations similarly identify health care as a fundamental right, including the Convention on the Rights of the Child, Convention against All Forms of Discrimination against Women, African Charter on Human and People's Rights, Additional Protocol to the American Convention on Human Rights, European Social Charter, and Cairo Declaration on Human Rights in Islam. Such international legal instruments demonstrate a growing consensus among the international community about the recognition of health care as a human right.

National Human Rights Standards Human rights law does not only encompass international treaties but also domestic legal standards. An overview of health care as a human right therefore entails considering how various countries approach the issue in their own legal systems.

Overall, national constitutions created since the 20th century reflect a relatively stronger commitment to socio-economic rights such as health care, education, or housing, as suggested by research from Sunstein, Avi Ben-Bassat, and Mohi Dahan. Still, there is not a statistically significant relationship between the age of a constitution and the recognition of socioeconomic rights, perhaps because most national constitutions can be amended rather easily based on rising support for such rights.

⊕ Impacts and Issues

In the modern Western world, health care generally is considered a fundamental human right in all countries except the United States, which stands out as the sole Western democracy having refused to ratify the ICESCR. Access to health care seldom is identified as a "human right" issue in the United States, unlike in European nations, Canada, Australia, and New Zealand. By contrast to the United States, these Western countries have had universal health-care systems for decades and generally regard medical treatment as a "human right," not only under international treaties or declarations but also under their own domestic laws.

This exception reflects a broader American pattern, as the concept of "human rights" has limited weight overall in domestic U.S. law compared to other Western democracies. In addition, due to the particularly significant suspicion of the welfare state in the United States, American jurists are warier of "positive rights" that oblige the government to provide social benefits. (By contrast, "negative rights" preclude government action, such as censorship or inhumane punishments.) The domestic legal principles of other Western democracies therefore give greater importance to social and economic rights such as access to medical treatment.

Beyond the Western world, diverse nations identify health care as a fundamental right in their national constitutions. The South African Constitution of 1996, ratified following the end of the apartheid regime, often is regarded as a model for its human rights provisions. It especially provides that "Everyone has the right to have access to ... health care services, including reproductive health care." The Constitution of Kenya, ratified in 2010 subsequent to a reform movement, followed this trend by stating that "Every person has the right to ... the highest attainable standard of health, which includes the right to health care services, including reproductive health care." Other examples illustrate this global pattern, as health care is identified either as a right or policy objective in the constitutions of India, Japan, and Mexico.

Implementing Access to Health Care The recognition of health care as a human right should be distinguished from actual access to medical treatment, which varies markedly depending on a country's degree of economic

Comparison of Global Estimated Life Expectancy at Birth in 1990 and in 2011

	Both sexes		Male		Female	
	1990	2011	1990	2011	1990	2011
Global	64	70	62	68	67	72
WHO region						
African Region	50	56	48	55	51	58
Region of the Americas	71	76	68	73	75	79
South-East Asia Region	59	67	58	65	60	69
European Region	72	76	68	72	76	79
Eastern Mediterranean Region	61	68	59	67	63	70
Western Pacific Region	70	76	68	74	72	78
Income group						
Low income	52	60	51	59	54	61
Lower middle income	59	66	58	64	61	68
Upper middle income	68	74	66	72	71	76
High income	76	80	72	78	79	83

SOURCE: World Health Organization, 2013.

Life expectancy is one way to measure the availability of access to health care and medical treatment. As measured by the graphic, specific regions and higher income countries fare better in this comparison, with the highest-income countries on average living 20 years more than those in low-income countries. However, between 1990 and 2011, there were greater advances in the lowest-income countries (eight years on average) as opposed to those in the highest-income countries (four years).

development and form of government. The WHO has emphasized that "while constitutional recognition of the right to access to essential medicines is an important sign of national values and commitment, it is neither a guarantee nor an essential step. This is shown by the many countries with failing health systems despite good constitutional language, and by those countries with good access to essential medicines without it."

The human right to health care generally is fulfilled in wealthy industrialized nations, most of whom have had universal health care systems for several decades. These systems can differ widely, however, because universal access to medical treatment can be implemented through diverse public policy frameworks.

Besides Germany, the Bismarck model exists in various forms in a diverse group of states, including Belgium, France, Japan, the Netherlands, Switzerland, Mexico, and to a degree in certain other Latin American countries. Health care under the Bismarck model usually is funded by a combination of payroll taxes on both employers and employees, out-of-pocket costs, nonprofit private insurance companies, and government subsidies.

A distinct policy approach to universal health care is a single-payer model under which the entirety or the vast majority of health care is funded by the government on the basis of tax revenue. This model notably is found in the United Kingdom, where patients do not have to pay a bill when they visit a medical doctor. Variations of the single-payer system exist in other countries, such as

Canada, although certain Canadian provinces additionally require premium payments.

The United States is again an exception, as it is the only wealthy industrialized nation without a genuine universal health-care system. A 2009 study by Andrew P. Wilper and other scientists found that up to 45,000 annual deaths in the United States were attributable to the lack of health insurance. Although the Obama administration's Affordable Care Act of 2010 expanded access to health care, approximately 31 million people in the country are projected to remain uninsured following the reform's full implementation according to the Congressional Budget Office. Most Americans with access to health insurance usually acquire it under a system akin to the Bismarck model. Yet universal health care essentially exists for seniors under the federal government's Medicare program, which covers all Americans once they turn 65 years old.

The case of the United States suggests that achieving universal access to health care may require regulating the cost of medical insurance, drugs, and services. Even though the United States has by far the most expensive health-care system worldwide, Americans have drastically less access to affordable care than the citizens of other industrialized countries, as well as generally worse health levels. This paradox is due to the fact that the United States is essentially the sole wealthy nation where health-care providers and insurance companies are authorized to make considerable profits over people's health problems, as illustrated by Steven Brill's investigative reporting on highly lucrative hospitals. Millions of Americans thus cannot afford the substantial cost of medical treatment in the United States, from expensive insurance premiums and deductibles, to the exorbitant out-of-pocket costs incurred when people are either uninsured or underinsured.

In European nations, Canada, Australia, New Zealand, and Japan, for instance, basic health care is not considered primarily a for-profit business but rather a public health imperative. As T. R. Reid notes in his comparative analysis, these countries therefore regulate the cost of medical drugs and services, unlike the United States. They also do not allow health insurance companies to profit from basic medical coverage. Their approach reflects ethical norms against profiteering by health-care providers and insurance companies that have been influenced partly by the notion that medical treatment is a fundamental human right.

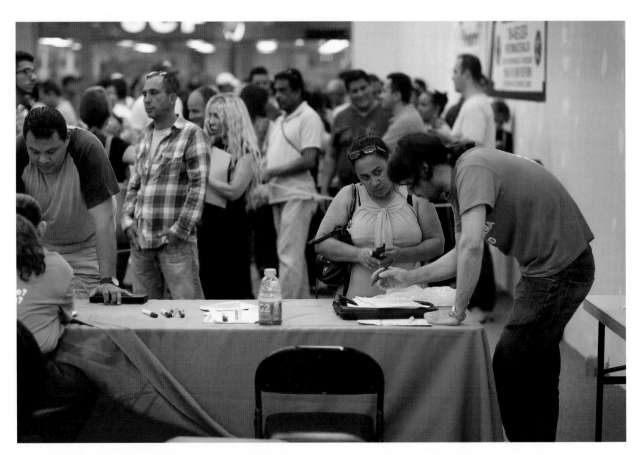

A woman speaks with an adviser as she, along with others in line, register to meet with Sunshine Life and Health Advisors that are selling insurance under the Affordable Care Act (ACA) at a store set up in the Mall of the Americas on March 31, 2014, in Miami, Florida. It was the last day for the first yearly sign-up period for the ACA plans, and saw a wait of four hours or more for people to see a health insurance adviser. © *Joe Raedle/Getty Images.*

Nonindustrialized countries lack universal health care systems. Consequently, health care typically is paid fully out-of-pocket—namely without any insurance or government support—and often accessible solely to the most privileged citizens. Reid underlines that "in rural regions of Africa, India, China, and South America, hundreds of millions of people go their whole lives without ever seeing a doctor…. Out-of-pocket payments account for 91 percent of total health spending in Cambodia, 85 percent in India, and 73 percent in Egypt."

Certain developing countries report lower out-of-pocket spending, such as Kenya, with approximately 36 percent, as the government draws upon funding from international aid. However, the national health-care spending in developing countries is commonly focused in their capital cities to the detriment of rural regions. Cuba stands out as an exception in the developing world in light of its universal health-care system modeled on the Soviet Union's state-run hospital system.

In addition to the poor, other vulnerable persons are prone to being denied access to medical treatment in countries without universal health-care systems. Discrimination can affect the availability of treatment for girls and women, who are also liable to being denied access to basic reproductive care in certain parts of the world. Inequity likewise can hinder access to treatment for racial, ethnic, religious or sexual minorities, as well as prisoners.

⊕ Future Implications

A substantial gap continues to exist between the recognition of health care as a human right and access to care in practice. Whereas wealthy nations have made great

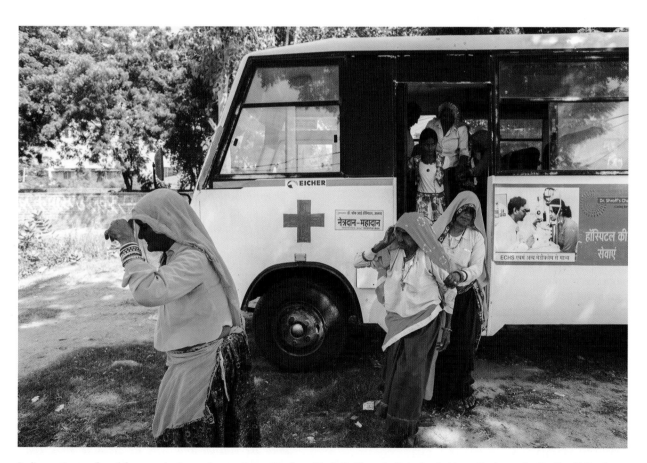

Indian patients referred for consultation and treatment arrive from Nagledi village, in Rajasthan's Alwar district, at the Dr Shroff Charity Eye Hospital, which operates a network of hospitals and vision centers in towns and villages in an attempt to tackle avoidable blindness. Offering low-cost or pro-bono treatment for conditions like cataracts and glaucoma, staff travel to remote areas to provide check-ups at field camps and work in vision centers in towns and villages, referring certain cases to larger hospitals. The network aims extend access to low-cost, high-quality eye care to those who might not normally be able to access or afford it. More women than men suffer problems with eyesight, according to staff, because of societal roles. Women traditionally spend a greater amount of time working outdoors, exposed to harsh sunlight and UV rays. They often feed male family members and children first, consuming less-nutritious meals after others have eaten, and cook over naked flames where they are exposed to smoke from animal dung, leaves, or coal used as fuel. Women also earn less and live in more unhygienic conditions, which can lead to infections, while male family members often relocate to towns or cities for work, where conditions and salaries are better. *© Rebecca Conway/AFP/Getty Images.*

strides toward achieving universal health care, much of the world's population lacks access to basic medical treatment. A vast number of developing countries have ratified the International Covenant on Economic, Social and Cultural Rights but remain far from meeting its provisions regarding medical treatment. The right to health care under numerous national constitutions likewise is contradicted by the situation on the ground. For instance, the Kenyan Constitution enacted in 2010 emphasized that "Every person has the right to ... health care services," although only an estimated 20 percent of the Kenyan population—9 million out of 44 million people—had access to health care as of 2014. The infant mortality rate, a revealing health indicator, is 48 per 1,000 annual births in Kenya, compared to 5 and 2, respectively, in industrialized countries such as New Zealand and Japan.

Despite relative progress, partly attributable to the UN Millennium Development Goals initiative, the situation remains particularly dire in the world's poorest countries, where scores lack access to basic drugs and medical services. Millions of people die each year from HIV/AIDS, malaria, tuberculosis, tropical diseases, malnutrition, and various other preventable or curable medical problems.

Public health is undermined critically by broader development problems such as inadequate infrastructure, extreme poverty, malnutrition, and the lack of safe drinking water. Corruption can undermine access to health care further by impeding the proper investment of national resources. Armed conflicts and population displacements into substandard refugee camps can have an equally catastrophic impact on access to health care.

Achieving universal health care further depends on the implementation of an adequate public policy framework. As exemplified by the case of the United States, a significant tension exists between the profit motive in the medical sector and realizing universal health care, which entails regulating the cost of medical insurance, drugs, and services to make them affordable to all as a human right.

PRIMARY SOURCE

International Covenant on Economic, Social and Cultural Rights

SOURCE *"Article 12," from* International Covenant on Economic, Social and Cultural Rights. *United Nations General Assembly, December 16, 1966 (entry into force January 3, 1976).* http://www.ohchr.org/EN/ProfessionalInterest/Pages/CESCR.aspx

INTRODUCTION *This primary source is taken from a 1966 United Nations international covenant recognizing the basic human right of full health and access to health care.*

Article 12

1. The States Parties to the present Covenant recognize the right of everyone to the enjoyment of the highest attainable standard of physical and mental health.

2. The steps to be taken by the States Parties to the present Covenant to achieve the full realization of this right shall include those necessary for:

   (a) The provision for the reduction of the still-birth-rate and of infant mortality and for the healthy development of the child;

   (b) The improvement of all aspects of environmental and industrial hygiene;

   (c) The prevention, treatment and control of epidemic, endemic, occupational and other diseases;

   (d) The creation of conditions which would assure to all medical service and medical attention in the event of sickness.

SEE ALSO *Global Health Initiatives; Social Theory and Global Health; Universal Health Coverage*

BIBLIOGRAPHY

Books

Holtz, Carol, ed. *Global Health Care: Issues and Policies*, 2nd ed. Burlington, MA: Jones and Bartlett Learning, 2012.

Lipset, Seymour Martin. *American Exceptionalism: A Double-Edged Sword*. New York: Norton, 1996.

Reid, T. R. *The Healing of America: A Global Quest for Better, Cheaper, and Fairer Health Care*. New York: Penguin, 2010.

Sachs, Jeffrey D. *The End of Poverty: Economic Possibilities for Our Time*. New York: Penguin, 2006.

Sunstein, Cass R. *The Second Bill of Rights: FDR's Unfinished Revolution and Why We Need It More Than Ever*. New York: Basic Books, 2004.

Periodicals

Ben-Bassat, Avi, and Mohi Dahan. "Social Rights in the Constitution and in Practice." *Journal of Comparative Economics* 36, no. 1 (March 2008): 103–119.

Himmelstein, David U., et al. "Medical Bankruptcy in the United States, 2007: Results of a National

Study." *American Journal of Medicine* 122, no. 8 (August 2009): 741–746.

Jouet, Mugambi. "The Exceptional Absence of Human Rights as a Principle in American Law." *Pace Law Review* 34, no. 2 (Spring 2014): 688–735.

Knaul, Felicia Marie, et al. "The Quest for Universal Health Coverage: Achieving Social Protection for All in Mexico." *The Lancet* 380, no. 9849 (October 6, 2012): 1259–1279.

New York Times Editorial Board. "The Race to Improve Global Health." *New York Times* (September 11, 2013): A26. Available online at http://www.nytimes.com/2013/09/11/opinion/the-race-to-improve-global-health.html?_r=0 (accessed February 4, 2015).

Wilper, Andrew P., et al. "Health Insurance and Mortality in US Adults." *American Journal of Public Health* 99, no. 12 (December 2009): 2289–2295.

Websites

Brill, Steven. "Bitter Pill: Why Medical Bills Are Killing Us." *Time*, February 20, 2013. http://time.com/198/bitter-pill-why-medical-bills-are-killing-us/ (accessed February 5, 2015).

"Health Systems." *Civitas*. http://www.civitas.org.uk/nhs/health_systems.php (accessed February 5, 2015).

"How Does Corruption Affect Health Care Systems, and How Can Regulation Tackle It?" *World Health Organization*. http://www.euro.who.int/en/data-and-evidence/evidence-informed-policy-making/publications/hen-summaries-of-network-members-reports/how-does-corruption-affect-health-care-systems,-and-how-can-regulation-tackle-it (February 5, 2015).

Klein, Ezra, "Why an MRI Costs $1,080 in America and $280 in France." *Washington Post*, March 15, 2013. http://www.washingtonpost.com/blogs/wonkblog/wp/2013/03/15/why-an-mri-costs-1080-in-america-and-280-in-france/ (accessed February 5, 2015).

"The Millennium Development Goals Report 2014." *United Nations*. http://www.un.org/millenniumgoals/2014%20MDG%20report/MDG%202014%20English%20web.pdf (accessed February 5, 2015).

"Mortality Rate, Infant (per 1,000 Live Births)." *World Bank*. http://data.worldbank.org/indicator/SP.DYN.IMRT.IN?order=wbapi_data_value_2013+wbapi_data_value+wbapi_data_value-last&sort=asc (accessed February 5, 2015).

"Rapport Annuel 2013/2014 de Médecins Sans Frontières 43e Assemblee Generale." *Médecins Sans Frontières*, 14–15 Juin, 2014. http://www.msf.fr/sites/www.msf.fr/files/rapannuel2013-2014.pdf (accessed February 5, 2015).

Sachs, Jeffrey D. "The End of Poverty, Soon." *New York Times*, September 24, 2013. http://www.nytimes.com/2013/09/25/opinion/the-end-of-poverty-soon.html (accessed February 5, 2015).

"UNHCR Global Report 2013." *Office of the United Nations High Commissioner for Refugees*. http://www.unhcr.org/gr13/index.xml (accessed February 4, 2015).

"Updated Estimates of the Effects of the Insurance Coverage Provisions of the Affordable Care Act, April 2014." *Congressional Budget Office*, April 2014. http://www.cbo.gov/sites/default/files/cbofiles/attachments/45231-ACA_Estimates.pdf (accessed February 4, 2015).

"Why Is Health Spending in the United States So High?" *Organisation for Economic Co-operation and Development*. http://www.oecd.org/unitedstates/49084355.pdf (accessed February 5, 2015).

"The World Medicines Situation 2011: Access to Essential Medicines as Part of the Right to Health." *World Health Organization*. http://apps.who.int/medicinedocs/documents/s18772en/s18772en.pdf (accessed February 5, 2015).

Mugambi Jouet

Health in the WHO African Region

🌐 Introduction

The World Health Organization (WHO) African Regional Office (AFRO) is one of six WHO regional offices, each of which is responsible for monitoring and improving public health, implementing WHO policies, and administering WHO programs and campaigns within the defined region. AFRO covers 47 African nations, which includes all of Africa with the exception of Djibouti, Egypt, Libya, Morocco, Somalia, Sudan, and Tunisia, which are covered by the Eastern Mediterranean Regional Office (EMRO).

AFRO faces many challenges in meeting WHO priorities and improving public health within the region because of geographic location, high levels of poverty, poor governance, inadequate health-care infrastructure, and relatively low levels of public education in many member states. The substantial issues confronting AFRO in its region include communicable (infectious and transmissible) diseases, noncommunicable (non-infectious and non-transmissible) diseases, neglected tropical diseases (NTDs), maternity and child health, malnutrition, degraded physical environments, and lifestyle risks.

Despite the challenges faced within AFRO, the WHO has made significant progress in combating many communicable diseases, issues with maternal health, and childhood mortality within the region. The WHO and the international community have dedicated significant attention and financial resources to many of these public health issues under the United Nations (UN) Millennium Development Goals (MDGs). The MDGs are a set of eight goals adopted by UN member states in 2000 to improve global public health and sustainable development by 2015. Despite the improvement within many areas of public health achieved within AFRO nations since 2000, many nations will require additional years and resources to achieve the MDG public health goals.

🌐 Historical Background

In 1946, all 51 member states and 10 nonmember states of the newly established UN created a specialized UN agency to address global health concerns. The World Health Assembly (WHA), held its first annual meeting in July 1948. Health ministers from each member nation serve on the WHA, which sets the priorities and policies of the WHO. Representatives of the first annual meeting of the WHA established the initial public health priorities of the WHO as maternal and infant health, nutrition, and the prevention of certain communicable diseases such as malaria, sexually transmitted diseases, and tuberculosis.

The first WHA also tasked the WHO with compiling complete, accurate statistics about the occurrence of disease. WHO epidemiological research (focusing on the occurrence, distribution, and control of diseases and factors associated with health and illness) about communicable and noncommunicable diseases continues to form an important part of the WHO's mission and assists the WHA, UN, and national health ministries in establishing and evaluating public health priorities.

From 1949 through 1952, the WHA created regional offices designed to meet the specific public health needs of a particular area of the world. As of 2014, the WHO had six regional offices: AFRO; the Regional Office for the Americas (AMRO, also known as the Pan American Health Organization [PAHO]); the Regional Office for South-East Asia (SEARO); the Regional Office for Europe (EURO); EMRO; and the Regional Office for the Western Pacific (WPRO).

Each regional office of the WHO is governed by a regional committee, which meets annually. Each regional committee is composed of the health ministers from each UN member state and non-UN member states within that particular region. The regional committees are tasked with implementing the policies and guidelines adopted by the WHA. Regional committees also monitor the effectiveness of WHO projects and policies within its region. In addition, each regional committee elects a regional director, who oversees daily operations within the region. The regional director serves a five-year team and may be reelected to one additional five-year term.

AFRO covers 47 African nations that constitute most of Africa with the exception of a few North African countries that are located in EMRO. AFRO is located in Brazzaville, Republic of the Congo. Additionally, AFRO operates country offices in the following nations: Algeria, Angola, Benin, Botswana, Burkina Faso, Burundi, Cameroon, Cape Verde, the Central African Republic, Chad, Comoros, the Republic of the Congo, Ivory Coast (Côte d'Ivoire), the Democratic Republic of the Congo, Equatorial Guinea, Ethiopia, Eritrea, Gabon, the Gambia, Ghana, Guinea, Guinea-Bissau, Kenya, Lesotho, Liberia, Madagascar, Malawi, Mali, Mauritania, Mauritius, Mozambique, Namibia, Niger, Nigeria, Rwanda, São Tomé and Principe, Senegal, the Seychelles, Sierra Leone, South Africa, South Sudan, Swaziland, Togo, Uganda, Tanzania, Zambia, and Zimbabwe.

⊕ Impacts and Issues

AFRO is responsible for implementing WHO policies within the region and collecting and monitoring public health information within its nations. In "The Role of the WHO in Public Health" the WHO defines its core functions in monitoring and improving public health as the following:

> Providing leadership on matters critical to health and engaging in partnerships where joint action is needed; shaping the research agenda and stimulating the generation, translation and dissemination of valuable knowledge; setting norms and standards and promoting and monitoring their implementation; articulating ethical and evidence-based policy options; providing technical support, catalyzing change, and building sustainable institutional capacity; and monitoring the health situation and assessing health trends.

During the decade from 2005 to 2015, AFRO has instituted organizational and management reforms intended to improve organizational efficiency and effectiveness. For example, AFRO provided guidance and technical support to assist member states to improve their national health systems so they would be better able to realize the MDGs by 2015. AFRO also created the African Health Workforce Observatory and African Health Observatory, which enable production, collection, and dissemination of information, evidence, and knowledge among the member states.

Communicable Diseases

Communicable diseases account for two-thirds of the total disease burden within the AFRO region. Nations within the AFRO region experience some of the highest rates of HIV/AIDS, tuberculosis, malaria, and NTDs in the world.

The HIV/AIDS epidemic is one of the greatest public health threats faced in the AFRO region. In 2012, the region accounted for 71 percent of the global HIV/AIDS burden. The HIV/AIDS prevalence (the number of cases of a disease or condition present in a particular population at a given time), in 2011, was 4.6 percent among adults aged 15 to 49 years old in the AFRO region. The next highest prevalence within a WHO region was in the Americas at 0.5 percent. In 2011, the prevalence of HIV/AIDS among adults equaled or exceeded 10 percent in nine AFRO nations: Swaziland (26 percent), Botswana (23.4 percent), Lesotho (23.3 percent), South Africa (17.3 percent), Zimbabwe (14.9 percent), Namibia (13.4 percent), Zambia (12.5 percent), Mozambique (11.3 percent), and Malawi (10 percent).

The high HIV/AIDS prevalence in some AFRO nations, combined with low treatment rates, is responsible in large part for the decline in life expectancy in some AFRO nations to some of the lowest levels in the world. In 2011, life expectancy at birth in six AFRO nations was 50 years or lower. These countries are Sierra Leone (47 years), Central African Republic (48), Democratic Republic of the Congo (49), Guinea-Bissau (50), Lesotho (50), and Swaziland (50). The life expectancy in these countries is at least 20 years less than the global average of 70 years.

The AFRO countries also bear a disproportionately high prevalence of tuberculosis (TB). The region has the highest prevalence (per 100,000 population) of TB in the world, accounting for 27 percent of the 1.3 million new TB cases diagnosed worldwide in 2012. As of 2011, countries within the AFRO region reported 293 cases of TB per 100,000 population. This rate far exceeds the global prevalence of 170 cases per 100,000 population.

Malaria is another disease that disproportionately affects nations within AFRO. An infectious disease caused by protozoans transmitted to humans through the bite of mosquitos that carry the protozoa, malaria may induce fever, vomiting, and fatigue. Severe cases of malaria may cause seizures, jaundice (yellow skin), and death. Infants and children are particularly susceptible to more severe forms of malaria.

Globally, an estimated 207 million cases of malaria occurred in 2012, with 80 percent of these cases occurring within the AFRO region. The incidence (the number of new cases of a disease or condition that develop during a specific period) rate (per 100,000 population) of malaria in AFRO countries in 2010 was 20,913 cases, meaning that more than a fifth of the population within the region suffered from malaria within that year. The malaria incidence rate within AFRO countries was about nine times higher than the next highest WHO region, EMRO, which had an incidence rate of 2,491 cases per 100,000.

MILLENNIUM DEVELOPMENT GOALS IN AFRICA

Much of the progress in public health issues in the WHO African Region (AFRO) has been a result of the World Health Organization (WHO), nongovernmental organization (NGO), and governmental action to achieve the Millennium Development Goals (MDGs). At the United Nations (UN) Millennium Summit in 2000, all United Nations (UN) member states and 23 international organizations committed to reach eight development goals by 2015. In order to achieve the MDGs, the G8, World Bank, International Monetary Fund, African Development Bank, and other organizations agreed to forgive up to US$55 billion in debt owed by heavily indebted poor countries. The WHO, NGOs, and the international community spend additional billions of dollars to assist developing countries achieve the MDGs.

Three of the eight MDGs relate directly to improving public health, while many of the others have elements that address health concerns. MDG 4 seeks to reduce child mortality. Specifically, MDG Target 4A aims to reduce the 1990 under-five mortality by two-thirds by 2015. MDG 5 seeks to improve maternal health. Target 5A sets a goal of reducing the maternal mortality rate by three-quarters of the 1990 rate by 2015, and Target 5B aims to make reproductive health available to all women by 2015. MDG 6 seeks to combat HIV/AIDS, malaria, and other diseases. Target 6A aims at halting and reversing the spread of HIV/AIDS, and Target 6B seeks to make antiretroviral (ARV) treatment available to all HIV/AIDS patients. Target 6C seeks to halt and begin the reversal of the incidence of malaria, tuberculosis, and other major diseases.

Parts of MDG 7 also relate to health, as it sets a variety of targets to improve environmental sustainability, including improving access to clean water and sanitation, promoting sustainable development, reducing biodiversity loss, and improving the lives of people living in slums. A portion of this goal was met in 2010, five years earlier than the goal, when the proportion of the population without sustainable access to drinking water was met. However, in 2012 an estimated 748 million people still lived without access to improved drinking water sources.

The remaining MDGs are dedicated to targets that promote sustainable development, equality, and lifestyles. MDG 1 seeks to eliminate extreme poverty and hunger. Target 1A seeks to halve the proportion of people (based on the 1990 rate) living on $1.25 or less per day, while Target 1B aims to improve employment opportunities. Target 1C seeks to halve the proportion of people suffering from hunger (between the 1990 and 2015 rates). MDG 2 aims for universal primary school education for all children. MDG 3 promotes gender equality and the empowerment of women by calling for elimination of gender disparity at all levels of education. MDG 8 seeks to promote international partnerships that facilitate growth and progress in developing countries. Target 8E seeks to provide access to what the WHO calls "essential medicines" by working with pharmaceutical companies.

Despite the efforts of the WHO and other organizations within the WHO African Region, many nations within the region will fail to reach the MDG health goals. According to the African Regional Office (AFRO), in 2014, 16 nations (out of the region's 47 nations) were on track to meet MDG 4A, 4 for MDG 5A, 7 for MDG 5B, 34 for MDG 6A, 10 for MDG 6B, and 12 for MDG 6C.

Malaria remains a major cause of death within the AFRO countries. An estimated 90 percent of global malaria deaths occur within the region. In 2010, the malaria mortality rate (per 100,000 population) within AFRO countries was 72 compared to the global rate of 12. Despite the relatively high malaria mortality rate in AFRO nations in 2010, the rate represented a significant improvement compared to the 2006 mortality rate of 104.

Children represent a disproportionately high number of the total malaria deaths within AFRO nations. In 2012, children under age five accounted for 462,000 out of the estimated 564,000 malaria deaths in the region.

Noncommunicable Diseases

Noncommunicable diseases pose an increasing threat to public health in Africa. Cancer, cardiovascular diseases, chronic respiratory diseases, and diabetes are the most common noncommunicable diseases. According to the WHO, noncommunicable diseases result in 38 million deaths annually worldwide. About 75 percent of all noncommunicable disease deaths occur in low- and middle-income countries. Individuals in low- and middle-income countries are more likely to die prematurely (before the age of 70) from noncommunicable diseases, with 82 percent of such deaths occurring in low- and middle-income countries.

A variety of genetic, environmental, and behavioral risk factors contribute to noncommunicable diseases. Although people cannot readily modify or reduce specific genetic and environmental risk factors, they can decrease the risk of developing noncommunicable diseases by making healthy lifestyle choices. The WHO reports that tobacco use, physical inactivity, excessive alcohol consumption, and unhealthy diets are the four most common behavioral risk factors for developing noncommunicable diseases.

Although just 30 percent of the population in the African region consume alcohol, among those who consume alcohol, the average per capita consumption is high. As much as 36 percent of African youth use tobacco and nearly half (48 percent) are exposed to secondhand smoke. In many countries in the region, undernutrition and underweight among children persist as a result of food shortages and poor feeding practices. At the same time, there is

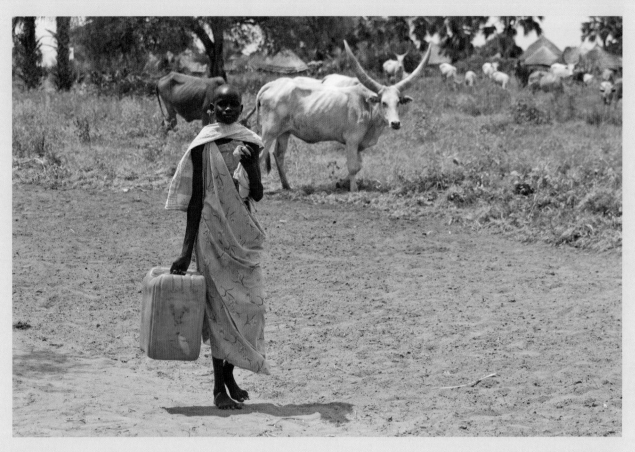

A woman carries a large water jug to get water from the Nile in South Sudan. Access to water and improved sanitation are limited in many AFRO countries, a concern addressed by MDG 7. © *John Wollwerth/Shutterstock.com.*

growing overweight and obesity, especially in urban centers, as diets high in sugar, salt, and fat have replaced traditional diets that were rich in fruits and vegetables. Physical inactivity, especially among women and children in urban centers also increases risk for noncommunicable diseases.

Within the AFRO countries, noncommunicable diseases are expected to increase by 27 percent by 2025. AFRO reports that this increase will result in an additional 28 million deaths per year at the end of the period. Noncommunicable diseases already account for more than 50 percent of all deaths in three AFRO nations: Mauritius, Namibia, and Seychelles. By 2030, however, AFRO estimates that noncommunicable diseases will account for more deaths within the region than all communicable, maternal, neonatal, and nutritional diseases combined.

Maternal, Neonatal, and Childhood Diseases

Nations within the WHO African region have some of the highest levels of maternal, neonatal, and childhood disease and mortality rates in the world. The lack of access to skilled health personnel during childbirth poses a significant risk to women giving birth within the region. Between 2005 and 2012, skilled health personnel attended less than half of all births in the region. The lack of access to health care during and after birth results a lifetime risk of maternal death in the WHO African region that is more than four times higher than the global average. In 2010, women within AFRO nations had a 1 in 42 lifetime risk of maternal death compared to the global rate of one in 180.

According to WHO statistics released in 2014, although the AFRO region constitutes only about 12 percent of the world's population, the region accounts for one-third of global neonatal (within 28 days of birth) deaths with more than 1 million neonatal deaths in 2013. Three-quarters of all neonatal deaths within the region occur within one week of birth, including one-half of all neonatal deaths within 24 hours of birth. The leading causes of neonatal deaths in the region are premature birth and birth trauma, which each accounting for about one-third of neonatal deaths.

Even after the neonatal period, infants and children under five face significant health risks within AFRO

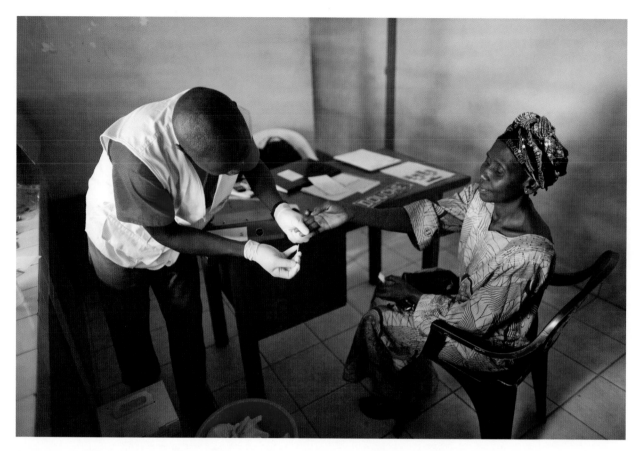

A woman with HIV/AIDS is treated by a Médicins Sans Frontières (Doctors Without Borders) worker in the Central African Republic.
© Ton Koene / Horizons WWP / Alamy.

nations from communicable diseases, malnutrition, and other factors. In 2012, the infant mortality rate (deaths within the first year of life, per 1,000 live births) within the region was 63. Although this number exceeds the global infant mortality rate of 35, it represents a significant improvement from the AFRO rate of 105 in 1990.

Globally, 6.3 million children under the age of five died in 2013. Childhood (under the age of five) mortality in African region is the highest in the world. The childhood mortality rate in 2012 was 95 deaths per 1,000 live births—nearly double the global rate of 48 deaths per 1,000 live births. The leading causes of childhood death within the WHO African region are pneumonia (15.9 percent of all childhood deaths), malaria (14.9 percent), and diarrheal diseases (10.1 percent).

Neglected Tropical Diseases

Nations within the AFRO region also suffer a disproportionately high burden of neglected tropical diseases (NTDs). NTDs are a group of 17 diseases that primarily affect people in developing nations. Because NTDs seldom are experienced in the developed countries, they have received relatively low levels of research and funding until recent years. The WHO estimates that 1.4 billion people in 149 countries are at risk for at least one NTD.

Every country within the WHO African region is endemic (disease found in or confined to a particular region) for at least one NTD, and more than three-quarters of the countries within the region are at risk for five or more NTDs. Lymphatic filariasis threatens the greatest number of people within the AFRO area with 470 million people at risk. Lymphatic filariasis, also known as elephantiasis, is caused by mosquito-borne parasitic worms that damage the lymphatic system and may result in massive swelling of the arms, legs, or other parts of the body. More than 330 million people in the AFRO region are at risk of developing soil-transmitted helminthiasis, a disease caused by parasitic worms, resulting in intestinal problems, delays in physical and cognitive development, and low energy levels. An estimated 250 million people within the region are at risk of trachoma, a bacterial infection that may result in blindness; and 220 million are at risk of schistosomiasis, a potentially fatal disease caused by parasitic worms.

Many NTDs are easily preventable or treatable. The WHO has focused its NTD eradication efforts in the AFRO region on the mass administration of preventive medicines for some diseases, including lymphatic filariasis, schistosomiasis, and soil-transmitted helminthiasis, as well as on early detection and treatment of other

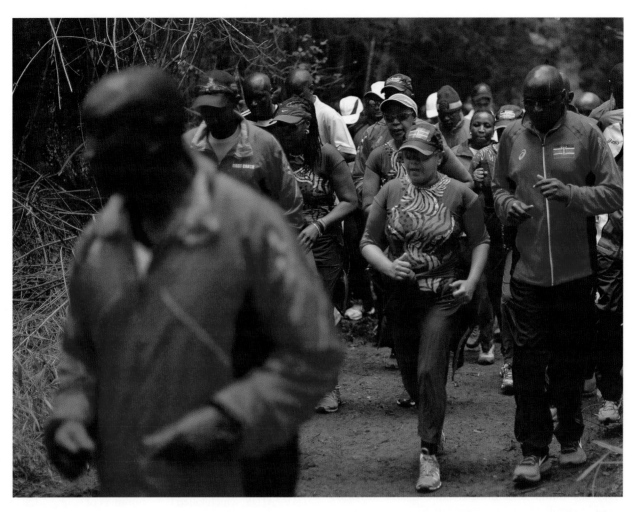

First Lady Margaret Kenyatta (center) of Kenya takes part on October 19, 2014, with other participants to a run to raise awareness of her "Beyond Zero" campaign to create access to maternal care in Kenya, where 15 women die every day due to pregnancy-related complications. A 2014 UNICEF report, "Committing to Child Survival," places Kenya among the countries with the lowest coverage of postnatal care in the world, and high newborn deaths, most occurring in the first 28 days of life and during birth (intrapartum), followed by preterm births.   © *Tony Karumba/Getty Images.*

NTDs, such as Buruli ulcer, African trypanosomiasis, leprosy, leishmaniasis, and yaws.

⊕ Future Implications

Despite some of the highest burdens of communicable, noncommunicable, maternal, neonatal, and childhood diseases in the world, the WHO African region has made significant strides in reducing the prevalence of certain diseases within the region. In partnership with local and foreign governments, NGOs, and nonprofit organizations, the WHO has implemented relatively successful programs to combat HIV/AIDS, malaria, TB, maternal mortality, and neonatal and childhood mortality. Many of the improvements in public health in the region are the result of increased focus and financial resources dedicated to particular health issues under the UN MDGs.

The AFRO region has made significant progress in reducing the childhood mortality rate but will miss the MDG target of a two-thirds reduction in the 1990 rate by 2015. The 1990 childhood mortality rate in the region was 173 per 1,000 live births. In 2012, the AFRO childhood mortality rate stood at 95 per 1,000 live births, which does not meet the MDG target requirement of 57.7 deaths per 1,000 live births.

Countries within the AFRO region also have improved maternal mortality rates but most will fail to meet the MDG target of a three-quarters reduction over the 1990 rate. In 1990, the AFRO region had a maternal mortality rate of 960 deaths per 100,000 live births. By 2013, the rate had fallen to 500, which remains twice as high as the MDG target.

Despite the devastating toll of the HIV/AIDS epidemic within the AFRO region, the WHO and international aid organization have made significant improvements in the region's HIV/AIDS public health outlook. Between 2001 and 2011, the HIV/AIDS incidence rate (per 100,000 population) within the AFRO region fell from 351 to 205. During the same period, the HIV/AIDS mortality rate (per 100,000 population) within the region dropped from 219 to 139.

The declining HIV/AIDS prevalence and mortality rate in the AFRO region largely is attributable to the efforts of the WHO, foreign governments, and international aid organizations to increase the availability and use of antiretroviral (ARV) treatment. Between 2007 and 2011, the percentage of people with advanced HIV receiving ARVs in the region increased from 44 percent to 57 percent. Only the Americas WHO region (at 68 percent) exceeds the AFRO region in ARV treatment.

The WHO also has targeted the use of ARV treatment at pregnant women in the region to reduce mother-to-child HIV transmission. Because of an increase in the percentage of pregnant women receiving ARV from 34 percent in 2009 to 63 percent in 2012, the rate of mother-to-child HIV transmission fell 37 percent within the period.

The number of malaria deaths in the region has declined compared to 1990 rates primarily through the prevention of child deaths from malaria, which decreased by 54 percent between 2000 and 2012. The decrease in malaria infections and deaths in the region results from the increased availability and use of insecticide-treated bed nets for children, increased malaria diagnosis and antimalarial drug treatment, and increased vector control. These improvements have been possible through massive international government, NGO, and WHO expenditures on malarial control and treatment measures. Between 2000 and 2013, expenditures on malaria control increased from less than $100 million to $1.93 billion.

The 2011 TB prevalence rate of 293 cases marks a significant improvement compared to the 2002 rate of approximately 370 cases per 100,000 population. AFRO implemented the Stop TB Strategy adopted by the WHO in 2006. The program focuses on increased detection rates, integrating TB and HIV/AIDS diagnosis and treatment, and strengthening local primary health care. The decline in TB prevalence in the AFRO region is attributable mostly to a near doubling of the TB case-detection rate within the region between 1990 and 2011. Earlier detection allows for more rapid treatment and a decrease in the spread of TB.

Countries within the AFRO region have made significant progress in improving public health since the 1990s, but the region continues to experience some of the highest disease burdens in the world. The UN and WHO aim to continue the progress achieved under the MDGs by intensifying collective efforts and continuing programs and partnerships to improve public health.

PRIMARY SOURCE

WHO in the African Region

SOURCE *"Introduction," from* The Health of the People: What Works—The African Regional Health Report 2014. *Brazzaville, Republic of the Congo: World Health Organization Regional Office for Africa (AFRO), 2014, 7–9. http://apps.who.int/iris/ bitstream/10665/137377/4/9789290232612. pdf?ua=1 (accessed February 2, 2015).*

INTRODUCTION *This primary source is taken from the introduction to a 2014 World Health Organization Regional Office for Africa publication that describes the progress that the region has experienced in tackling some of its health challenges in the preceding 20 years.*

Progress on health outcomes

The Region has seen marked improvements in health outcomes during the past decade. There has been a considerable decline in child, maternal and adult mortality rates, and substantial decreases in the burdens of several diseases. In the period 1990–2011, the Region has struggled with, and begun to overcome, one of the most devastating epidemics in human history—that caused by HIV.

Between 1990 and 2008, adult mortality rates increased—largely as a result of the havoc wreaked by HIV/AIDS, which killed large numbers of young adults. However, by 2011, efforts to curb HIV led to a drop in adult mortality to 339 per 1000 adults. Despite the catastrophic effects of the HIV/AIDS epidemic, which peaked in 2004, the Region has managed to achieve an overall increase in life expectancy at birth—from 50 years in 1990 to 56 years in 2011. However, there is still a long way to go to catch up with the rest of the world. The mean global life expectancy in 2011 was 70 years: thus a child born in Africa in 2011 still cannot expect to live as long a life as his or her peers in the rest of the world.

None the less, it should be remembered that this life expectancy is an average…. [S]ome countries within the Region have made outstanding progress, raising life expectancies considerably….

In the two decades since 1990, HIV-related diseases—particularly tuberculosis—became the dominant causes of death in the Region. Other major causes of death were diarrhoeal diseases, malaria, pneumonia, meningitis, malnutrition, preterm birth complications, injuries and violence. Noncommunicable diseases (NCDs), including cancer, cardiovascular disorders and diabetes, are increasing in significance as a cause of death throughout Africa, particularly in the southern African region….

There has been impressive progress in reducing mortality rates in children less than 5 years of age. Improving access to treatment for infectious diseases such as pneumonia, diarrhoea, malaria and HIV/AIDS, greater use of preventive measures such as insecticide-treated nets (ITNs), and immunization and nutrition interventions have all had an impact on child survival. Improved management and coverage of severe acute malnutrition has also contributed to the reduction in child deaths.

Between 1990 and 2012, the under-five mortality rate in the Region fell from 173 to 95 per 1000 live births. During the same period, the global mean mortality rate for children less than 5 years of age fell from 90 to 48 per 1000 live births. Infant mortality rate has also been reduced in the Region, falling from 105 to 63 per 1000 live births between 1990 and 2012. Although the death rate has fallen, one third of these deaths are occurring in the neonatal period (the first 28 days after birth), mainly due to complications of prematurity, birth asphyxia and infections.

Worldwide, there has been a marked reduction in the maternal death rate. This has also been achieved in sub-Saharan Africa, which has seen a decline in the maternal death rate of 48% between 1990 and 2013.

SEE ALSO *HIV/AIDS; Malaria; Noncommunicable Diseases (Lifestyle Diseases); Tuberculosis (TB); World Health Organization: Organization, Funding, and Enforcement Powers*

BIBLIOGRAPHY

Books

Falola, Toyin, and Matthew M. Heaton, eds. *HIV/AIDS, Illness, and African Well-Being.* Rochester, NY: University of Rochester Press, 2007.

Stein, Howard. *Gendered Insecurities, Health and Development in Africa.* London: Routledge, 2012.

Viterbo, Paula, and Kalala J. Ngalamulume, eds. *Medicine and Health in Africa: Multidisciplinary Perspectives.* East Lansing: Michigan State University Press, 2011.

Sambo, Luis Gomes. *A Decade of WHO Action in the African Region: Striving Together to Achieve Health Goals.* Brazzaville: World Health Organization, 2015.

Periodicals

Kebede, Derege, et al. "The Way Forward: Narrowing the Knowledge Gap in Sub-Saharan Africa to Strengthen Health Systems." *Journal of the Royal Society of Medicine* 107, supp. 1 (May 2014): 10–12.

Keita, Bah, Jean-Baptiste Roungou, and Yacouba Toloba. "Introduction de l'enseignement de la tuberculose et de la lutte contre la tuberculose dans les écoles de médecine des pays francophones de la région africaine: Leçons apprises et perspectives." *African Health Monitor,* no. 18 (November 2013): 32–35.

Musango, Laurent, Riku Elovainio, and Bokar Toure. "AFRO Support for a Policy Dialogue to Develop Health Financing Systems and Move towards Universal Health Coverage in Africa." *African Health Monitor,* no. 17 (July 2013): 2–3.

Websites

"Atlas of African Health Statistics 2014: Health Situation Analysis in the African Region." *World Health Organization (WHO). Regional Office for Africa,* 2014. http://www.aho.afro.who.int/sites/default/files/publications/921/AFRO-Statistical_Factsheet.pdf (accessed January 27, 2015).

"The Health of the People: What Works—The African Regional Health Report." *World Health Organization (WHO).* http://www.aho.afro.who.int/sites/default/files/publications/1786/ARHR-2014-en.pdf (accessed January 27, 2015).

"Opening Address of Dr. L. G. Sambo at the Multi-stakeholders' Dialogue on Addressing Risk Factors for Noncommunicable Diseases in the African Region: 18–20 March, 2013, Johannesburg, South Africa." *World Health Organization (WHO),* March 2013. http://www.afro.who.int/en/rdo/speeches/3801-opening-address-of-dr-l-g-sambo-at-the-multi-stakeholders-dialogue-on-addressing-risk-factors-for-noncommunicable-diseases-in-the-african-region.html (accessed March 14, 2015).

"World Health Statistics 2014." *World Health Organization (WHO).* http://apps.who.int/iris/bitstream/10665/112738/1/9789240692671_eng.pdf (accessed January 27, 2015).

Joseph P. Hyder

Health in the WHO Americas Region

🌐 Introduction

The World Health Organization (WHO) Regional Office for the Americas (AMRO) is one of six WHO regional offices and became known as the Pan American Health Organization (PAHO) in 1958. AMRO and PAHO are used interchangeably, but PAHO is more commonly used. The WHO is a specialized United Nations (UN) agency under the United Nations Development Group that is tasked with improving public health around the world. PAHO works with the national health organizations of its 35 member states to implement WHO policies, monitor public health, and coordinate health programs in the WHO Americas region.

Although most health indicators in the Americas exceed global averages, access to health care and public health resources are distributed inequitably among the region's citizens. More affluent citizens have increased access to high-level and preventive health care in many PAHO nations that less affluent citizens lack. North American member states have better overall health indicators than member states in Central America or part of the Caribbean. The region's least economically developed countries struggle with a higher disease burden of communicable (infectious and transmissible) diseases; their wealthier neighbors face greater health burdens with noncommunicable (noninfectious and non-transmissible), chronic diseases, such as cardiovascular and respiratory diseases, cancer, and diabetes. However, chronic disease incidence (the number of new cases of a disease or condition that develop during a specific period) is increasing across the PAHO region. As the graphic on page 253 displaying the leading causes of death in the Americas region reveals, seven of the ten leading causes of death in the region are chronic diseases.

PAHO also bolsters its primary mission by promoting universal access to health care and health coverage, community participation in health programs, human rights and nondiscrimination, and gender equality. Other PAHO efforts focus on the health needs of indigenous communities and traditionally neglected or marginalized populations.

🌐 Historical Background

The League of Nations, the predecessor organization to the UN, established a Health Organization to promote public health across national lines. The Health Organization directed the League of Nations' public health initiatives with a primary focus on preventing the spread of leprosy, malaria, typhus, and yellow fever. After the end of World War II (1939–1945), the newly formed UN sought to transfer the duties of the Health Organization to a new UN agency. In 1946, all 51 UN member states and 10 non-member states signed an agreement to create a specialized agency of the UN to address global health concerns. The new agency, known as the World Health Organization (WHO), began operations in April 1948 after a majority of signatory nations ratified its constitution.

The World Health Assembly (WHA) sets global health policies, priorities, and goals for the WHO. Health ministers from each UN member state serve on the WHA. Representatives of the first annual meeting of the World Health Assembly in July 1948 established maternal and infant health, nutrition, and the prevention of certain communicable diseases (malaria, sexually transmitted diseases, and tuberculosis) as the initial public health priorities of the WHO. These public health issues remain priorities for the WHO worldwide.

The first WHA also tasked the WHO with the compilation of complete and accurate statistics on life expectancy, mortality, and morbidity of disease. WHO research on the prevalence and morbidity of communicable and noncommunicable diseases continues to form an important part of the WHO's mission and assists the WHA and government health ministries in establishing and evaluating public health priorities.

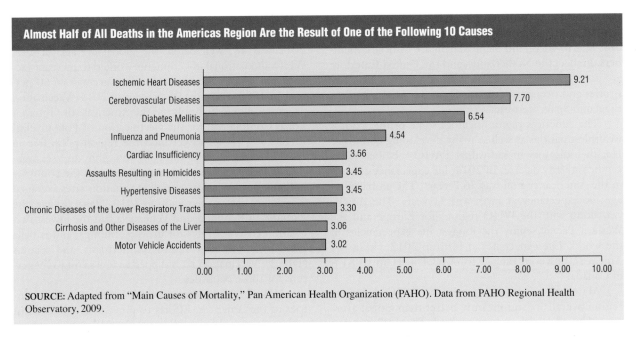

Almost Half of All Deaths in the Americas Region Are the Result of One of the Following 10 Causes

Cause	Value
Ischemic Heart Diseases	9.21
Cerebrovascular Diseases	7.70
Diabetes Mellitis	6.54
Influenza and Pneumonia	4.54
Cardiac Insufficiency	3.56
Assaults Resulting in Homicides	3.45
Hypertensive Diseases	3.45
Chronic Diseases of the Lower Respiratory Tracts	3.30
Cirrhosis and Other Diseases of the Liver	3.06
Motor Vehicle Accidents	3.02

SOURCE: Adapted from "Main Causes of Mortality," Pan American Health Organization (PAHO). Data from PAHO Regional Health Observatory, 2009.

According to WHO, ischemic heart disease is the main cause of death in the Americas region.

In the mid-2010s, the WHA is composed of the health ministers from almost all UN member states (except Lichtenstein). Several nongovernmental organizations (NGOs) and nonmember states of the UN participate as observers at WHA meetings. The Holy See (Vatican City), the Palestinian Authority, Taiwan (as Chinese Taipei), the Inter-Parliamentary Union, the International Committee of the Red Cross, the International Federation of Red Cross and Red Crescent Societies, and the Order of Malta all maintain observer status within the WHA.

During the period from 1949 through 1952, the WHA created regional offices to meet the specific public health needs of various areas of the world. The WHO has six regional offices: the Regional Office for Africa (AFRO); AMRO, now most commonly known as PAHO; the Regional Office for South-East Asia (SEARO); the Regional Office for Europe (EURO); the Regional Office for the Eastern Mediterranean (EMRO); and the Regional Office for the Western Pacific (WPRO).

PAHO was established in 1902 as the International Sanitary Bureau (ISB). The ISB administration was staffed primarily by health officials from the United States, but also included representatives from Chile, Costa Rica, Cuba, and Mexico. The U.S. surgeon general also served as the ISB chairman. The first decade of the ISB focused on advancing U.S. health and quarantine interests surrounding the construction of the Panama Canal. Sanitation and health efforts reduced canal worker deaths dramatically: 5,609 canal workers, primarily West Indians, died of diseases and accidents during the U.S. construction period (1904–1914), a significant reduction from the estimated 18,000–22,000 who died during the previous French construction efforts in the period 1881–1894.

At the Fifth International Conference of American States in Santiago, Chile, in 1923, representatives changed the name of the ISB to the Pan American Sanitary Bureau. In 1924, 21 member states adopted the Pan American Sanitary Code. The code provided for basic sanitation and health initiatives and made the Pan American Sanitary Bureau the primary coordinating agency for international health programs across the Americas. In 1947, the bureau became the executive agency of the Pan American Sanitary Organization. Two years later, the WHO designated the Pan American Sanitary Organization as its regional office in the Americas. The office became known as the Pan American Health Organization (PAHO) in 1958.

⊕ Impacts and Issues

PAHO is headquartered in Washington, D.C., in the United States. PAHO is responsible for monitoring health in all North, Central, South American, and Caribbean countries. The member countries and territories of the PAHO include: Antigua and Barbuda, Argentina, Bahamas, Barbados, Belize, Bermuda, Bolivia, Brazil, Canada, Chile, Colombia, Costa Rica, Cuba, Dominica, the Dominican Republic, Ecuador, El Salvador, Grenada, Guatemala, Guyana, Haiti, Honduras, Jamaica, Mexico, Nicaragua, Panama, Paraguay, Peru, Saint Kitts and Nevis, Saint Lucia, Saint Vincent and the Grenadines, Suriname, Trinidad and Tobago, the United States, Uruguay, and Venezuela. Aruba, Curaçao, Puerto Rico, and Saint Martin are associate members. France, the Netherlands, and the United Kingdom are participating states in PAHO because they have territories and overseas departments in the Americas. Portugal and Spain are observer states.

The Americas region includes some of the world's wealthiest nations as well as many developing countries. Health indicators in individual PAHO member states can be similarly diverse. In 2014, life expectancy at birth in the Americas region was 76.7 years. The global average life expectancy at birth was 71 years. The Americas, along with the WHO regions for Europe and the Western Pacific, enjoy the longest life expectancies in the world. Life expectancy at birth in 2012 within the Americas, however, ranged from 63.4 in Haiti to 81.6 in Canada.

Maternal and infant care in the WHO Americas region overall are significantly better than global averages. Skilled health-care personnel attend 93 percent of all births, and 95 percent of women receive at least some prenatal health care. However, infant mortality rates also reveal the considerable inequalities that exist within the region. The average infant mortality rate (deaths before one year of age per 1,000 live births) among all PAHO nations in 2012 was 12.7. However, North America's infant mortality rate was only 5.9 whereas the Latin Caribbean subregion rate was 33.9. Every member state in the region except for Haiti has an infant mortality rate lower than the global average of 35 deaths per 1,000 live births. Latin America and the Caribbean have the lowest infant mortality rates of any of the world's developing regions. The Americas region had an under-five mortality rate (deaths before age five per 1,000 live births) of 15.6 in 2013. Haiti's under-five mortality rate was 88.

In 2012, 6.5 million childhood deaths (under age five) occurred globally. The Latin American and Caribbean subregions of the PAHO, where most childhood deaths occur, made significant progress against the problem with the aid of Millennium Development Goal (MDG) programs. Worldwide, the under-five mortality rate declined by half between 1990 and 2014. The PAHO region as a whole reported 15.6 under-five deaths per 1,000 live births in 2013.

Health and sanitation infrastructure in the PAHO region is fairly robust. More than 96 percent of PAHO region inhabitants use an improved drinking water source, and 89 percent have regular access to improved sanitation facilities. However, sanitation remains a public health problem in ad hoc settlements, disaster areas, and underdeveloped regions. Haiti, for example, has some of the world's worst rates for access to sanitation: only 24 percent of people in Haiti live with improved sanitation infrastructure. Waste frequently pollutes water sources, spreading disease.

The Americas region mortality rate (deaths per 100,000 population) from communicable diseases in 2012 was 48, well below the global average of 147. WHO and national governments worked to increase vaccination rates in the region from an average of 60 percent in 1980 to almost 95 percent in 2014. Vaccination programs eliminated polio in the Americas: the International Commission for the Certification of Poliomyelitis Eradication (ICCPE) certified the region polio-free in 1994. However, for some communicable diseases, vaccination rates can vary dramatically among the countries in the region. Whereas overall vaccination rates averaged 93 percent across the region in 2010, Haiti, Bolivia, the Dominican Republic, and Venezuela had the lowest vaccination coverage rates for measles, mumps, and rubella (MMR vaccine) and diphtheria, pertussis, and tetanus (DPT3). Vaccination rates dipped as low as 60 to 79 percent for those countries.

HIV/AIDS remains a health burden on the countries of the Americas. Efforts to prevent new infections, educate the public, and improve HIV-patient access to health care aim to reduce incidence of the disease. Compared to other low-to-middle-income countries worldwide, Latin America has highest percentage of HIV-positive people who receive HIV/AIDS treatment in the form of antiretroviral (ARV) drugs. Around 75 percent of HIV-positive people in the region have had access to ARV treatment. The global treatment rate is 61 percent.

Because part of the Americas region lies in the tropics, public health efforts also target neglected tropical diseases (NTDs) and malaria. These illnesses disproportionately strike rural citizens, neglected or marginalized populations, and children. With increased public health efforts to combat NTDs in the Americas, leprosy, Chagas disease, onchocerciasis, trachoma, and helminth infection have declined significantly. However, filariasis and leishmaniasis have increased. PAHO officials estimate that the burden of NTDs in the Americas exceeds the disease burden of malaria or tuberculosis. Zoonotic diseases (diseases with animal or insect vectors) are controlled for the most part, but remain a health problem. Chikungunya, a mosquito-borne virus, was identified for the first time in the Americas in December 2013.

Access to universal, government-provided, or government-subsidized general health care varies widely across the PAHO member countries. Some countries, such as Canada, offer comprehensive universal health care for citizens. A few PAHO countries have only ad-hoc health systems or rely on foreign aid workers as significant providers of health care. The PAHO region has the highest per-capita health-care expenditures in the world at an average of US$3,483 in 2011. Health-care expenditures within the region are among the most inequitable within any WHO region, however. The per-capita health-care expenditure in Bolivia in 2012,

CHOLERA IN HAITI

On January 12, 2010, a magnitude 7.0 earthquake caused catastrophic damage in the Haiti's capital of Port-au-Prince and the surrounding region. Crowded neighborhoods and makeshift construction practices increased the devastation. With the country already lacking reliable infrastructure and sufficient health-care facilities to support the population, the quake and its immediate aftermath killed an estimated 160,000 people.

In October 2010, 10 months after the quake, foreign nongovernmental organizations (NGOs) working in the Artibonite River region north of Port-au-Prince identified the first cases of cholera. Caused by drinking and irrigation water fouled by the bacterium *Vibrio cholera*, cholera is a diarrheal illness that can cause rapid dehydration and death. Cholera kills more than 100,000 people globally each year and takes it greatest toll in the world's poorest regions.

A scourge for centuries in many world cities, cholera is controlled most successfully through the construction of public sanitation systems to carry away, isolate, and treat human waste. Systems that allow for easy access to water from a clean source or that treat the water to make it safe further reduce the risk of cholera. Without functional sanitation systems (even those as simple as adequately maintained latrines) and routine access to clean water, waterborne diseases are difficult to control. The cholera epidemic that began in Haiti in 2010 eventually spread to three additional countries (with isolated cases related to travel identified in others): the Dominican Republic, Cuba, and Mexico. Haiti recorded 717,203 cases of cholera as of November 2014. Neighboring Dominican Republic identified 31,681, primarily in the region along the border with Haiti. Cuban officials recorded 678 cases and 190 were counted in Mexico. Without infrastructure, and with three of four Haitians lacking continuous access to an improved water source and sanitation system, cholera flourished in Haiti. Infrastructure, as well as geographic remoteness from the epicenter of the epidemic, limited related cases elsewhere.

Lack of adequate health care increases cholera mortality. Even before the earthquake, Haiti's population already had been critically underserved in health care, with its health system reliant on foreign aid workers. After the earthquake,

foreign aid efforts intensified. Evidence from genetic testing of the cholera strain that took hold in Haiti suggests that it may have been reintroduced to Haiti after the earthquake by foreign peacekeepers and aid workers encamped near the Artibonite River just 62 miles (100 kilometers) north of Haiti's capital city.

Intense cholera symptoms appear and worsen quickly, making access to health care critical. With basic health care, cholera mortality drops. Routine cases are fairly easy to treat with early medical intervention to administer fluids, oral rehydration salts, and antibiotics. Of the 9,197 people who had died of cholera as of November 2014, 8,721 died in Haiti. The other countries—all with better health systems—recorded 476 dead combined, with 472 of those deaths occurring in the Dominican Republic.

When cholera reached Port-au-Prince in November 2010, most of the urban population lived in large, dense, temporary settlements. Pan American Health Organization (PAHO) researchers predicted that cholera rapidly would become epidemic and infect 270,000 people within a year of its reemergence. The country's Ministry of Public Health and Population established a National Cholera Surveillance System (NCSS) with the help of PAHO and the World Health Organization. The NCSS and PAHO reported 350,000 cases of cholera from November 2010 through the end of 2011. The annual number of cases has declined since its 2011 peak—just over 50,000 cases were reported during 2013—but cholera remains endemic in Haiti. Working with PAHO and the United Nations (UN), Haiti's government introduced its 10-Year National Plan for the Elimination of Cholera in 2013. PAHO and the UN humanitarian office continue to identify a lack of sanitation systems as the major cause of the persistence of cholera. However, because Haiti still trails the rest of the Americas region in almost every health indicator, health efforts have focused primarily on providing acute care and public education. PAHO officials also recommended in 2012 that a cholera vaccination be made universally available in Haiti and the Dominican Republic. PAHO workers began administering a vaccine to the most at-risk populations in Haiti in September 2014.

---

for example, was around $100. Spending in the United States averaged approximately $7,400. Bermuda had the highest per-capita expenditure in health in the Americas, around $10,830.

Although communicable diseases remain a significant health threat in many PAHO subregions, noncommunicable diseases pose the most significant growing health threat to the region. Noncommunicable diseases are chronic conditions that are non-transmissible between individuals. According to the WHO, noncommunicable diseases kill 38 million people each year worldwide. The four most common noncommunicable diseases globally

are cardiovascular disease, cancer, respiratory diseases, and diabetes. Major risk factors for developing noncommunicable diseases include smoking, physical inactivity, excessive alcohol consumption, and unhealthful diets. Ischemic heart disease (IHD) is the first cause of death in the Americas.

The increasing prevalence of noncommunicable diseases within the WHO Americas region, combined with the high health-care costs associated with such diseases, has highlighted health-care inequalities within the region based on geography and relative income level.

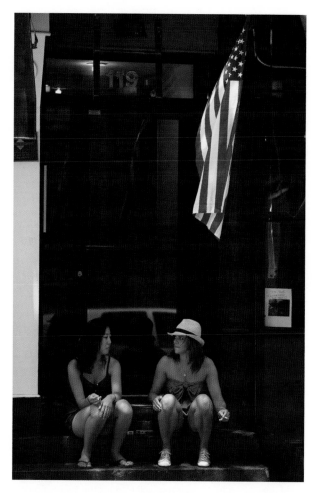

Two women smoke cigarettes outside an apartment building. The Pan American Health Organization (PAHO) has been working to decrease the number of smokers in the region to combat the biggest noncommunicable killers, many of which are related to tobacco use. Dr. Carissa F. Etienne, director of PAHO, stated in 2015 that this was being done by implementing the Framework Convention on Tobacco Control, a treaty signed by 30 of the 35 PAHO countries "establishing smoke-free environments, requiring graphic warnings on tobacco packages, banning tobacco advertising, promotion and sponsorship, and increasing tobacco taxes." Tobacco use was the leading cause of preventable death in PAHO countries in 2014, killing 1 million people annually. © *Don Emmert/Getty Images.*

⊕ Future Implications

The Americas region population is aging. In 2006, around 100 million people in the region were over 60 years of age. The regional over-60 population will double by 2020. In North America, almost 70 percent of those over 60 years old in 2020 will live beyond age 80. Fifty percent of those in Latin America and the Caribbean will live beyond age 80. As more of the population ages and lives longer, health officials expect to see a rise in diagnosis and incidence of health issues more common in people of advanced age, such as diabetes, heart disease, cancer, and dementia. An aging population also will require improvements in elder-care health systems in many countries. PAHO officials state that countries should aim for "self-management and self-care" programs for older residents to improve social inclusion and quality of life for people over 60.

Economic development is the most significant global indicator of overall improvements in public health. The Americas region will continue its trend of development, with the Latin America and Caribbean (LAC) subregion of the Americas remaining one of the fastest-developing regions in the world. More than 60 million people emerged from poverty in LAC countries in 2010 alone. However, according to the United Nations Economic Commission for Latin America and the Caribbean, the LAC subregion will remain one of the world's most economically inequitable regions through 2025. Health outcomes, access to health care, and health-promoting infrastructure correspondingly will vary dramatically throughout the region.

While the global trend toward urbanization will continue, the Americas region is already the world's most urbanized region. More than 80 percent of all Americans lived in urban areas in 2012. By 2025, 9 of the 30 most populous cities in the world will be in the Americas. The relative incidence of urban poverty decreased by 12 percent from 1990 to 2007, but the total number of urban poor increased by 5 million (from 122 million to 127 million people) during the same period. Researchers anticipate that the total number of inhabitants exposed to poor air quality will increase, along with air-quality-related health conditions and deaths. In the mid-2010s, air pollution is associated with nearly 133,000 deaths per year in the Americas.

As the WHO region with the greatest range in climate zones, from subarctic and subantarctic to tropical, the Americas region is vulnerable to global climate change. PAHO reports assert that 25 percent of the burden of disease in the region already is associated with environmental degradation. This is likely to increase with climate change. Furthermore, sub-regions are likely to see an increase in various diseases or the introduction of new diseases that previously were absent. Tropical diseases such as dengue fever, once limited to the tropics, have spread to warming subtropical areas of the Americas. PAHO studies anticipate significant increases in vector-borne and waterborne diseases in the region.

As the population, economic landscape, and climate of the Americas region changes in the coming decades, PAHO will continue to monitor regional health indicators and assist national governments in the creation of locally responsive health systems.

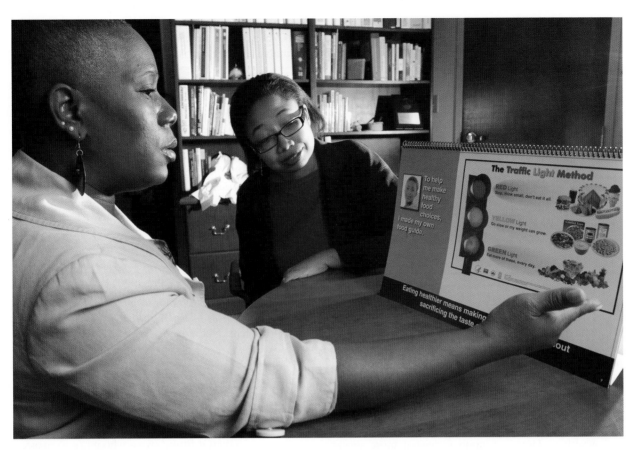

A diabetic woman listens to a community health worker familiar with the necessary diet needed to maintain control over the detrimental effects of diabetes. In the Pan American Health Organization (PAHO) region, rates of obesity and diabetes were steadily increasing for people at all income levels in 2014, however, income levels did affect outcomes when it came to managing diabetes and its complications. In 2012 PAHO officials called diabetes an "epidemic," especially in Latin America and the Caribbean. PAHO estimated the number of those in the region with diabetes was 62.8 million in 2011 and projected it would reach 91.1 million by 2030. *Amanda Mills/U.S. Centers for Disease Control and Prevention.*

PRIMARY SOURCE

Health in the Americas: 2012 Edition

SOURCE *"Chapter 1: A Century of Public Health in the Americas," in* Health in the Americas: 2012 Edition: Regional Volume, *Pan American Health Organization, 2012, 1–4. http://www.paho.org/saludenlasamericas/ index.php-option=com_docman&task=doc_ view&gid=155&Itemid= (accessed January 25, 2015).*

INTRODUCTION *This primary source is an excerpt from the introduction of a volume published by the Pan American Health Organization branch of the World Health Organization. It gives an overview of progress achieved in public health of the Americas during the 20th and early 21st centuries.*

INTRODUCTION

The Region of the Americas has made remarkable strides in population health. In the last 110 years, the infant mortality rate decreased from 167.4 per 1,000 live births in 1900 (229.1 in Latin America and the Caribbean; 145.0 in North America) to 15.2 in 2010 (20.3 in Latin America and the Caribbean; 6.6 in North America): that is, on average, an astounding 11-fold reduction (22-fold in North America) in the absolute risk of dying before reaching age 1. In simpler terms, in 1900, one out of every four babies born in Latin America and the Caribbean and one out of every seven babies born in North America would not live to see their first birthday. A century and a decade later, 99% of babies in North America and 98% of babies in Latin America and the Caribbean have already survived beyond their first year of life and have a very good chance of making it through childhood, adolescence, adulthood, and old age.

Life expectancy at birth rose from 40.9 years in 1900 (48.0 in North America; 29.2 in Latin America and the Caribbean) to 75.8 years in 2010 (78.6 in North

America; 74.2 in Latin America and the Caribbean): that is, a solid absolute gain of 35 years in the expectation of life at birth (31 in North America; 45 in Latin America and the Caribbean), which is, on average, just 15% short of doubling it from the previous century. In other words, a baby born in the Americas in 1900 had only 41 years to live, learn, work, start a family, and contribute to society; a baby born this very day in our Region will live almost twice that long and will probably be able to see his children and perhaps even his grandchildren grow and become parents themselves....

These gains notwithstanding, the Americas also experiences—simultaneously and contrastingly—persistent inequities both in its health and in its social realms. In fact, there is plentiful evidence currently available that points to the latter as being determinants of the former: persistent social inequities are determinants of persistent health inequities. With this understanding, unambiguously advanced by the WHO Commission on Social Determinants of Health, comes the realization that the reduction and elimination of health inequities only can be attained by acting on the social determinants of health across the whole spectrum of the social gradient....

Upon reflecting on the sweep of changes experienced in the Americas over the last 110 years, it is possible to be convinced that the Region's countries have collectively succeeded in making this part of the world healthier and wealthier. However, upon reviewing more recent developments in the population's health and its determinants in the Americas—as documented in this publication's chapters—the picture does not seem quite so rosy. The Pan American Health Organization, working hand in hand with the countries' governments, leaders, and communities, and with our partners, must now "walk the walk" and march forward to make this Region a more equitable and sustainable home.

SEE ALSO *Health in the WHO African Region; Health in the WHO Eastern Mediterranean Region; Health in the WHO European Region; Health in the WHO South-East Asian Region; Health in the WHO Western Pacific Region; World Health Organization: Organization, Funding, and Enforcement Powers*

BIBLIOGRAPHY

Books

Benatar, Solomon R., and Gillian Brock, eds. *Global Health and Global Health Ethics.* Cambridge, UK: Cambridge University Press, 2011.

Fairman, David, et al. *Negotiating Public Health in a Globalized World: Global Health Diplomacy in Action.* Dordrecht, Netherlands: Springer, 2012.

Websites

"Global Burden of Disease." *World Health Organization (WHO).* http://www.who.int/topics/global_burden_of_disease/en (accessed February 18, 2015).

"Governance: The Executive Board." *World Health Organization (WHO).* http://www.who.int/governance/eb/en/ (accessed February 18, 2015).

Pan American Health Organization (PAHO). http://www.paho.org/hq/ (accessed February 18, 2015).

Joseph P. Hyder

Health in the WHO Eastern Mediterranean Region

⊕ Introduction

The Eastern Mediterranean Regional Office (EMRO) of the World Health Organization (WHO) coordinates public health initiatives and campaigns within an area that covers North Africa, the Middle East, and parts of Central and South Asia. EMRO is one of six WHO regional offices that addresses the particular health concerns and needs within its area of administration. Staff, governments, public health agencies, nongovernmental organizations (NGOs) and others that work with the regional offices of the WHO, therefore, gain specialized technical knowledge applicable to the diseases and health-care delivery issues involved in each particular WHO region.

EMRO faces challenges unique to its mission to coordinate and deliver health care in one of the most ethnically diverse and conflict-afflicted regions of the world. The WHO, physicians, and public health organizations working within the area under EMRO's direction must monitor the efficacy of public health campaigns in the region constantly and respond quickly to health-care emergencies related to wars and conflicts in the region. As of 2015, more than a dozen conflicts within EMRO's region have produced millions of refugees and internally displaced persons with urgent and varied public health needs.

The WHO navigates a complex array of public health issues within the EMRO region. These range from noncommunicable (noninfectious and non-transmissible) diseases, also known as diseases of affluence, in wealthy nations around the Persian Gulf to the scourge of preventable and treatable communicable (infectious and transmissible) diseases, also known as diseases of poverty, in some of the world's poorest countries. Furthermore, cultural differences among some ethnic groups in the region have complicated global public health efforts, such as the eradication of poliomyelitis (polio). In fact, in Pakistan and Afghanistan—two of the three countries in the world with endemic polio—health-care workers carrying out vaccination campaigns have been targeted by Islamist militant groups. Wars in other areas under EMRO's control, such as Somalia and Syria, have seen the return of polio to those countries in recent years. EMRO also is responsible for monitoring and containing emerging health threats in the region, such as the 2012 emergence of the highly virulent Middle East respiratory syndrome coronavirus (MERS CoV).

⊕ Historical Background

The constitution of the WHO was opened for signatures on July 22, 1946, and became the first specialized agency of the United Nations (UN) to have every UN member state join. The WHO was officially formed in April 1948 by combining the League of Nations Health Organization and the epidemiological service of the Office International d'Hygiène Publique (OIHP).

The WHO initially sought to tackle the spread of widely recognized global health issues, including malaria, child and maternal health, sexually transmitted diseases, and tuberculosis. Article 44 of the WHO Constitution allows the World Health Assembly (WHA), the forum through which the 194 member states of the WHO govern the agency, to define geographic areas and "establish a regional organization to meet the special needs of such area." Article 44, therefore, allowed the WHA to create regional offices of the WHO to address the specific health and development needs unique to particular geographic areas.

Between 1949 and 1952, the WHA created six regional offices of the WHO. The WHO regional offices include the following: Africa (AFRO); Europe (EURO); Southeast Asia (SEARO); EMRO; Western Pacific (WPRO); and the Americas (AMRO; also known as the Pan American Health Organization [PAHO]).

In 1997 UN Secretary-General Kofi Annan (1938–) reorganized all UN agencies dedicated to working on development issues in order to promote efficiency and sharing of technical knowledge. With the approval of the UN General Assembly, Annan created the United Nations Development Group, which coordinates activities between the WHO, UNICEF, the United Nations Development Programme, the World Food Programme, the Food and Agriculture Organization, and about a dozen other UN agencies and programs. The UN Development Operations Coordination Office (DOCO) coordinates strategic support on UN development issues across UN bodies and in cooperation with national governments and nongovernmental organizations. A key area of concern for DOCO has been coordinating UN action toward meeting the UN Millennium Development Goals (MDGs).

EMRO is headquartered in Cairo, Egypt, and provides services to one nonmember state (the occupied Palestinian territory—the West Bank and Gaza Strip) and 21 member states: Afghanistan, Bahrain, Djibouti, Egypt, Iran, Iraq, Jordan, Kuwait, Lebanon, Libya, Morocco, Oman, Pakistan, Qatar, Saudi Arabia, Somalia, Sudan, Syria, Tunisia, the United Arab Emirates, and Yemen. EMRO serves a population of nearly 583 million people.

Historically, chief among the many challenges EMRO has faced are obtaining data to conduct disease surveillance (monitoring) and report of vital health statistics. A 2012 survey found that nearly half (40 percent)

of EMRO counties have inadequate or weak reporting systems, which means that they have little to no ability to track the causes of morbidity (disease) and mortality (deaths). Just one-quarter of EMRO countries have satisfactory data gathering and reporting systems. This widespread deficiency hampers public health efforts. As noted by Dr. Ala Alwan, the regional director for EMRO, in a 2014 report, "Reliable and timely health information is essential for policy development, proper health management, evidence-based decision-making, rational resource allocation and monitoring and evaluation."

EMRO also continues to contend with the results of conflicts throughout the region that damage and destroy health-care delivery systems; health and humanitarian crises; sanitation, vector-borne diseases and food-borne illnesses; maternal and child health issues; and a rise in noncommunicable diseases at least in part fueled by tobacco use. The graphic shows that nearly one-quarter (22 percent) of the population over age 15 in the region uses tobacco. The region trails the Western Pacific and Europe but has a higher rate of tobacco use by males than Africa, South-East Asia and the Americas; it is only exceeded the Western Pacific region, with 47 percent. It also must prepare for other threats to health security such as pandemic (global epidemic) influenza and other disease outbreaks as well as the accidental or deliberate release of chemical or biological agents that harm health.

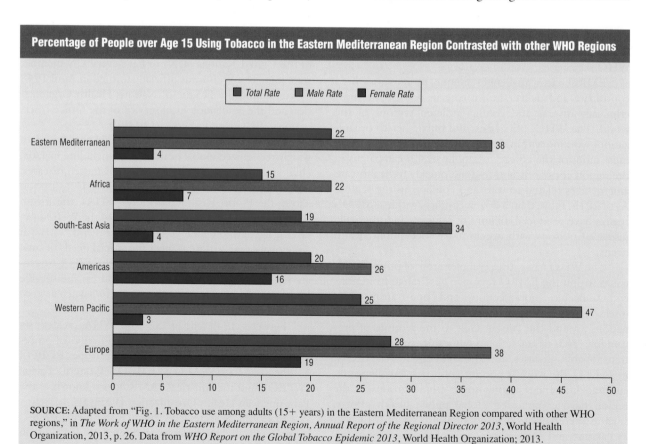

Percentage of People over Age 15 Using Tobacco in the Eastern Mediterranean Region Contrasted with other WHO Regions

■ Total Rate　■ Male Rate　■ Female Rate

Eastern Mediterranean: 22, 38, 4
Africa: 15, 22, 7
South-East Asia: 19, 34, 4
Americas: 20, 26, 16
Western Pacific: 25, 47, 3
Europe: 28, 38, 19

SOURCE: Adapted from "Fig. 1. Tobacco use among adults (15+ years) in the Eastern Mediterranean Region compared with other WHO regions," in *The Work of WHO in the Eastern Mediterranean Region, Annual Report of the Regional Director 2013*, World Health Organization, 2013, p. 26. Data from *WHO Report on the Global Tobacco Epidemic 2013*, World Health Organization; 2013.

⊕ Impacts and Issues

EMRO faces a wide range of public health and development issues in its territory. EMRO's region stretches over 6,000 miles (10,000 kilometers) from the Saharan Desert of Morocco in North Africa to the Himalayan Mountains in northwest Pakistan in South Asia. EMRO's region covers nearly 580 million people. These characteristics of EMRO's mandate region present challenges in dealing with and communicating about complex health issues across numerous languages and cultures. These complications have hindered the WHO's efforts in vital public health campaigns, such as polio eradication, and preventing the spread of novel infectious diseases, such as MERS-CoV. Numerous wars and armed conflicts throughout the region further complicate efforts to monitor and improve public health in EMRO's coverage area.

Language and Cultural Barriers

EMRO's diverse region encompasses dozens of languages and more than 100 dialects spoken by members of dozens of ethnic groups. Arabic, English, and French are the official languages of the WHO in the Eastern Mediterranean region. All official communications are published in one or more of these languages and EMRO's monthly medical journal, *Eastern Mediterranean Health Journal*, publishes articles in all of these languages. EMRO, however, also has adopted other languages, including Dari, Pashto, Persian, Somali, and Urdu to communicate with local health organizations and individuals.

Cultural differences place some ethnic groups or tribes within the region at greater health risk as they may be less receptive to EMRO's mission to promote public health care. The proliferation of militant groups in areas of Pakistan and Afghanistan—two of three countries in the world where polio remains endemic—has led to strict bans on vaccination teams in some areas. In 2012, militants in Pakistan began targeting WHO-affiliated polio vaccination teams. A WHO-UNICEF polio vaccination campaign in Pakistan was suspended in December 2012 following the killing of nine health workers. In May 2014, militants in Pakistan's Khyber Agency launched one of the deadliest anti-vaccination attacks to that date by targeting two vans carrying members of a polio vaccination team. The attack, which included roadside bombs and small arms fire, killed 11 people.

In July 2014, Taliban militants announced that polio vaccination teams would not be allowed to operate in

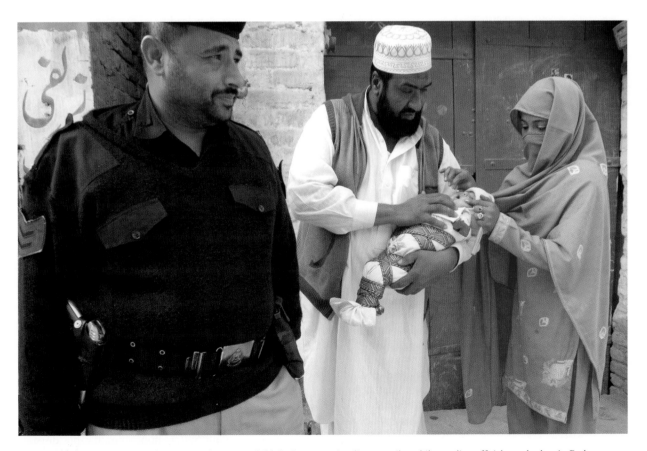

A health worker administers polio-vaccine drops to a child during an anti-polio campaign while a police official stands alert in Peshawar, Pakistan. © *Asianet-Pakistan/Shutterstock.com.*

CIA LOCATES OSAMA BIN LADEN, UNDERMINES POLIO VACCINATION CAMPAIGN IN PAKISTAN

In the months leading up to the raid on al-Qaeda leader Osama bin Laden's compound near Abbottabad, Pakistan, in May 2011, the U.S. Central Intelligence Agency (CIA) worked with a local Pakistani physician, Shakil Afridi (1962–), to coordinate a fake hepatitis B vaccination campaign. In the summer of 2010, U.S. intelligence agencies had tracked Abu Ahmad al-Kuwaiti (died 2011), an al-Qaeda courier, to a compound near Abbottabad. The CIA suspected that a high-level al-Qaeda target, possibly including bin Laden, was located at the compound.

To verify the presence of bin Laden in Abbottabad, the CIA crafted the fake vaccination campaign in hopes of collecting DNA samples from bin Laden's children. U.S. intelligence agencies planned on comparing the DNA collected from the vaccination program with DNA from bin Laden's estranged sister, who died in Boston in 2010.

Afridi set up the fake vaccination campaign in a poor section of Abbottabad to lend greater credence to program. The hepatitis B vaccine typically is given in three doses, spaced out over several months. After administering the first doses in the poorer area of Abbottabad, however, Afridi moved the campaign to the affluent suburb of Bilal Town, where the bin Laden compound was located. The children who received the initial doses of the hepatitis B vaccine never received the remaining two doses of the series. While in Bilal Town, a nurse gained access to the bin Laden compound to administer vaccines to children at that location.

DNA collected from the fake vaccination campaign did not confirm the presence of bin Laden in the Abbottabad area. In the early morning hours of May 2, 2011, however, U.S. special forces raided the suspected bin Laden compound and shot and killed bin Laden.

Pakistani authorities arrested Afridi shortly after the May 2 raid on the bin Laden compound. On May 23, 2012, Afridi was sentenced to 33 years in prison. Initial reports indicated that Afridi's sentence was related to his cooperation with U.S. agencies leading to the bin Laden raid, but later reports from the Pakistani government claim that his conviction and sentence stem from ties to the Lashkar-e-Islam militant group. A Lashkar-e-Islam commander, however, stated that the organization never had contact with Afridi and would kill him if given the opportunity.

The CIA received widespread condemnation from the international health community for using a fake vaccination campaign to gain intelligence, particularly in a country where many people were already skeptical of vaccination campaigns. Acknowledging that the Abbottabad fake vaccination campaign may have harmed efforts to eradicate polio and control other diseases, in May 2014 the administration of U.S. President Barack Obama (1961–) stated that the CIA would no longer use fake vaccination campaigns to gain intelligence information.

Afghanistan's Helmand Province. The Taliban had previously allowed vaccination teams in the area, but in its July 2014 announcement it stated that it views vaccination workers as spies. The revelation in July 2011 that the U.S. Central Intelligence Agency (CIA) had used a fake vaccination campaign in northern Pakistan to gather DNA evidence to identify the location of al-Qaeda leader Osama bin Laden (1957–2011) increased mistrust of vaccination campaigns among many in the Pakistani-Afghan border area.

Disease Eradication and Prevention

In 1988, the WHO, UNICEF, and the Rotary Foundation launched a massive public health campaign to eradicate polio by 2000. Although the organizations missed their original target date, they did succeed in reducing the number of global polio cases from an estimated 350,000 in 1988 to fewer than 3,000 by 2000 and 291 cases in 2012. In 2012, Pakistan reported 58 cases of wild polio. After militants began targeting vaccination workers in late 2012, however, Pakistan saw an increase in the number of cases, with 91 cases reported in 2013. Afghanistan saw the number of wild polio cases in the country fall from 80 in 2011 to 37 in 2012 and 13 in 2013. The effect of the Taliban's July 2014 prohibition of vaccination health workers in some areas of the country, however, may lead to an increase in the number of cases.

In 2012, EMRO faced an emergence of a new disease within its territory—MERS CoV. MERS patients generally present the symptoms of fever, cough, and shortness of breath. Affected patients may develop acute respiratory distress syndrome, which often results in death. In the two years following the discovery of MERS in Saudi Arabia, the country reported 688 cases resulting in 282 deaths for a case fatality rate of more than 40 percent.

Public Health Issues and Income Disparity

The wealth disparity between countries in EMRO's coverage area also highlights the varied health needs among their member states. In the Persian Gulf state of Qatar, for example, the per-capita gross domestic product (GDP) exceeds $92,000 per year, and annual health-care expenditures in the country are almost $1,800 per capita. In the East African nations of Somalia, Sudan, and South Sudan, however, per-capita GDP is US$284, $1,234, and $1,972, respectively. Per-capita health expenditures in these countries range from virtually nonexistent in Somalia to US$104 in Sudan.

The disparities in income and health-care expenditures in these countries compel EMRO to address a wide range of public health and development issues. In the prosperous Gulf States, noncommunicable diseases (NCDs), which are typically associated with affluent societies, are a major concern. NCDs include diseases and conditions such as obesity, cancer, cardiovascular disease, diabetes, and high blood pressure.

In East Africa and poorer, rural areas in the Middle East, Afghanistan, and Pakistan, EMRO must address communicable diseases such as diarrheal diseases, cholera, malnutrition, tuberculosis, and neglected diseases. While many of these diseases of poverty are easily preventable or treatable, access to adequate infrastructure and health-care facilities limits progress. Diarrheal diseases, for example, claim more than 760,000 lives of children under the age of five annually around the world, making diarrheal diseases the second-leading cause of childhood deaths. Diarrheal diseases are easily preventable with access to improved water supplies and sanitation. EMRO estimates that only 29 percent of Somalis and 50 percent of South Sudanese had access to improved water sources in 2008. In Pakistan—the most populous country covered by EMRO—only 56 percent of the population had access to improved water sources in 2009, leaving more than 83 million Pakistanis without access to clean freshwater. Access to improved sanitation is even more dire in many countries. In South Sudan, Yemen, Sudan, and Somalia, for example, only 7, 23, 27, and 30 percent of their populations, respectively, have access to improved sanitation.

⊕ Future Implications

EMRO's efforts to improve public health in its region will be compromised in the coming years by numerous armed conflicts across North Africa, the Middle East, and Central and South Asia. As of 2014, more than one dozen armed conflicts in the region under EMRO's oversight hampered efforts to deliver preventive and emergency medical care to hundreds of thousands of people in the region.

The Syrian Civil War, which began in 2011, had resulted in an estimated 260,000 deaths—mostly civilians—as of 2014. The conflict has also resulted in more than 3 million refugees seeking safety near the borders areas of Lebanon, Turkey, Jordan, and Iraq. An additional 4.5 million to 5 million Syrians have been internally displaced as they seek safer areas within their own country. The fighting, which pits numerous militant groups against the Syrian government (and against one another), makes the delivery of emergency and routine medical care virtually impossible in many areas.

The Iraqi insurgency, which escalated in 2011 following the withdrawal of U.S. troops, has pitted insurgents against the central government of Iraq. Sectarian violence also increased. In January 2014, a radical Sunni militant and terrorist group known as the Islamic State in Iraq and the Levant (ISIL) or the Islamic State in Iraq and al-Sham (ISIS) emerged from the chaos of the Syrian Civil War. Within months, ISIS had claimed large swaths of eastern Syria and northwestern Iraq. In June 2014, ISIS occupied Mosul, Iraq's second-largest city,

and had taken control of Iraq's border areas with Jordan and Syria. ISIS had moved to within 56 miles (90 kilometers) of the Iraqi capital of Baghdad, before the Iraqi Army launched a meaningful counteroffensive.

The rapid ISIS advance through Syria and Iraq was accompanied by extreme brutality toward those who disagreed with the group's radical version of Islam. (In February 2014, al-Qaeda severed ties with ISIS, in large part, over the brutality of ISIS.) More than 1 million people, including virtually all members of religious and ethnic minorities, fled the ISIS advance and sought refuge in the Kurdish-controlled areas of Iraq and Turkey. These refugees and internally displaced persons added to the already considerable burden of the WHO and other organizations providing emergency and medical supplies to those displaced by the neighboring Syrian Civil War.

In addition to the health-care needs of war refugees and internally displaced persons, conflicts in the Middle East are undermining the WHO's polio eradication campaign. The inability to get polio vaccines to children in the conflict zones led to a polio outbreak in Syria in 2013 in which 36 cases were reported. Furthermore, conflict in Somalia resulted in a drop in vaccination levels, leading to the reintroduction of polio to the country, which had been declared polio-free in 2007. In 2013, however, Somalia reported 185 cases of polio—more than half of the cases reported in the world for the year. The strain of polio found in Somalia had been imported from Nigeria, one of three countries in the world with endemic polio. After the rapid spread of polio in Somalia, Somali emigrants spread polio to Ethiopia and Kenya. In response, the WHO increased polio vaccination campaigns in the affected countries, as well as Djibouti and Yemen.

Since the first confirmed case of MERS in Saudi Arabia in 2012, the disease has been reported in 22 countries. Infected persons traveling out of Saudi Arabia, however, exported most of the cases recorded outside of Saudi Arabia. Although many early media reports likened MERS to severe acute respiratory syndrome (SARS), taxonomical analysis (the description, identification, naming, and classification of organisms based on shared characteristics) revealed that MERS CoV is linked most closely to the bat coronaviruses HKU4 and HKU5. Despite its close taxonomical links to bat coronaviruses (and initial suspicions that certain bat species transmitted the virus to humans), research published in March 2014 identified camels as the primary source of human infections. Researchers believe that African or Australian bats carrying the coronavirus transmitted the virus to camels, which were then sold in the Middle East.

The threats to public health in the Eastern Mediterranean region are varied, and many require intensive and often complex interventions. In the coming years, continued conflict in the region will continue to pose one of the greatest threats to the efforts of the WHO and other public health organizations to improve public health and human development in the region.

WHO Events Addressing Public Health Priorities

SOURCE *"WHO Events Addressing Public Health Priorities," from* Eastern Mediterranean Health Journal (EMHJ) *20, no. 8 (August 2014): 521–523. World Health Organization (WHO). http://applications.emro.who.int/emhj/v20/08/ EMHJ_2014_20_8_521_523.pdf (accessed January 25, 2015).*

INTRODUCTION *This primary source on the subject of health diplomacy was a produced by the World Health Organization Regional Office for the Eastern Mediterranean. It gives an overview of the topic, and also touches on several specific public health challenges in the area.*

WHO EVENTS ADDRESSING PUBLIC HEALTH PRIORITIES

Moving health diplomacy forward

Why is health diplomacy important?

Increasingly, health challenges can no longer be resolved at the technical level only—they require political negotiations and solutions, and often need to involve a wide range of actors. Thus diplomacy plays an ever growing and crucial role in shaping and managing the policy environment for health. Health diplomacy refers to the negotiation processes that shape and manage that environment and is important for the countries of the WHO Eastern Mediterranean Region because many of the development issues they face relate directly to health and because it is disproportionately affected by man made and humanitarian crises.

Health diplomacy is gaining even further relevance as the Region seeks to find solutions to issues that require global action and collaboration across borders, such as Middle East Respiratory Syndrome (MERS), humanitarian health relief, noncommunicable diseases and antimicrobial resistance. But health diplomacy at the national and regional level is also critical for the implementation of health programmes through complex partnerships. For example, polio eradication in the Region is dependent on successful negotiations with many players, whose trust has to be gained, to be able to carry out safe and secure vaccination campaigns.

...

Health diplomacy in action

There are several health challenges in the Region that currently require health diplomacy efforts.

Polio: In the final push to eliminate polio from the world, including in the two remaining endemic countries in the Eastern Mediterranean Region, the success of the polio programme has become a foreign and domestic policy issue. Diplomacy at national and international levels can help build political and community will and engagement, coordinate response and improve access to children.

Insecurity: The displacement and migration of populations across the Region, due to natural and manmade disasters, have resulted in significant risks to health, but populations left behind are often at equal or greater risk. In the Syrian Arab Republic, for example, a decade of human development is estimated to have been lost because of the ongoing conflict. In these situations, foreign policy, health diplomacy and humanitarian diplomacy intersect at many levels to protect populations and health workers, as well as to gain support for humanitarian action.

Noncommunicable diseases: The rapidly increasing epidemic in the Region threatens to have huge impact on the health systems and economies of Member States in the coming decades. Tobacco use, unhealthy diet and physical inactivity are the main risk factors and are very prevalent in the Region. Health diplomacy is needed at a national level to engage all the sectors and stakeholders that can have an influence in reducing deaths due to these diseases, while it is equally important to be engaged at the international level in negotiations that affect countries' ability to set standards for imported food products, among other things.

SEE ALSO *Conflict, Violence, and Terrorism: Health Impacts; Poliomyelitis (Polio); SARS, MERS, and the Emergence of Coronaviruses; Vaccines; Viral Diseases*

BIBLIOGRAPHY

Books

Buettner, Dan. *The Blue Zones: Nine Lessons for Living Longer from the People Who've Lived the Longest,* 2nd ed. Washington, DC: National Geographic Society, 2014.

Perry, Megan A., ed. *Bioarchaeology and Behavior: The People of the Ancient Near East.* Gainesville: University Press of Florida, 2012.

Promoting a Healthy Diet for the WHO Eastern Mediterranean Region: User-Friendly Guide. Cairo: World Health Organization. Regional Office for the Eastern Mediterranean, 2012.

Razzak, Junaid A. *Eastern Mediterranean Status Report on Road Safety: Call for Action.* Cairo: World Health Organization, Regional Office for the Eastern Mediterranean, 2012.

The Work of WHO in the Eastern Mediterranean Region: Annual Report of the Regional Director 2012. Cairo: World Health Organization, Regional

Office for the Eastern Mediterranean, 2013. Available online at http://apps.who.int/iris/handle/10665/124619 (accessed October 23, 2014).

Periodicals

Arvanitakis, Constantine, and Nurdan Tozun. "Mediterranean Diet: Health and Culture." *International Journal of Anthropology* 28, no. 4 (2013): 207–235.

Bustreo, Flavia. "Less than 1000 Days to Go for MDGs 4 and 5: Where Are We and What Needs to be Done." *Eastern Mediterranean Health Journal* 20, no. 1 (January 2014): 3–4.

Martelli, P. "Working Together for Public Health." *Transcultural Psychiatry* 46, no. 2 (2009): 316–27.

Tourlouki, Eleni. "The 'Secrets' of the Long Livers in Mediterranean Islands: The Medis Study." *European Journal of Public Health* 20, no. 6 (2010).

Websites

"Demographic, Social and Health Indicators for Countries of the Eastern Mediterranean: 2013." *World Health Organization (WHO), Regional Office for the Eastern Mediterranean (EMRO)*. http://applications.emro.who.int/dsaf/EMROPUB_2013_EN_1537.pdf?ua=1 (accessed October 24, 2014).

"Eastern Mediterranean Region: Framework for Health Information Systems and Core Indicators for Monitoring Health Situation and Health System Performance 2014." *World Health Organization (WHO), Regional Office for the Eastern Mediterranean (EMRO)*. http://applications.emro.who.int/dsaf/EMROPUB_2014_EN_1792.pdf?ua=1 (accessed October 24, 2014).

"From Kebabs to Fattoush—Keeping Lebanon's Food Safe." *World Health Organization (WHO). Regional Office for the Eastern Mediterranean*. http://www.emro.who.int/lbn/lebanon-news/from-kebabs-to-fattoush-keeping-lebanons-food-safe.html (accessed March 16, 2015).

"Global Health Security—Challenges and Opportunities with Special Emphasis on the International Health Regulations (2005)." *World Health Organization (WHO), Regional Office for the Eastern Mediterranean (EMRO)*. http://applications.emro.who.int/docs/RC61_Resolutions_2014_R2_15554_EN.pdf (accessed March 16, 2015).

"Regional Health Observatory." *World Health Organization (WHO), Regional Office for the Eastern Mediterranean (EMRO)*. http://rho.emro.who.int/rhodata/ (accessed October 24, 2014).

"Regional Office for the Eastern Mediterranean." *World Health Organization (WHO)*. http://www.who.int/about/regions/emro/en/ (accessed October 24, 2014).

"Save Lives: Recommit to Implementing WHO's Framework Convention on Tobacco Control." *World Health Organization (WHO), Regional Office for the Eastern Mediterranean*. http://www.emro.who.int/tobacco/tfi-news/10-years-fctc.html (accessed March 16, 2015).

"Seasonal Influenza (Flu): WHO Eastern Mediterranean Region (EMR)." *U.S. Centers for Disease Control and Prevention (CDC)*. http://www.cdc.gov/flu/international/program/emr.htm (accessed October 2, 2014).

Joseph P. Hyder

Health in the WHO European Region

⊕ Introduction

The World Health Organization (WHO) European Regional Office (EURO) is one of six WHO regional offices. The WHO is a specialized United Nations (UN) agency under the United Nations Development Group that is tasked with improving public health around the world. EURO is responsible for implementing WHO policies, monitoring public health, and coordinating public health initiatives and programs within the region's 53 nations.

Headquartered in Copenhagen, Denmark, EURO is responsible for monitoring health in most European countries, as well as Israel and Central Asian countries that were part of the Soviet Union. The countries covered by EURO are: Albania, Andorra, Armenia, Austria, Azerbaijan, Belarus, Belgium, Bosnia and Herzegovina, Bulgaria, Croatia, Cyprus, the Czech Republic, Denmark, Estonia, Finland, France, Georgia, Germany, Greece, Hungary, Iceland, Ireland, Israel, Italy, Kazakhstan, Kyrgyzstan, Latvia, Lithuania, Luxembourg, Malta, Monaco, Montenegro, the Netherlands, Norway, Poland, Portugal, Moldova, Romania, the Russian Federation, San Marino, Serbia, Slovakia, Slovenia, Spain, Sweden, Switzerland, Tajikistan, Macedonia, Turkey, Turkmenistan, Ukraine, the United Kingdom, and Uzbekistan. EURO does not cover the Holy See (Vatican City), which has only permanent observer status at the United Nations, or Lichtenstein, which is the only UN member state that is not a member of the WHO.

Many nations within EURO enjoy high standards of economic development, well-funded health infrastructure, and low burdens of many diseases. At the same time, many nations within EURO have relatively high burdens of noncommunicable (noninfectious and nontransmissible) diseases, such as cardiovascular disease, cancer, diabetes, and respiratory diseases. Noncommunicable diseases are chronic conditions that often result from lifestyle choices, such as tobacco use, excessive alcohol consumption, physical inactivity, and poor diet. These chronic conditions place a heavy financial burden on health-care systems because they are ongoing and often require decades of disease management. The increasing prevalence of noncommunicable diseases in EURO likely will increase health-care costs in the region in the coming decades.

EURO also faces issues related to the inequitable distribution of health care within nations and between the region's nations. Lower-income residents in many EURO nations are not entitled to the same high-level care available to more affluent citizens. Many nations within EURO, particularly those that were part of the Soviet Union, have lower life expectancies and higher disease burden than other EURO nations. EURO has implemented programs to reduce inequalities related to the availability of health care in the region and reduce the prevalence of noncommunicable diseases in all EURO nations.

⊕ Historical Background

The UN's predecessor, the League of Nations, had the Health Organization as one of its principal bodies. The Health Organization oversaw the League of Nations' public health initiatives with a primary focus on preventing the spread of leprosy, malaria, typhus, and yellow fever. Following the dissolution of the League of Nations, the newly formed UN transferred the duties of the Health Organization to a new UN agency in 1948, the World Health Organization (WHO).

The World Health Assembly (WHA) sets policies, priorities, and goals for the WHO. Health ministers from each UN member state serve on the WHA. Representatives at the first annual meeting of the World Health Assembly in 1948 established maternal and infant health, nutrition, and the prevention of certain communicable diseases (namely malaria, sexually transmitted diseases, and tuberculosis) as the initial public health priorities of the WHO. These public health issues remain priorities for many of the WHO member countries.

The first World Health Assembly also tasked the WHO with compiling complete, accurate statistics on the life expectancy, mortality, and morbidity of disease. WHO research on the prevalence and morbidity of communicable (infectious and transmissible) and noncommunicable diseases continues to form an important part of the WHO's mission and assists the WHA and government health ministries in establishing and evaluating public health priorities.

In the mid-2010s, the WHA is composed of the health ministers from all UN member states except Lichtenstein. In addition to UN member states, several nongovernmental organizations and nonmember states of the UN participate as observers at WHA meetings. The Holy See (Vatican City), the Palestinian Authority, Taiwan (as Chinese Taipei), the Inter-Parliamentary Union, the International Committee of the Red Cross, the International Federation of Red Cross and Red Crescent Societies, and the Order of Malta have observer status at the WHA.

From 1949 until 1952, the WHA exercised its authority under Section 44 of the WHO constitution to create regional offices designed to meet the specific public health needs of designated areas of the world. The WHO has six regional offices: the Regional Office for Africa (AFRO); the Regional Office for the Americas (AMRO, also known as the Pan American Health Organization [PAHO]); the Regional Office for South-East Asia (SEARO); the Regional Office for the Western Pacific (WPRO); the Regional Office for the Eastern Mediterranean (EMRO); and EURO.

Initially EURO was housed in the main WHO headquarters in Geneva, Switzerland, but in 1957 it was relocated to Copenhagen, Denmark. Although European countries were undergoing rapid economic development EURO maintained its focus on basic public health issues—communicable diseases, maternal and child health, occupational health, and nursing. There was also an emphasis on sharing experience and intercountry initiatives. For example, in 1960 Bulgaria and France hosted seminars about health-care delivery in rural areas.

From the late 1950s through the following decade EURO shifted its focus in response to the decline in communicable diseases and the rise of noncommunicable diseases and conditions—accidents and trauma, cardiovascular diseases, cancer, diabetes, water, soil, air and noise pollution as well as mental health problems. It also emphasized education and training and preventive strategies.

In 1960 EURO created a chronic disease and gerontology unit. It promoted early detection programs and health screening, and considered ways to improve care for older adults. EURO joined forces with the United Nations Children's Fund (UNICEF) to offer training in maternal and child health services throughout Europe. School doctors and nurses became agents for improving children's health and EURO also developed educational and training programs to enhance awareness and understanding of the effects of disability.

During the 1970s and 1980s, EURO launched three long-term programs—cardiovascular diseases, mental health, and environmental health emphasizing prevention as well as treatment. The mental health program pioneered a comprehensive model for service delivery that included preventive treatment and rehabilitation services delivered in the community by multidisciplinary teams of health professionals. The environmental health program addressed water supply and sanitation, waste treatment and disposal, chemical and food safety, radiation protection, and occupational health.

EURO was active in policy development, drafting the European strategy to deliver health for all, which was based on equity, solidarity, and participation. Equity was defined as ensuring equal opportunity for people to achieve their health potential. Solidarity implied the collective efforts of society should be brought to bear to promote the health of its members and participation called upon all stakeholders to have a voice in decisions aimed at improving health and health-care systems.

In 1990, EURO created EUROHEALTH, a program intended to meet the needs of countries in Eastern Europe. EUROHEALTH had six priorities: health policy, health-care reform, women and children's health, infectious diseases, noncommunicable diseases and health promotion, and environmental health. During the 1990s EURO responded to armed conflicts in Yugoslavia and Kosovo and developed rapid responses to humanitarian crises such as refugee health programs. It also worked to help new member states repair and restore their health-care delivery systems.

In the first decade of the 21st century, EURO responded to other health emergencies. In January 2006 Turley reported a possible outbreak of avian influenza (bird flu) and, working with the Turkish government, the WHO, the European Centre for Disease Prevention and Control, UNICEF, and the World Organisation for Animal Health, an epidemic was averted. In the winter of 2007–2008, EURO responded to a health emergency created by unusually frigid weather in Tajikistan and helped to implement much needed reforms in the country's health-care system.

EURO also enhanced its communication programs, providing access to reliable, evidence-based information for health professionals and the lay public. Its website (http://www.euro.who.int) informs about 10,000 visitors a day.

PUBLIC HEALTH IN NATIONS OF THE FORMER SOVIET UNION

Following the dissolution of the Soviet Union in December 1991, 15 post-Soviet states ultimately came into existence. The Russian Federation became the primary successor state and assumed all of the rights and obligations under international agreements ratified by the Soviet Union. Russia also assumed the Soviet Union's seat as a permanent member on the United Nations Security Council. In addition to Russia, the post-Soviet states of Armenia, Azerbaijan, Belarus, Estonia, Georgia, Kazakhstan, Kyrgyzstan, Latvia, Lithuania, Moldova, Tajikistan, Turkmenistan, Ukraine, and Uzbekistan emerged from the fallen empire. Even though many of the post-Soviet states are located entirely within Central Asia, all post-Soviet states are members of the WHO Regional Office for Europe.

Under the Soviet Union, citizens had access to universal health care. The Soviet health-care system had quickly turned around a population that significantly trailed Western Europe and the United States in life expectancy and other health indicators. A child born in the Soviet Union in 1927 had a life expectancy of 44.4, compared to about 60.5 years in the United States. By the 1960s, however, life expectancy in the Soviet Union approached that of the United States before declining throughout the 1970s and 1980s, largely as a result of noncommunicable diseases related to excessive alcohol consumption.

Since the fall of the Soviet Union, many post-Soviet states have enjoyed increased economic prosperity. According to EURO, however, this financial prosperity has not translated into more comprehensive and effective health care. Declining state funding for health care combined with outdated policies and programs have undermined public health in post-Soviet states.

Statistics on life expectancy, mortality, and morbidity reflect the declining standard of public health in post-Soviet states. Out of the 53 nations in the WHO European Region, the 10 nations with the lowest life expectancy at birth and the lowest life expectancy at age 65 are all post-Soviet states. Furthermore, the top 10 EURO nations with the highest incidence of premature deaths (before age 70) are also all post-Soviet states.

Post-Soviet states do not fare much better in terms of maternal, infant, and childhood health when compared to their EURO neighbors. Eight of the top 10 EURO nations in the incidence of maternal deaths (per 100,000 live births) and nine out of the top 10 in the incidence of infant deaths are post-Soviet states.

The poor health statistics from post-Soviet states relative to other EURO nations result from underinvestment in health-care infrastructure and high rates of noncommunicable diseases caused primarily by high smoking and alcohol consumption rates. Numerous WHO and EURO policies, including Health 2020; the Moscow Declaration; the *Action Plan for Implementation of the European Strategy for the Prevention and Control of Noncommunicable Diseases, 2012–2016*; and the WHO Framework Convention on Tobacco Control, are designed to strengthen the health-care infrastructure and decrease risk factors for noncommunicable diseases.

⊕ Impacts and Issues

According to most health indicators compiled by the United Nations, EURO places at or near the top in almost every category of public health and economic development. In 2012, life expectancy at birth in the European region was 76 years, which tied the region with the WHO regions for the Americas and the Western Pacific for longest life expectancy. The global average life expectancy at birth was 70 years in 2012. Life expectancy at birth in 2012 within the EURO region, however, ranged from 68 in Kazakhstan to 83 in Switzerland and San Marino. Along with geographic variation, the region shows significant gaps in life expectancy between sexes from 1980 to 2010. (See graphic.) In 2010, the average life expectancy at birth was 73 years for men and 80 years for women.

The infant mortality rate (deaths before one year of age per 1,000 live births) among EURO nations in 2012 was 10, which was the lowest rate for any WHO region and less than one-third of the global average of 35. The EURO region performed even better in the under-five mortality rate (deaths before age five per 1,000 live births) with a rate of 12, which was one-quarter of the global average of 48.

The long life expectancies, low infant mortality, and low childhood mortality rates in EURO indicate a low burden of communicable disease and a strong health-care system. The EURO mortality rate (deaths per 100,000 population) from communicable diseases in 2012 was 45, which was the lowest rate for any WHO region and well below the global average of 147. Only 136,000 of the 6.5 million childhood (under age five) deaths that occurred globally in 2012 were in the EURO region, representing only about 2 percent of all childhood deaths globally (despite EURO nations accounting for more than 12 percent of the global population). Nations within EURO fare particularly well in low prevalence of many childhood diseases. In 2012, the percentage of childhood (under age five) deaths caused by HIV/AIDS, diarrheal diseases, measles, and malaria were 0, 4, 0, and 0 percent respectively.

Maternal and infant care in the WHO European Region are also among the best in the world. Within EURO nations, skilled health-care personnel attend 98 percent of all births, which represents the highest rate in the world. In addition, the WHO European Region has the highest global rates of immunization among one-year-olds for measles, diphtheria, tetanus, and pertussis.

Despite the low burden and high level of treatment of communicable diseases within the WHO European Region, the region lags behind other parts of the world in the treatment of HIV/AIDS despite the region's widely available health-care treatment and relatively low level of stigma associated with the disease. The region had a low prevalence of HIV/AIDS, at 244 cases per 100,000 population in 2012, which was less than half of the global prevalence of 511 per 100,000. Within EURO

Changes in Life Expectancy at Birth from 1980–2010 in the WHO European Region

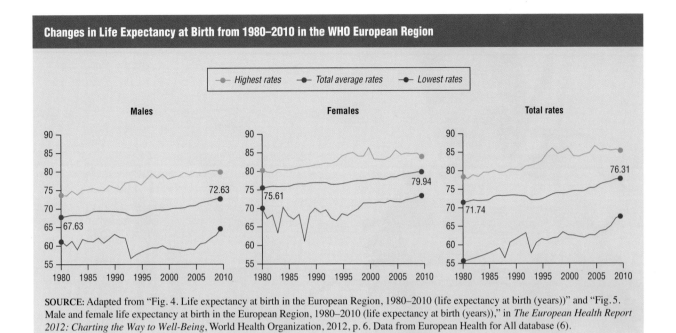

SOURCE: Adapted from "Fig. 4. Life expectancy at birth in the European Region, 1980–2010 (life expectancy at birth (years))" and "Fig. 5. Male and female life expectancy at birth in the European Region, 1980–2010 (life expectancy at birth (years))," in *The European Health Report 2012: Charting the Way to Well-Being*, World Health Organization, 2012, p. 6. Data from European Health for All database (6).

Total change of life expectancy rates in Europe from 1980 to 2010 has increased five years overall.

nations, however, the percentage of eligible HIV/AIDS infected individuals receiving antiretroviral (ARV) treatment was only 38 percent, which was the second-lowest rate among any WHO region after EMRO at 15 percent. The global ARV treatment rate was 61 percent.

Many EURO nations, particularly in Western Europe, have universal or highly subsidized health care provided by the state. In 2011, government expenditures on health care accounted for 73.9 percent of all health-care expenditures in the region, compared to 25.8 percent in private expenditures. The EURO region has the second-highest per capita health-care expenditures in the world at an average of US$2,370 in 2011, which placed it behind only AMRO/PAHO at $3,483 per capita. Health care expenditures in the region are among the most inequitable within any WHO region, however. The per capita health-care expenditure in Tajikistan in 2011, for example, was only $48, compared to $9,908 per capita in Norway.

The WHO European Region has the highest concentration of physicians and nurses in the world, with 33.1 physicians and 80.5 nurses per 10,000 population. The global average is 14.1 physicians and 29.2 nurses per 10,000 population. EURO nations also have widely available psychiatric care with 1.1 psychiatrists per 10,000 population, which is more than double the rate found in the next closest region and almost four times higher than the global average of 0.3 psychiatrists per 10,000 population.

Despite the relatively low level of communicable diseases in WHO European Region, noncommunicable diseases pose a major public health threat within the region. According to the WHO, noncommunicable diseases kill

38 million people each year worldwide. The four most common noncommunicable diseases globally are cardiovascular disease, cancer, respiratory diseases, and diabetes. Major risk factors for developing noncommunicable diseases include smoking, physical inactivity, alcohol consumption, and unhealthy diets.

According to EURO, in its *Action Plan for Implementation of the European Strategy for the Prevention and Control of Noncommunicable Diseases, 2012–2016*, noncommunicable diseases are the leading cause of disease and death within the region. Noncommunicable diseases account for 77 percent of the disease burden with EURO nations and 86 percent of all deaths compared to 68 percent of global deaths. Because noncommunicable diseases are chronic, patients often require decades of health care to manage symptoms. The high prevalence of noncommunicable diseases in EURO, therefore, places an increasing economic strain on national health-care systems and increases the cost of health care throughout the region.

The growing prevalence of noncommunicable diseases within the WHO European Region, combined with the high health-care costs associated with such diseases, has highlighted health-care inequalities within the region based on geography and relative income level. In order to control noncommunicable diseases throughout the WHO European Region, the EURO Regional Committee adopted Europe 2020, a comprehensive plan to strengthen health-care capacity throughout the region by 2020. EURO also contributed to the adoption of the Moscow Declaration at the First Ministerial Conference on Healthy Lifestyles and Noncommunicable Disease Control in 2011. The Moscow Declaration calls on

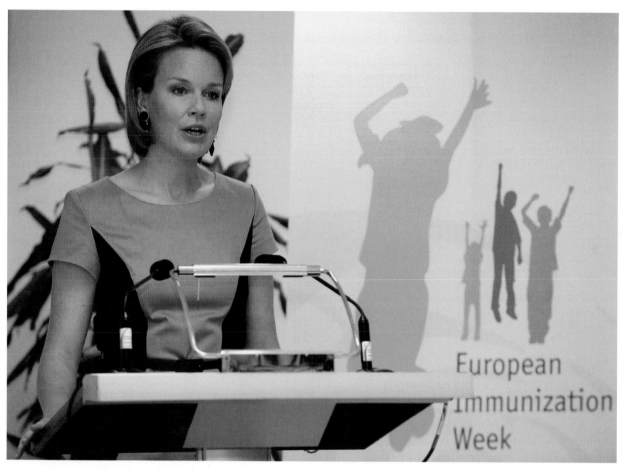

Princess Mathilde of Belgium speaks on April 26, 2011, during the launch of the sixth World Health Organization (WHO) European Immunization Week in Brussels.   © *Dirk Waem/AFP/Getty Images.*

WHO regions and local offices to develop and implement plans to address the rise of noncommunicable diseases around the world. In 2012, EURO adopted an action plan to implement the Moscow Declaration within the WHO European Region.

⊕ Future Implications

Despite its relatively high level of economic development and robust health-care systems, the WHO European Region faces a number of public health challenges, particularly those related to the prevalence of noncommunicable diseases and inequalities of health care available between nations in the region. An aging population in the region caused by declining birthrates and an increase in life expectancy poses challenges to the region's health-care systems as health problems related to mobility and dementia become more common. Furthermore, the burden of noncommunicable diseases among aging populations will lead to significant increases in the cost of health care in the region.

In 2010, the EURO Regional Committee began a consultative process with health ministers and professionals from EURO member states and the international community. This consultative process was designed to improve public health and strengthen public health systems in the region. Specifically, the consultative process sought to analyze the changing health context within the region related to changing demographic, economic, environmental, and social conditions in order to implement a framework health policy that would benefit people of different economic status throughout the region.

In September 2012, after two years of consultation, the 53 member states of the WHO Regional Committee for Europe adopted Health 2020: The European Policy for Health and Well-Being. Health 2020 seeks to "significantly improve the health and well-being of populations, reduce health inequalities, strengthen public health and ensure people-centered health systems that are universal, equitable, sustainable and of high quality."

In order to achieve Health 2020's goal, the initiative establishes seven key components for EURO and its member nations. First, Health 2020 acknowledges the WHO Constitution's guarantee of high standard of health as a human right. Second, the initiative recognizes that high-quality health of individuals makes societies

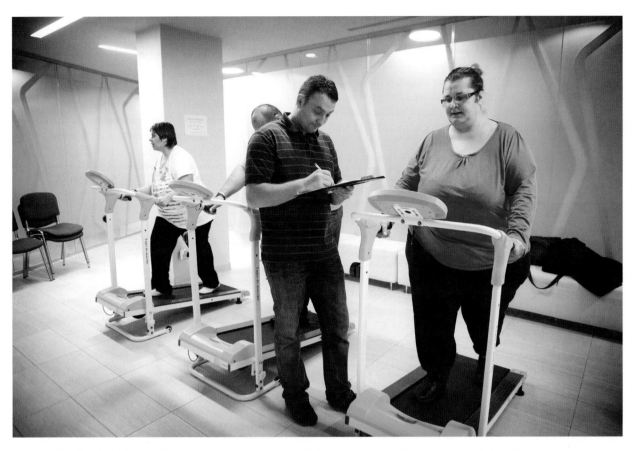

At an obesity clinic in Mulhouse, France, patients engage in a physical exercise session with a masseur-physiotherapist. Patients must attend these sessions before and after surgery for obesity. The aim is to get the patient used to doing regular physical exercise again. In developed nations, increased rates of obesity correspond with increasing rates of noncommunicable diseases like cardiovascular disease and type 2 diabetes.   ©: *BSIP/UIG via Getty Images.*

more productive by increasing economic productivity and diverting resources from social disability programs and health-care costs. Third, Health 2020 provides a flexible framework within which policy makers may respond to changing demographic, epidemiological, financial, and social factors. Fourth, Health 2020 aims to remove existing barriers and increase future cooperation among health partners, including the WHO, national and local governments, nongovernmental organizations, private health-care industry, nonprofit organizations, and other stakeholders. Fifth, Health 2020 seeks to achieve equality in health care by identifying gaps in health-care systems focusing the attention of stakeholders on these deficiencies. Notably, Health 2020 aims to provide equality in health care by promoting strong public health care and safety nets funded by sustainable public expenditures. Sixth, Health 2020 will utilize and share evidence of the efficacy and efficiency of existing and developing health-care practices and technologies. Finally, Health 2020 encourages governments to work across all levels to achieve two strategic objectives: improving health for all citizens and reducing inequalities in health care; and improving national leadership and participatory governance on health issues.

In addition to these seven key components, the Health 2020 framework sets four priority areas for national governments to build upon and strengthen global and regional WHO action plans. First, governments within the EURO region should invest in health care at all levels of life development, including maternal, infant, childhood, and elderly health issues. Second, Health 2020 calls on national governments to address the region's major disease burdens, particularly in the area of noncommunicable diseases. Third, Health 2020 requests that national governments increase public health capacity, including emergency preparedness and response. Finally, Health 2020 sets the creation of supportive environments as a national public health priority.

While Health 2020 sets broad policies and priority areas, the WHO Regional Office for Europe aims to assist governments in setting specific, attainable public health goals related to the Health 2020 framework that are most suitable for each nation. EURO admits, however, that some of the goals and priorities of Health 2020 may be too general to associate benchmarks with government policies or actions. Regardless, EURO will assist member nations in achieving the goals of the Health 2020 framework by supporting governments through provision of health data to assist policy makers in establishing or modifying goals and priorities, distributing policy-relevant health information collected by EURO in partnership with other member states or organizations, and investigating how government health indicators should be interpreted to show improvement in public health, such as health-care system performance, morbidity, and mortality.

The priorities and goals set forth in the Health 2020 policy framework take into account other WHO and EURO public health initiatives. EURO's Action Plan for Implementation of the European Strategy for the Prevention and Control of Noncommunicable Diseases, 2012–2016 seeks to decrease the number of deaths in member nations caused by noncommunicable diseases. Like Health 2020, the initiative contains broad action areas, including fostering alliances between health-care stakeholders, improving health surveillance (monitoring) and research, promoting health and preventing disease, and refocusing the health-care industry in EURO to focus on chronic diseases. EURO's noncommunicable disease action plan, however, also contains several concrete priority intervention areas for the WHO, governments, and other stakeholders. First, the plan calls for the use of government and fiscal policy controls to limit marketing and, consequently, public demand for tobacco, alcohol, and foods high in saturated fat, trans fats, salt, and sugar. Second, it requires the elimination of trans fats from foods through national and international agreements. Third, the action plan aims to reduce individual daily sodium intake to less than 5,000 milligrams per day by regulating sodium levels in processed foods. Fourth, the plan calls for the assessment and reduction of cardio-metabolic risk scores to lower the risk of diabetes and cardiovascular disease. EURO hopes to achieve this goal through increased support to primary care providers to assess and manage these risks through better education programs. The final objective of EURO's noncommunicable disease action plan is earlier detection of cancer through better organized screening campaigns and increased public awareness.

PRIMARY SOURCE

Action Plan for Implementation of the European Strategy for the Prevention and Control of Noncommunicable Diseases, 2012–2016

SOURCE Action Plan for Implementation of the European Strategy for the Prevention and Control of Noncommunicable Diseases, 2012–2016. *Copenhagen, Denmark: World Health Organization (WHO) Regional Office*

for Europe, 2012, 1–2. http://www.euro.who. int/__data/assets/pdf_file/0019/170155/ e96638.pdf?ua=1 (accessed January 25, 2015).

INTRODUCTION *This primary source is from the introduction to a publication setting out the action plan of the World Health Organization Regional Office for Europe with regard to non-communicable diseases. The excerpt is from the* Action Plan for Implementation of the European Strategy for the Prevention and Control of Noncommunicable Diseases, 2012–2016.

Mandate

In 2006, the WHO Regional Committee for Europe at its fifty-sixth session adopted a comprehensive, action-oriented strategy for the prevention and control of noncommunicable diseases (NCDs) (resolution EUR/RC56/R2). This was a Europe-specific response to the Global Strategy for the Prevention and Control of Noncommunicable Diseases adopted by the World Health Assembly in 2000. A global action plan followed in 2008.

In September 2010, the Regional Committee at its sixtieth session called for the development of a new European policy for health, Health 2020, and for public health capacities and services in Europe to be strengthened. The WHO Regional Director for Europe was requested to maintain a commitment to strengthening health systems, to rejuvenate the commitment to public health capacity and to work hand in hand with Member States to support them in their development of comprehensive national health policies and plans (resolution EUR/RC60/R5).

Health 2020 responds to the changing context in Europe: the glaring health inequities within and between countries, the re-emergence of infectious disease threats, the impact of globalization and new technologies, the ageing population, concerns about the financial sustainability of health systems, the changing role of citizens, and the particularly alarming growth of NCDs....

Epidemiological context

NCDs are the leading cause of death, disease and disability in the WHO European Region. The four major NCDs (cardiovascular disease, cancer, chronic obstructive pulmonary diseases and diabetes) together account for the vast majority of the disease burden and of premature mortality in the Region. In Europe, NCDs (more broadly defined) account for nearly 86% of deaths and 77% of the disease burden, putting increasing strain on health systems, economic development and the well-being of large parts of the population, in particular people aged 50 years and older. At the same time, NCDs are responsible for many of the growing health inequalities that have been observed in many countries, showing a strong socioeconomic gradient and important gender differences. The same is true for the widening health gap between countries in Europe. However, the social gradient and/or distribution of risk vary for different risk factors and in different Member States. In addition, there has recently been great concern that NCD risk factors increasingly affect younger age groups, with considerable consequences for public health trends in Europe in the future.

As individuals age, NCDs become the leading causes of morbidity, disability and mortality, and a great proportion of health care needs and costs are concentrated in the latter years of people's lives. European women live around eight years longer than men, with a greater share of their lives in poor health. An ageing population and the NCD disease burden risk imposing substantial costs on society. Dealing with chronic diseases and their risk factors comprises a significant proportion of a country's gross domestic product, while treatment costs, reduced income, early retirement and increased reliance on welfare support may be faced by the sufferer and/or their career(s). Employers, and society as a whole, bear the burden of absenteeism, reduced productivity and increased employee turnover.

SEE ALSO *Health in the WHO African Region; Health in the WHO Americas Region; Health in the WHO Eastern Mediterranean Region; Health in the WHO South-East Asian Region; Health in the WHO Western Pacific Region; World Health Organization: Organization, Funding, and Enforcement Powers*

BIBLIOGRAPHY

Books

Benatar, Solomon R., and Gillian Brock, eds. *Global Health and Global Health Ethics.* Cambridge, UK: Cambridge University Press, 2011.

Fairman, David, et al. *Negotiating Public Health in a Globalized World Global Health Diplomacy in Action.* Dordrecht, Netherlands: Springer, 2012.

Websites

"Global Burden of Disease." *World Health Organization (WHO).* http://www.who.int/topics/global_burden_of_disease/en (accessed January 31, 2015).

"Governance: The Executive Board." *World Health Organization (WHO).* http://www.who.int/governance/eb/en/ (accessed January 31, 2015).

"Sixty Years of WHO in Europe." *World Health Organization (WHO).* http://www.euro.who.int/__data/assets/pdf_file/0004/98437/E93312.pdf (accessed March 14, 2015).

"WHO European Office for Investment for Health and Development." *World Health Organization Regional Office for Europe (EURO).* http://www.euro.who.int/ihd (accessed January 31, 2015).

World Health Organization Regional Office for Europe (EURO). http://www.euro.who.int/ (accessed January 31, 2015).

Joseph P. Hyder

Health in the WHO South-East Asia Region

⊕ Introduction

The World Health Organization (WHO) Regional Office for South-East Asia is responsible for implementing WHO policies within its member states. The South-East Asia Regional Office (SEARO) is one of six WHO regional offices worldwide, which collect statistical data on public health, partner with national governments and other health-care stakeholders to identify and address unmet health-care needs, improve public health systems, and conduct public health education, prevention and promotion campaigns. Today, the SEARO countries are home to 1.8 billion people—one-quarter of the world's population.

The WHO health indicators show that the SEARO region faces significant public health challenges. In its 2006 publication "Department of Communicable Diseases: Profile and Vision," SEARO stated that the region "suffers disproportionately from the global burden of communicable diseases." For example, in terms of communicable (contagious) diseases, measles and rubella persist as considerable causes of morbidity (illness) and mortality (death) in the region; in 2011 about half of the global deaths attributed to measles occurred in the region, though only 25 percent of the world's population lives in the region covered by SEARO. About 38 percent of the global burden of tuberculosis (TB) cases are in the region. In addition to these challenges, SEARO also seeks to combat other communicable diseases, including human immunodeficiency virus/acquired immune deficiency syndrome (HIV/AIDS), malaria, dengue, and other vector-borne diseases, and other emerging infectious diseases, such as severe acute respiratory syndrome (SARS).

SEARO also has the highest noncommunicable disease mortality rate of any WHO region, at 656 deaths per 100,000, and the second-highest injury mortality rate, at 99 deaths per 100,000. The region has some of the highest noncommunicable disease mortality rates for cardiovascular (heart) diseases, cancers, chronic respiratory diseases and diabetes of any WHO regional office, despite an average or below-average prevalence of associated behavioral risk factors. The region's high noncommunicable disease mortality rate is associated with the its low expenditures on health care. SEARO ranks last in per capita health expenditures. Many people with noncommunicable diseases do not receive adequate health care to manage their chronic conditions.

Furthermore, in some member countries in the SEARO region, access to treatment is sharply limited because direct, out-of-pocket expenses, largely for the purchase of medicine, can impoverish households. These out-of-pocket expenses prevent persons with noncommunicable diseases from obtaining treatment that would reduce morbidity and premature mortality associated with these chronic diseases.

Rapid economic development and urbanization in many SEARO nations has already served to increase the burden of noncommunicable diseases over the next several decades, and this increase is projected to continue, which will stretch the region's limited health resources. In response, SEARO is partnering with governments and other stakeholders to develop health-care systems that reduce geographic inequalities in health care between rural and urban areas.

⊕ Historical Background

After World War II (1939–1945) and the creation of the United Nations (UN) in 1946, the 51 UN member states and 10 nonmember states signed an agreement to create a specialized agency of the UN to address global health concerns. The first global health entity, the WHO, was established in 1948. The first World Health Assembly convened that year and placed the countries of the world into six geographically-defined regions—Eastern Mediterranean (EMRO), Western Pacific (WPRO), Europe (EURO), Africa (south of the Sahara; AFRO), the Americas (AMRO or Pan American Health Organization

[PAHO]), and South-East Asia (SEARO). The member countries in the regions were only similar in terms of geography and were often quite varied in terms their politics, economic and industrial development, religions, cultures, and resources, as well as the health challenges they faced.

According to the SEARO website, initially, it had five member countries: Afghanistan, Burma (renamed Myanmar in 1988), Ceylon (Sri Lanka), India, and Siam (Thailand), and the countries responsible for international relations for the member countries also were permitted to attend regional meetings. As a result, France and Portugal represented the territories in India they governed, and the United Kingdom represented the Maldive Islands. In 1954 the French territories became part of India, and the Portuguese territories followed in 1961. Shortly thereafter, in 1965, the Maldive Islands gained independence.

Although at first Indonesia was placed in the Western Pacific Region, when Indonesia joined the WHO in 1950, it requested and was granted entry to the South-East Asian Region. The Republic of Vietnam and the Kingdoms of Cambodia and Laos also were originally included in the South-East Asia Region but in 1951, when WPRO opened, they chose to join that region.

The Kingdom of Nepal joined the South-East Asia Region in 1953, and the Maldive Islands joined the region in 1965.

In 1969, Afghanistan, one of the original members of SEARO, requested and was granted transfer to EMRO because of geographical proximity to that region and for political reasons. In 1971, Bangladesh (formerly East Pakistan and officially, the People's Republic of Bangladesh) joined the South-East Asia Region, and in 1973 the Democratic People's Republic of Korea (North Korea) joined the South-East Asia Region. The Kingdom of Bhutan joined in 1982. With the 2003 addition of the Republic of Timor-Leste to the region, its number of member states rose to 11.

⊕ Impacts and Issues

Headquartered in New Delhi, India, SEARO includes 11 UN member states: Bangladesh, Bhutan, Democratic People's Republic of Korea, India, Indonesia, the Maldives, Myanmar, Nepal, Sri Lanka, Thailand, and Timor-Leste. SEARO covers a geographically, politically, and socioeconomically diverse region, stretching from the tropical areas of Bangladesh, India, Myanmar, and Thailand to the mountainous Himalayan nations of Bhutan

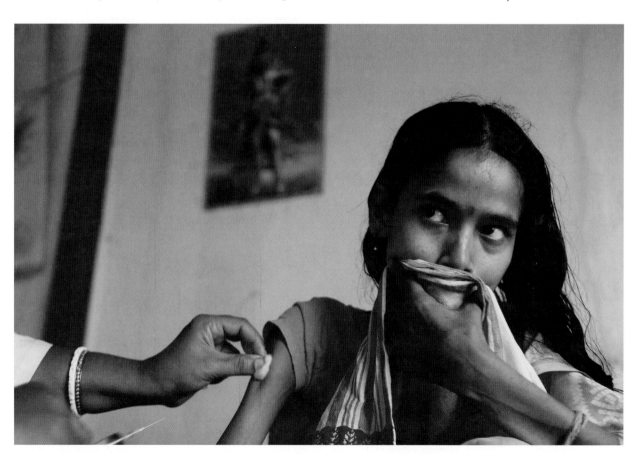

A nurse administers a shot to a tuberculosis (TB) patient at the state TB hospital in Gauhati, India. TB is a major problem in the region. © *Anupam Nath/AP Images.*

and Nepal. SEARO also must balance serving the sprawling megacities of India and Indonesia with rural areas located throughout the region. The isolationist nations of Bhutan and North Korea present additional challenges in terms of effectively monitoring public health and implementing SEARO policies.

The average life expectancy at birth (in 2012) in the SEARO region was 67 years, which places the region below the global average of 70. The region experienced an eight-year increase in life expectancy at birth from 1990 to 2012, however, which ties the region with the WHO African Region for the greatest improvement in life expectancy during the period. Life expectancy within the region ranges from 66 years in India, Myanmar, and Timor-Leste to 77 years in the Maldives.

The SEARO region exceeds the global average in mortality rates (deaths per 100,000 population) for communicable diseases, noncommunicable diseases, and injuries. The region has the second-highest communicable disease mortality rate of any WHO region, at 232 deaths per 100,000.

According to SEARO, TB is one of the communicable diseases of major concern in the region. SEARO estimates there are 3.4 million new cases of TB in the region each year, and the region has 38 percent of the world's TB cases. India alone represented 21 percent of all global deaths from the disease. In 2013, an estimated 440,000 died from the disease in the region. In addition, of the more than 3 million who acquire the disease every year, SEARO estimates about 33 percent do not receive treatment.

The SEARO region also exceeds the global average in neonatal, infant, and childhood mortality rates. The region's neonatal mortality rate (death within 28 days per 1,000 live births) was 27 in 2012 compared to the global rate of 21. The infant mortality rate (death before age one per 1,000 live births) in the region was 39 in 2012, which was higher than the global rate of 35. The SEARO childhood mortality rate (death before age five per 1,000 live births) in 2012 was 50, which was also slightly above the global rate of 48. The graph displaying childhood mortality rates in the SEARO region shows the relatively low rates in Sri Lanka, the Maldives, and Thailand and the higher than the global average rates in Myanmar, India, and Timor-Leste. Despite the relatively high mortality rates in parts of the region in 2012, the SEARO nations have made significant improvements since 1990 when the neonatal, infant, and childhood mortality rates stood at 47, 83, and 118, respectively.

Childhood health in the SEARO region suffers because of low immunization rates, inadequate sanitation, a lack of access to regular medical care, and poor nutrition. Of the six WHO regions, SEARO has the second-lowest childhood immunization rates for measles, diphtheria, tetanus, and pertussis. The region is tied for the lowest childhood immunization rate for

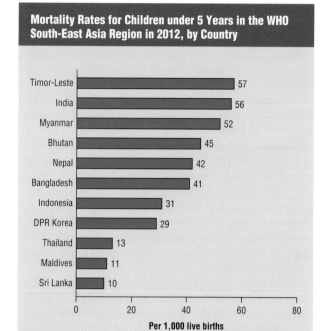

Mortality Rates for Children under 5 Years in the WHO South-East Asia Region in 2012, by Country

Country	Per 1,000 live births
Timor-Leste	57
India	56
Myanmar	52
Bhutan	45
Nepal	42
Bangladesh	41
Indonesia	31
DPR Korea	29
Thailand	13
Maldives	11
Sri Lanka	10

SOURCE: Adapted from "Under-five mortality rates (2012)," in *Situation of Newborn and Child Health in South-East Asia Progress towards MDG 4*, World Health Organization, Regional Office for South-East Asia, 2014. Data from *The UN Inter-agency Group for Child Mortality Estimation (IGME). Levels and Trends in Child Mortality: Report 2013*.

According to the WHO report on child mortality in the South-East Asia Region in 2012, Timor-Leste and India have the highest mortality rates for children under five years of age.

hepatitis B. In 2012, only 45 percent of the population within SEARO had access to improved sanitation. Lack of access to improved sanitation can result in a number of potentially fatal diseases, including diarrheal diseases, which cause 10 percent of all under-five deaths in the region. Finally, the region has the highest percentage of underweight children of any WHO region: More than one-quarter of children under five in the region—an estimated 71 million children—are underweight and more than one-third experience stunting (early growth retardation).

The WHO observes that undernutrition, frequently attributable to a shortage of quality food, contributes to about one-third of all child deaths and impairs healthy development and serves to increase noncommunicable diseases. Children with stunted growth and early malnutrition are at increased risk of developing chronic diseases like heart disease and diabetes. Simple, inexpensive measures such as exclusively breast-feeding infants until they are six months old and adding safe, appropriate foods at six months with continued breast-feeding until age two is advised to prevent the long-range health consequences of malnutrition.

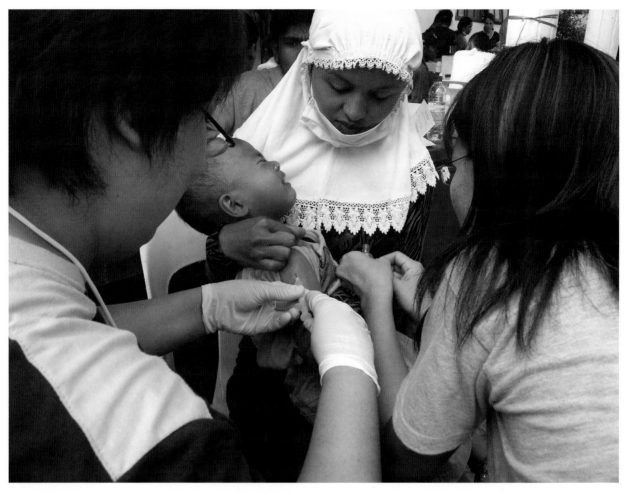

Red Cross volunteers help tsunami refugees in Aceh, Indonesia, by delivering vaccines to children.   © *A.S. Zain/Shutterstock.com.*

The SEARO region's relatively poor health indicators are attributable largely to the region's poor health-care infrastructure and low levels of health-care expenditures. The region has the second-lowest density of physicians of any WHO region, with only 5.9 physicians and 15.3 nurses per 10,000 population. The SEARO region also has the lowest level of health expenditure, both as a percentage of gross domestic product (GDP) and in total per capita expenditures. In 2011, the total expenditure on health care in the region was only 3.7 percent of GDP compared to the global average of 9.1 percent. The per capita health-care expenditure in 2011 was US$69 in 2011, which was far below the global average of $1,007.

As a result of the lack of health-care expenditures, surveillance (monitoring), prevention, and treatment of noncommunicable diseases has been neglected and underfunded. Despite the fact that many behavioral risk factors associated with noncommunicable diseases within the region are at or below the global average, SEARO has the highest noncommunicable disease mortality rate (deaths per 100,000 population) of any WHO

region. Noncommunicable diseases are chronic, nontransmissible conditions. Globally, noncommunicable diseases kill more than 38 million people annually and an estimated 8 million of these deaths occur in the SEARO region. The four leading noncommunicable diseases are cancer, cardiovascular diseases, diabetes, and chronic respiratory diseases, which combined account for more than 80 percent of all noncommunicable disease deaths. Thalassemia (inherited blood disorders involving underproduction of the oxygen-carrying protein hemoglobin), chronic kidney disease, and chronic liver disease also are prevalent in some countries in the region.

One-third of deaths from noncommunicable diseases in the region are of people less than age 60. More than 40 percent of all deaths caused by noncommunicable diseases globally are considered premature deaths, that is, a death that occurs before age 70. Premature deaths result in huge social and economic losses.

Among health indicators for noncommunicable diseases, the region's prevalence (the number of cases of a disease or condition present in a particular population at a given time) of elevated blood glucose,

THE WHO SOUTH EAST-ASIA REGION ACHIEVES POLIO-FREE CERTIFICATION

The eradication of poliomyelitis (polio) is the largest international public health effort in human history. Before 1985, polio paralyzed more than 350,000 people per year worldwide. Polio disproportionately affects children under five. The most severe, paralytic form of the disease often causes paralysis of the legs but can also cause death if breathing muscles are affected. The paralytic form of the disease represents only a fraction of polio cases. One case of paralytic polio may represent as many as 200 to 1,000 less severe or silent cases. The vaccines that prevent polio are inexpensive and easy to administer.

Various agencies within the United Nations, including the World Health Organization (WHO), along with Rotary International, the U.S. Centers for Disease Control and Prevention, and other international health organizations, nongovernmental organizations (NGOs), and national health systems began the Global Polio Eradication Initiative to eliminate polio through vaccination campaigns, sanitation improvement, and coordinated disease surveillance. In 1995, the international community developed a formal certification process for recognizing various world regions as "polio-free." The Global Certification Commission certifies areas as free of polio only after there are no registered cases of wild polio for three years. Certification requires careful and thorough disease monitoring to ensure that no new cases have occurred. Three WHO regions achieved polio-free status before 2014: the Americas (1994), Western Pacific (2000), and Europe (2002).

When the global initiative against polio began in 1988, India recorded more than 200,000 cases of the disease annually. The country was the world's largest reservoir of paralytic polio, averaging 50,000 to 100,000 cases per year between 1978 and 1995. Outbreaks of polio frequently were exported from India through travel and migration. At the outset of the Global Polio Eradication Initiative and the Universal Immunization Program, health experts initially anticipated that India would be the most difficult country from which to eradicate polio because of the nation's geographic size, large population, and underdeveloped sanitation infrastructure. However, vaccination initiatives began to reduce the occurrence of polio cases dramatically within the first decade of the anti-polio campaign.

In January 2011, 18-month-old Rukhsar Khatoon contracted paralytic polio in her home village of Shapara, near Kolkata, West Bengal State. She survived and later regained the ability to walk. Khatoon was India's last registered case of polio: The WHO declared India polio-free in January 2014. Several months later, the WHO South-East Asia Region also was declared polio-free.

With the certification of the WHO South-East Asia Region as polio-free, an estimated 80 percent of the global population lives in polio-free areas. However, the WHO African Region and the Eastern Mediterranean Region continue to combat polio. Efforts to eliminate polio from Afghanistan, Nigeria, and Pakistan have yet to succeed. Conflict regions once free of polio, such as Syria, reported outbreaks of polio reintroduced into the local population in 2013 by foreign fighters from polio-endemic countries.

---

increased blood pressure, and smoking are at or slightly below the global average. The region's obesity rate is the lowest in the world, and its alcohol consumption is the second lowest behind only EMRO. Nevertheless, noncommunicable diseases are the leading cause of death in the SEARO region, claiming nearly 8 million lives annually.

Major behavioral risk factors associated with noncommunicable diseases include tobacco use, physical inactivity, excessive consumption of alcohol, and unhealthful diets. In the SEARO region as much as 26 percent of the population does not meet global guidelines for physical activity; nearly 250 million people smoke and an equal number use smokeless tobacco products; the majority (80 percent) do not consume adequate quantities of fruits and vegetables; and childhood and adult obesity are increasing. The WHO observes that SEARO region has the double burden of undernutrition and overweight. These behavioral risk factors may lead to high blood, pressure, diabetes, cancer, respiratory ailments, and other conditions associated with noncommunicable diseases.

⊕ Future Implications

SEARO is dedicated to reducing the noncommunicable disease burden within the region in the 21st century. SEARO adopted the *Action Plan for the Prevention and Control of Noncommunicable Diseases in South-East Asia, 2013–2020.* SEARO's noncommunicable disease action plan is based on the *Action Plan for the Global Strategy for the Prevention and Control of Noncommunicable Diseases* adopted by the World Health Assembly in May 2008. The World Health Assembly (WHA) sets policies, priorities, and goals for the WHO.

SEARO's noncommunicable disease action plan adopts 10 public health targets. First, the plan calls for a 25 percent reduction in overall mortality from cancer, cardiovascular disease, diabetes, and respiratory diseases. Second, it seeks a 10 percent relative reduction in the harmful use of alcohol. Third, the plan aims for a 30 percent reduction in tobacco use among persons over age 15. Fourth, SEARO has set a goal of a 10 percent relative reduction in the prevalence of physical inactivity. Fifth, the SEARO action plan specifies a

30 percent relative reduction in sodium intake. Sixth, the plan targets a 25 percent reduction in the prevalence of raised blood pressure. Seventh, the plan calls for a halt in the rise of obesity and diabetes rates. The eighth SEARO target is a 50 percent reduction in proportion of households using solid fuels, such as wood or charcoal, as a primary source of cooking. Ninth, the plan sets a goal of 50 percent of eligible people receiving drugs and counseling for heart attacks and strokes. Tenth, the plan calls for basic technologies and medicines needed to treat and control noncommunicable diseases to be made available to 80 percent of the people in the region.

This final noncommunicable disease target touches on one of the most pressing public health needs in the SEARO region: strengthening the region's health systems and services. In 2004, the South-East Asia Public Health Initiative was launched to assist countries in the region in identifying the most essential public health services based on each country's situation and needs. This initiative allows each nation to focus limited resources on it most pressing public health needs.

Given the low level of health expenditures in the region, SEARO also has promoted self-care and family care programs. Self-care and family care is based on the principle that individuals can take care of many of their (or their families') health-care needs. Through education campaigns, people learn how to identify and treat certain conditions. They also learn to identify more serious conditions that may require a trip to a clinic or hospital, which often results in earlier detection and professional health intervention, which often increases the likelihood that treatment will be successful. Additionally, SEARO has launched telemedicine systems in some nations. The telemedicine programs improve access to care by enabling physicians and other health professionals to connect to prospective patients in remote areas to provide diagnosis and treatment advice.

Although primary prevention programs are necessary to stem the rising tide of noncommunicable diseases in the region, the health care system requires the cooperation of other governments, other industries, and education to effectively address the many issues involved in modifying behavioral risk factors and reducing disease-causing environmental exposures. For example, the food and agriculture sector could reduce salt and sugar in processed foods and governments could subsidize fruits and vegetables to promote their consumption. Environmental issues such as air pollution and elimination of lead in paint require industry and government cooperation. Other strategies some countries in the region have undertaken to prevent and reduce noncommunicable diseases include increasing taxes and banning advertising of tobacco and alcohol to discourage their use and involving the media and schools to educate children and adults about the importance of healthful diets and physical activity.

PRIMARY SOURCE

Action Plan for the Prevention and Control of Noncommunicable Diseases in South-East Asia, 2013–2020

SOURCE *"Situational Analysis," in* Action Plan for the Prevention and Control of Noncommunicable Diseases in South-East Asia, 2013–2020, *World Health Organization (WHO) Regional Office for South-East Asia, 2013, 1–4. http:// www.searo.who.int/entity/noncommunicable_ diseases/documents/sea-ncd-89(reduced). pdf?ua=1 (accessed January 25, 2015).*

INTRODUCTION *This primary source document was prepared by the World Health Organization Regional Office for South-East Asia. It is the introductory section from a report on the noncommunicable disease epidemic and describes the problem in that specific geographic area.*

SECTION 1. SITUATION ANALYSIS

1.1 Regional burden of noncommunicable diseases

Noncommunicable diseases (NCDs) are the leading cause of death in the WHO South-East Asia Region. Each year, an estimated 7.9 million lives are lost due to NCDs, accounting for 55% of all deaths. Furthermore, NCDs claim lives at a younger age in the South-East Asia Region compared to the other WHO regions. In 2008, the proportion of NCD deaths occurring among people under the age of 60 was 34%, compared to 23% in the rest of the world. Cardiovascular diseases are the most frequent cause of NCD deaths, followed by chronic respiratory diseases, cancers, and diabetes.

…

Besides being an enormous health burden, NCDs have serious socioeconomic implications. They disproportionately affect the poor, leading to loss of household income from unhealthy behaviours, poor physical capacity and loss of wages. Due to long-term treatment costs and high out-of-pocket costs, NCDs can result in catastrophic health expenditures and impoverishment....

1.2 Determinants and risk factors for NCDs

The increasing burden of NCDs is attributed to determinants such as population ageing, rapid and unplanned urbanization, negative effects of globalization (such as trade and irresponsible marketing of unhealthy products), low literacy, and poverty. From 2000 to 2025, it is projected that the proportion of the population aged above 65 years will increase from

3.6% to 6.6% in Bangladesh, from 4.4% to 7.7% in India and from 6.3% to 12.3% in Sri Lanka. As the prevalence of NCDs increases with age, these progressively aging populations will result in a corresponding increase in NCD cases.

Urbanization in the South-East Asia Region is occurring at a rapid rate and increased from 26% in 1990 to 33% in 2009. It is projected that the percentage of populations residing in urban areas will more than double by 2050 in most Member States. Several studies in the Region show that behavioural, anthropometric and biochemical risk factors for NCDs are more prevalent in urban than rural areas. Unplanned urbanization reduces options for physical activity and increases exposure to air pollution.

Globalization has brought processed foods and diets high in total energy, fats, salt and sugar into millions of homes. Nearly 30% of the Region's population remains non-literate. Low levels of literacy affect health behaviours and lifestyle choices. Poor levels of awareness can also result in high consumption of salt, as well as saturated fats and trans fats, and thus aggravate development of NCDs. Studies in Bangladesh, India, Indonesia, Sri Lanka and Thailand have revealed that both smoking and smokeless tobacco use are more prevalent among the less educated.

Globalization and underlying social determinants are driving unhealthy lifestyle behaviours. Four modifiable lifestyle-related risk behaviours, namely tobacco use, unhealthy diet, insufficient physical activity and harmful use of alcohol, are responsible for the majority of NCDs. The prevalence of these unhealthy risk behaviours is very high in the Region.

SEE ALSO   *Health in the WHO African Region; Health in the WHO Americas Region; Health in the WHO Eastern Mediterranean Region; Health in the WHO European Region; Health in the WHO Western Pacific Region; World Health Organization: Organization, Funding, and Enforcement Powers*

BIBLIOGRAPHY

Books

Birn, Anne-Emanuelle, Yogan Pillay, and Timothy H. Holtz. *Textbook of International Health: Global Health in a Dynamic World*, 3rd ed. New York: Oxford University Press, 2009.

Bliss, Katherine Elaine, ed. *Key Players in Global Health: How Brazil, Russia, India, China, and South Africa Are Influencing the Game*. Washington, DC: Center for Strategic and International Studies, 2010.

Jacobsen, Kathryn H. *Introduction to Global Health*, 2nd ed. Burlington, MA: Jones and Bartlett Learning, 2014.

Websites

The Global Polio Eradication Initiative. http://www.polioeradication.org (accessed February 1, 2015).

"Health Systems." *World Health Organization (WHO).* http://www.who.int/entity/healthsystems/en (accessed February 1, 2015).

"History of the WHO South-East Asia Region." *World Health Organization (WHO), South-East Asia Region (SEARO).* http://www.searo.who.int/about/history/en/ (accessed March 13, 2015).

"Regional Office for South-East Asia." *World Health Organization (WHO), South-East Asia Region (SEARO).* http://www.searo.who.int/ (accessed February 1, 2015).

"WHO Highlights Key Health Issues in South-East Asia." *World Health Organization (WHO).* http://www.searo.who.int/mediacentre/releases/2013/pr1560/en/ (accessed March 13, 2015).

"WHO Raises the Alarm over Nutrition Problems." *World Health Organization (WHO).* http://origin.searo.who.int/mediacentre/releases/2011/pr1528/en/ (accessed March 13, 2015).

"WHO World Health Report 2013: Research for Universal Health Coverage." *World Health Organization (WHO).* http://www.who.int/whr/ (accessed February 1, 2015).

Joseph P. Hyder

Health in the WHO Western Pacific Region

🌐 Introduction

The World Health Organization (WHO) Western Pacific Regional Office (WPRO) is tasked with implementing the WHO policies within its 37 nations/areas, which covers the Western Pacific and Oceania. WPRO is one of six WHO regional offices worldwide. The WHO regional offices collect and evaluate statistical data on public health, partner with national governments and other health-care stakeholders to improve public health systems, and conduct education campaigns on health issues.

WHO health indicators show that the region is relatively healthy compared to other WHO regions. High-income countries in the region, such as Australia and Japan, have well-funded health-care systems. China—the region's most populous nation—has state-subsidized health care that reaches the majority of its population. The quality and availability of health care, however, varies greatly throughout the WPRO region and even within many of its nations.

The increase of noncommunicable (noninfectious and non-transmissible) diseases will present a formidable challenge for health-care systems in the region over the coming decades. Rapid economic development in China, Malaysia, and other WPRO countries has resulted in an increasing frequency of the behavioral risk factors associated with noncommunicable diseases, such as increased tobacco use, physical inactivity, and unhealthful diets.

🌐 Historical Background

The United Nations' predecessor, the League of Nations, had the Health Organization as one of its principal bodies. The Health Organization oversaw the League of Nations' public health initiatives, which primarily focused on preventing the spread of communicable (infectious and transmissible) diseases such as leprosy,

malaria, typhus, and yellow fever. Following the dissolution of the League of Nations in 1946, the newly formed United Nations (UN) sought to transfer the duties of the Health Organization and the Office International d'Hygiène Publique, an international organization designed to monitor disease and quarantine ships to prevent the spread of disease, to a new UN agency. In 1946, all 51 UN member states, and 10 nonmember states, signed an agreement to create a specialized agency of the UN to address global health concerns. The constitution of the new agency, known as WHO, entered into effect in April 1948 following its ratification by a majority of signatory nations. In the mid-2010s, the WHO is a specialized agency under the UN Development Group. Every UN member state except Lichtenstein is a member of the WHO.

The World Health Assembly (WHA) sets policies, priorities, and goals for the WHO. Health ministers from each UN member state serve on the WHA, which generally meets annually. The WHA concluded its first annual meeting in July 1948, at which the WHA established maternal and infant health, nutrition, and the prevention of certain communicable diseases—malaria, sexually transmitted diseases, and tuberculosis—as the initial public health priorities of the WHO. These public health issues along with prevention of noncommunicable diseases remain priorities for the WHO.

From 1949 to 1952, the WHA created regional offices designed to meet the specific public health needs of particular areas of the world. Currently, the WHO has six regional offices: the Regional Office for Africa (AFRO); the Regional Office for the Americas (AMRO, also known as the Pan American Health Organization [PAHO]); the Regional Office for South-East Asia (SEARO); the Regional Office for Europe (EURO); the Regional Office for the Eastern Mediterranean (EMRO); and WPRO.

The third World Health Assembly approved the establishment of WPRO, and its office was initially located in Hong Kong. In 1951 the regional office was relocated to Manila, Philippines. The Philippine

EMERGENCY RESPONSE IN THE WHO WESTERN PACIFIC REGION

Many member states of the World Health Organization (WHO) Western Pacific Region sit along the western edge of the Pacific Ocean's Ring of Fire—an area with significant and frequent earthquake and volcanic activity. The WPRO therefore faces a constant threat of emergency response and public health support in the event of a natural disaster. The WPRO states that 10 of the world's top 20 nations at greatest risk of natural disaster lie within the WPRO region. In addition to the loss of life caused by a natural disaster itself, survivors of the disaster face an immediate need for freshwater and food supplies along with continued public health monitoring and support in the absence of basic sanitation.

In 2014, the WPRO stated in the *Report of the Regional Director: The Work of WHO in the Western Pacific Region* that more than 7,000 natural disasters had occurred around the world in the preceding two decades. These natural disasters affected more than 4.3 billion people, including 2.7 billion within the WHO Western Pacific Region. The economic cost of natural disasters within the region during this period exceeded $2.2 trillion, representing more than 40 percent of the global burden.

The world map on page 284 shows how the WPRO member countries have been disproportionately affected by natural disasters that have displaced millions of the region's residents. Despite the excessively high number of natural disasters (and the related economic impact) within the WPRO region, only 15 percent of global deaths from natural disasters occurred in the region within the period. WPRO credits this relatively low percentage to well-planned and coordinated disaster response. National governments and nongovernmental organizations (NGOs) within the region, including the WHO, work together to ensure a rapid and efficient response to disasters.

The emergency response of government and NGOs within the region was tested in 2013 when Typhoon Haiyan (known as Yolanda in the Philippines) made landfall near Tacloban, Philippines, on November 8. Typhoon Haiyan was the strongest tropical storm ever recorded at landfall, with one-minute sustained winds of 195 miles per hour (315 kilometers per hour) just before landfall. The typhoon destroyed more than 90 percent of the structures in Tacloban. It is estimated that between 6,000 and 7,000 people died, and more than 1.9 million people were left homeless by Typhoon Haiyan.

Damage to virtually all infrastructure in the region, including electricity, mobile phone service, roads, and damage to Tacloban's airport, hampered relief efforts. The Philippine government noted that the extent of devastation caused by the storm caused a breakdown in local government, which typically coordinates aid efforts on the ground. Five days after landfall, many residents of Tacloban still struggled to find drinking water and food while many rural areas received no aid at all. Health concerns about uncollected dead bodies and lack of food, water, and shelter mounted in the weeks following the storm. Beginning on November 10, the U.S. military began a humanitarian operation that delivered more than 4 million pounds (1.8 million kilograms) of supplies and evacuated more than 20,000 people. Typhoon Haiyan caused in excess of $2 billion in damage.

---

government donated the site for a new building to house the office to the WHO, and WPRO opened in September 1958.

WPRO is organized into six divisions—Communicable Diseases, Health Security and Emergencies, NCD [Noncommunicable Disease] and Health through the Life-Course, Health Sector Development, Pacific Technical Support, and Administration and Finance. Its 15 country offices offer support, guidance and collaborative efforts to meet the health-care needs of the region's 1.8 billion people.

🌐 Impacts and Issues

WPRO covers 37 countries and areas along the rim of the Western Pacific and within Oceania. The countries covered by WPRO range from China—the most populous nation in the world with more than 1 billion people—to a collection of small, sparsely populated island nations, including the Pitcairn Islands with a population of less than 60. The nations and areas covered by WPRO are: American Samoa, Australia, Brunei Darussalam, Cambodia, China, Cook Islands, Fiji, French Polynesia, Guam, Hong Kong, Japan, Kiribati, Laos, Macao, Malaysia, Marshall Islands, Federated States of Micronesia, Mongolia, Nauru, New Caledonia, New Zealand, Niue, Northern Mariana Islands, Palau, Papua New Guinea, the Philippines, Pitcairn Islands, the Republic of Korea (South Korea), Samoa, Singapore, Solomon Islands, Tokelau (as an associate member), Tonga, Tuvalu, Vanuatu, Vietnam, and Wallis and Futuna.

WPRO is unique among the six WHO regional offices in that other UN member states are responsible for more than one-quarter of WPRO members. The responsible UN member states and their WPRO affiliates are: China (Hong Kong and Macao); France

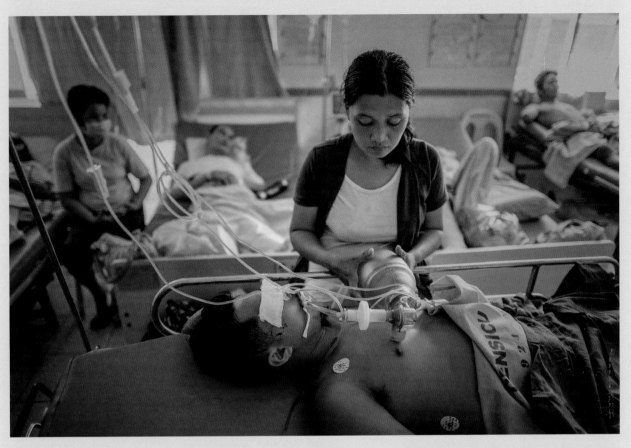

A woman checks on her husband as she keeps him alive by manually pumping air into his lungs following a leg amputation that led to an infection. The hospital was still operating without electrical power one week after Typhoon Haiyan hit the Philippines on November 8, 2013. © *Philippe Lopez/AFP/Getty Images.*

(French Polynesia, New Caledonia, and Wallis and Futuna); the United Kingdom (Pitcairn Islands); and the United States (American Samoa, Guam, and the Northern Mariana Islands).

WPRO faces unique concerns in setting and implementing public health policies and initiatives across its region because of the income disparity between WPRO members and the varied public health concerns the region faces. The disparate public health issues are largely attributable to geographic and demographic differences between the member countries. The public health concerns presented in some of the world's largest megacities in China differ greatly from those faced in remote, sparsely populated island nations. In fact, only 12 of the WPRO region's 37 nations/areas have a population of 250,000 or greater.

The WHO Western Pacific Region as a whole, however, is at or near the top of WHO regions in many leading health indicators. Average life expectancy at birth in 2012 in WPRO nations was 76 years, tying the region with AMRO/PAHO and EURO for highest life expectancy. The WPRO life expectancy in 2012 represents a major increase from life expectancy in the region at birth in 1990, which stood at 69 years. The average life expectancy among WPRO nations varies greatly, however, from 62 years at birth in Papua New Guinea (in 2012) to 84 years in Japan.

Between 1990 and 2012, WPRO experienced significant improvements in reducing neonatal, infant, and childhood mortality. The neonatal mortality rate (deaths within the first month of life per 1,000 live births) declined in the WPRO region from 23 to 9. The infant mortality rate (deaths before age one per 1,000 live births) declined from 40 in 1990 to 14 in 2012. The under-five mortality rate (deaths before age five per 1,000 live births) in the WPRO region declined from 52 in 1990 to 16 in 2012. Overall, the WPRO region experienced the greatest reduction in neonatal, infant,

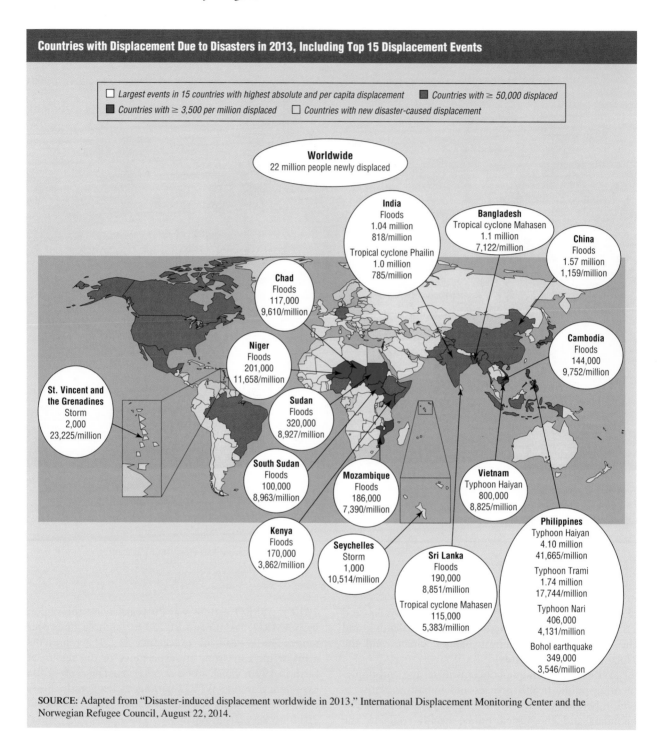

Countries with Displacement Due to Disasters in 2013, Including Top 15 Displacement Events

□ *Largest events in 15 countries with highest absolute and per capita displacement*   ■ *Countries with ≥ 50,000 displaced*

■ *Countries with ≥ 3,500 per million displaced*   □ *Countries with new disaster-caused displacement*

Worldwide
22 million people newly displaced

India
Floods
1.04 million
818/million

Tropical cyclone Phailin
1.0 million
785/million

Bangladesh
Tropical cyclone Mahasen
1.1 million
7,122/million

China
Floods
1.57 million
1,159/million

Chad
Floods
117,000
9,610/million

Niger
Floods
201,000
11,658/million

Cambodia
Floods
144,000
9,752/million

St. Vincent and the Grenadines
Storm
2,000
23,225/million

Sudan
Floods
320,000
8,927/million

South Sudan
Floods
100,000
8,963/million

Mozambique
Floods
186,000
7,390/million

Vietnam
Typhoon Haiyan
800,000
8,825/million

Kenya
Floods
170,000
3,862/million

Seychelles
Storm
1,000
10,514/million

Sri Lanka
Floods
190,000
8,851/million

Tropical cyclone Mahasen
115,000
5,383/million

Philippines
Typhoon Haiyan
4.10 million
41,665/million

Typhoon Trami
1.74 million
17,744/million

Typhoon Nari
406,000
4,131/million

Bohol earthquake
349,000
3,546/million

SOURCE: Adapted from "Disaster-induced displacement worldwide in 2013," International Displacement Monitoring Center and the Norwegian Refugee Council, August 22, 2014.

and childhood mortality (as a percentage of 1990 rates) of any WHO region. Like life expectancy in the region, the neonatal, infant, and under-five mortality rates also show considerable disparity between WPRO nations. Comparing Japan and Papua New Guinea again shows that the neonatal, infant, and under-five mortality rates in the two nations (as of 2012) range from 24, 48, and 63, respectively, in Papua New Guinea, compared to 1, 2, and 3, respectively, in Japan.

The WPRO region also has made significant improvements in maternal health since 1990. Between 1990 and 2010, the region's maternal mortality rate (deaths per 100,000 live births) fell from 110 to 45, which is the second-lowest rate among WHO regions (behind only EURO). The decline in the maternal mortality rate in China from 97 in 1990 to 32 in 2012 was a major driving factor in the overall decline in the region because China comprises more than two-thirds of the region's total population. Again, the region has a great discrepancy in maternal mortality rates between the region's more developed nations and its developing nations. The 2012 maternal mortality rate in Papua New Guinea and Laos (at 220) is more than 36 times the maternal mortality rate in Japan (at 6).

Communicable Diseases

The WHO Western Pacific Region has relatively low levels of life-threatening communicable diseases, particularly those targeted for global reduction under the UN Millennium Development Goals (MDGs). The MDGs specifically target human immunodeficiency virus/acquired immune deficiency syndrome (HIV/AIDS), malaria, and tuberculosis for reduction. According to the WHO's *World Health Statistics 2014*, WPRO has the second-lowest HIV/AIDS mortality rate (deaths per 100,000 population) of any WHO region, trailing only EMRO. The HIV/AIDS mortality rate in WPRO nations more than tripled between 2001 and 2012: In 2001, WPRO had an HIV/AIDS mortality rate of 2.1 deaths per 100,000 population; in 2012, the HIV/AIDS mortality rate in the region had increased to 6.8. Between 2001 and 2012, the prevalence of HIV/AIDS (cases per 100,000 population) increased from 43 to 75, also ranking the region second behind EMRO.

The HIV/AIDS mortality and prevalence statistics released by the WHO, however, do not present a complete picture of HIV/AIDS in the region. Notably, the statistics from the WHO's *World Health Statistics 2014* do not include HIV/AIDS prevalence or mortality statistics for China or Japan, the region's two most populous nations. (Together China and Japan account for about 85 percent of WPRO's total population.) The Central Intelligence Agency's *World Factbook* lists the HIV/AIDS prevalence rate for both China and Japan at around 0.1 percent, or about 10 cases per 100,000 population, ranking China and Japan 130th and 120th in the world, respectively, in HIV/AIDS prevalence. Reliable statistics on the HIV/AIDS mortality rates in China and Japan are difficult to verify. Both nations, however, have aggressive HIV/AIDS public health policies. China, for example, provides free HIV/AIDS testing, along with free antiretroviral drugs for pregnant women and people living in rural areas. Despite these efforts, in February 2009, China announced that HIV/AIDS had become the nation's leading cause of death from infectious diseases.

The WPRO region has had success in controlling the spread of tuberculosis and malaria. As of 2014, 9 out of the 10 WPRO low- and middle-income countries (LMICs) with populations of 250,000 or more were on track to meet the MDG target of successfully treating more than 85 percent of tuberculosis cases. Only Malaysia apparently will miss the MDG tuberculosis target. All WPRO LMICs with endemic malaria were progressing as planned to meet the MDG target of reducing the malaria mortality rate by 60 percent.

The WPRO region also excels in health indicators related to maternal and child health. The region has the highest rates of met needs for family planning and contraceptive use in the world at 94 percent and 80 percent, respectively. The region also has a high percentage (93 percent) of births attended by health professionals, and at least 94 percent of women receive some form of prenatal (during pregnancy) health care. Additionally, the WPRO region has the highest worldwide rates of vaccination for measles, diphtheria, tetanus, pertussis, and hepatitis B.

However, more work remains to be done in terms of child nutrition. Malnutrition, which contributes to one-third of all global child deaths and also affects morbidity and mortality throughout life, has been targeted by WPRO with the Action Plan to Reduce the Double Burden of Malnutrition in the WHO Western Pacific Region from 2015 to 2020. The double burden includes undernutrition, which contributes to wasting, stunting, and micronutrient deficiencies, and hinders children's abilities to progress physically and mentally, and overweight, which can coincide with malnutrition and over the life course lead to some noncommunicable diseases. As with many other issues in the WPRO countries, there are disparities in this burden; countries such as Australia have little to no stunting due to malnutrition in children under five, however, most countries in the region do report levels of stunting, and Cambodia, Laos, and Papua New Guinea show rates over 40 percent. (See graphic.)

Noncommunicable Diseases

According to the WHO, noncommunicable diseases kill 37 million people annually worldwide and are projected to claim 44 million lives in 2020. More than 25 percent of these 44 million deaths (12.3 million) will occur in the WHO Western Pacific Region. The four most common noncommunicable diseases are cancer, cardiovascular diseases, diabetes, and respiratory diseases, which combined account for more than 82 percent of all noncommunicable disease deaths. Noncommunicable diseases often result from lifestyle choices or exposure to environmental factors. The four leading risk factors for developing noncommunicable diseases are tobacco use, physical inactivity, excessive alcohol use, and unhealthful diets.

Noncommunicable diseases often have significant socioeconomic costs for individuals, families, and society. Because noncommunicable diseases are chronic conditions, persons with noncommunicable diseases may require decades of health care to manage the symptoms of disease and decrease the likelihood of premature death (death before age 70). This places a

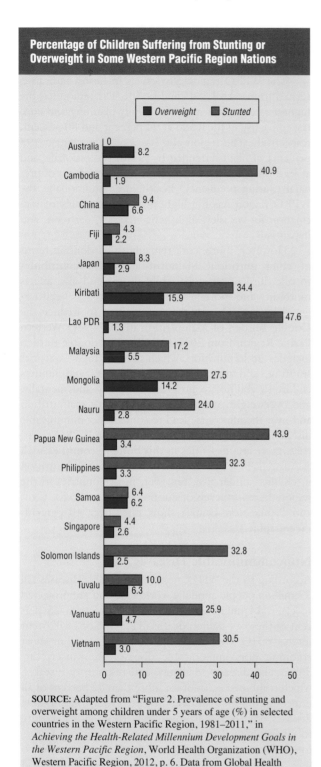

Percentage of Children Suffering from Stunting or Overweight in Some Western Pacific Region Nations

Legend: Overweight, Stunted

Country	Overweight	Stunted
Australia	0	8.2
Cambodia	40.9	1.9
China	9.4	6.6
Fiji	4.3	2.2
Japan	8.3	2.9
Kiribati	34.4	15.9
Lao PDR	47.6	1.3
Malaysia	17.2	5.5
Mongolia	27.5	14.2
Nauru	24.0	2.8
Papua New Guinea	43.9	3.4
Philippines	32.3	3.3
Samoa	6.4	6.2
Singapore	4.4	2.6
Solomon Islands	32.8	2.5
Tuvalu	10.0	6.3
Vanuatu	25.9	4.7
Vietnam	30.5	3.0

SOURCE: Adapted from "Figure 2. Prevalence of stunting and overweight among children under 5 years of age (%) in selected countries in the Western Pacific Region, 1981–2011," in *Achieving the Health-Related Millennium Development Goals in the Western Pacific Region*, World Health Organization (WHO), Western Pacific Region, 2012, p. 6. Data from Global Health Observatory database, WHO.

noncommunicable diseases, and economic productivity decreases due to disability or underemployment of individuals with noncommunicable diseases. In 2011, the World Economic Forum and the Harvard School of Public Health released *The Global Economic Burden of Noncommunicable Diseases* report, which states that cardiovascular disease alone cost WPRO more than $107 billion in 2010, including more than $50 billion in lost productivity.

Noncommunicable diseases are the leading cause of death in the WPRO region and the leading cause of premature deaths. According to WPRO, noncommunicable diseases account for more than 80 percent of deaths in the region and half of all premature deaths. WPRO estimates that about 40 percent of all cancers and about 80 percent of premature heart attacks, strokes, and type 2 diabetes could be prevented through regular exercise, smoking cessation, and healthful diets. Unfortunately, WPRO estimates that these risk factors are becoming more prevalent in the region because of the effects of increased urbanization and economic development on lifestyles.

⊕ Future Implications

Combating Noncommunicable Diseases

Reducing the prevalence (the number of cases of a disease or condition present in a particular population at a given time) of risk factors associated with noncommunicable diseases is the most pressing public health issue in the WHO Western Pacific Region. In May 2008, the WHA adopted the Action Plan for the Global Strategy for the Prevention and Control of Noncommunicable Diseases at its 61st annual meeting. The WHA encouraged the WHO regional offices to adopt concomitant action plans tailored to reduce noncommunicable diseases within each region. WPRO adopted a noncommunicable disease action plan in 2009 and its revised plan in 2014. WPRO hopes to achieve a reduction in noncommunicable diseases in the region through the implementation of the Western Pacific Regional Action Plan for the Prevention and Control of Noncommunicable Diseases (2014–2020).

WPRO's noncommunicable disease action plan sets six objectives for its member nations. First, place a higher priority on the prevention and control of noncommunicable diseases. Second, strengthen national capacity and foster partnerships to accelerate national response to noncommunicable diseases. Third, reduce risk factors associated with noncommunicable diseases. Fourth, strengthen national health systems and emphasize the prevention of noncommunicable diseases. Fifth, promote national capacity to conduct research and development for noncommunicable disease prevention. Sixth, monitor noncommunicable disease trends and

burden on individual and family resources, which, particularly in low- and middle-income countries, contributes to a cycle of poverty. Society meanwhile often bears some of the high health-care costs associated with

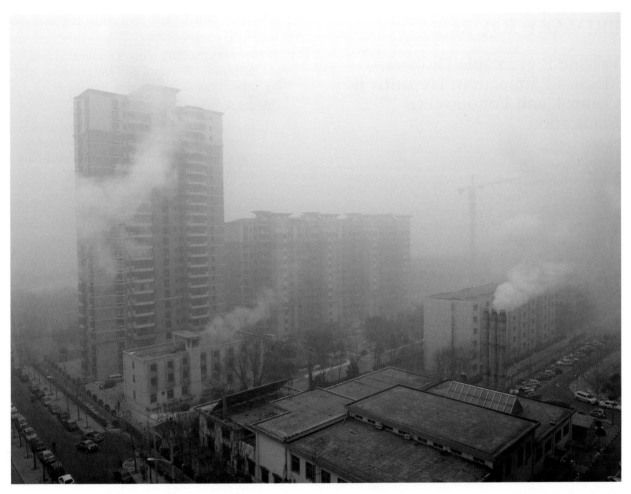

Severe air pollution on January 12, 2013, in Beijing, China, when air-quality index levels were classed as "Beyond Index" (PM 2.5 of over 700 micrograms per cubic meter). Urban and indoor air pollution are major problems in the Western Pacific Regional Office countries, contributing to an estimated 860,000 deaths annually.   © *Hung Chung Chih/Shutterstock.com.*

evaluate the effectiveness of noncommunicable disease prevention and control programs.

In addition to the six objectives, the WPRO noncommunicable diseases action plan establishes voluntary public health targets. First, the plan calls for a 25 percent reduction in premature deaths from the four leading noncommunicable diseases. Second, the WPRO aims for at least a 10 percent reduction in the harmful use of alcohol. Third, the plan sets a goal of a 10 percent reduction in the prevalence of insufficient physical activity, which is defined as at least 150 minutes of moderate physical activity per week. Fourth, the WPRO action plan specifies a 30 percent reduction in sodium intake. The fifth target is a 30 percent reduction in tobacco use among persons aged 15 or over. The WPRO region has the highest rate of tobacco use in the world with 47 percent prevalence among males aged 15 or over. Sixth, the plan seeks a 25 percent reduction in the prevalence of raised blood pressure. Finally, the WPRO noncommunicable action plan calls for a halt of the increase in obesity and diabetes rates.

Reducing Inequalities in Health Coverage

WPRO also faces great disparity between health-care expenditures among its member states, which affects the quality of health care. For example, the high-income countries of Australia, Japan, and New Zealand have per capita health-care expenditures of US$5,991, US$4,656, and US$3,715 per year. In the low-income countries of Cambodia, Papua New Guinea, and the Philippines, however, per capita health expenditures are only US$49, US$74, and US$105, respectively.

To improve public health within the region, WPRO is working toward the WHO goal of access to universal health coverage. WPRO's Health Care Financing unit cooperates with national governments and other stakeholders to improve health-care policy and build national health-care capacity to enable universal health coverage. WPRO states that it will continue to facilitate high-level health-care policy dialogue and promote the importance of universal health coverage as an area of national priority for each member state.

PRIMARY SOURCE

Vaccine Preventable Diseases: Measles Elimination, Hepatitis B Control, and Poliomyelitis Eradication

SOURCE *"Vaccine Preventable Diseases: Measles Elimination, Hepatitis B Control, and Poliomyelitis Eradication." World Health Organization (WHO) Regional Office for the Western Pacific, October 14, 2010. http://www2. wpro.who.int/NR/rdonlyres/A001CD03-976E-4770-859F-178BD8D37F7D/0/ R7Vaccinepreventablediseases.pdf (accessed January 25, 2015).*

INTRODUCTION *This primary source is a resolution by the Regional Committee for the Western Pacific of the World Health Organization. It addresses the public health issue of vaccine-preventable diseases in that part of the world, including background, current situation, and goals.*

WPR/RC61.R7

VACCINE PREVENTABLE DISEASES: MEASLES ELIMINATION, HEPATITIS B CONTROL, AND POLIOMYELITIS ERADICATION

The Regional Committee,

Noting resolution WPR/RC56.R8 that called for the elimination of measles by 2012 and a reduction in the seroprevalence of hepatitis B surface antigen (HBsAg) to less than 2% in 5-year-old children by 2012 as an interim milestone towards the final regional goal of less than 1% HBsAg;

Aware of the ongoing risk that importations of wild poliovirus pose to the maintenance of poliomyelitis-free status in the Western Pacific Region;

Noting resolution WPR/RC54.R3 that calls for the use of measles elimination and hepatitis B control strategies as means to strengthen the Expanded Programme on Immunization and other public health programmes, such as those intended to prevent the spread of congenital rubella syndrome;

Mindful of the positive impact of poliomyelitis eradication, measles elimination and hepatitis B control strategies in the Western Pacific Region on child health, immunization systems and overall health;

Recognizing that many countries and areas have made dramatic progress towards the achievement of the 2012 goals of measles elimination and the reduction in seroprevalence of HBsAg to less than 2%, but that many others face substantial financial and operational challenges to achieve the 2012 goals,

1. REAFFIRMS the 2012 measles elimination goal and the hepatitis B control goal and milestone, and the maintenance of poliomyelitis-free status;

URGES Member States:

1. to commit the human and financial resources necessary to achieve and sustain the measles elimination and hepatitis B control goals, and to maintain poliomyelitis-free status;

2. to develop and implement workplans to ensure high immunization coverage against measles, hepatitis B and poliomyelitis, and sensitive and timely epidemiologic and laboratory surveillance to achieve measles elimination and maintain poliomyelitis-free status;

3. to report measles and poliomyelitis, and where feasible rubella, surveillance data to the Regional Office in a regular and timely manner;

4. to establish an independent national verification process for measles elimination following the establishment by the WHO Regional Office for the Western Pacific of standardized regional verification mechanisms;

5. to accelerate control of rubella and the prevention of congenital rubella syndrome;

6. to vigorously implement all activities to maintain poliomyelitis-free status;

REQUESTS the Regional Director:

1. to establish Regional verification mechanisms for measles elimination;

2. to strengthen technical cooperation with Member States to achieve regional immunization goals;

3. to seek additional resources to achieve regional goals utilizing frequent interagency coordination committee meetings and other mechanisms;

4. to report progress periodically to the Regional Committee.

Seventh meeting WPR/RC61/SR/7

14 October 2010

SEE ALSO *Health in the WHO African Region; Health in the WHO Americas Region; Health in the WHO Eastern Mediterranean Region; Health in the WHO European Region; Health in the WHO South-East Asia Region; World Health Organization: Organization, Funding, and Enforcement Powers*

BIBLIOGRAPHY

Books

Birn, Anne-Emanuelle, Yogan Pillay, and Timothy H. Holtz. *Textbook of International Health: Global Health in a Dynamic World.* New York: Oxford University Press, 2009.

Bliss, Katherine Elaine, ed. *Key Players in Global Health: How Brazil, Russia, India, China, and South Africa Are Influencing the Game.* Washington, DC: Center for Strategic and International Studies, 2010.

Jacobsen, Kathryn H. *Introduction to Global Health,* 2nd ed. Burlington, MA: Jones and Bartlett Learning, 2014.

Websites

"Founding of the Western Pacific Regional Office." *World Health Organization (WHO). Western Pacific Region.* http://www.wpro.who.int/about/in_brief/history/en/ (accessed March 14, 2015).

"Health Systems." *World Health Organization (WHO).* http://www.who.int/entity/healthsystems/en (accessed February 1, 2015).

"WHO in the Western Pacific: Divisions." *World Health Organization (WHO). Western Pacific Region.* http://www.wpro.who.int/about/administration_structure/en/ (accessed March 14, 2015).

"WHO World Health Report 2013: Research for Universal Health Coverage." *World Health Organization (WHO).* http://www.who.int/whr/ (accessed February 1, 2015).

World Health Organization Regional Office for the Western Pacific. http://www.wpro.who.int/ (accessed March 1, 2015).

Joseph P. Hyder

Health-Care Worker Safety and Shortages

⊕ Introduction

Health-care workers face daily risks while performing their jobs. Health-care services are provided in a variety of settings, including hospitals, doctors' offices, outpatient surgery centers, homes, nursing homes, and war zones, and each presents a range of risks, threats, and hazards. Health-care workers may be exposed to life-threatening infections and chemicals as well as physical and psychological threats to their well-being. Stress, burnout, and workplace violence are acknowledged hazards in the health-care industry. Shortages of health-care workers and staffing issues can exacerbate these safety risks.

In the United States, health care is the fastest-growing sector of the economy and employs more than 18 million workers. Health-care workers suffer more injuries and illnesses—about 650,000 per year—than workers in any other industry. In 2010, health-care workers sustained approximately 152,000 more injuries and illnesses than those in manufacturing. And while there are more than twice as many health-care workers as construction workers, the U.S. Occupational Safety and Health Administration (OSHA), the agency responsible for worker safety, conducts nearly 20 times more inspections of construction sites than it does of health-care facilities.

In addition to work-related illnesses and injuries, health-care workers also encounter more nonfatal violence than any other profession—nearly three-quarters of all workplace assaults that result in days away from work are attacks on health-care workers. A 2014 survey of more than 5,000 registered nurses found that during the year prior to the survey, about one-third of the nurses had experienced physical violence or abuse from hospital patients or visitors.

⊕ Historical Background

Hospitals and other health-care facilities have long been frequent sites of workplace injuries. Similarly, violence against health-care workers, particularly those in areas of conflict and war zones, is not new. It has been documented since the 1800s. In the Second Italo-Ethiopian War (1935–1936) and in World War II (1939–1945), members of the Red Cross were targeted by military forces. An airplane affiliated with the International Committee of the Red Cross was shot down in 1969 during the Nigerian Civil War. From 1955 to 1975, many health-care workers were injured or killed in the Vietnam War. In 1996, the murder of six members of the International Committee of the Red Cross during the First Chechen War reinforced the belief that violence against health-care workers was growing.

International humanitarian law (IHL) is a law instituted to protect health-care missions and other humanitarian workers during times of conflict or peace. IHL is based on the Geneva Conventions of 1949, and though it is applicable only in international armed conflict, it is considered rule of law in all medical missions.

Health-Care Safety Standards

In 1970, the U.S. Congress established OSHA to improve workplace safety and health. OSHA was created to provide training and education and enforce standards to maintain the health and safety of workers. It writes regulations for workplace safety, ensures compliance by conducting reviews, and takes action against those violating the regulations. Since its creation, there has been a more than 60 percent decrease in work-related injuries, illnesses, and deaths. Other regulatory agencies responsible for enforcing safety standards in the health-care arena include The Joint Commission (formerly the Joint Commission on Accreditation of Healthcare Organizations) and Medicare.

During the 1980s, when the human immunodeficiency virus (HIV) came to the forefront, the role of this key regulatory agency in the health-care field expanded to include policy recommendations. In accordance with OSHA recommendations, the Blood Borne Pathogens Act of 1991 was enacted to limit health-care worker exposure to blood and body fluids.

The Blood Borne Pathogens Act requires employers to establish an exposure control plan that makes universal precautions and use of personal protective equipment mandatory.

Another part of the plan requires measures to prevent needlesticks, also known as sharps accidents. According to reports by the U.S. Centers for Disease Control and Prevention (CDC), approximately 385,000 hospital workers are injured in sharps accidents each year. All health-care facilities must have a plan in place to help prevent these injuries, and this plan must be updated annually. The Blood Borne Pathogens Act requires health-care institutions to initiate necessary precautions to protect health-care workers from hepatitis C, HIV, hepatitis B, and other blood-borne pathogens. These precautions include the use of needle-less systems, needle shield devices, and avoidance of recapping needles.

More recent legal actions include the Nurse and Health Care Worker Protection Act of 2013, which the U.S. Congress passed to help reduce injuries to health-care workers. This act requires facilities to develop and implement a program for safe patient handling, mobility, and injury prevention, and to acquire the appropriate equipment and technology to support those objectives. Another requirement of the act is that health-care workers be provided with education and training in patient and employee safety. Health-care facilities also must provide surveillance and preventive measures to protect workers and patients.

Health-care workers have the right to safe work environments, and laws in the United States enforce this provision. Should health-care workers believe their facilities do not adhere to OSHA standards, they can file complaints and request workplace inspections.

⊕ Impacts and Issues

Health-Care Staffing Shortages

According to a 2006 World Health Organization (WHO) report, unsafe working conditions have contributed to the reduction in numbers of health-care workers in many countries. The WHO reports severe health-care worker shortages in 57 countries, most notably in Africa and Asia. Protecting health-care workers from occupational hazards is essential to improving and maintaining adequate supplies of workers. A November 2013 WHO report estimates that in 2013 there was a global shortfall of 7.2 million health-care workers; it also predicts that by 2035 the global shortfall will be 12.9 million health-care workers.

An aging workforce is one cause of shortages in the health-care field, and there are too few people training and entering the industry. Demanding work and relatively

Health Workforce Density per 10,000 Population, Global, Regional, and Income Group

	Physicians (2006–2013)	Nursing and midwifery personnel (2006–2013)	Dentistry personnel (dentists, dental technicians/assistants and related occupations) (2006–2013)	Pharmaceutical personnel (pharmacists, pharmaceutical technicians/assistants and related occupations) (2006–2013)	Psychiatrists (2006–2010)
Global	14.1	29.2	2.7	4.3	0.3
Ranges of country values					
Minimum	0.1	1.1	<0.05	<0.05	<0.05
Median	12.8	28.4	2.9	2.4	2.0
Maximum	77.4	173.6	40.0	27.1	4.1
WHO region					
African Region	2.6	12.0	0.5	0.9	<0.05
Region of the Americas	20.8	45.8	6.9	6.7	0.5
South-East Asia Region	5.9	15.3	1.0	3.8	<0.05
European Region	33.1	80.5	5.0	5.1	1.1
Eastern Mediterranean Region	11.4	16.1	1.9	6.1	0.1
Western Pacific Region	15.3	25.1	—	4.5	0.2
Income group					
Low income	2.4	5.4	0.3	0.5	<0.05
Lower middle income	7.8	17.8	1.2	4.2	0.1
Upper middle income	15.5	25.3	—	3.1	0.2
High income	29.4	86.9	5.8	8.4	1.0

SOURCE: Adapted from "Table 6. Health Systems," in *World Health Statistics 2014*, World Health Organization (WHO), 2014. Data from *Mental Health Atlas 2011*, WHO, 2011, *WHO Global Health Workforce Statistics*, WHO, 2014; World Population Prospects database, United Nations Population Division.

A basic threshold of 23 skilled health professionals per 10,000 people is the recommended target, according to the WHO, however not enough workers are being trained for current and future demand.

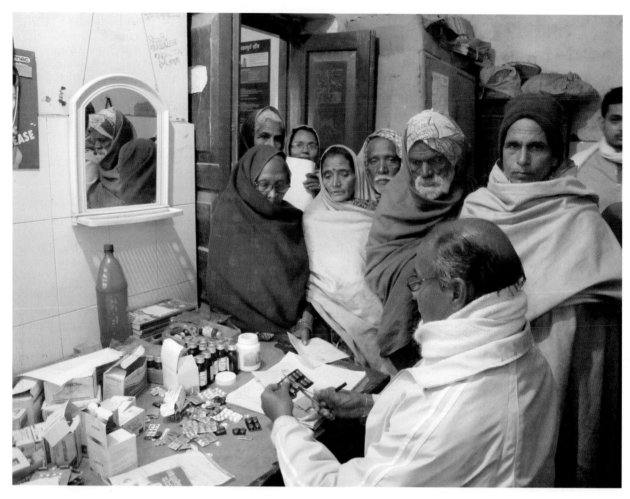

At a primary health-care center in a rural subdistrict in Bihiya, India, a filing clerk doubles up as a pharmacist. In a nation of over 1.2 billion people, India faces a crippling shortage of health-care workers that contributes to high infant mortality and chronic malnutrition and clouds India's economic prospects. The shortage ranges from doctors, nurses, anesthetists, and radiologists to village-level public health workers who battle infectious diseases like malaria, leprosy, and tuberculosis. In 2013, the World Health Organization estimated that there was a shortage of 7.2 million health-care workers around the globe, a figure predicted to rise to 12.9 million by 2035.   © *Rama Lakshmi/The Washington Post via Getty Images.*

low pay contribute to the loss of workers and discourage young people from entering the health-care workforce.

Health workforce density refers to the number of health-care workers in the active labor force. The WHO table shows the differences in health workforce density from 2006 to 2013 by region and type of health-care worker as well as the relationship between income and workforce density. A basic threshold of 23 skilled health professionals per 10,000 people is the recommended target, according to the WHO, however, not enough workers are being trained for current and future demand. The WHO predicts that by 2025 the greatest numerical shortages will be in parts of Asia, though the density is expected to stay lowest in Africa. The WHO encourages all nations to evaluate their needs and train people accordingly, concentrating on developing multidisciplinary teams of physicians, nurses, and allied health professionals to deliver primary care.

Workplace Violence

The causes for the shortages in the number of health-care workers are many, however, work hazards, including violence against health-care workers, are often cited as factors. One cause of violence in health-care settings is stress. Feelings of frustration and vulnerability can cause patients and families to feel out of control, leading to violent outbursts. Health-care workers in closest contact with patients—doctors, nurses, and nursing assistants—are usually at the highest risk, as are workers in psychiatric departments, emergency departments, and geriatric units. Reception areas and waiting rooms are also common sites for violent threats or victimizations. Patients or visitors who are intoxicated or under the influence of drugs, or have a history of violence, may pose greater threats. Understaffing, overcrowding in waiting rooms, and long wait times also may be contributing factors.

To effectively prevent and reduce violence in health-care settings, the CDC identifies the key issues that health-care organizations and facilities must address: access to and availability of skilled crisis intervention and workplace safety policies and education for employees on recognizing potential risks, as well as broader societal issues such as stricter access to guns and decreasing the culture of violence.

By 2015, more than half of the 50 U.S. states had passed laws designating penalties for the assault of nurses, and seven additional states required employers to run workplace violence prevention programs. For example, as of January 2015, California law requires hospitals to regularly assess their staffing levels to determine whether inadequate staffing poses a safety risk for health-care workers. The law also requires hospitals to conduct campus-wide security audits to identify and evaluate security risks.

Violence against health-care workers also affects patients and employers. In addition to any physical injury sustained, workers who experience violence or threats of violence may suffer from psychological problems such as loss of sleep, nightmares, and flashbacks. In some cases, victims may develop serious, life-limiting conditions such as post-traumatic stress disorder (PTSD is a condition in which people feel stressed or fearful even when they are no longer in danger). The consequences of violence can persist and affect quality of life for workers for years after the event. The workers may also have to deal with lost wages and legal fees, adding to the stress they are already feeling.

Immediate intervention, such as counseling after a traumatic event, can provide a needed support system for victims of workplace violence. Implementation of a critical-incident stress debriefing (CISD) may prevent serious long-term complications from exposure to violent events. CISD allows the employee to process the event and put it into proper perspective. Many hospitals have CISD teams in place to help employees following terrifying or traumatic events.

Workplace violence also has an impact on employers. It can increase staff turnover, absenteeism, and employee health-care costs and may result in property damage and litigation.

Violence against Health-Care Workers in Conflict Zones

The International Committee of the Red Cross (ICRC) reports that between 2012 and 2014, there were more than 2,300 instances of violence aimed at health-care workers and health-care facilities and observes that many more occur but are unreported. In addition to violence against local health-care workers, there has been a surge of violence against volunteer workers such as the international volunteers that provide medical services with humanitarian aid organizations such as Médecins Sans Frontières (MSF; also known as Doctors Without Borders). In 2012 alone, the ICRC reported in *Violent*

Incidents Affecting Health Care: January to December 2012 that 150 health-care workers were killed and 73 kidnapped. Many others were threatened.

In 2014, a United Nations General Assembly meeting focused on the problem of increasing violence in health-care settings around the world with a session titled "Health Care and Violence: The Need for Effective Protection," which was led by the head of the WHO, Dr. Margaret Chan, and the head of the ICRC, Dr. Peter Maurer.

Health-Care System Safety Measures

Though many challenges faced by health-care workers are similar globally, some issues are unique to a country or region. In addition, attempts by various countries to create solutions and provide safe work environments have varied.

Canada The Canadian health-care system has several safety initiatives underway, including use of a comprehensive systems approach to promote health-care safety. The Occupational Health and Safety Agency for Healthcare (OHSAH) in British Columbia has spearheaded development and implementation of safety initiatives.

The OHSAH in British Columbia is jointly governed by health-care unions and employers, with the shared goal of improving working conditions for the profession. Approximately 40 percent of all violence-related claims in British Columbia come from health-care workers, who constitute only 5 percent of the workforce. With these statistics in mind, the Workers' Compensation Board of British Columbia established a program to train the health-care workforce about violence. Their research demonstrates that reducing physical and psychological hazards for health-care workers will, in turn, improve patient safety.

United Kingdom In the United Kingdom (UK), the Health and Safety at Work Act (HASWA) of 1974 set forth general laws to protect health-care workers. The Health and Safety Executive (HSE) is the UK's governing agency with legislative power to investigate and prosecute breaches in safety regulations. Failure to comply with HASWA can result in fines and/or imprisonment; a civil suit may follow to aid those affected by the breach. Settlements in civil suits are often much higher than the fines imposed by the courts.

The UK has been working to reduce risk of violence for its National Health Service (NHS) staff. From 2008 to 2009 there were 54,758 reported acts of violence against NHS staff in England, which equates to four times more workplace violence and aggression than experienced by other workers. Through an approach called safe systems of work, risk assessment and risk management assess both the probability of an adverse event and the consequences of that event. The time, effort, and resources needed to reduce that risk can then be addressed. An evaluation of antiviolence training in the health-care setting showed

HEALTH-CARE WORKERS ATTACKED IN PAKISTAN AFTER CIA FALSE VACCINE PLOY

In July 2011, intense global media coverage revealed that the U.S. Central Intelligence Agency (CIA) orchestrated a hepatitis B vaccination program in the Pakistan and Afghanistan border regions as cover to collect DNA samples from relatives of Osama bin Laden in an effort to help locate the internationally wanted terrorist. Though the ploy did not give the CIA the information they needed, the publicity surrounding the operation angered local populations and led to distrust of vaccination teams, including those trying to eradicate polio in the two countries, where it remains endemic. (Bin Laden, who claimed responsibility for the September 11, 2001, attacks on the United States, was eventually found hiding in Abbottabad, Pakistan, and killed in a raid by U.S. Special Forces in May 2011.)

The CIA operation, which tied a spying operation with humanitarian efforts in regions in which creating and maintaining relationships with those who need health care is an ongoing concern, was widely condemned by health officials and public health officers worldwide. Médecins Sans Frontières (MSF; also known as Doctors Without Borders) president Unni Karunakara spoke out immediately against the operation. MSF officials said that such an operation was a significant breach of trust that could threaten future field-workers and reduce effectiveness of vaccination programs that require community involvement and confidence in those delivering health care.

This was indeed the case, and many international aid organizations were forced to move health workers out of Pakistan because of violence against workers. From 2011 through 2014 in Pakistan, attacks on health-care workers and security personnel protecting them resulted in 60 deaths. In December 2012 during a three-day polio vaccination drive, five female polio vaccination workers, including a 17-year-old volunteer, were killed by gunmen. Four were killed in Karachi, and the teenaged volunteer was shot in Peshawar. The killings led the World Health Organization and the United Nations Children's Fund to call on community leaders to protect vaccination workers. In November 2014, four health-care workers in western Pakistan's province of Balochistan were killed while administering polio vaccinations. The Pakistani Taliban struck again in March 2015, killing two female workers and a police guard in the Mansehra district in Khyber-Pakhtunkhwa Province.

Increasing numbers of Pakistanis have become suspicious of the workers and have refused to have their children vaccinated. In addition to beliefs about vaccination workers being spies, some believe that polio vaccination campaigns are plots to sterilize Muslims by Western governments. In early 2015, the Pakistani government began jailing parents who refused to allow their children to receive the vaccine.

In 2013, the deans of 12 U.S. public health schools wrote U.S. President Obama to protest "collateral consequences" of the CIA operation. In May 2014, a White House official stated that the CIA will no longer use vaccination campaigns or vaccination workers as part of CIA operations. Lynn Goldman, one of the deans who wrote to the White House, responded to the changed policy in a statement in a May 19, 2014, article in the the *Washington Post*: "People involved as vaccination workers need to be able to do their work safely. They need to be protected by all people globally."

---

that use of proactive measures such as risk assessment and control methods was more effective in reducing acts of violence than just training alone. Failure to use risk assessment is now a breach of regulations.

Africa With over 20,000 cases of Ebola reported in eight African countries from 2014 to early 2015, the safety of health-care workers there is of utmost importance. Workers can become infected by touching a patient's body fluids or equipment and supplies that have been contaminated with body fluids. The spread of Ebola can be prevented by appropriate infection control measures and proper personal protective equipment. It is essential for health-care workers caring for Ebola patients to be provided with the appropriate training and equipment. In addition to Ebola, health-care workers must take precautions against all blood-borne pathogens and other contagious disease that are prevalent on the continent of Africa.

Violence against health-care workers has long been a problem in Africa and is now on the increase. Incidents of violence against health-care workers and people seeking treatment have been reported during conflicts in the Central African Republic. Violent victimization of health-care workers further jeopardizes the already precarious public health in many countries because when workers and health-care facilities cannot be kept safe, lifesaving services to those in need cannot be delivered.

China During the 20th century, China's health-care system suffered as the state no longer assumed responsibility for providing health-care services. Hospitals and doctors struggled to remain financially viable, and doctors, especially, feel overworked and underpaid. Most doctors see far more patients per day than their U.S. and European counterparts; one study found that an average patient visit lasted just seven minutes. Doctors' salaries are generally low, and many doctors supplement their earnings by selling prescription drugs; some even accept bribes from patients seeking specialized medical treatment or surgery.

Understandably, these conditions create considerable patient dissatisfaction. Although hospitals do handle patient complaints and grievances, and patients can sue doctors and hospitals for medical malpractice, many Chinese people do not trust the legal system and choose to resolve differences with hospitals and doctors privately.

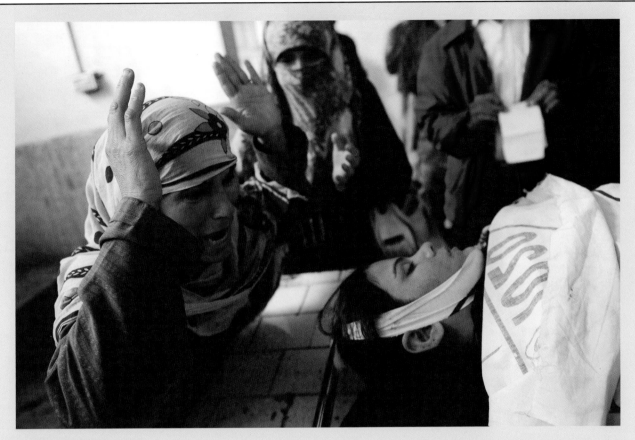

A mother mourns her daughter, a polio vaccine worker, killed by gunmen on motorbikes in Karachi, Pakistan, December 18, 2012. Five female Pakistani polio vaccination workers were killed during a three-day drive against the disease. © *Rizwan Tabassum/AFP/Getty Images.*

When patients feel wronged or do not receive the treatment or compensation they seek, they sometimes take matters into their own hands, staging public protests or resorting to violence. From 2002 to 2012, attacks on doctors and other health-care workers rose nearly 23 percent each year and the average number of assaults per hospital spiked from 20.6 per year in 2008 to 27.3 in 2012. Although medical centers with more than 2,000 beds are supposed to have 100 security guards, many doctors, nurses, and other health-care workers feel there are few or no provisions in place to protect them from violent victimizations. Some observers believe that until people feel confident about China's legal channels and their ability to receive fair rulings on medical malpractice claims violence directed at physicians will continue.

⊕ Future Implications

Health-care workers face a multitude of health and safety risks every day, from biological risks such as needlesticks to psychosocial and stress-related challenges and deliberate violence by patients and combatants in conflict zones. Such risks must be addressed to encourage more workers to enter the health-care profession and limit the projected shortages in health-care workers in the coming decades. The WHO states that the global shortage of health-care workers has "serious implications for the health of billions of people across all regions of the world."

It is critical that prevention and management of violence be a concerted, global priority in all health-care settings. Workplace violence is a complicated issue in all health-care settings. Workers acting on their own have little effect on prevention. In the United States, laws intended to protect health-care workers have been enacted and strengthened; in many states, assaults on health-care workers in the performance of their duties are no longer considered simple assaults, they are considered aggravated assaults. Higher penalties result for those committing such assaults. In 31 states, battery against a health-care worker is a felony. However, many countries around the world do not have such protections for health-care workers, and more must be done to increase

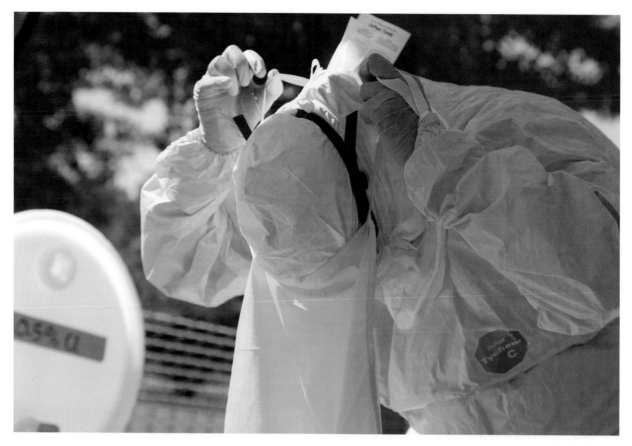

A health-care worker dons the final article of personal protective equipment (PPE), a plastic apron, to complete the protective uniform as part of participation in the U.S. Centers for Disease Control and Prevention's (CDC) 2014 Domestic Ebola Treatment Unit Training Course. The course was designed to educate participants who would be deployed as members of the West African Ebola Response team, where there was a shortage of trained health-care workers during the epidemic. The CDC course trained physicians, nurses, and other providers in proper safety protocols when treating Ebola patients. According to the CDC, "The primary purpose of the course is to ensure that clinicians intending to provide medical care to patients with Ebola have sufficient knowledge of the disease, and its transmission routes in order to work safely and efficiently in a well-designed Ebola treatment unit." *Nahid Bhadelia, M.D./U.S. Centers for Disease Control and Prevention.*

safe working conditions for all workers in health-care fields. Future research will to help identify the best practices for preventing violence against health-care workers.

SEE ALSO *Conflict, Violence, and Terrorism: Health Impacts; Health as a Human Right and Health-Care Access; Médecins Sans Frontières; Post-Traumatic Stress Syndrome; Vulnerable Populations; Workplace Health and Safety; World Health Organization: Organization, Funding, and Enforcement Powers*

BIBLIOGRAPHY

Books

Fried, Bruce J., and Myron D. Fottler, eds. *Fundamentals of Human Resources in Healthcare.* Chicago: Health Administration Press, 2012.

Injury and Illness Prevention Programs: White Paper, Occupational Safety and Health Administration (OSHA), U.S. Department of Labor, 2012. Available online at https://www.osha.gov/dsg/topics/safetyhealth/OSHAwhite-paper-january2012sm.pdf (accessed March 1, 2015).

Lemiere, Christoph, et al. *Reducing Geographical Imbalances of Health Workers in Sub-Saharan Africa: A Labor Market Prospective on What Works, What Does Not, and Why.* Washington, DC: World Bank Group, 2010.

Tulchinsky, Theodore H., and Elena Varavikova. *The New Public Health,* 3rd ed. Amsterdam: Academic Press, 2014.

Tweedy, James T. *Healthcare Hazard Control and Safety Management,* 3rd ed. Boca Raton, FL: CRC Press/Taylor and Francis, 2014.

Zerwekh, JoAnn, and Ashley Zerwekh Garneau, eds. *Nursing Today: Transition and Trends,* 7th ed. Maryland Heights, MO: Elsevier/Saunders, 2014.

Websites

Goldberg, Stephanie. "Attacks on Hospital Nurses Trigger State Laws to Protect Them." *Business Insurance*, November 23, 2014. http://www.businessinsurance.com/article/20141123/NEWS08/311239978/attacks-on-hospital-nurses-trigger-state-laws-to-protect-them?tags=|84|92|304 (accessed March 1, 2015).

"Guidelines for Protecting the Safety and Health of Health Care Workers." *U.S. Centers for Disease Control and Prevention (CDC)*. http://www.cdc.gov/niosh/docs/88–119/ (accessed February 1, 2015).

"Health Care: Risks for Health Care Workers." *European Agency for Safety and Health at Work.* https://osha.europa.eu/en/faq/what-are-the-main-occupational-health-and-safety-risks-for-health-care-workers (accessed February 1, 2015).

"Health Care Worker Safety." *World Health Organization (WHO)*. http://www.who.int/injection_safety/toolbox/en/AM_HCW_Safety_EN.pdf (accessed February 1, 2015).

"Health Care Workers Suffer Highest Total Worker Injury Toll While Having Few Federal Safety Protections, Study Shows." *Public Citizen*, July 17, 2013. http://www.citizen.org/pressroom/pressroomredirect.cfm?ID=3940 (accessed February 1, 2015).

"Healthcare." *U.S. Department of Labor.* https://www.osha.gov/SLTC/healthcarefacilities/ (accessed February 1, 2015).

Jacobson, Roni. "Epidemic of Violence against Health Care Workers Plagues Hospitals." *Scientific American*, December 31, 2014. http://www.scientificamerican.com/article/epidemic-of-violence-against-health-care-workers-plagues-hospitals/ (accessed March 1, 2015).

Klibanoff, Eleanor. "Awful Moments In Quarantine History: Remember Typhoid Mary?" *NPR*, October 30, 2014. http://www.npr.org/blogs/goatsandsoda/2014/10/30/360120406/awful-moments-in-quarantine-history-remember-typhoid-mary (accessed January 30, 2015).

Langfitt, Frank. "In Violent Hospitals, China's Doctors Can Become Patients." *NPR*, November 6, 2013. http://www.npr.org/blogs/parallels/2013/11/06/242344329/in-violent-hospitals-chinas-doctors-can-become-patients (accessed March 1, 2015).

"Occupational Health for Healthcare Providers." *National Institutes of Health.* http://www.nlm.nih.gov/medlineplus/occupationalhealthforhealthcareproviders.html (accessed February 1, 2015).

Rauhala, Emily. "Why China's Doctors Are Getting Beat Up." *Time.com*, March 7, 2014. http://time.com/15185/chinas-doctors-overworked-underpaid-attacked/ (accessed March 1, 2015).

Speroni, Karen Gabel, et al. "Incidence and Cost of Nurse Workplace Violence Perpetrated by Hospital Patients or Patient Visitors." *Journal of Emergency Nursing*, 40, no. 3 (May 2014): 218–228. Available online at http://www.jenonline.org/article/S0099-1767(13)00216-X/abstract?cc=y (accessed March 1, 2015).

Sun, Lena H. "CIA: No More Vaccination Campaigns in Spy Operations." *Washington Post*, May 19, 2014. http://www.washingtonpost.com/world/national-security/cia-no-more-vaccination-campaigns-in-spy-operations/2014/05/19/406c4f3e-df88-11e3-8dcc-d6b7fede081a_story.html (accessed March 10, 2015).

"Violent Incidents Affecting Health Care: January to December 2012." *International Committee of the Red Cross (ICRC)*, March 15, 2013. https://www.icrc.org/eng/resources/documents/report/2013-05-15-health-care-in-danger-incident-report.htm (accessed April 1, 2015).

Lisa Lehmann
Elisabeth Lee Rennie

Health-Related Education and Information Access

⊕ Introduction

Health education is a way of providing individuals, groups, and communities with the knowledge necessary to make informed decisions when it comes to health and well-being. This can include information about disease, nutrition, hygiene, and reproduction, as well as life skills necessary to maintain good physical, mental, and social health.

Health education can also include communication of information concerning underlying social, economic, and environmental conditions impacting health, as well as individual risk factors, risk behaviors, and use of the health-care system, according to the World Health Organization (WHO).

People access this information in a variety of ways, such as searching books, journals, and the Internet; getting formal education, attending workshops and classes; visiting clinics; and having discussions with family members, health-care professionals, community leaders, and social service agencies.

In developing nations, access to quality health education has been a challenge for a number of reasons. Infrastructure and literacy skills necessary to access the information in books or the Internet are often lacking. Health-care workers are often trained using outdated or inadequate materials, if trained at all, leaving them unable to provide adequate information and treatment to the populations they serve. In some countries, religious, cultural, or social mores and conventions can restrict certain members of society from accessing this information. Research shows that lack of access to quality lifesaving information has a tremendous impact on the high number of deaths from preventable diseases among children.

Even developed countries have had their troubles accessing quality health information. In some parts of the United States, for example, religious and political beliefs can restrict the teaching of reproductive health in schools. In other cases, protestors driven by these same ideals can prevent women from seeking out reproductive information in clinics. This can have a detrimental effect in terms of unwanted pregnancies and proliferation of sexually transmitted infections (STIs).

⊕ Historical Background

There is evidence to show that even the earliest civilizations had some form of health education. Writings of the Babylonians, Egyptians, and Old Testament Israelites indicate that various health promotion techniques were utilized, according to James A. Johnson and Donald J. Breckon in *Managing Health Promotion Programs: Leadership Skills for the 21st Century.* This included development of community systems to provide safe drinking water and sewage disposal, advocacy for personal cleanliness, and warnings against troublesome intoxication. While the means of catching a disease was not known, the earliest civilizations advocated ways to avoid and cure them, including the use of quarantine and herbal medicines.

Early organized religions sponsored many of the first health-care facilities and practiced the healing arts. In many cultures, gods were considered the cause of good or ill health.

The ancient Greeks championed the benefits of proper diet and physical exercise. The Pythagoreans, for example, placed a premium on hygiene and developed the Pythagorean way of living. This model emphasized the idea of health as a condition of perfect equilibrium. Preserving equilibrium meant practicing moderation as well as maintaining self-control and a sense of calm. Diet, gymnastics, and music were all ways to achieve these goals and restore balance when there was an upset in the equilibrium.

The modern concept of health education and promotion has its beginnings in the Industrial Revolution. Abysmal work conditions led to labor laws and work site programs that for the first time took workers' health and safety into account. The evolution of labor unions brought change not only in advocacy for healthy work

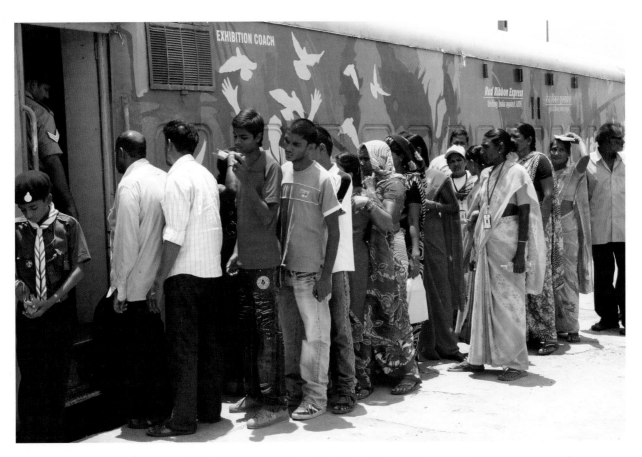

Local people wait outside the Red Ribbon Express to see the exhibits of the Indian Railways HIV/AIDS awareness campaign in Secunderabad, India. The train traveled through many districts and territories to spread awareness and promote safe sex practices. India has the world's third-largest population living with HIV/AIDS. © *reddees/Shutterstock.com.*

environments but for insurance programs that eventually would include the concept of prevention.

Scientific discovery and technological advances also had an effect on health education. Scientists were discovering the causative role of pathogens and learning the value of prevention. This concept led to programs that tackled everything from the benefits of diet and exercise to the ills of substance abuse and chronic disease.

Myriad public health campaigns targeting maternal health and infectious disease followed. According to Don Nutbeam in his article, "Health Literacy as a Public Health Goal: A Challenge for Contemporary Health Education and Communication Strategies into the 21st Century," for the journal *Health Promotion International*, in campaigns of the 1960s and 1970s in developed countries, the message shifted to the prevention of noncommunicable diseases by promoting healthy lifestyles. The campaigns were somewhat single-minded in that the goal was simply to transmit the message of the campaign and not, as would be the case later, to offer explanation or cure the underlying causes.

By the 1980s, that started to change. These programs started to focus on the social context of behavioral decisions, and on helping people develop the personal and social skills required to make positive behavior choices. Nutbeam goes on to write, "These theories have helped to identify and explain the complex relationships between knowledge, beliefs and perceived social norms, and provide practical guidance on the content of educational programs to promote behavioural change in a given set of circumstances."

By the 1990s and into the next decade, health education morphed one more time and as a result broadened its reach. Health promotion has shifted toward improving people's control over all modifiable determinants of health, Nutbeam asserts. And not just when it comes to personal behavior, but public policy. For example, where an old smoking cessation campaign may have simply communicated the benefits of not smoking, a contemporary campaign would give that information along with a campaign showing that it is not socially acceptable to smoke, information on ways to sustain a nonsmoking lifestyle, and access to support groups in a community to help a person get at the root cause of why he or she is smoking. Another new component of a modern campaign, continuing with the smoking example, would be giving advice on how to promote nonsmoking in a community and even how to advocate

HEALTH PROMOTION AND SOCIAL MEDIA

Researchers and public health officials are increasingly trying to harness the power of popular social media sites to not only track infectious disease but to disseminate information to the public.

For example, food-borne illness affects more than 105 million people in the United States alone each year and costs an average of US$2 billion to $4 billion each year. Health officials have long realized that this is just the tip of the iceberg. Millions of people in the United States experience gastroenteritis (food poisoning) every year, but many people do not seek treatment. This leaves health agencies lacking vital information regarding actual numbers of cases and cost of illness. One way to reduce the number of food-borne illnesses is to identify the source of the problem, such as food from a particular restaurant, food cart, or grocery store. Although most people do not report the business or the incident to their local health department, they do talk about it on social media.

An article in the U.S Centers for Disease Control and Prevention (CDC's) weekly *Morbidity and Mortality Weekly Report* from 2014 describes one instance in which a city began to use social media to track such illnesses. The Chicago Department of Public Health and nongovernmental partners started FoodBorne Chicago, "a website aimed at improving food safety in Chicago by identifying and responding to complaints on Twitter about possible foodborne illnesses." Using a specialized algorithm, FoodBorne Chicago staff tracked Twitter messages originating in Chicago that included the phrase "food poisoning" to identify specific instances. Once the tweets were identified, staff members reviewed them, looking for mention of symptoms such as stomach cramps, diarrhea, or vomiting from food prepared outside the home.

For tweets meeting the criteria, staff members used Twitter to tell potential food poisoning victims what they could do to lodge a complaint and get access to information on food-borne illness. For example, Tweet: "Guess who's got food poisoning? This girl!" Reply: "That doesn't sound good. Help us prevent this and report where you ate here (link to Foodborne Chicago and a web form to report the illness)."

Between March 2013 and January 2014, FoodBorne Chicago identified 2,241 food poisoning tweets originating from Chicago and neighboring suburbs. From these, staff members identified 270 tweets describing specific instances of persons with complaints of food-borne illness. Eight of the 270 tweets mentioned a visit to a doctor or a hospital emergency department. A total of 193 complaints of food poisoning were submitted through the FoodBorne Chicago web form.

Social media has also been used to share information in times of disaster. During the devastating 2010 earthquake and hurricane in Haiti, health-care workers were able to map out the worst-hit areas and send help based on the number of social media messages from a particular area.

Social media has also been used in recent years to track infectious diseases such as flu, cholera, and yellow fever. In the case of cholera, researchers discovered during the 2010 outbreak in Haiti that followed the earthquake that cases were reported on Twitter by doctors in the field a full two weeks before the official record showed the outbreak had started. In this way, for those who have access to mobile technology, which about two-thirds of the world does, social media can be used as an early warning system to the public. Many researchers and scientists believe that as developing nations connect to the Internet, it can ultimately be a great tool for health promotion and disease prevention.

---

for legislative or policy changes. Nutbeam writes, "This more comprehensive approach is not only addressing the individual behaviour, but also some of the underlying social and environmental determinants of that behaviour."

⊕ Impacts and Issues

Health education and access to correct and updated health information have a direct relationship to positive health outcomes. However, in many developing countries people lack access to vital health information for a variety of reasons.

One major hurdle to overcome for many is that the health-care workers providing the information lack the knowledge themselves. In a 2009 review for the journal *Human Resources for Health,* authors Neil Pakenham-Walsh and Frederick Bukachi examined 35 studies assessing the information and learning needs of health-care

providers in developing countries. Of their findings they wrote, "The studies suggest a gross lack of knowledge about the basics on how to diagnose and manage common diseases, going right across the health workforce and often associated with suboptimal, ineffective and dangerous health care practices."

This lack of information hurts the patients in the care of these health-care workers. One study referenced in the review examined the management of severely malnourished children at two rural district hospitals in South Africa. The study found that the combined case fatality rate for severe malnutrition was 32 percent, which was a high rate that could have been much lower with sufficient training of the health workers. According to the study, many of the children died during the first few days of treatment because of missed infections, hypoglycemia due to lack of night feedings, hypothermia, cardiac failure due to overhydration from intravenous fluids, and electrolyte imbalance due to use of diuretics.

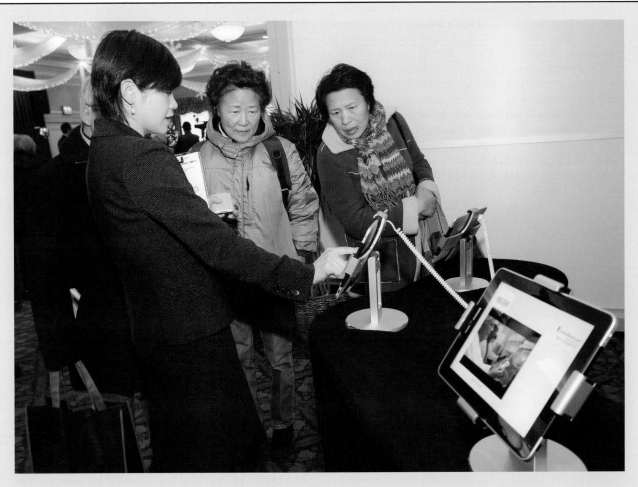

A UnitedHealthcare representative demonstrates how Medicare beneficiaries can use the latest technology, including social media, to access health information online. © *Rick Maiman/AP Images for UnitedHealthcare.*

Furthermore, this lack of knowledge means they are not passing on proper information to patients. A study from Egypt showed that 90 percent of diabetic patients had poor knowledge of their disease. Eighty percent were not fully informed about the complications of the disease, and 96 percent were not aware of how to control the disease. The researchers of the study asserted that more research was needed to determine what types and how much information was most helpful and what methods were most efficient for delivering the information to diabetics and their families. In addition, better training was crucial for health workers so that they could implement these best practices into their discussions with patients.

However, a study from South Africa that quoted a health-care worker suggests that for some that is next to impossible. "You only have an average of six minutes per patient. By the time you've examined them and found out that they're diabetic and what their glucose level is, you cannot possibly educate somebody in three minutes [or less]."

These gaps in knowledge not only leave patients with a dearth of information but with a fear of seeking out health services. The studies seem to indicate this results in patients seeing hospitals as a place one goes to die, not a place for treatment or information. Pakenham-Walsh and Bukachi conclude that, "If this level of knowledge and practice is representative, as it appears to be, it indicates that modern medicine, even at a basic level, has largely failed the majority of the world's population. The information and learning needs of family caregivers and primary and district health workers have been ignored for too long. Improving the availability and use of relevant, reliable health care information has enormous potential to radically improve health care worldwide."

It is not that these health-care workers are not bright, diligent, or caring. There are considerable barriers to accessing the information they need, and these challenges mimic the troubles the general population has in getting the same information.

One of the major challenges is a lack of infrastructure. The hospitals may have some access to the Internet and a working phone line, but in some places, service is sporadic or nonexistent. This is crucial, because medical information can change rapidly. So if doctors are relying on journal articles and outdated textbooks for information, as opposed to the latest research or health alerts those in the developed world can access on their mobile devices, they are at a distinct disadvantage. And while there have been investments in technology in the developing world, the research indicates much of it has gone to the wealthier sectors of the countries and rarely trickles down to the health workers in the smaller, rural, and more impoverished areas of the countries.

There are also some major cultural and religious restrictions that can keep people, particularly women, from accessing health care. For example, a woman may fear reprisal from a spouse or even her community if it is discovered she has a disease; in this case, she may just refuse to seek out medical treatment or information. This is true particularly of women who are HIV positive, many of whom never return for follow-up care after receiving an initial diagnosis.

Furthermore, many of these countries have gone through, or are in the midst of, brutal and bloody civil wars and political upheaval. This leaves many of their inhabitants deeply mistrustful of those in authority, as a health-care worker may be perceived to be. Workers with an nongovernmental agency who are there to deliver information on vaccines might be considered outsiders and met with mistrust and fear.

Meanwhile, while not on the order of what developing nations are experiencing, even developed countries have seen some access issues in the past few decades. This primarily has revolved around the debate of whether sexual education should be a part of a school-based health curriculum and, if it is, whether it should be comprehensive or abstinence-only education.

In recent years, the latter has become a more common option in the United States, primarily because of federal funding put toward the effort. Abstinence-only education is a curriculum that only promotes abstinence from sexual activity until marriage. By contrast, the comprehensive approach would include information about abstinence as well as contraception, STIs, HIV/AIDS, abortion, and high-risk behaviors.

Advocates for abstinence-only curriculum assert that this is the only way to keep middle- and high-school-age children from engaging in behaviors that lead to teenage pregnancy and disease. However, critics say that abstinence-only education has the exact opposite effect and does not teach young people how to responsibly handle sexual activity.

And at least one study shows that science may be on their side. In a 2011 study by Kathrin F. Stanger-Hall and David Hall, titled "Abstinence-Only Education and Teen Pregnancy Rates: Why We Need Comprehensive Sex Education in the U.S.," published in the journal *PLoS ONE*, the authors found that the states with abstinence-only curriculum had higher teen pregnancy rates than those that had comprehensive sexual education. The authors went on to recommend that schools "adopt an integration of comprehensive sex and STD [sexually transmitted disease] education into the biology curriculum in middle and high school science classes and a parallel social studies curriculum that addresses risk-aversion behaviors and planning for the future."

⊕ Future Implications

Health education is critical to stopping the spread of disease and encouraging people to live a healthy lifestyle. Life expectancy remains low in impoverished countries, and children continue to die by the millions from preventable diseases such as diarrhea and pneumonia. It is generally accepted that providing children and their caregivers with information on proper self-care, hygiene, and disease prevention and management can drastically reduce those numbers.

Though public health agencies have launched in-school health campaigns across the developing world, they remain inadequate due to cultural and economic barriers and lack of resources, among other reasons. In a 2012 article for the *Stanford Social Innovation Review*, titled "Redefining Education in the Developing World," authors Mark J. Epstein and Kristi Yuthas assert that curricula in schools across the developing world need to do a better job teaching and building life skills such as financial literacy, entrepreneurship, and basic health and self-care.

They further pose that the health curriculum should draw on the work of the WHO and focus on preventing disease, caring for sick children, and obtaining medical care. Students should be expected to put into practice what they learn at school, such as washing their hands and wearing shoes near latrines. The authors suggest that children could learn other important behaviors, such as boiling drinking water and using malaria nets.

Health education in schools is part of a larger growing movement known as health literacy. According to the WHO, health literacy represents the "cognitive and social skills which determine the motivation and ability of individuals to gain access to, understand and use information in ways which promote and maintain good health.... [It] means more than being able to read pamphlets and successfully make appointments." Both of these are important skills; but a growing number of public health officials are beginning to believe that health literacy is critical to empowerment.

Research shows that health literacy skills are low worldwide, and, according to Ilona Kickbusch and others, in the 2013 WHO publication "Health Literacy:

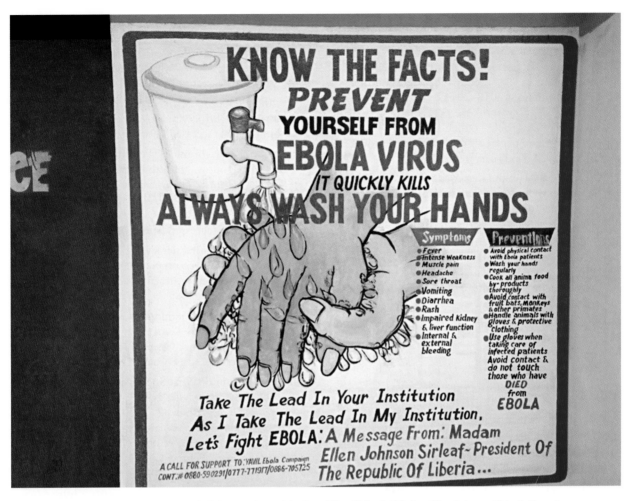

A public service poster produced on behalf of the President of the Republic of Liberia, Madam Ellen Johnson Sirleaf, disseminates an educational message telling viewers that washing their hands helps protect them against the spread and acquisition of the Ebola virus. The poster lists symptoms associated with Ebola HF, and protocols that, if followed, hamper viral spread. A number is included at the bottom, directing viewers to make a phone call if they have any questions about Ebola HF.   *Sally Ezra/U.S. Centers for Disease Control and Prevention.*

The Solid Facts," this lack of knowledge leads to "riskier behaviour, poorer health, less self-management and more hospitalization and costs." They also note that "strengthening health literacy has been shown to build individual and community resilience, help address health inequities, and improve health and well-being."

Public health officials are continuing to build health literacy with the belief that by building these skills it could greatly impact the reduction of disease burdens due to noncommunicable diseases, the effective management of public health emergencies such as pandemic influenza, as well as the development of worldwide actions to combat issues that pose a threat to sustainable development, such as climate change.

SEE ALSO   *Centers for Disease Control and Prevention (CDC); Health as a Human Right and Health-Care Access; World Health Organization: Organization, Funding, and Enforcement Powers*

BIBLIOGRAPHY

Books

Allensworth, Diane, Elaine Lawson, Lois Nicholson, and James Wyche, eds. *Schools and Health: Our Nation's Investment.* Washington, DC: National Academies Press, 1997.

Johnson, James A., and Donald J. Breckon. *Managing Health Promotion Programs: Leadership Skills for the 21st Century,* 2nd ed. Sudbury, MA: Jones and Bartlett, 2007.

Periodicals

Epstein, Marc J., and Kristi Yuthas. "Redefining Quality in Developing World Education." *Innovations: Technology, Governance, Globalization* 8, nos. 3–4 (2013): 197–211.

Haque, Monirul, et al. "Barriers to Initiating Insulin Therapy in Patients with Type 2 Diabetes Mellitus in

Public-Sector Primary Health Care Centres in Cape Town." *South African Medical Journal* 95, no. 11 (2005): 94.

Harris, Jenine K., et al. "Health Department Use of Social Media to Identify Foodborne Illness—Chicago, Illinois, 2013–2014." *Morbidity and Mortality Weekly Report* 63, no. 32 (August 15, 2014): 681–685. Available online at http://www.cdc .gov/mmwr/preview/mmwrhtml/mm6332a1. htm (accessed February 11, 2015).

Nutbeam, Don. "Health Literacy as a Public Health Goal: A Challenge for Contemporary Health Education and Communication Strategies into the 21st Century." *Health Promotion International* 15, no. 3 (2000): 259.

Pakenham-Walsh, Neil. "Towards a Collective Understanding of the Information Needs of Health Care Providers in Low-Income Countries, and How to Meet Them." *Journal of Health Communication* 17 (2012): 9–17.

Pakenham-Walsh, Neil, and Frederick Bukachi. "Information Needs of Health Care Workers in Developing Countries: A Literature Review with a Focus on Africa." *Human Resources for Health* 7 (2009): 30.

Puoane, T., et al. "Evaluating the Clinical Management of Severely Malnourished Children—a Study of Two Rural District Hospitals." *South African Medical Journal* 91, no. 2 (2001): 137–141.

Stanger-Hall, Kathrin F., and David W. Hall. "Abstinence-Only Education and Teen Pregnancy Rates: Why We Need Comprehensive Sex Education in the U.S." *PloS ONE* 6, no. 10 (October 14, 2011). Available online at http://journals.plos.org/plosone/ article?id=10.1371/journal.pone.0024658 (accessed March 31, 2015).

Tountas, Yannis. "The Historical Origins of the Basic Concepts of Health Promotion and Education: The Role of Ancient Greek Philosophy and Medicine." *Health Promotion International* 24, no. 2 (2009): 185–192.

Websites

Epstein, Mark J., and Kristi Yuthas. "Redefining Education in the Developing World." *Stanford Social Innovation Review*, Winter 2012. http://www.ssireview .org/articles/entry/redefining_education_in_the_ developing_world (accessed February 11, 2015).

"Global School Health Initiative." *World Health Organization.* http://www.who.int/school_youth_health/ gshi/en/ (accessed February 11, 2015).

"Health Literacy." *National Network of Libraries of Medicine.* http://nnlm.gov/outreach/consumer/ hlthlit.html (accessed February 11, 2015).

Kickbusch, Ilona, Jürgen M. Pelikan, Franklin Apfel, and Agis D. Tsouros. "Health Literacy: The Solid Facts." *World Health Organization (WHO), Regional Office for Europe (EURO)*, 2013. http://www.euro .who.int/__data/assets/pdf_file/0008/190655/ e96854.pdf (accessed April 10, 2015).

"Learn about Health Literacy." *U.S. Centers for Disease Control and Prevention (CDC).* http://www.cdc .gov/healthliteracy/learn/ (accessed February 11, 2015).

Levine, Adam. "Staff Training Is Crucial for Third World Health." *Brown University*, January 16, 2013. https://news.brown.edu/articles/2013/01/ Rwanda (accessed February 11, 2015).

McNab, Christine. "What Social Media Offers to Health Professionals and Citizens." *Bulletin of the World Health Organization* 87 (2009): 566. doi: 10.2471/ BLT.09.066712. Available online at http://www .who.int/bulletin/volumes/87/8/09-066712/ en/ (accessed February 11, 2015).

"Quick Guide to Health Literacy." *U.S. Department of Health and Human Services.* http://www .health.gov/communication/literacy/quickguide/ (accessed February 11, 2015).

Steakley, Lia. "Promoting Health in Developing Nations with Social Media." *Scope*, May 13, 2011. http:// scopeblog.stanford.edu/2011/05/13/using_ social_me/ (accessed February 11, 2015).

"Track 2: Health Literacy and Health Behavior." *World Health Organization (WHO).* http://www.who .int/healthpromotion/conferences/7gchp/track2/ en/l (accessed April 11, 2015).

Melanie R. Plenda

Hemorrhagic Diseases

⊕ Introduction

Hemorrhagic diseases are caused by viruses or bacteria. Viral diseases are also known as viral hemorrhagic fevers. Bacterial hemorrhagic disease (e.g., scrub typhus) does occur but is much more rare.

The onset of a hemorrhagic fever or disease can produce a range of symptoms from mild to unalterably lethal, with both internal and extrusive bleeding a common hallmark of a hemorrhagic disease. The most well-known hemorrhagic diseases are infamous because of the speed that some infections take hold and the ferocity of their symptoms. Many hemorrhagic maladies, such as Ebola, have high mortality rates.

⊕ Historical Background

Hemorrhagic diseases are zoonotic diseases, ones that occur by the transfer of the disease-causing agent from a nonhuman to a human. For some of the hemorrhagic viruses, the reservoir host is known. They include the cotton rat, deer mouse, house mouse, arthropod ticks, and mosquitoes. However, for viruses such as the Ebola and Marburg viruses, the natural host still is not definitively known. Outbreaks with these two viruses have involved transfer of the virus to human via primates. Whether the primate is the natural reservoir host, or whether primates acquire the virus as the result of contact with the true natural reservoir host, is yet another aspect of hemorrhagic diseases that is not clear.

Hemorrhagic Viruses

Four main groups of viruses exist that cause hemorrhagic disease or fever: arenaviruses, filoviruses, bunyaviruses, and flaviviruses.

Arenaviruses cause Argentine hemorrhagic fever, Bolivian hemorrhagic fever, Sabia-associated hemorrhagic fever, lymphocytic choriomeningitis, Venezuelan hemorrhagic fever, and Lassa fever. Members of the filovirus group cause Ebola hemorrhagic fever and Marburg hemorrhagic fever. Bunyaviruses cause Crimean-Congo hemorrhagic fever, Rift Valley fever, and hantavirus pulmonary syndrome. Lastly, flaviviruses cause tick-borne encephalitis, yellow fever, dengue hemorrhagic fever, Kyasanur Forest disease, and Omsk hemorrhagic fever.

These viruses differ in structure and in the severity of the symptoms they can cause. They all, however, share common features. All hemorrhagic viruses contain ribonucleic acid (RNA) as their genetic material. The RNA is protected and confined in a membrane called the viral envelope. The envelope is typically made of lipid. Another feature of hemorrhagic viruses, and indeed of all viruses, is the requirement for a host in which to live and produce new viral particles. Hemorrhagic viruses can live in some nonhuman mammals, such as primates, and in insects. The primates and insects are described as being natural reservoirs of the particular virus. Humans are not a natural reservoir. Epidemiologists (disease trackers) suspect that initial infections of humans occur only accidentally when a human and a host primate or insect come into close contact.

In contrast to the reservoir host, the presence of the hemorrhagic virus in humans typically produces a serious illness. The symptoms can rapidly progress from mild to life threatening (i.e., in only hours). While catastrophic for the victims and difficult for health personnel to treat, the rapid nature of the outbreaks has an advantage. Because victims succumb quickly, the transmission of the virus from human to human generally is limited. An outbreak can appear in a local population and run its course through susceptible victims within a relatively short time, usually within days or a few weeks.

The viruses that cause the various hemorrhagic fevers and diseases do not survive in the host following the disease (the human immunodeficiency virus, or HIV, in contrast, is able remain latent in the host and survive for prolonged periods before symptoms of infection appear). However, people who are recovering

HEMORRHAGIC FEVERS

Hemorrhagic diseases typically begin with a fever, a feeling of tiredness, and a generalized aching of muscles. In rare instances, symptoms may not progress any further, in which case recovery is rapid. For unknown reasons, however, more serious damage often occurs. Here, symptoms include bleeding from the mouth, eyes, and ears. Internal bleeding also occurs, as organs are attacked and destroyed by the infection. Death is typically the result of the overwhelming damage to the organs and from the failure of the nervous system. Often, victims have seizures and lapse into a coma prior to death.

A hemorrhagic fever is a viral infection that features a high fever and a high volume of (copious) bleeding. The bleeding is caused by the formation of tiny blood clots throughout the bloodstream. These blood clots—also called microthrombi—deplete platelets and fibrinogen in the bloodstream. When bleeding begins, the factors needed for the clotting of the blood are scarce. Thus, uncontrolled bleeding (hemorrhage) ensues.

Symptoms of the various diseases vary, but common symptoms are a high fever, fatigue, dizziness, muscle aches, and loss of strength. As the patient deteriorates, marked bleeding under the skin (internally) and from body orifices (like the mouth, ears, and eyes) develops.

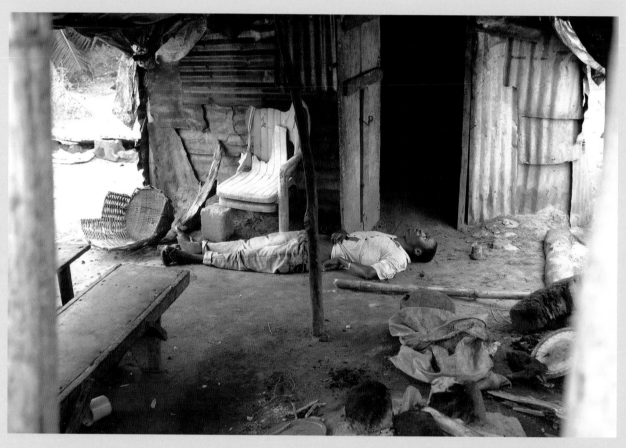

A man infected with the Ebola virus lies unconscious in his house in the small city of Banjol, 18 miles (30 kilometers) from Monrovia, Liberia.   © *Dominique Faget/Getty Images.*

from infections caused by hantavirus and Argentine hemorrhagic fever can excrete infectious viruses in their urine.

In some cases, the viruses do not damage their primate or insect hosts as they do a human who acquires the microorganisms. The reasons for this difference are unknown. Researchers are attempting to discover the basis of the natural resistance, as this would help in finding an effective treatment for human hemorrhagic diseases.

The sporadic appearance of hemorrhagic outbreaks and the fact that they often occur in geographically isolated regions (e.g., the interior of Africa) has made the study of the diseases difficult. It is known that there is not any timetable to the appearance of a hemorrhagic fever, such as in one season of the year relative to another season. The only factor that is known clearly is that the viruses are passed from the natural host to humans. For many hemorrhagic fevers, how this transfer occurs and why it occurs sporadically are not known.

The devastating infection caused by the hemorrhagic viruses is remarkable given the very small amount of genetic material that the viruses contain. For example, Ebola viruses can produce fewer than 12 proteins. Exactly how the viruses are able to evade the host immune responses and establish infections is unknown but two cellular enzymes that the Ebola virus must have to reproduce were found in 2005. The virus may commandeer the host's genetic material to produce proteins that the virus itself is unable to produce. Or, hemorrhagic viruses may be exquisitely designed infection machines, containing only the resources needed to evade the host and establish an infection. Sequencing of the genetic material of Ebola-Sudan, Ebola-Zaire, Ebola-Bundibugyo, and Ebola-Reston is complete, and clues in the genomes of these hemorrhagic viruses could help distinguish between these two possibilities.

Hemorrhagic Diseases

Hemorrhagic diseases are difficult to treat. One reason is because of the rapid progression of the disease. Another reason is because vaccines exist for only a few of the diseases (i.e., yellow fever and Argentine hemorrhagic fever). For the remaining diseases, supportive care such as keeping the infected person hydrated is often the only course of action.

Ebola virus disease (EVD) is caused by the Ebola virus, named after a river located in the Democratic Republic of the Congo (DRC), where the virus was first discovered in 1976. The first identified EVD outbreak occurred in the western part of the African nation of Sudan and in nearby Zaire (present-day DRC), giving rise to the name Ebola-Zaire for virus type or species. The worst Ebola outbreak to date began in Guinea in 2014, quickly spreading to several other West African countries, with cases exported to other countries around the world, including the United States. As of March 18, 2015, the WHO reported that 24,701 cases of Ebola had been reported, and there had been 10,194 deaths linked to the outbreak. The spread of this hemorrhagic disease was unprecedented.

There are five species of Ebola virus. These differ in their arrangement of their genetic material and in the severity of the infection they cause. Zaire ebolavirus, Sudan ebolavirus, Bundibugyo ebolavirus, and Taï Forest ebolavirus (also called Côte d'Ivoire ebolavirus) cause disease in humans. The fifth species, Reston ebolavirus, causes disease in primates.

Ebola spreads by intimate contact with body fluids. Other hemorrhagic viruses can be spread by air. These include the Marburg, Lassa, Congo-Crimean, and hantaviruses. In 2005, one of the largest outbreaks of

Marburg Hemorrhagic Fever Outbreaks from 1967–2014

Year	Country	Cases	Deaths	Case fatality rate
1967	Germany	29	7	24%
1967	Yugoslavia	2	0	0%
1975	South Africa	3	1	33%
1980	Kenya	2	1	50%
1987	Kenya	1	1	100%
1998–2000	Democratic Republic of the Congo	154	128	83%
2005	Angola	374	329	88%
2007	Uganda	4	2	50%
2008	USA (exported from Uganda)	1	0	0%
2008	Netherlands (exported from Uganda)	1	1	100%
2012	Uganda	20	9	45%
2014	Uganda	1	1	100%

SOURCE: Adapted from "Table: Chronology of major Marburg Haemorrhagic Fever outbreaks," in "Marburg Haemorrhagic Fever," Fact Sheet, November 2012, World Health Organization (WHO), 2012. Additional data from "Marburg Haemorrhagic Fever in Uganda – Update," November 23, 2012, and "Marburg Virus Disease – Uganda," November 13, 2014, WHO.

hemorrhagic fever ever recorded occurred in Uige Province of Angola, where more than 320 people died of Marburg hemorrhagic fever, including mostly children, 14 nurses, and 2 physicians. (See table.)

The Junin virus causes the hemorrhagic fever known as Argentine hemorrhagic fever. The virus was discovered in 1955, during a disease outbreak among corn harvesters in Argentina. It was later determined that the virus was spread to the workers by contact with rodent feces that had dried in the cornfields. The same route of transmission is used by the Machupo virus, which causes Bolivian hemorrhagic fever.

Congo-Crimean viral hemorrhagic fever (CCVHF) is transmitted to people by ticks. The tick is likely not the natural reservoir host of the virus but acquires the virus when it feeds on the natural reservoir host. The identity of this host is not known. This hemorrhagic fever occurs in Crimea and in regions of Africa, Asia, and Europe. CCVHF is transmitted to other humans only by direct contact with infected blood or body fluids. In autumn 2012, health officials documented the first laboratory-confirmed case of CCVHF in the United Kingdom. The man fell ill upon arriving in Glasgow, Scotland, after traveling by commercial airline from Kabul, Afghanistan, via Dubai. He later died after being transferred to a London hospital for specialist treatment.

Another hemorrhagic fever, Rift Valley fever, occurs mainly in Africa. Like Ebola, it causes explosive outbreaks of disease.

The first description of hantavirus disease occurred around the time of World War II (1939–1945), in Manchuria. The disease sickened United Nations troops stationed in Korea during the Korean War (1950–1953).

A lung infection caused by the virus, which can progress rapidly to death, became prominent because of an outbreak in the southwestern region of the United States in the mid-1990s, and scientists linked a subsequent outbreak to visitor cabins in Yosemite National Park in 2012. As with some of the other hemorrhagic fevers, the cause of hantavirus pulmonary syndrome is inhalation of dried rodent feces.

Many of the above hemorrhagic fevers were discovered between the mid-20th and early 21st centuries. Other hemorrhagic fevers have a longer history. For example, the causative agent for yellow fever was discovered in the first decade of the 20th century, when a disease outbreak occurred among workers who were constructing the Panama Canal.

The diagnosis of hemorrhagic fevers often requires knowledge of the recent travel of the patient. This helps to clarify natural hosts with which the patient may have come in contact.

At the present time, the best methods for preventing the spread of infection for hemorrhagic fevers are minimizing contact with the source of infection, isolation of the infected person, and care when handling the patient. For example, health-care workers should be dressed in protective clothing, including gloves and protective facemasks. Also, any material or equipment that comes into contact with the patient should be sterilized to kill any virus that may have adhered to the items.

A yellow fever vaccine exists that consists of live virus particles that have been modified so as not to be capable of growth or of causing an infection. The virus is capable of stimulating the immune system to produce antiviral antibodies. The vaccine must be taken by those who are traveling to areas of the world where yellow fever is actively present (areas of Africa and South America). The vaccine may have some potential in protecting people from the virus that causes Bolivian hemorrhagic fever.

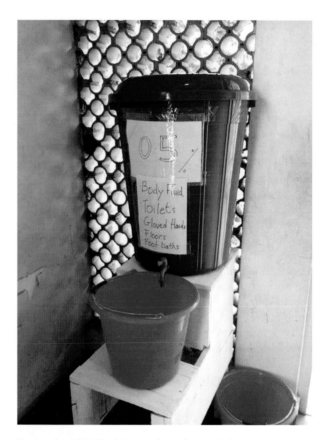

During the 2014 Ebola hemorrhagic fever (Ebola HF) outbreak, a decontamination station sits near a new Ebola isolation ward equipped with upgraded facilities, ready for Ebola HF patients in Lagos, Nigeria. The signage indicates that contained within is a 0.5% antiseptic solution used to decontaminate fomites (anything capable of carrying infections organisms) suspected of harboring the Ebola virus, including toilets, gloved hands, floors, and foot baths that had been contaminated with patient bodily fluids. Ebola HF is one of numerous viral hemorrhagic fevers. *Sally Ezra/U.S. Centers for Disease Control and Prevention.*

⊕ Impacts and Issues

In the known outbreaks of hemorrhagic fever, the disease usually flares up, wreaking havoc in the community where the outbreak occurs, and then disappears. Why the viral agents of hemorrhagic fevers are so devastating is not understood, nor is it yet understood why the diseases do not persist for long in a population. For highly lethal forms such as Ebola, one explanation is that the disease essentially works so quickly—and with such a high lethality—that if it occurs in an isolated population, it can destroy all available hosts. The lack of available hosts then inhibits the spread of the virus.

The speed at which hemorrhagic fevers appear and end in human populations, combined with their frequent occurrence in relatively isolated areas of the globe has made detailed study difficult. Even though some of the diseases, such as Argentine hemorrhagic fever, have been known for almost 50 years, knowledge of the molecular basis of the disease is lacking. For example, while it is apparent that some hemorrhagic viruses can be transmitted through the air as aerosols, the pathway of infection once the microorganism has been inhaled is still largely unknown.

As mentioned, hemorrhagic fevers can rapidly spread through a human population. This is due to human-to-human transmission. This transmission occurs easily, often via body fluids that accidentally come into contact with a person who is caring for the afflicted person. Funeral practices of handling and washing the bodies of the deceased have contributed to human-to-human transmission of Ebola during outbreaks in Africa.

The best strategies for dealing with hemorrhagic fevers at the present time is to limit human contact with the animal or insect hosts of the viruses and to ensure that the home and workplace is free from potential viral hosts, like rodents. Researchers are striving to develop better containment and treatment strategies, including vaccines, for the viral agents of hemorrhagic fevers. Another goal is to devise rapid detection techniques utilizing immunologic and molecular tools.

⊕ Future Implications

To prevent outbreaks, the most effective policy is to curb human interaction with the natural reservoir of the microbe in question.

Hemorrhagic fevers are significant, not only because of the human suffering they cause, but because some of the viral agents could be exploited as bioweapons. For these reasons, a great deal of research effort is devoted toward understanding the origins and behaviors of the viruses.

The WHO consistently stresses that the risk for regional and global infectious disease epidemics is increasing. Major infectious diseases such as Ebola and other hemorrhagic fevers increased their spread in the early 21st century. In 2007, a WHO report, *A Safer Future*, stated that the rate of emerging infectious diseases discoveries was "historically unprecedented." Since the start of the 21st century, continuing conflict was credited with destroying the public health infrastructure in areas of Angola and the DRC that, in turn, allowed outbreaks of Marburg and Ebola hemorrhagic fevers to flourish with little or delayed response. The report also noted alarming increases in diseases such as yellow fever since the 1990s. Globally, almost 40 new diseases (and the agents that cause them, such as the Ebola and Marburg viruses) were identified between the 1970s and the first decade of the 21st century. Additional factors cited included increased levels and interconnectedness of global airline travel, and lack of full international cooperation in sharing of data, technology, and other efforts to develop effective vaccines and other countermeasures.

SEE ALSO *Ebola Virus Disease; Epidemiology: Surveillance for Emerging Infectious Diseases; Health-Care Worker Safety and Shortages; Insect-Borne Diseases; Isolation and Quarantine; Médicins Sans Frontières; NGOs and Health Care: Deliverance or Dependence; Viral Diseases; Zoonotic (Animal-Borne) Diseases*

BIBLIOGRAPHY

Books

Beltz, Lisa A. *Emerging Infectious Diseases: A Guide to Diseases, Causative Agents, and Surveillance.* San Francisco: Jossey-Bass, 2011.

Biehl, João, and Adriana Petryna. *When People Come First: Critical Studies in Global Health.* Princeton, NJ: Princeton University Press, 2013.

Calisher, Charles H. *Lifting the Impenetrable Veil: From Yellow Fever to Ebola Hemorrhagic Fever and SARS.* Red Feather Lakes, CO: Rockpile Press, 2013.

Centers for Disease Control and Prevention (U.S.). *West Africa Ebola Outbreak.* Atlanta: U.S. Department of Health and Human Services, 2014.

Evans, David, et al. *The Economic Impact of the 2014 Ebola Epidemic: Short- and Medium-Term Estimates for West Africa.* Washington, DC: World Bank Group, 2014.

Garrett, Laurie. *Ebola: Story of an Outbreak.* New York: Hachette Books, 2014.

Gubler, Duane J., Eng Eong Ooi, Subhash Vasudevan, and Jeremy Farrar, eds. *Dengue and Dengue Hemorrhagic Fever*, 2nd ed. Wallingford, UK: CABI, 2014.

Kaslow, Richard A., Lawrence R. Stanberry, and James W. LeDuc, eds. *Viral Infections of Humans: Epidemiology and Control*, 5th ed. New York: Springer, 2014.

McDowell, Mary Ann, and Sima Rafati, eds. *Neglected Tropical Diseases—Middle East and North Africa.* New York: Springer, 2014.

Okeke, Iruka N. *Divining without Seeds: The Case for Strengthening Laboratory Medicine in Africa.* Ithaca, NY: ILR Press, 2011.

Quammen, David. *Ebola: The Natural and Human History of a Deadly Virus.* New York: Norton, 2014.

Singh, Sunit K., and Daniel Ruzek, eds. *Viral Hemorrhagic Fevers.* Boca Raton, FL: CRC Press, 2013.

Periodicals

Feldmann H., and T. W. Geisbert. "Ebola Hemorrhagic Fever." *The Lancet* 377, no. 9768 (2011): 849–862.

Kuhn, J. H., P. B. Jahrling, and S. R. Radoshitzky. "Viral Hemorrhagic Fevers." *Infectious Disease and Therapy* 50 (2010): 328–343.

Kutsuna S., and N. Ohmagari. "Dengue Fever." *Internal Medicine* 53, no. 15 (2014) 1.

Olugasa, Babasola O., et al. "Development of a Time-Trend Model for Analyzing and Predicting Case-Pattern of Lassa Fever Epidemics in Liberia, 2013–2017." *Annals of African Medicine* 14, no. 2 (2015): 89.

Parviainen, Markku, et al. "Detection of Acute Hantavirus Infections Using Novel Instrument-Readable Rapid Tests." *European Infectious Disease* 5 (2011): 35–37.

Roddy, P., et al. "Filovirus Hemorrhagic Fever Outbreak Case Management: A Review of Current and Future Treatment Options." *Journal of Infectious Diseases* (2011): S791–S2011.

Sharts-Hopko, N. "Ebola." *American Journal of Nursing* 115, no. 3 (2015): 13.

Wilkinson, Annie, and Melissa Leach. "Briefing: Ebola-Myths, Realities, and Structural Violence." *African Affairs: The Journal of the Royal African Society* 114, no. 454 (2015): 136–148.

Websites

"Hemorrhagic Fevers." *Medline Plus.* http://www.nlm.nih.gov/medlineplus/hemorrhagicfevers.html (accessed March 18, 2015).

"Hemorrhagic Fevers, Viral." *World Health Organization (WHO).* http://www.who.int/topics/haemorrhagic_fevers_viral/en/ (accessed March 18, 2015).

Preston, Richard. "The Ebola Wars." *New Yorker*, October 27, 2014. http://www.newyorker.com/magazine/2014/10/27/ebola-wars (accessed March 18, 2015).

Viral Hemorrhagic Fever Consortium. http://vhfc.org (accessed March 18, 2015).

"Viral Hemorrhagic Fevers." *U.S. Centers for Disease Control and Prevention (CDC).* http://www.cdc.gov/ncidod/dvrd/spb/mnpages/dispages/vhf.htm (accessed March 18, 2015).

"The World Health Report 2007 - A Safer Future: Global Public Health Security in the 21st Century." *World Health Organization (WHO)*, 2007. http://www.who.int/whr/2007/en/ (accessed May 30, 2015).

K. Lee Lerner

High Blood Pressure

⊕ Introduction

Blood pressure is created by the force of blood against the wall of the blood vessel when it is pumped around the body by the heart. It is measured in millimeters of mercury (mmHg) and is recorded as two figures. The systolic blood pressure (upper figure) is the pressure created when the heart contracts or beats, and the diastolic blood pressure (lower figure) is that created when the heart relaxes, between beats. According to the National Heart and Lung Institute, a normal adult blood pressure reading for adults consists of a systolic pressure of less than 120 mmHg and a diastolic pressure of less than 80 mmHg. High blood pressure (HBP), clinically known as hypertension, is a blood pressure of 140/90 mmHg or more. Often known as the "silent killer" because it usually has no symptoms, high blood pressure can cause long-term damage to the body and is a major risk factor for serious health problems.

High blood pressure is a leading global public health issue and was the cause of 9.4 million deaths and 162 million years of lives lost in 2010. Around one-third of adults in most countries in the world have high blood pressure, with those in middle- and low-income countries being most affected. In many cases, people are either unaware they have the condition or are not being treated for it. Hypertension is the most common chronic condition with which health-care professionals have to deal.

To complicate matters, most people with elevated blood pressure also have other risk factors, such as obesity or diabetes, which further increase the risk of serious health consequences. High blood pressure is the cause of 50 percent of heart disease, stroke, and heart failure and is responsible for 13 percent of deaths overall. Most cases of hypertension are essential, or primary, hypertension, caused by lifestyle factors such as unhealthful diet, including excessive salt consumption; smoking; excess alcohol consumption; and lack of exercise. Because these factors are modifiable, high blood pressure can be prevented by lifestyle change. The condition also is treatable by a variety of effective medications that are more cost effective to health-care systems than treating the complications of uncontrolled blood pressure.

⊕ Historical Background

Measuring Blood Pressure

Blood pressure was first referred to in the Egyptian text known as the Edwin Smith Papyrus, dating from 1600 BCE, which discusses the examination of the pulse. However, it was not until 1860 that blood pressure itself was measured in humans, when French physiologist Étienne-Jules Marey (1830–1904) devised a device that could do so. His sphygmograph amplified and recorded the pulse wave in the radial artery, located near the wrist, onto a smoked paper.

British physician Frederick Mahomid (1849–1884) adapted Marey's device into clinical practice and from then a number of technical advances resulted in routine measurement of systolic blood pressure. Another significant development was Nikolai Korotkoff's (1874–1920) discovery, in 1905, of specific sounds that occur when the arm is compressed by the cuff of the blood pressure measuring device. Manual measurements of blood pressure continue to rely on Korotkoff's sounds, which also form the basis of routine measurement of diastolic blood pressure.

High Blood Pressure and Health

Discoveries in the late 19th and 20th centuries led to further understanding of the roles blood pressure plays in human health and how to treat high blood pressure. One significant discovery, made in 1889, was of the hormone renin, which plays a significant role in regulating blood pressure. Blood pressure drugs that target renin remain the mainstay of treatment. In 1904, researchers linked high blood pressure to kidney disease and high salt intake. Physicians long considered hypertension an inherited disorder, but British physician Sir George Pickering

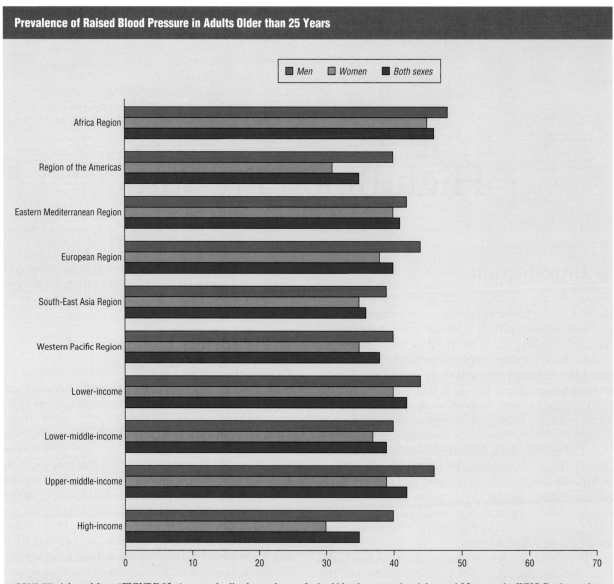

Prevalence of Raised Blood Pressure in Adults Older than 25 Years

Men · Women · Both sexes

SOURCE: Adapted from "FIGURE 03. Age-standardized prevalence of raised blood pressure in adults aged 25+ years by WHO Region and World Bank income group, comparable estimates, 2008," in *A Global Brief on Hypertension: Silent Killer, Global Public Health Crisis* World Health Organization (WHO), 2013, p. 10. Data from *Global Status Report on Noncommunicable Diseases 2010*, WHO, 2011.

(1904–1980) challenged this traditional view in the second half of the 20th century. He used epidemiological studies to demonstrate that hypertension is in fact a condition arising from the interaction of environmental, lifestyle, and genetic disorders.

⊕ Impacts and Issues

Global Patterns

Factors such as the aging of the population, rapid urbanization, and the spread of unhealthy lifestyles have led to a profound shift in patterns of disease worldwide. No longer is infection the leading cause of mortality, even in less developed nations: it is the noncommunicable diseases, including cancer, cardiovascular disease, diabetes, and chronic lung disease, that claim the most lives. High blood pressure, which affects 1 billion people around the world, is a major risk factor in cardiovascular disease and therefore plays a key role in the increasing toll from noncommunicable disease.

Overall, high-income countries have a lower prevalence of hypertension, at 35 percent of the population aged 25 and above, compared with middle and low-income countries at 40 percent. The prevalence of hypertension is highest in the African region, affecting 46 percent, and lowest in the Americas at 35 percent. The impact of hypertension also is greater in the less developed countries, because not only is the prevalence higher but the populations are larger too, meaning that the absolute numbers affected are greater than they are in richer countries. Furthermore, because health-care systems are weaker, people in middle- to low-income countries with hypertension are more likely to go undiagnosed and untreated. In the long term, this means a significantly higher burden of ill health from the consequences of uncontrolled high blood pressure in these countries.

Behavioral Risk Factors

Tackling the global public health challenge of high blood pressure starts with understanding the underlying risk factors for the condition. A diet containing too much fat and salt and too few fruits and vegetables is a major contributor to hypertension, as is physical inactivity and lack of exercise. Poor stress management, excessive alcohol consumption, and tobacco use are also known risk factors. In addition, genetic factors may play a role in the development of high blood pressure.

There are a number of socioeconomic influences that drive the behaviors described above. Income, education, and housing all can have an adverse effect on healthy behavior. For instance, poor living and working conditions may increase stress and may also be associated with poor access to health care. Rapid, unplanned urbanization often goes hand in hand with unhealthy lifestyle factors such as sedentary behavior, alcohol and tobacco use, and fast-food consumption. Finally, populations worldwide are aging, and hypertension increases with age due to hardening of the blood vessels.

Impact on Health

Research has shown a close relationship between blood pressure levels and the risk of cardiovascular events, strokes, and kidney disease. The risk of these adverse outcomes is lowest at a blood pressure of around 115/75 mmHg. Thereafter, for each increase of 20 mmHg in systolic blood pressure or 10 mmHg increase in diastolic blood pressure, the risk of heart attack or stroke doubles. This is why systolic blood pressures between 120 and 139 mmHg and diastolic pressures between 80 and 89 mmHg sometimes are termed prehypertension. A person identified with prehypertension should be encouraged to undertake lifestyle changes that may delay or prevent hypertension proper.

Globally, cardiovascular disease accounts for around 17 million deaths per year, of which 9.4 million can be attributed to high blood pressure. According to the World Health Organization (WHO), high blood pressure is responsible for at least 45 percent of deaths from heart disease and 51 percent of deaths from stroke. Nearly 80 percent of cardiovascular deaths occur in low- and middle-income countries. These are the countries that can least afford the economic costs associated with such a high burden of ill health and mortality.

Screening and Diagnosis

High blood pressure is diagnosed readily by the use of electronic, aneroid, or mercury-based devices. The WHO recommends the use of affordable and electronic devices with the option to take manual readings in resource-poor settings. Early detection of high blood pressure minimizes the risk of long-term health problems, so all adults should have regular checks as advised by their primary care providers and be aware of their blood pressure numbers and what they mean.

Cholesterol, fasting blood glucose, and urine albumin also should be analyzed to determine the patient's overall cardiovascular and kidney health. If hypertension has been present and undetected for some time, then health complications already may have set in and should be dealt with as soon as possible. Many people diagnosed with hypertension do indeed have additional cardiovascular risk or already have evidence of blood pressure-related damage; these conditions need to be identified.

Lifestyle Changes

Improving diet, losing weight, increasing physical activity, lowering salt and alcohol consumption, reducing stress, and quitting use of tobacco are the main lifestyle changes that individuals can adopt to avoid or help control high blood pressure. Meeting these challenges successfully involves investment of time and money on the part of many different stakeholders, including policy makers, health-care workers, and individuals. It is important that policies and approaches are evidence-based and cost effective.

Examples of evidence-based policy intervention for prevention of high blood pressure include salt reduction in processed foods, replacement of trans-fats with polyunsaturated fats in a range of foods, and public awareness programs on diet and physical activity. Much has been accomplished regarding tobacco use including the introduction of smoke-free indoor workplaces and public places, bans on advertising, and excise tax increases. Similar policy measures been applied to reduce harmful alcohol use.

Workplace Wellness Programs In 2011, the United Nations high-level meeting on prevention and control of noncommunicable disease called upon the private sector to promote and create an enabling environment for healthy behaviors among workers. Where appropriate, this should include workplace wellness programs, with emphasis on physical activity and healthy diet, as well as health insurance and occupational health support, including hypertension screening. The workplace approach can support those who feel they are too busy to see the doctor for preventive checkups.

The wellness approach also has been implemented in the public sector. For instance, the United Kingdom National Health Service (NHS) has committed to helping its employees keep to a healthy weight. Given that the

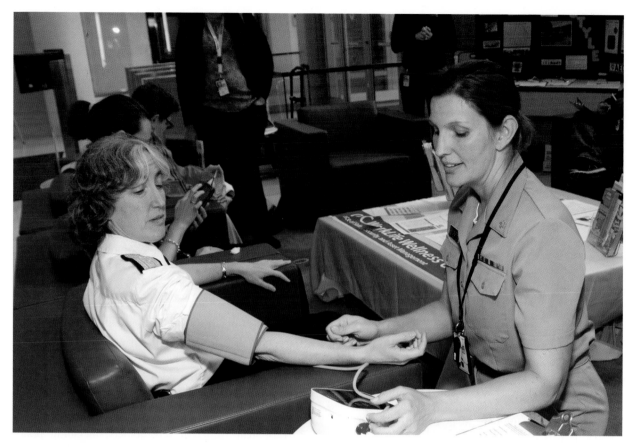

Anne Schuchat, MD, the U.S. assistant surgeon general, has her blood pressure checked by a member of the Public Health Service using an electronic sphygmomanometer (blood pressure cuff). According to the U.S. National Health Service, 1 in 3 adults in the United States has high blood pressure, which can lead to coronary heart disease, heart failure, stroke, kidney failure, and other health problems. Globally, the overall prevalence of raised blood pressure in adults aged 25 and over was around 40 percent in 2008, according to the World Health Organization. *Becky Rentz/U.S. Centers for Disease Control and Prevention.*

NHS is the world's fifth-largest employer, with a workforce of 1.7 million, this pledge, were it to be achieved, could have a significant impact on hypertension prevention and control in the British population.

Dietary Approaches to Stop Hypertension The Dietary Approaches to Stop Hypertension (DASH) eating plan as developed in research sponsored by the U.S. National Institutes of Health has the aim of lowering blood pressure without medication. Numerous studies have indicated that the DASH diet not only lowers blood pressure, but also improves insulin sensitivity and reduces cholesterol. Those who adopt the diet also reduce their risk of heart disease, stroke, diabetes, kidney stones, and some cancers, as well as promote weight loss.

The DASH diet eating plan is rich in fruits and vegetables, and includes low-fat or nonfat dairy products. It also includes grains (especially whole grains), lean meat, fish and poultry, nuts, and beans. The diet is high in fiber and low-to-moderate in fat. The Dietary Guidelines for Americans recommend the DASH plan as a model of healthful eating for everyone. It works by providing plenty of potassium, magnesium, and calcium, all of which help to lower blood pressure.

Blood Pressure Medication

Unless blood pressure is very high, most doctors will advise lifestyle changes and ongoing monitoring before putting a patient on medication. There are nine classes of medications that can lower blood pressure, and they all work in different ways. The choice of medication depends on many factors, including age, ethnicity, and the presence of other conditions or risk factors. Generally, medications that are long acting are preferable to those that need to be taken more often. Often, a patient will need to take more than one medication in order to keep blood pressure under control.

The choice of a blood pressure–lowering drug is further influenced by its availability and affordability. Even among generic drugs, which are usually cheaper than branded products, there can be a big variation in cost. For those in low- and middle-income countries, where high blood pressure is more of an issue, it is essential that these drugs are made more widely available.

GLOBAL SALT CONSUMPTION

Salt is sodium chloride, and the kidneys need a certain amount of sodium to maintain proper fluid balance in the body. However, too much sodium can cause water retention, both in the circulation and inside the cells. This situation leads to high blood pressure, particularly so when the balance of sodium to potassium is in excess, for potassium has the opposite effect on fluid balance, and lowers the blood pressure.

Scientists have long assumed that high salt intake is a risk factor in developing high blood pressure and also that salt should be avoided by all those who have been diagnosed with hypertension. However, studies on the genes involved in high blood pressure suggest that some people are more sensitive to the impact of salt intake on high blood pressure than others. In the future, it may be possible to pair diagnosis of high blood pressure with a genetic test to determine whether an individual is salt sensitive and should be particularly careful to avoid salt consumption. It is already known that black people are more likely to be salt sensitive. However, research has shown that a modest reduction in salt consumption reduces blood pressure in both those with hypertension and those with normal blood pressure, whatever their racial/ethnic group, although the level of reduction does vary between populations.

Like sugar, salt is used widely in the Western diet to make food more palatable. Salt use also is common in non-Western, traditional diets. Therefore, average consumption around the world is high, at between 9 and 12 grams per person per day. People may stop adding salt at the table in an attempt to avoid high blood pressure, but they may not realize the high levels of salt present in many prepared foods, some of which do not taste particularly salty. People may also dislike the taste of food cooked with little or no salt and may need time and persuasion to accustom themselves to this altered dietary approach.

Bread typically contains 250 milligrams of salt per 100 grams of bread, whereas processed meats such as bacon contain as much as 1.5 grams of salt per 100 grams. Snack foods, such as chips, peanuts, and pretzels, and sauces, including soy sauce and stock cubes, also tend to have a high salt content. High salt consumption seems to be a product of modern living. The Yanomamo Indians, who live in Brazil and Venezuela, have a traditional diet that includes hardly any salt. They have been much studied by medical researchers who found they do not have high blood pressure or blood pressure that rises with age.

The WHO recommends that adults not consume more than 2 grams of sodium (equivalent to 5 grams of salt) per day. Furthermore, adults should counterbalance their sodium consumption with potassium, consuming at least 3.5 grams of potassium per day. Potassium-rich foods include bananas, dates, papayas, peas, beans, and vegetables such as cabbage and spinach.

Reducing salt consumption requires action from individuals, government, the food industry, and nongovernmental organizations. Voluntary reduction of salt content in foods and condiments already is occurring in many countries and widespread food labeling is helpful to the consumer, who can look for low or no-salt products.

Several countries have shown that reduction of salt intake among their populations is possible. In Finland, health officials initiated a systematic approach to this challenge in the late 1970s through a mass media campaign, cooperation with the food industry, and the implementation of legislation on salt labeling. As a result, there were declines in both systolic and diastolic blood pressure of 10 mmHg or more among the population. This in turn had a real impact on health, with reductions in both heart disease and stroke mortality in Finland following these initiatives.

There also have been salt reduction programs in the United Kingdom and the United States, based upon voluntary cooperation with the food industry. More recently there has been development of salt reduction initiatives in a number of less-developed countries. Several research studies have shown that reducing salt intake is one of the most cost-effective interventions for reducing heart disease and stroke at the population level.

Individual Responsibility

Ultimately, it is up to the individual to adopt a lifestyle that will reduce the odds of developing high blood pressure and thereby avoid its adverse consequences. Key to this is a healthful diet, with reduced salt, saturated fat, and total fat intake. Regular physical activity, with 30 minutes per day five days per week as a minimum goal, is important too, as is avoiding tobacco and harmful alcohol use. Stress management is also key to avoiding high blood pressure. People may need public health information and support from health-care professionals to put these measures into place and to keep following them.

Individuals who already have been diagnosed with high blood pressure can participate in managing their condition by adopting, or continuing with, healthy lifestyle measures. Regular blood pressure checks as advised by a health-care professional should be attended, supplemented by home blood pressure monitoring where appropriate. Those who are on medication should take it as prescribed. If side effects are a problem, then the physician usually can prescribe a more acceptable alternative. It is important not to discontinue a blood pressure medication without informing one's physician.

⊕ Future Implications

The International Society of Hypertension has laid down a number of recommendations for its national counterparts to help meet the global challenge of high blood pressure. First, there needs to be a strategic plan, in each country, for prevention and control. These are already in place in many countries, but more needs to be done.

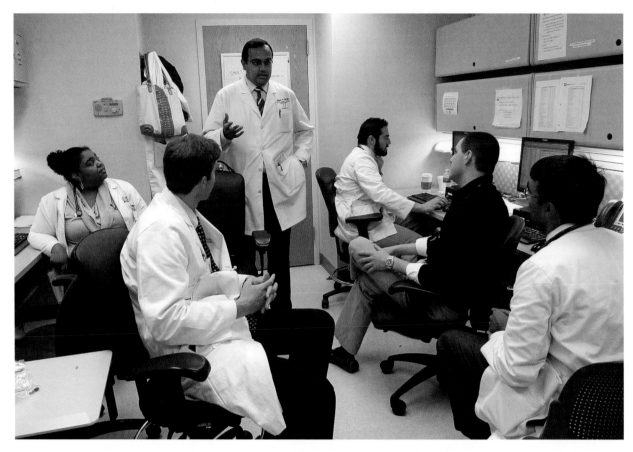

Dr. Manesh Patel, an interventional cardiologist at Duke Heart Center, speaks with resident doctors at Duke University Hospital in Durham, North Carolina. Patel is participating in a research study to treat high blood pressure by threading a catheter to the kidney and zapping nearby nerves that fuel blood pressure. Duke is one of more than 60 hospitals taking part in the clinical trial of what is called renal denervation. *© Gerry Broome/AP Photo.*

National hypertension organizations also should advocate for public health policies around issues such as salt reduction and smoking cessation. There are international hypertension guidelines available, and national organizations should do all they can to ensure these are taken up and adapted to their country's population. They also should develop strong partnerships with organizations that represent health-care providers involved in hypertension diagnosis and management. Finally, it is important to make sure efforts to prevent and control hypertension are monitored and evaluated properly.

Health-Care Professionals

Health-care professionals are one of the first lines of defense in the fight against high blood pressure and its related risks. Health-care professionals can encourage their patients know their blood pressure numbers, their blood pressure reduction target where appropriate, and what to do to achieve this. Sometimes, they may recommend that a patient take blood pressure measurements at home using a monitoring device. Readings can be downloaded to a computer or smartphone app, which then can be conveyed to the health-care professional for discussion at the next consultation. In patients with hypertension, doctors and practice nurses also evaluate the overall cardiovascular risk to patients with additional testing. Health-care professionals also can advocate for public health policies and encourage community blood pressure screening programs.

Key Messages

High blood pressure is a growing global health threat but is largely preventable. Policies that facilitate healthier choices could be implemented and may go a long way toward prevention. These would need to be adapted to different countries. Although they may require investment, the payback in terms of reduced adverse health outcomes would make the expense worthwhile.

It is easy to screen for, and diagnose, high blood pressure. However, only around half of those who have the condition are aware of it, meaning there is an urgent need to improve awareness. Once the condition is known to exist, lifestyle changes and effective medication usually are able to control high blood pressure and reduce adverse outcomes among most people who have the condition.

SEE ALSO *Cardiovascular Diseases; Noncommunicable Diseases (Lifestyle Diseases); Nutrition; Obesity*

BIBLIOGRAPHY

Books

Cruickshank, John M. *Essential Hypertension.* Shelton, CT: Peoples Medical Publishing House, 2013.

Moore, Thomas J., et al. *The DASH Diet for Hypertension.* New York: Pocket Books, 2003.

Rubin, Alan. *High Blood Pressure for Dummies*, 2nd ed. New York: Wiley, 2007.

World Health Organization. *A Global Brief on Hypertension: Silent Killer, Global Public Health Crisis.* Geneva: World Health Organization, 2013. Available online at http://www.who.int/cardiovascular_diseases/publications/global_brief_hypertension/en/ (accessed January 9, 2015).

World Health Organization. *Guideline: Sodium Intake for Adults and Children.* Geneva: World Health Organization, 2012. Available online at http://www.who.int/nutrition/publications/guidelines/sodium_intake/en/ (accessed January 9, 2015).

Periodicals

Weber, Michael A., et al. "Clinical Practice Guidelines for the Management of Hypertension in the Community: A Statement by the American Society of Hypertension and the International Society of Hypertension." *Journal of Hypertension* 32, no. 1 (January 2014): 3–15.

Websites

Freedman, David A., and Diana B. Petitti. "Salt and Blood Pressure: Conventional Wisdom Reconsidered." *University of California, Berkeley, Department of Statistics*, November 16, 2012. http://www.stat.berkeley.edu/~census/573.pdf (accessed January 9, 2015).

"High Blood Pressure." *U.S. Centers for Disease Control and Prevention (CDC).* http://www.cdc.gov/bloodpressure/index.htm (accessed April 1, 2015).

Mayo Clinic Staff. "Diseases and Conditions: High Blood Pressure (Hypertension)." *Mayo Clinic.* http://www.mayoclinic.org/diseases-conditions/high-blood-pressure/basics/definition/con-20019580?p=1 (accessed January 9, 2015).

"What Is High Blood Pressure?" *National Heart, Lung, and Blood Institute (U.S.).* http://www.nhlbi.nih.gov/health/health-topics/topics/hbp/ (accessed January 9, 2015).

Susan Aldridge

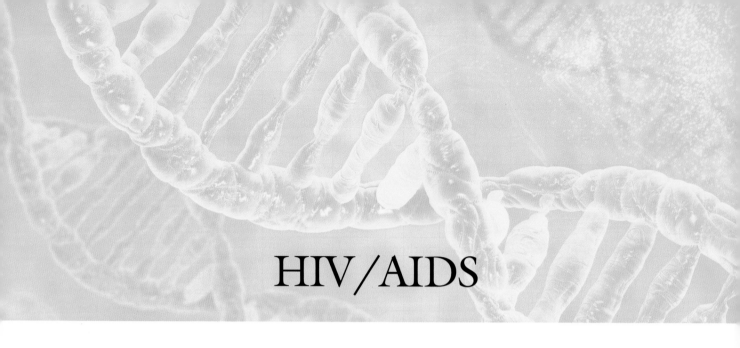

HIV/AIDS

⊕ Introduction

The human immunodeficiency virus (HIV) is a zoonotic infection that targets the immune system. Zoonotic diseases are infectious diseases of animals that can naturally be transmitted to humans. Acquired immune deficiency syndrome (AIDS) is the final stage of HIV and is a disease in which there is a severe loss of the body's cellular immunity, greatly lowering the resistance to infection and malignancy.

HIV is transmitted through an exchange of bodily fluids such as blood, breast milk, semen, or vaginal secretions from infected individuals. Those at greater risk of contracting HIV, according to the World Health Organization (WHO), are people who have unprotected sex; have another sexually transmitted infection such as syphilis, herpes, chlamydia, gonorrhea, or bacterial vaginosis; are intravenous drug users who share contaminated needles, syringes, other injecting equipment or drug solutions; have received unsafe injections, blood transfusions, and medical procedures that involve unsterile cutting or piercing; and have experienced accidental needlestick injuries.

The symptoms of HIV vary depending on stage of infection. Some people do not experience any symptoms at all in the first few weeks after infection, while others report experiencing a flulike illness including fever, headache, rash, or sore throat, according to the WHO. As a person's immune system weakens, he or she may experience swollen lymph nodes, weight loss, fever, diarrhea, and cough. Without treatment, those infected become susceptible to AIDS-related diseases as well as opportunistic diseases, which are those caused by pathogens that normally would not result in disease in an otherwise healthy host.

HIV infection can be diagnosed through a blood test for the presence or absence of HIV antibodies. There is currently no cure for HIV infection. However, treatment with antiretroviral (ARV) drugs has been effective in controlling the virus so that that people with HIV can maintain fairly normal lives.

HIV is a retrovirus, or one of a group of RNA viruses that have a genetic code comprised of RNA rather than DNA. Such viruses use the DNA of the infected host cells to replicate. As a virus, HIV is also unique in that it changes over time through mutations and recombinations. This is one of the reasons why finding an effective treatment and a vaccine for the disease have proven difficult.

Once a person is infected, HIV destroys the function of immune cells, causing a person to become immunodeficient. This means the body loses some or all of its ability to fight infectious disease. A person with an immunodeficiency is more susceptible to a wide range of infections and diseases than someone with a healthy immune system, which would fend off such infections.

Immune function is typically measured by CD4 cell count. CD4 count refers to the number of CD4 or T-helper cells (white blood cells) in the body. T cells help B cells, which produce antibodies (a blood protein produced in response to and counteracting a specific antigen). Antibodies are proteins with special shapes that identify and bind to foreign substances, such as bacteria or viruses. Scavenger cells then destroy the substances and flush them out of the body.

If a person's T-cell count falls below 200 cells per microliter, this is considered stage 3 infection or AIDS. At that point, the infected person has a much higher risk for contracting AIDS-defining illnesses, which can include bacterial, fungal, and viral infections as well as some cancers. It can take anywhere from 2 to 15 years and sometimes longer for HIV to develop into AIDS.

As of 2014, the WHO estimated that HIV/AIDS had infected more than 75 million people and killed more than 39 million. It remains a major global health concern. There were approximately 35 million people living with HIV at the end of 2013, with 2.1 million people becoming newly infected that year. Sub-Saharan Africa accounts for almost 70 percent of the global total of new HIV infections, according to the WHO.

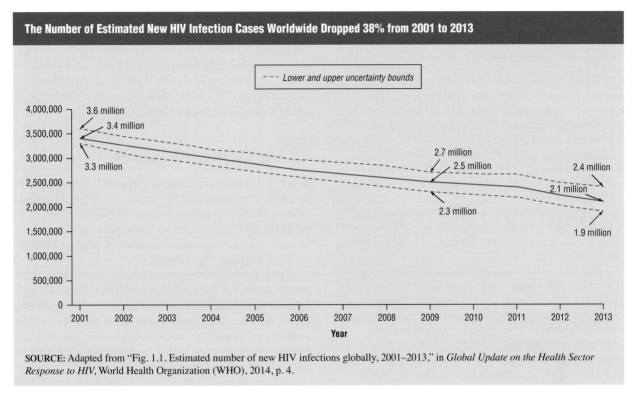

The Number of Estimated New HIV Infection Cases Worldwide Dropped 38% from 2001 to 2013

- - - *Lower and upper uncertainty bounds*

SOURCE: Adapted from "Fig. 1.1. Estimated number of new HIV infections globally, 2001–2013," in *Global Update on the Health Sector Response to HIV*, World Health Organization (WHO), 2014, p. 4.

Though the number of new HIV cases worldwide dropped 38% from 2001 to 2013, HIV and AIDS remains a global health concern with approximately 35 million people living with HIV at the end of 2013 and 2.1 million people becoming newly infected in 2013.

⊕ Historical Background

Scientists have been stymied by the origins of HIV/AIDS since reports of the disease first started emerging in the early 1980s. Early on, scientists determined that there are two species of HIV, known as HIV-1 and HIV-2. HIV-1 seems to have evolved from an immune deficiency found in chimpanzees, known as simian immunodeficiency virus (SIV). The second species of virus, also an SIV, came from the sooty mangabey, which is a type of monkey. While HIV-2 has largely remained in western Africa where it originated, HIV-1 is much more virulent and is responsible for 90 percent of HIV/AIDS infections worldwide.

The first known case of HIV infection comes from a man who died in Leopoldville, Belgian Congo (now Kinshasa, Democratic Republic of the Congo), in 1959. For years, the blood sample taken from this patient was kept in a freezer. In 1998, with the advent of advanced methods of testing for HIV, the sample was tested and determined to be HIV positive.

Current research indicates HIV-1 likely made the jump from chimpanzees to humans before the 1920s, with primate hunters. Those who butchered bushmeat would naturally have been exposed to the blood and other bodily fluids of chimps, and thus SIVs. That blood could be introduced through any open wound, even a small cut, into the hunters' bodies. People of western Africa not only hunted primates but kept them as pets,

including the sooty mangabey, and so were likely exposed to SIVs through feces, blood, or saliva.

With the disease established in human hosts, the problem was amplified with the urbanization of places like Kinshasa. Laborers were flocking to the city for work, and with them came a growing sex trade in the city. This situation, coupled with a public health campaign encouraging injections (likely with dirty needles due to cost constraints) to ward off or cure infectious disease and a railway that carried 1 million people in and out of Kinshasa per year by the 1940s, created the right conditions, researchers think, for the birth of a pandemic.

By the 1960s, an extensive railroad system seems to have promoted the spread of the virus to mining areas in southeastern Congo and beyond, according to the 2014 study "The Early Spread and Epidemic Ignition of HIV-1 in Human Populations" led by researcher Nuno Faria with the Department of Zoology, University of Oxford in the United Kingdom. Based on that study, researchers assert that HIV eventually crossed the Atlantic with Haitian teachers returning home.

On June 5, 1981, the U.S. Centers for Disease Control and Prevention (CDC) issued its first warning about an outbreak of a rare form of pneumonia among a small group of young homosexual men in Los Angeles, California, in the United States. Though this is probably not the start of the current global AIDS crisis, it marks the beginning of public awareness.

VIRAL MYSTERIES

Back in 1981, a devastating virus seemed to appear out of nowhere; however, scientists suspected the virus existed long before then. Studies done in the beginning of the 21st century have started to shed some light on when, where, and possibly how the virus started to spread.

There are two species of human immunodeficiency virus (HIV) and three groups within those species. The more virulent of the two species, and the one responsible for the vast majority of illnesses, is HIV-1. By contrast, HIV-2 is not as tough and has largely been confined to western Africa where it originated. In the HIV-1 species, there are three groups: M (major), N (new), and O (outlier). The N and O groups are much rarer than the M group.

In 2000, Dr. Bette Korber, with the Los Alamos National Laboratory in New Mexico, was able to calculate the age of the HIV-1 virus. With the help of a sample from the first known case of HIV-1, Korber and her team employed a model that determines the age of a virus based on its mutations. From this, Korber was able to estimate that the pandemic strain of HIV first showed up in humans just before 1931.

A 2006 study led by Beatrice Hahn, a researcher with the Departments of Medicine and Microbiology at the University of Alabama at Birmingham in Alabama, and published in the journal *Science*, resulted in researchers pinpointing the natural reservoir (long-term host of a pathogen of an infectious disease) for the virus. The researchers collected and analyzed 600 fecal samples from wild chimpanzees in and around the Democratic Republic of the Congo, looking for evidence of simian immunodeficiency virus (SIV), the strain most closely related to HIV-1.

Of the fecal samples taken from three populations of chimps, two were carrying SIV that was virtually indistinguishable, molecularly, from HIV-1 M. Furthermore, many of the chimps in the third population carried SIV, molecularly very similar to HIV-1 N. The study was able to establish the chimpanzee subspecies *Pan troglodytes troglodytes* as the natural reservoir of HIV-1.

Finally, in "The Early Spread and Epidemic Ignition of HIV-1 in Human Populations," researchers described how they were able to reconstruct HIV-1's genetic family tree by working backward from mutations. In this way they were able to discover that the disease mostly likely made the jump to humans before 1920 with chimpanzee hunters and then worsened with urbanization and mass transit from the 1930s to the 1960s.

While some of these theories are still being debated, information and discoveries about the origins of HIV could hold the keys to unlocking a vaccine or creating even more effective drug therapies for treatment.

Over the next 30 years, a disease that was a certain death sentence for those infected has become a manageable chronic disease. This is due in large part to the development of drug therapies that control the virus for a time.

The spread of HIV/AIDS seems to have slowed during the early 2010s in more developed countries, but it remains a crisis in other parts of the world, particularly in sub-Saharan Africa. World leaders have called for action and funding from across the globe to address the issue and get HIV/AIDS medications into the hands of the sick people who need them.

⊕ Impacts and Issues

Roughly 1.5 million people died from HIV-related causes in 2013. The worst affected region is sub-Saharan Africa where, of the 35 million people worldwide infected as of 2013, 24.7 million reside. Treatment for the disease, though not a cure, is effective; however, it is not available to many of those who have HIV.

The primary form of treatment for HIV is ARV drugs (known as ART when referring to the antiretroviral treatment itself). The treatment consists of combining three or more ARV drugs. These drugs control the virus replication within the body and allow an individual's immune system to strengthen and regain the capacity to fight off infections.

However, once a person has slipped into stage 3 or AIDS, he or she is more susceptible to AIDS-defining illnesses. These diseases are serious but become severe and very deadly for a person with a compromised immune system. There are myriad AIDS-defining illnesses; some of the more common, identified by the CDC, include *Pneumocystis carinii* pneumonia, which is caused by a funguslike protozoan; Kaposi's sarcoma, a cancer of the connective tissues that support blood vessels; toxoplasmosis, which is caused by *Toxoplasma gondii*, a parasite that infects the brain and sometimes the heart and lungs; lymphoma, a form of cancer that starts in the lymph nodes; tuberculosis, a contagious airborne communicable disease; and cryptosporidiosis, a protozoal infection.

Contraction and spread of HIV can be prevented by limiting exposure to certain risk factors. One of those risk factors is unprotected sex. The WHO states that "correct and consistent use of male or female condoms during vaginal or anal sex can protect against the spread of sexually transmitted infections, including HIV." Research estimates suggest that using male latex condoms gives an 85 percent or greater protective effect against sexually transmitted infections, including HIV.

Another mode of prevention that has emerged in recent years is voluntary medical male circumcision. According to the WHO, this procedure can reduce the risk of heterosexually acquired HIV infection in men by approximately 60 percent. This preventive method is typically recommended in areas where male circumcision rates are low but HIV prevalence is high.

However, male circumcision, whether of a child or an adult, is usually rife with controversy. Many critics point to previous erroneous claims that circumcision would cure mental illness, tuberculosis, excessive masturbation, and schistosomiasis. Though circumcision is common around the world and generally considered safe, the debate is ongoing as to whether it should be promoted to prevent the spread of HIV without definitive proof of its benefit for all males.

While ARV drugs have been used to treat HIV for decades, their use for prevention is relatively new. A 2011 trial confirmed that if an HIV-positive person adheres to an ART regimen, the risk of transmitting the virus to an uninfected sexual partner can be reduced by 96 percent, according to the WHO. When a person who has HIV takes the ARV drugs, it reduces the amount of HIV in their bodies, leaving less of the virus to pass on to another person. The research is very promising; the problem, according to WHO officials, is that for every person who starts treatment, another two are newly infected. The WHO has recommended further scale-up and strategic use of the medicines.

Researchers have also found that pre-exposure prophylaxis, or daily use of ARV drugs by a partner who is not infected with HIV, may block acquisition of HIV

from an infected partner. Research also shows that post-exposure prophylaxis (PEP), the use of ARV drugs within 72 hours of exposure to HIV, can be effective in preventing infection. According to the WHO, "PEP includes counselling, first aid care, HIV testing, and depending on risk level, administering of a 28-day course of antiretroviral drugs with follow-up care." This is particularly pertinent to people who engage in high-risk behavior such as unprotected sex or intravenous drug use. According to the CDC, "when someone is exposed to HIV through sex or injection drug use, these medicines can work to keep the virus from establishing a permanent infection." If they are taken consistently, they reduce risk by 92 percent.

Another way that HIV can be transmitted is from mother to child. Known as vertical transmission or mother to child transmission (MTCT), rates of this form of transmission range from 15 to 45 percent. However, scientists now say that MTCT can be virtually eliminated if mother and child are provided with ARV drugs throughout pregnancy, labor, delivery, and the postnatal period. The WHO further recommends offering lifelong

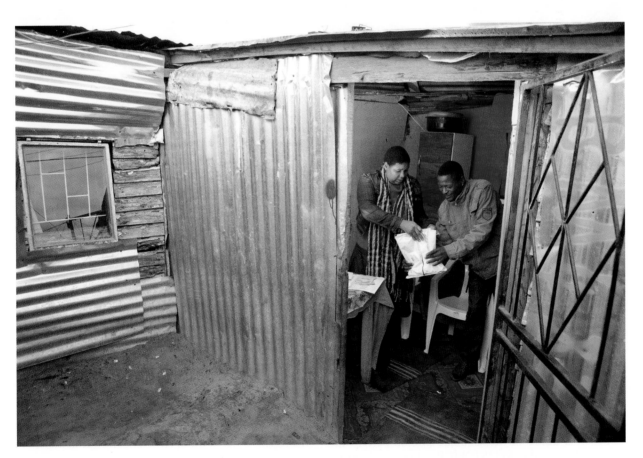

An HIV-positive patient is given a two-month supply of antiretroviral (ARV) drugs by a drug club facilitator during a support group meeting in the patient's house in Kayelitsha township, Cape Town, South Africa. The clubs are called adherence clubs, meant for stable patients diagnosed with HIV. The clubs were the idea of Médicins Sans Frontières (Doctors Without Borders) to provide a quicker method for stable patients diagnosed with HIV to meet at a private home or meeting place to get quick checkups and receive their ARV drugs and to provide peer support. The groups meet once every two months. *© Melanie Stetson Freeman/The Christian Science Monitor via Getty Images.*

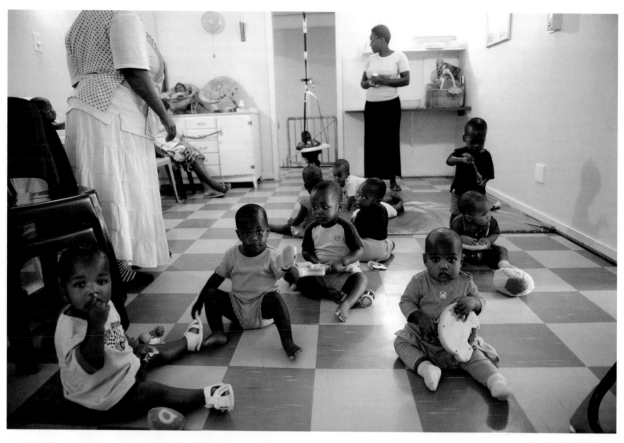

Orphans sit on the floor in an orphanage in Bulembu, Swaziland. In 2011, Swaziland had the world's highest rate of HIV infection, with at least one in four adults carrying the virus. About 120,000 children have been orphaned in Swaziland, constituting more than 10 percent of the total population. Canadian entrepreneur Volker Wagner bought the entire town of Bulembu in 2006, five years after it was abandoned, helping to create a private community developed around the orphanage. *© Stephane de Sakutin/AFP/Getty Images.*

treatment to HIV-positive women who become pregnant, regardless of their CD4 count.

The number of women in low- and middle-income countries receiving treatment is increasing. In 2013, 67 percent of the estimated 1.4 million HIV-positive pregnant women living in these countries received effective ARV drugs to avoid transmission to their children. This was up from 47 percent in 2009.

Without treatment, more than half of all babies born with HIV will die within the first two years of life, according to the United Nations Children's Fund (UNICEF). In high-burden countries in southern Africa, HIV contributes to between 10 and 28 percent of all deaths among children younger than five years of age.

HIV also contributes to a significant portion of maternal deaths, especially in southern Africa, where HIV-related maternal deaths range from 26.8 percent of all maternal deaths in Mozambique to 67.3 percent in Swaziland, according to UNICEF. Reaching the women in need of services in this region presents a challenge. Many of these women do not have access to services. In 2010, of those who did access them, fewer than half received an HIV test. Of those who did and tested

positive, many dropped out of the program for fear of discrimination and rejection by their male partners and families, according to UNICEF.

⊕ Future Implications

HIV/AIDS remains a significant public health challenge, particularly in low- and middle-income countries. However, because more people have access to ART, more people are living longer and healthier lives than ever before. Drug therapies have significantly reduced the transmission of HIV.

Progress has also been made in preventing MTCT and keeping mothers alive. In 2013, nearly 7 out of 10 pregnant women living with HIV, roughly 970,000 women, received ARV drugs. However, coverage for infants and children is still lacking. Only one in four children is on ART, compared to one in three adults, according to the WHO. Of adults living with HIV, 37 percent were receiving treatment, whereas just 23 percent of all children living with HIV were receiving these medications in 2013.

The reasons for this are many but come down mainly to lack of access to ARV treatment for children. To date, there is a lack of cheap and feasible diagnostic tests for those younger than 18 months, as well as lack of trained staff to administer tests and drugs.

A truly child-friendly ARV treatment has yet to be developed. Drugs have been developed for adults, allowing them to take one or two pills of fixed dose combinations of ARV drugs. But such a simplified treatment for children is not available, mainly because countries have difficulties getting simple and affordable combinations of the drugs, according to the WHO. Generic fixed dose drugs for children were in clinical trials as of 2014, but further work is needed.

Adults also have difficulty gaining access to ARTs, due to expense and for logistical reasons. The changing drug regimens make the program hard for clinics to manage. Also, it is hard to predict quantities of the drugs that will be needed to supply the population, which often leads to clinics running out of stock. When the restock process alone takes up to one year, many people can be left without their medicine for a considerable amount of time. Further exacerbating the problem is lack of staff to administer the programs, inadequate storage for the drugs they do have, and delays and interruptions in grant funding. Interrupted supply of ARV drugs not only puts individual patients at risk of disease progression and death but jeopardizes public health due to development of ARV drug resistance. These problems hamper progress toward universal access and diminish credibility of ART programs in the eyes of patients, the community, and health-care providers.

Possible improvements include increasing national stock of the drugs from three months to a minimum of six months' supply; establishing a national buffer supply of medicine; hiring and establishing a dedicated full-time team for supply management of HIV commodities; and establishing a fund that will lend money to HIV programs.

Despite the effectiveness of ARV drugs on HIV suppression, these drugs do not cure HIV, nor are they a vaccine. However, they are helping to stem the tide of transmission and helping more people live productive lives while HIV positive. According to the WHO, approximately 11.7 million people living with HIV in low- and middle-income countries were receiving ART at the end of 2013. About 740,000 of those were children.

Scientists are continuing to work on an HIV vaccine. However, there are several scientific challenges to developing an effective vaccine, according to a presentation at the Global Vaccine Immunization Research Forum on March 4, 2014, in Bethesda, Maryland.

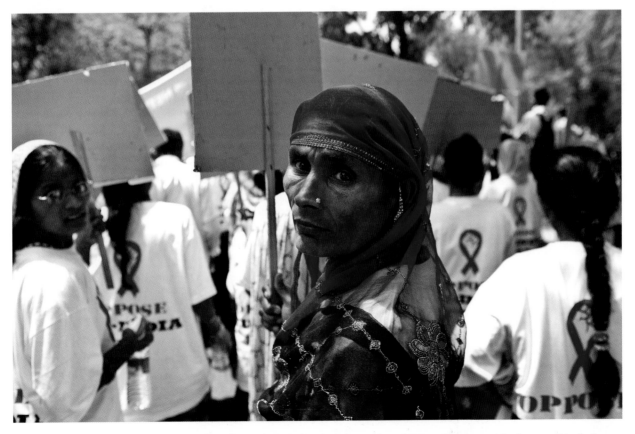

HIV/AIDS campaigners carry placards during a protest rally in New Delhi on April 10, 2013, against the negative impact of the India–European Union Free Trade Agreement on affordable medicines across developing countries. © Manan Vatsyayana/AFP/Getty Images.

Among them are the variability of the virus, the lack of an ideal animal model, and the fact that natural immunity fails to clear HIV, according to Wayne C. Koff, chief scientific officer of the International AIDS Vaccine Initiative. Further, since HIV is a retrovirus, it integrates into the host genome, and there is only a short window of opportunity to control it. Also, because the disease is transmitted sexually, transmission needs to be blocked at mucosal surfaces. According to Koff, "HIV targets cells of the immune system" and "has evasion mechanisms for induction of broadly neutralizing antibodies."

Koff asserts that a vaccine is feasible, but several factors must be in place to accelerate progress. These include additional investments in innovation and technology development to enable rapid, small, hypothesis-driven clinical research studies; analytics and process development; and manufacturing.

The WHO, along with the Joint United Nations Programme on AIDS (UNAIDS), is working toward several goals for the future. They aim to implement strategic use of ARV drugs for HIV treatment and prevention; eliminate HIV in children and expand access to pediatric treatment; improve the health sector response to HIV among key populations; support innovation in HIV prevention, diagnosis, treatment, and care; gather strategic information for effective scale-up; and build stronger links between HIV and related health outcomes.

PRIMARY SOURCE

AIDS 2014 Conference

SOURCE *"The Last Climb: Ending AIDS, Leaving No One Behind," 20th International AIDS Conference Opening Session, July 20, 2014. Copyright © 2014 UNAIDS. http://www.unaids.org/sites/default/files/media_asset/20140720_SP_EXD_AIDS2014opening_en.pdf (accessed January 25, 2015).*

INTRODUCTION *The primary source is the speech given by Michel Sidibé, the executive director of UNAIDS, at the opening session of the 20th International AIDS Conference in 2014. In his address, Sidibé lays out goals and targets for ending AIDS by 2030.*

THE LAST CLIMB

A Vision for Ending AIDS

Over the past 20 years, activists, researchers and policymakers have united at this international conference to bring hope and extend the lives of millions of people. AIDS 2014 calls on us to be bold.

Today, I am calling for ending AIDS by 2030.

My vision for ending AIDS looks like this: voluntary testing and treatment reaching everyone, everywhere; each person living with HIV reaching viral suppression; no one dies from an AIDS-related illness or is born with HIV; and people living with HIV live with dignity, protected by laws and free to move and live anywhere in the world.

This is not just my own vision. It is the one of my friend and mentor Joep Lange. His vision will stay with me until it becomes a reality.

Globally, the AIDS response has averted 10 million new infections since 2002 and avoided more than 7 million deaths. Today, almost 14 million people are on life-saving HIV treatment. What a great collective achievement.

But, to quote Nelson Mandela: "After climbing a great hill, we find that there are many more hills to climb."

We have been climbing this epidemic one hill at a time. Now we must finish our journey with a final climb, and we cannot lose anyone along the way.

Leaving No One Behind

We all agree on what ending AIDS by 2030 means: we will bring the HIV epidemic under control so that it is not a public health threat to any country, village, family or individual.

And for the millions of people living with HIV, your health and quality of life will remain our first priority.

As we saw in the new UNAIDS *Gap report*, our challenge boils down to one painful truth: too many are being left behind today. If the world wants stability, peace and sustainable development, we cannot run away from the needs of lesbian, gay, bisexual, transgender and intersex people, sex workers, people who inject drugs, prisoners, migrants, women and girls, and people with disabilities.

We cannot run away from the harm caused by criminalizing populations. Ahead of the United Nations General Assembly Special Session on Drugs in 2016, we must implement the recommendations of the Global Commission on HIV and the Law.

We cannot run away from the crisis in paediatric AIDS. We must ensure 100% treatment coverage for all children living with HIV. No child should die of an AIDS-related illness.

We cannot run away from the tuberculosis epidemic among people living with HIV. All our efforts to keep people living with HIV alive will be lost if they die from tuberculosis.

We cannot run away from adolescents. HIV is the leading cause of adolescent mortality in Africa—especially among young women. This is a moral injustice. I am calling on young people to lead the new All In initiative, alongside the United Nations Children's Fund and UNAIDS, to end the adolescent AIDS epidemic.

We cannot accept the high cost of second- and third-line regimens, drugs for hepatitis C and viral load tests.

These prices are out of reach and out of control. We urgently need an easy-to-use viral load test that costs no more than US$5. This is my special request to President Clinton, with the support of the Clinton Health Access Initiative and UNITAID: let us seal this deal.

Now, more than ever, we must concentrate our limited resources on where most infections occur and on where most people die. The world needs a new "catch-up" plan for the 15 countries that account for 75% of new HIV infections and AIDS-related deaths.

For the G20, the BRICS countries and the private sector, ending AIDS will be a litmus test for global solidarity and shared responsibility.

I am grateful for the leadership of the United States President's Emergency Plan for AIDS Relief (PEPFAR), including its focus on public health and human rights. There is complete solidarity between the leadership of PEPFAR, the Global Fund to Fight AIDS, Tuberculosis and Malaria and UNAIDS. This gives me great hope for rapid acceleration to end this epidemic.

A New HIV Treatment Target

We have a fragile, five-year window of opportunity. If we are smart and scale up fast by 2020, we will be on track to end the epidemic by 2030.

This is why I am calling on the world to adopt a new, ambitious target: 90% of people tested, 90% of people living with HIV on treatment and 90% of people on treatment with suppressed viral loads.

90–90–90 is not just a numeric target. It is a moral and economic imperative. It will keep people living with HIV alive and healthy, protect future generations from infection, provide economic value over the long term and drive the AIDS epidemic into history.

Our return on investment will be measured in millions of lives saved.

We need to use every tool we have to encourage voluntary testing and retesting for everyone. This means investing more in communities and building strong, accountable, community-based treatment literacy and adherence programmes.

Today, an undetectable viral load is the closest we have to a cure.

But let me be clear: HIV treatment alone will not get us to the top of this mountain or to the end of the epidemic. We need new, bold and achievable targets for HIV prevention as well. We must maximize our arsenal of existing tools. With support from the Bill & Melinda Gates Foundation and other partners, we must keep the promise alive for new prevention tools that benefit and focus on people still left behind—like the female-controlled microbicide ring. And, of course, the race for a vaccine and cure is moving ahead, especially here in Melbourne.

Ending AIDS Advances Development

I am pleased to share with you the latest good news from New York. The Open Working Group just concluded its final session and agreed to the target of "ending the epidemics of AIDS, tuberculosis and malaria by 2030." This is an unfinished agenda of the Millennium Development Goals.

What I am calling for today requires new approaches. First, the post-2015 agenda should explicitly embrace human rights. Second, we must be brave enough to stop public hypocrisy on sex, and promote universal sexual and reproductive health, education and rights. Third, by 2020 we must achieve our target of 90–90–90.

Arm in Arm, We Will Reach the Summit

My friends, let us not leave Melbourne thinking that it will be easy to reach the summit. Complacency will cause us to stumble. Will future generations say that we squandered the opportunity of a lifetime?

I know the path will be steep and the obstacles many.

Let us do this in memory of our colleagues who died en route to Melbourne and the millions who have died of AIDS-related illnesses and of the tens of millions of people living with HIV.

If every person here tonight, and everyone working to end the epidemic, acts with the same sense of urgency, the same hope and the same commitment to fight for those left behind, we will scale this mountain.

But only if we go arm in arm will we reach the top and the end.

SEE ALSO *Epidemiology: Surveillance for Emerging Infectious Diseases; Global Health Initiatives; Health in the WHO African Region; Health-Related Education and Information Access; Viral Diseases*

BIBLIOGRAPHY

Books

Bell, Sigall K., Kevin J. Selby, and Courtney L. McMickens. *AIDS*. Santa Barbara, CA: Greenwood, 2011.

Institute of Medicine (U.S.). *HIV Screening and Access to Care: Exploring Barriers and Facilitators to Expanded HIV Testing*. Washington, DC: National Academies Press, 2010.

Joint United Nations Programme on HIV/AIDS. *UNAIDS World AIDS Day Report 2011*. Geneva: UNAIDS, 2011. Available online at http://www.unaids.org/sites/default/files/en/media/unaids/contentassets/documents/unaidspublication/2011/JC2216_WorldAIDSday_report_2011_en.pdf (accessed February 19, 2015).

Pepin, Jacques. *The Origins of AIDS.* Cambridge, UK: Cambridge University Press, 2011.

UNAIDS. *AIDS at 30: Nations at the Crossroads.* Geneva: UNAIDS, 2011.

Periodicals

Faria, Nuno R., et al. "The Early Spread and Epidemic Ignition of HIV-1 in Human Populations." *Science* 346, no. 6205 (October 3, 2014): 56–61.

Websites

"AIDSinfo." *U.S. National Institutes of Health (NIH).* http://aidsinfo.nih.gov (accessed February 14, 2015).

"Child Survival: HIV/AIDS." *UNICEF.* http://www.unicefusa.org/mission/survival/hiv-aids (accessed February 14, 2015).

"HIV/AIDS." *U.S. Centers for Disease Control and Prevention (CDC).* http://www.cdc.gov/hiv/ (accessed February 14, 2015).

"HIV/AIDS." *World Health Organization (WHO).* http://www.who.int/topics/hiv_aids/en/ (accessed February 14, 2015).

"HIV/AIDS Basics." *AIDS.gov, U.S. Department of Health and Human Services.* https://www.aids.gov/hiv-aids-basics/ (accessed February 14, 2015).

"HIV/AIDS Definition." *Mayo Clinic.* http://www.mayoclinic.org/diseases-conditions/hiv-aids/basics/definition/con-20013732 (accessed February 14, 2015).

Koff, Wayne C. "Status of HIV Vaccine Research & Development," Presentation to Global Vaccine Immunization Research Forum, Bethesda, Maryland. *World Health Organization (WHO),* March 4, 2014. http://www.who.int/immunization/research/forums_and_initiatives/05_Koff_GVIRFHIV_Vaccine_Progress.pdf (accessed February 14, 2015).

Melanie R. Plenda

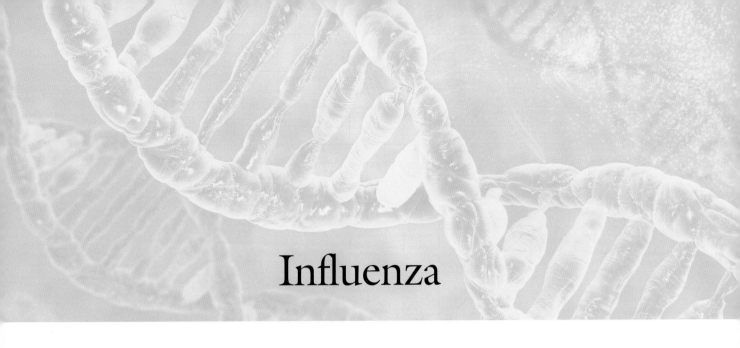

Influenza

⊕ Introduction

Influenza (flu) is a viral disease of global scope and distribution. The World Health Organization (WHO) estimates that influenza and diseases secondary to influenza inflection kill between 250,000 to 500,000 people around the world each year. In the United States, the National Institutes of Health estimates that there are 36,000 influenza related deaths each year. Even in countries with advanced research and treatment facilities, regular seasonal influenza is a deadly problem and a profound economic burden.

An influenza epidemic is a widespread outbreak within some group, area, country, or region. A pandemic is a worldwide outbreak of influenza that can cause large-scale illness and death. The extent of increase in illness, death, and hardship related to influenza epidemics and pandemics depends primarily on the novelty of the virus responsible for the influenza, transmissibility of the virus, and the lethality of the influenza, including lethality due to secondary complications of the influenza. Pandemic influenza is far more devastating in terms of numbers of cases, deaths, strain on health care delivery systems, economic loss, and geopolitical impacts.

⊕ Historical Background

Influenza pandemics normally occur several times during a century, but their exact timing is unpredictable. There have been four global pandemics since 1918. In July 2009, the WHO declared a pandemic of type A/H1N1 influenza (also known as "swine flu"). A low disease lethality and public health efforts—including rapid vaccine development, antiviral drug deployment, public education, and intense surveillance—are credited with keeping the death toll and economic impact of the 2009 pandemic to levels less than were observed during previous influenza pandemics.

1918 Spanish Influenza

The most lethal pandemic in recent modern history was the 1918 Spanish flu outbreak that killed as many as 40 million people worldwide. Other influenza pandemics occurred in 1957 and 1968. The 1918, 1957, and 1968 pandemics resulted from human influenza viruses sharing genetic material with an influenza virus that attacks birds. Human immune systems had never encountered the new or novel virus strain; as a result, in each case, the new virus swept rapidly through vulnerable populations around the globe.

In 2005, researchers from the U.S. Centers for Disease Control and Prevention (CDC) announced they had isolated the 1918 pandemic virus genetic code from the preserved lung tissue (and in one case, the frozen body) of pandemic victims. Scientists continue to investigate the genetics of the 1918 influenza virus in order to ascertain which aspects of the pathogen contributed to its virulence. In particular, whether specific mutations in current avian flu viruses might make them as infectious among humans as the 1918 virus.

Each year in the United States, 80 to 90 percent of the tens of thousands of deaths attributed to ordinary influenza occur among people older than 65 years of age. However, deaths during the 1918 influenza epidemic showed the opposite pattern, with the highest death rates among young, healthy adults. The reason is that vigorous immune responses among young, healthy people can produce heavy releases of cytokines, proteins produced by white blood cells that can rapidly kill infected cells. An explosive release of cytokines can also produce catastrophic damage to lung and other types of tissue, which in the case of the 1918 influenza pandemic, led to deaths from internal bleeding. Thus, people with immune systems that were less acutely reactive or even impaired actually had a better chance of surviving the 1918 pandemic than people expected to efficiently fight off an ordinary flu virus.

Scientists detected significant differences between the 1918 virus and the flu viruses that caused later human pandemics in 1957 and 1968. The latter viruses

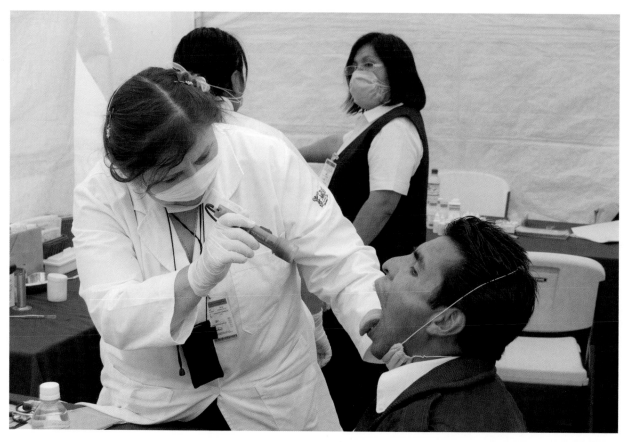

A doctor examines a patient for signs of H1N1 influenza at a clinic on April 29, 2009, in Mexico City, Mexico. Reports of approximately 148 cases existed in about nine countries at that time, but later that year it was declared a worldwide pandemic. By August 2010, when the pandemic was determined to be over by the World Health Organization, 18,000 people were suspected to have died worldwide from the strain of flu. © *Frontpage/Shutterstock.com.*

were human subtypes that had picked up a few genetic elements of avian flu but were not actual bird flu viruses. The 1918 flu virus appears to be more closely related genetically to current bird flu viruses such as H5N1 than existing human flu viruses, and also shows a similar pattern of deep lung tissue infection. It is estimated that only 25 to 30 amino acid sequences of more than 4,000 in the genetic code of the 1918 virus contributed to its transmissibility and lethality among humans.

The identification of the genetic code linked the pandemic to an avian flu just as the WHO issued warnings about the possibility of a future pandemic resulting from an emerging avian flu in Asia. These warnings caused governments around the world to stockpile antiviral drugs and begin to make plans for mass vaccination, shortages of antiviral medications, overtaxed health-care systems, and quarantines of entire regions.

However, the practical application of this information is that it should be possible to track mutations in H5N1 and other avian flu viruses to detect whether they are developing the capability to easily infect humans. This in turn could help scientists to proactively devise ways to disable the virus.

Influenza Types

Influenza viruses consist of three different major types known as A, B, and C. Of the three types, only A and B cause significant disease in humans. Both A and B types cause normal seasonal influenza, but at any one time there may be hundreds of different variations of each type circulating the globe. Both influenza A and B viruses change their structure often enough to prevent the development of long-lasting immunity. Influenza A, most commonly the cause of seasonal influenza outbreaks, generally causes more severe disease and is the most unpredictable. This multitude of subtle viral variations presents a challenge to human and animal immune systems and to researchers attempting to create effective vaccines and treatments.

An influenza A virus has two specific proteins on its surface that are important for infecting humans. These proteins, known as antigens, bear the names hemagglutinin (HA) and neuraminidase (NA). The HA and NA proteins vary in their chemical structure from year to year. This process, termed antigenic drift, results in virus particle proteins with subtle variations in structure. In 2014, 15 different HA subtypes were known to exist, with nine different NA subtypes. These subtypes receive

Percentage of Influenza–Positive Respiratory Specimens, with Virus Subtype, in Selected Geographical Areas, Week of November 9–15, 2014

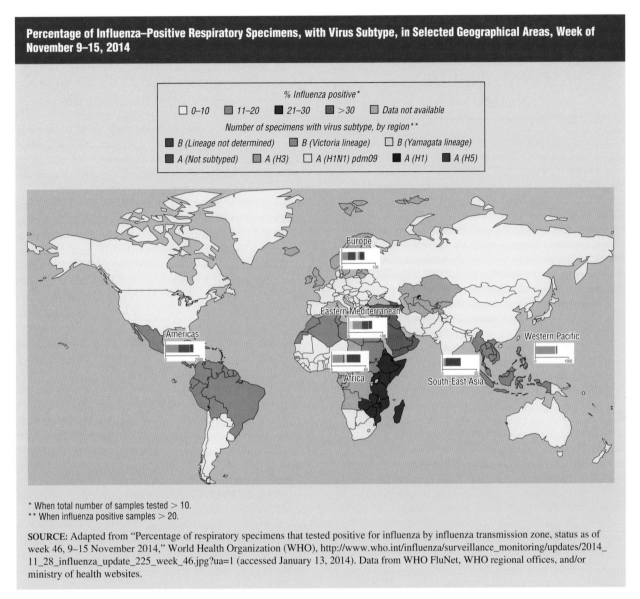

* When total number of samples tested > 10.

** When influenza positive samples > 20.

SOURCE: Adapted from "Percentage of respiratory specimens that tested positive for influenza by influenza transmission zone, status as of week 46, 9–15 November 2014," World Health Organization (WHO), http://www.who.int/influenza/surveillance_monitoring/updates/2014_11_28_influenza_update_225_week_46.jpg?ua=1 (accessed January 13, 2014). Data from WHO FluNet, WHO regional offices, and/or ministry of health websites.

Epidemiologists constantly monitor the global influenza situation in order to evaluate the prevalence and mortality rate of various influenza strains. Monitoring also helps anticipate the most likely upcoming seasonal strain in order to ensure effective vaccination.

different number designations, and the various influenza strains are named by the specific HA and NA proteins on the virus. For example, the H5N1 virus contains HA protein 5 and NA protein 1.

Other specific virus traits help them evade immune defenses. Influenza viruses also exist in animal populations, including domesticated birds and pigs. This allows virus strains to develop or evolve in animals and then leap to human populations. Humans and some animals usually have little to no protection against a new virus that arises due to a mutation, or to such novel viruses as the 2009 pandemic H1N1 virus, which is a unique mix of preexisting genes.

Influenza is highly contagious and primarily spreads from person to person in virus-laden droplets produced by sneezing or coughing. Alternatively, the droplets land on a surface and contaminate the hands that carry the virus to the mouth or nose. School-aged children are a key conduit in spreading influenza. Ten to 40 percent of school-aged children will usually contract a form of influenza in a particular flu season. Children swap viruses at school and bring them home, infecting family members. Children and others infected with most influenza viruses are contagious before they appear or feel ill, and the virus usually remains present in nasal mucous and cough droplets for about a week following apparent recovery from influenza.

In healthy adults and children, a case of influenza typically lasts from four days to a week. Milder forms may resemble a severe cold. However, influenza can be

DRUGS CURRENTLY AVAILABLE TO TREAT SEASONAL INFLUENZA IN ADULTS

As of early 2015, there are two classes of antiviral drugs available for the treatment of influenza in the United States. The drugs zanamivir (Relenza), oseltamivir (Tamiflu), and peramivir (Rapivab), are classified as neuraminidase inhibitors and have shown activity against influenza A and B. An older class of drugs, the adamantanes, which includes the drugs amantadine and rimantadine, is active only against influenza A. Due to marked increase in resistance to the adamantanes in recent years, the Advisory Committee on Immunization Practices no longer recommends the use of these drugs to treat influenza in the United States, except in special circumstances.

Treatment with the neuroaminidase inhibitors can lessen the duration of symptoms of influenza by as many three days in some people. However, the drugs must be administered within the first 24 to 30 hours of the onset of flu symptoms for the most beneficial effects to occur. The results of clinical trials show there is no benefit to taking the neuroaminidase inhibitors after two days or more of the onset of flu symptoms.

Results of other studies reveal that initiating antiviral therapy leads to a reduction in the amount and severity of flu-related complications, reduces the amount of time some patients diagnosed with influenza must remain in the hospital, and also decreases mortality rates associated with the flu. However, these results may not be the same for some patients with compromised immune systems who are diagnosed with influenza and who are treated with antiviral therapy.

unpredictable, and secondary complications sometimes occur that can kill otherwise healthy adults and children.

⊕ Impacts and Issues

Influenza vaccination provides the most effective treatment by preventing the disease, but the variability of influenza viruses poses a challenge for vaccine development. As the virus changes slightly from year to year, and more dramatically at unpredictable intervals, vaccines that are effective one year may not work the next. Each year, public health officials make an educated guess, based upon the patterns of influenza viruses that emerge mostly in tropical areas of Asia, as to what will be the prevalent strains circulating in the following season, and vaccine preparation commences targeting those strains.

The genetic makeup of the 2009 A/H1N1 pandemic virus, for example, has remained consistent—that is, the overwhelming majority of viruses tested around the world are highly similar to the virus first isolated and identified

in April 2009. Older populations continue to show some immunity to the A(H1N1)2009 virus because it is similar to a virus that circulated in the 1950s and 1960s.

By July 2010, the U.S. Food and Drug Administration (FDA) approved release of a seasonal flu vaccine with antigens offering protection against 2009 H1N1 pandemic flu. By 2012, however, another virus, A H2N3, became the dominant seasonal flu virus in many areas of the world. Evolution of viruses and such interplay between shifting dominant viruses from season to season is normal but also complicates production of the proper vaccine formulation.

In the first decade of the 21st century, a particularly virulent strain of avian flu known as H5N1 influenza emerged. Transmission of this virus between humans has occurred in only a few documented cases, and close contact with infected birds is usually required to catch this form of influenza. Experts fear that a mutation (a routine event in viruses) in the H5N1 virus that increases its transmissibility could spark a deadly global pandemic. Recognition of the stem portion of the HA molecule allows the production of antibodies that can fight, and potentially prevent, both H1N1 (swine flu) and H5N1 (avian flu) virus infections.

A United Nations Global Influenza Program routinely monitors global influenza cases and publishes updates of epidemiological data and assessments, releasing new epidemiological data every two weeks. As of January 2015, there were no confirmed reports of genetic changes in the A(H1N1)2009 virus that impact its transmissibility or lethality.

In March 2013, Chinese health authorities informed the WHO of the emergence of a new type of avian influenza that had infected humans. The first cases of influenza A subtype H7N9 occurred around Shanghai, China. The virus alarms international health officials because it can cause rapid, severe illness and multiple organ failures that may result in death.

⊕ Future Implications

Constant monitoring of the global influenza situation allows epidemiologists to evaluate the prevalence and mortality rate of various influenza strains. Monitoring emerging strains also allows public health officials to anticipate the most likely upcoming seasonal strain in order to ensure effective vaccination.

The trigger to the next global pandemic will be new types of genetic mutations that quickly alter currently existing influenza viruses. If, for example, an avian influenza virus mutates into a form that is easily transmissible from person to person the results could be globally catastrophic. For many scientists, the question is not if the virus will mutate into a form that allows human to human transmission, but rather when and how easily transmissible will the virus become?

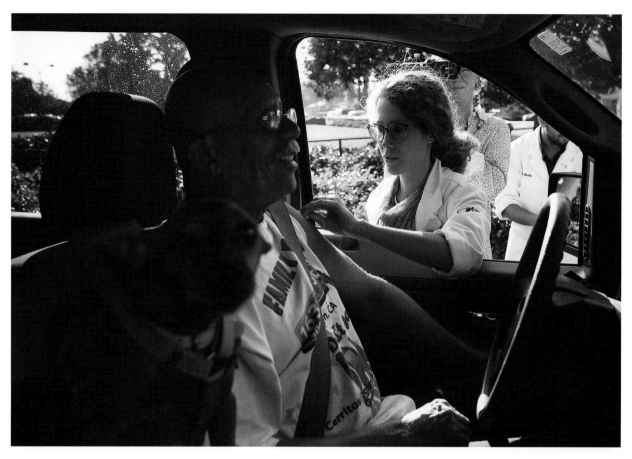

A medical school student administers a flu vaccine to a person in a car during a drive-through flu shot clinic in San Pablo, California. Doctors Medical Center hosted the drive-through flu shot clinic offering free vaccines for any community member over the age of 18. *© Justin Sullivan/Getty Images.*

Although humans are the primary viral "reservoir" (an animal population that harbors the virus) for most human influenza, other animal reservoirs such as swine and wild bird populations are probable sources of new human subtypes that emerge through genetic reassortment. Reassortment occurs when genes from one type of virus "jump" to a closely related virus subtype when they are both replicating in close proximity (e.g., within a human cell). Such new subtypes, with surface proteins that human immune systems have not encountered before, greatly increase the transmissibility of the virus and lower the effectiveness of the human immune system to recognize and combat the virus.

PRIMARY SOURCE

39 Steps Governments Should Take to Prepare for a Pandemic

SOURCE *"39 Steps Governments Should Take to Prepare for a Pandemic." Pandemic Influenza Contingency, United Nations*

Office for the Coordination of Humanitarian Affairs, December 2007. Copyright © 2007 United Nations. http://www.un.org/ influenza/39_steps.pdf (accessed January 25, 2015).

INTRODUCTION *This primary source is the full text of a 2007 paper prepared by the United Nations Office for the Coordination of Humanitarian Affairs. It lists 39 recommended actions for governments to take if an influenza pandemic should develop.*

39 STEPS GOVERNMENTS SHOULD TAKE TO PREPARE FOR A PANDEMIC

Experts at WHO believe the world is closer to an influenza pandemic than at any time since 1968. Experience with HIV/AIDS, malaria, SARS and previous influenza pandemics demonstrates that robust multi-sector support is needed to limit vulnerability and humanitarian consequences. Outbreaks of highly transmissible disease with high fatality rates are liable to trigger (through absenteeism) extreme adverse economic, governance, humanitarian and social impacts, including civil disruption, collapse of weak safety nets and impoverishment of vulnerable populations. Countries need to prepare adequately for the economic and social impacts of a pandemic. Minimising the disruption of vital services by planning for continuity of operations is of paramount importance.

This paper sets out a number of key actions which Governments and their partners should consider implementing in order to mitigate the 'beyond health' impacts of a pandemic.

A. Central Government planning and coordination

1) Pandemic preparedness should be integrated into national disaster management structures and approaches. An existing Government entity that is responsible for crisis management should coordinate the national response.

2) The roles and responsibilities of different Government entities and the command structure should be explicit.

3) A cross-Government Ministerial Committee should oversee preparations. There should be plenty of emphasis on the preparedness of many different sectors, in addition to human health and animal health.

4) Governments should articulate what budgets they are assigning to pandemic preparedness interventions from different Ministries.

5) Governments should review whether the legal and regulatory framework enables necessary actions in the event of a pandemic, for example relating to travel, quarantine, isolation, social distancing and closure of places of assembly.

6) The interests of vulnerable groups and migrants should be incorporated in planning.

7) Civil society and local communities should be involved in developing pandemic preparedness plans.

8) It is important to test contingency plans at all levels, including through simulation exercises, and learn lessons from such tests.

B. Local planning

9) It is important that planning extends to a local level, including the role of local authorities. Central authorities should provide advice to local authorities.

10) Local authorities and community groups should plan how to develop the capacity to deal with large numbers of deaths.

C. Actions in specific sectors

11) Governments should develop a comprehensive security plan to protect against theft, fraud, corruption, demonstrations, unrest, and illegal trade.

12) The Ministry of Defence should consider what military assets should be brought to bear in the event of a pandemic, how to mobilise them and how to intensively liaise with non-military partners in other sectors.

13) In countries dependent on electronic systems, ICT infrastructure and staff will be critical. Governments should consider how best to strengthen networks and prepare for surges in demand.

14) Transport operators and authorities need to minimise infection risks and staff absences in vital transport, air and sea ports, and loading and unloading facilities, to enable supply of medicines and food to continue even in WHO Phase 6.

15) The financial sector should plan business continuity, so as to be able to maintain essential cash, credit, banking, payment, salary, pension and regulation services in the face of significant absenteeism. Central banks, finance ministries and prudential regulators should conduct testing of systemic resilience to pandemic risks.

16) Governments should work with local and international humanitarian actors to develop plans as to who has the capacity where to meet which basic needs of vulnerable populations (food, health, shelter, water and sanitation) in a pandemic, so as to clarify responsibilities, identify gaps and avoid duplication.

D. Contingency planning for the maintenance of essential services

17) Essential services need to develop business continuity plans to limit disruption.

18) In business continuity plans, organisations should (a) consider how to deal with a high level of staff absenteeism and minimise its impact on their activities; (b) provide clear command structures, delegations of authority and orders of succession for workers; (c) assess the need to stockpile strategic reserves of supplies, material and equipment; (d) identify who is going to do what when and how; (e) identify the personnel, supplies and equipment vital to maintain essential functions; (f) assign and train alternates for critical posts; (g) establish guidelines for priority of access to essential services; (h) plan for security risks to their operations and supply chain; (i) prepare to enable staff to work from home; (j) consider the need for family and childcare support for essential workers; (k) consider the need for psychosocial support services to help workers to remain effective.

19) Specific individuals in organisations and businesses should be accountable for preparing for a crisis.

20) Organisations and businesses should prepare to face reduced travel, reduced face-to-face meetings, reduced accessibility of funds, disruptions in access to data systems, difficulty in procuring and distributing supplies and competition for skilled workers.

21) Employers should educate employees on prevention, health and safety and mitigation.

E. Information, education and communication

22) The Government should have a communication strategy to improve public awareness, including in remote rural areas.

23) The public should be informed and consulted about Government plans so as to manage expectations. Clear messages for citizens, media and international organisations about the threat and planned response should be delivered.

24) To maintain public confidence, Governments should demonstrate that they have robust preparedness plans; the power to take extraordinary measures if needed; the capacity to deliver essential services reliably; and arrangements to return to normal life quickly after the pandemic.

25) The Government should set up a national flu hotline and pandemic website as sources of advice and information and designate national and regional spokespersons.

26) Communication skills training should be provided to those expected to be involved in communicating.

27) Community groups and leaders should be used to build public confidence, disseminate information and identify people at risk.

28) Nominating pandemic preparedness representatives in minority populations can help to cross language and cultural barriers.

29) Communication should differentiate between avian flu and human flu, and be tailored to each WHO phase of the pandemic.

F. Social distancing

30) The Government should develop a strategy for how it will take and implement decisions on closure of schools, prisons, residential care homes and workplaces. Special care should be taken when considering school closures as it will then be necessary for adults in households to stay at home to take care of children, which may not be easy.

31) The Interior Ministry should develop a strategy regarding whether and how it will restrict mass gatherings.

32) At Phases 4–5, Governments should recommend reduced staff presence. Telecommuting and working from home should be encouraged. Non-critical staff should not come to work. Essential workers who come to work should stay at least one metre away from each other at all times.

33) Governments should consider introducing a 'pandemic severity index' with recommendations for communities to implement differentiated measures according to the evolving case fatality rate of the pandemic (as has been developed in the United States).

G. Movement and borders

34) Port and airport operators and carriers should consider how restrictions on international travel and additional entry or exit screening could be set in place quickly.

35) The Ministries of Transport and Interior should develop a strategy for whether and how they would impose and manage border control measures.

36) Governments should consider whether and how to restrict movement to and from affected areas.

37) Border control, quarantining, surveillance and screening measures should strike a balance between addressing containment and infection and limiting the impact on trade. Any measures to limit movement of people, animals or goods should not be maintained for longer than essential to achieve public health objectives; and should be driven by the science-based recommendations of international organisations.

H. Cross-border implications

38) Planning should be coordinated with other countries in the region whose actions could have a cross-border impact.

39) Governments should provide support to foreign nationals stranded by border closures, quarantine measures or transport disruption; and should have systems in place to identify dead foreigners and work with consulates to provide for burial or repatriation of bodies.

PRIMARY SOURCE

Global Action Plan for Influenza Vaccines: Global Progress Report, January 2006–September 2013

SOURCE *"Overview," in* Global Action Plan for Influenza Vaccines: Global Progress Report, January 2006–September 2013. *Geneva: World Health Organization (WHO), March 2014, 7–9. http://apps.who.int/iris/bitstr eam/10665/112307/1/9789241507011_eng .pdf?ua=1 (accessed January 25, 2015).*

INTRODUCTION *This primary source is from the overview of the World Health Organization's progress report on its global action plan for influenza vaccines. It categorizes progress under established objectives, and includes estimated vaccine data for potential pandemics.*

Overview

WHO's Global Action Plan for Influenza Vaccines (GAP) is a 10-year long (2006–2016) multi-stakeholder, multi-partner initiative aimed at ensuring the protection of populations worldwide through vaccination in the event of an influenza pandemic. Mathematical modelling shows that owing to the effects of herd immunity, vaccinating just 70% of the world's population with appropriate pandemic vaccines should be sufficient to protect the whole population. However, this will only be effective if sufficient pandemic vaccines are produced and distributed within 6 months of the transfer of the pandemic vaccine master seed to industry.

Gearing global production to provide timely and equitable access to pandemic influenza vaccines for 70% of the world's population is thus at the heart of the GAP mission. In order to achieve its mission, GAP advocates targeted action in three key areas:

- increasing evidence-based use of seasonal influenza vaccines;

- growing global pandemic vaccine production capacity and strengthening national regulatory competencies;

- fostering development of new influenza vaccines that are not only higher-yielding and faster to produce, but also broader in protection and of longer duration.

These lines of action form the basis of GAP's three core objectives. These were initially formulated in 2006 but have since been revised (in 2011) to their present form, as follows:

I. To increase evidence-based seasonal influenza vaccine use, ensuring that all countries have a policy in place, and are on track in its implementation, to vaccinate at least one at-risk population group.

Objective 1 can be achieved through:

- increasing knowledge about the burden of influenza, and vaccine performance and cost-effectiveness in different national and regional settings;

- strengthening disease and virological surveillance systems;

- developing regional and national plans for conducting seasonal influenza vaccination campaigns;

- increasing communication and awareness on the benefits and risks of influenza vaccination especially among health professionals and at-risk groups.

To increase pandemic vaccine production capacity and corresponding national regulatory competencies (to meet WHO criteria) towards the target of producing enough doses of vaccine to vaccinate at least 70% of the world's population in the event of a pandemic, and to spread production across the world to facilitate rapid and equitable access.

Objective 2 can be achieved by:

- Establishing and/or expanding pandemic influenza vaccine production in developing countries;

- developing surge production capacity;

- strengthening national regulatory authority capacities to license influenza vaccines which have either been imported or manufactured locally.

To develop more effective influenza vaccines with the aim to license, or to have in advanced clinical development, new influenza vaccines that are either higher yielding, and/or faster to produce, and/or broader in protection and/or of a longer duration of protection when compared with the current licensed vaccines.

Objective 3 can be achieved by:

- promoting research and development in new vaccine concepts (e.g. universal vaccines), correlates of protection, prototype pandemic seed strains and other new technologies that shorten influenza vaccine production timelines (e.g. potency testing, sterility testing);

- facilitating the exchange of information between researchers on new influenza vaccines.

SEE ALSO *Avian (Bird) and Swine Influenzas; Epidemiology: Surveillance for Emerging Infectious Diseases; Pandemic Preparedness; Vaccine-Preventable Diseases; Viral Diseases; Zoonotic (Animal-Borne) Diseases*

BIBLIOGRAPHY

Books

Abramson, Jon Stuart. *Inside the 2009 Influenza Pandemic.* Singapore: World Scientific, 2011.

Biehl, João, and Adriana Petryna. *When People Come First: Critical Studies in Global Health.* Princeton, NJ: Princeton University Press, 2013.

Bristow, Nancy K. *American Pandemic: The Lost Worlds of the 1918 Influenza Epidemic.* Oxford: Oxford University Press, 2012.

Crisp, Nigel. *Turning the World Upside Down: The Search for Global Health in the Twenty-First Century.* London: Royal Society of Medicine Press, 2010.

Dehner, George. *Global Flu and You: A History of Influenza.* London: Reaktion Books, 2012.

Dehner, George. *Influenza: A Century of Science and Public Health Response.* Pittsburgh, PA: University of Pittsburgh Press, 2012.

Food and Agriculture Organization of the United Nations. *Approaches to Controlling, Preventing and Eliminating H5N1 Highly Pathogenic Avian Influenza in Endemic Countries.* Rome: Food and Agriculture Organization of the United Nations, 2011.

Giles-Vernick, Tamara, Susan Craddock, and Jennifer Lee Gunn, eds. *Influenza and Public Health Learning from Past Pandemics.* London: Earthscan, 2010.

Honigsbaum, Mark. *A History of the Great Influenza Pandemics Death, Panic and Hysteria, 1830–1920.* New York: I.B. Tauris, 2014.

Humphries, Mark Osborne. *The Last Plague: Spanish Influenza and the Politics of Public Health in Canada*. Toronto: University of Toronto Press, 2013.

Jones, Esyllt Wynne, and Magdalena Fahrni, eds. *Epidemic Encounters: Influenza, Society, and Culture in Canada, 1918–20*. Vancouver: UBC Press, 2012.

Kapoor, Sanjay, and Kuldeep Dhama. *Insight into Influenza Viruses of Animals and Humans*. New York: Springer, 2014.

MacPhail, Theresa. *The Viral Network: A Pathography of the H1N1 Influenza Pandemic*. Ithaca, NY: Cornell University Press, 2014.

Matchett, Karin, Anne-Marie Mazza, and Steven Kendall. *Perspectives on Research with H5N1 Avian Influenza: Scientific Inquiry, Communication, Controversy: Summary of a Workshop*. Washington, DC: National Academies Press, 2013.

Oldstone, Michael B. A., and Richard W. Compans, eds. *Influenza Pathogenesis and Control*. New York: Springer, 2014.

Scoones, Ian, ed. *Avian Influenza Science, Policy and Politics*. Washington, DC: Earthscan, 2010.

Spackman, Erica, ed. *Animal Influenza Virus*. New York: Humana, 2014.

Van-Tam, Jonathan, and Chloe Sellwood. *Pandemic Influenza*, 2nd ed. Wallingford, UK: CABI, 2013.

Webster, Robert G., Arnold S. Monto, Thomas J. Braciale, and Robert A. Lamb, eds. *Textbook of Influenza*, 2nd ed. Chichester, UK: Wiley Blackwell, 2013.

Periodicals

Brockwell-Staats, Christy, Robert G. Webster, and Richard J. Webby. "Diversity of Influenza Viruses in Swine and the Emergence of a Novel Human Pandemic Influenza A (H1N1)." *Influenza and Other Respiratory Viruses* 3, no. 5 (2009): 207–213.

Carrico, Ruth M., et al. "Drive-Thru Influenza Immunization: Fifteen Years of Experience." *Journal of Emergency Management* 10, no. 3 (2012): 7–14.

Davies, Sara E., and Jeremy Youde. "The Politics of Disease Surveillance: Special Section." *Global Change, Peace & Security* 24, no. 1 (2012): 53–107.

Ferroni, E., and T. Jefferson. "Influenza." *American Family Physician* 86, no. 10 (2012): 958–960.

Institute of Biomedical Science. "A Panoply of Pathology: From Influenza to Modernization." *Biomedical Scientist* 55, no. 3 (2011).

Kamradt-Scott, Adam. "The Politics of Medicine and the Global Governance of Pandemic Influenza." *International Journal of Health Services* 43, no. 1 (2013): 105–121.

Souza, M. J. "Influenza." *Journal of Exotic Pet Medicine* 20, no. 1 (2011): 4–8.

Suarez, David L., and Erica Spackman. "Proceedings of the Eighth International Symposium on Avian Influenza." *Avian Diseases* 56, no. 4 (2012).

Vincent, A., et al. "Review of Influenza A Virus in Swine Worldwide: A Call for Increased Surveillance and Research." *Zoonoses and Public Health* 61, no. 1 (2014): 4–17.

Websites

"Avian Influenza A (H7N9)." *Global Early Warning System (GLEWS)*. http://www.glews.net/2013/10/avian-influenza-ah7n9-virus/ (accessed March 1, 2015).

Flu.gov. http://www.flu.gov (accessed March 1, 2015).

"Influenza." *World Health Organization (WHO)*. http://www.who.int/topics/influenza/en/ (accessed March 1, 2015).

"Influenza (Flu)." *U.S. Centers for Disease Control and Prevention (CDC)*. http://www.cdc.gov/flu/index.htm (accessed March 1, 2015).

"Update on Highly Pathogenic Avian Influenza in Animals (Type H5 and H7)." *World Organization for Animal Health*. http://www.oie.int/en/animal-health-in-the-world/update-on-avian-influenza/2015/ (accessed March 1, 2015).

K. Lee Lerner

Insect-Borne Diseases

⊕ Introduction

Insect-borne diseases, also called vector-borne diseases, are those caused by pathogens such as parasites, viruses, or bacteria transmitted between humans or from animals to humans by an insect, typically a bloodsucking insect. Though an insect-borne disease may cause illness in humans, it does not affect the organism that transfers it.

The disease usually is transferred when bloodsucking insects ingest blood that contains disease-producing microorganisms from an infected host, which can be a human or animal. When these insects subsequently bite another host for another meal, they inject the new host with the pathogen.

Examples of insect-borne diseases include malaria, dengue fever, West Nile virus, Lyme disease, filariasis, yellow fever, Chagas disease, chikungunya, leishmaniasis, human African trypanosomiasis, Japanese encephalitis, onchocerciasis, and schistosomiasis. According to the World Health Organization (WHO), mosquitoes are the best-known disease vector (carriers that transmit disease), however, others include ticks, flies, sand flies, fleas, triatomine bugs (large bloodsucking insects that exist mainly in Latin America), and some freshwater aquatic snails. Many of these diseases are preventable through protective measures, such as indoor and outdoor treatments with pesticides, insect repellents worn on the body, protective screens for households, and insecticide-treated bed nets.

According to the WHO, vector-borne diseases account for more than 17 percent of all infectious diseases and cause more than 1 million deaths annually. For example, more than 2.5 billion people in more than 100 countries are at risk of getting dengue fever, a debilitating viral disease transmitted by mosquitoes, which causes sudden fever and acute pains in the joints. Furthermore, malaria (also transmitted by mosquitoes) is a fever caused by a protozoan parasite that invades the red blood cells and kills more than 600,000 people globally each year, the majority of whom are children younger than the age of five.

Myriad and ever-changing environmental and social factors determine the distribution of these diseases. Factors affecting the impact of disease transmission include the globalization of travel and trade, climate change, and poor planning of urban areas.

⊕ Historical Background

As long as humans have existed, there have been insect-borne diseases exiting with them and causing problems. Though it was not known at the time, the plagues of the 14th century, including the Black Death and epidemics of yellow fever that hit the New World, were early examples of how insects could transmit severe and deadly diseases to humans.

Although early scholars had some sense there was a connection between certain insects and illness in humans and animals, the concept of arthropods (an invertebrate animal such as an insect, spider, or crustacean) transmitting disease is still relatively new. It was not until 1877 that Scottish physician Sir Patrick Manson (1844–1922) first proved a parasite, *Wuchereria bancrofti* (a human parasitic roundworm that is the major cause of lymphatic filariasis), could be transmitted between people by a mosquito.

Researcher Duane J. Gubler notes in his article "Resurgent Vector-Borne Diseases as a Global Health Problem," published in the journal *Emerging Infectious Diseases*, that "Historically, malaria, dengue, yellow fever, plague, filariasis, louse-borne typhus, trypanosomiasis, leishmaniasis, and other vector-borne diseases were responsible for more human disease and death in the 17th through the early 20th centuries than all other causes combined." In fairly short order, scientists discovered common transmission cycles for malaria (1898), yellow fever (1900), and dengue (1903). According to Gubler, by 1910, it was known that African sleeping sickness, plague, Rocky Mountain spotted fever, relapsing fever, Chagas disease, sandfly fever, and louse-borne

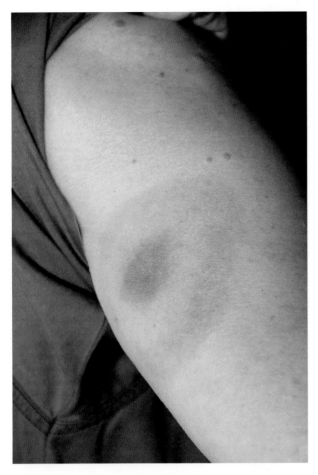

A rash (erythema migrans) in the pattern of a "bull's-eye" is manifested at the site of a tick bite in a patient who subsequently contracted Lyme disease. Approximately 80 percent of those who acquire the disease have such a rash. Lyme disease is caused by the bacterium *Borrelia burgdorferi* and is transmitted to humans by the bite of infected *Ixodes* ticks. Lyme disease patients who are diagnosed early and receive proper antibiotic treatment usually recover rapidly and completely, according to the U.S. Centers for Disease Control and Prevention. Typical symptoms of Lyme disease include rash, fever, headache, and fatigue. If left untreated, infection can spread to joints, the heart, and the nervous system. It is the most common insect-borne disease in the United States and Europe. It also appears in Russia, China, and Japan. Different subspecies of *Borrelia* may cause infection outside the United States and patients may have different symptoms depending on the subspecies. *James Gathany/U.S. Centers for Disease Control and Prevention.*

typhus were all vector-borne diseases transmitted from arthropods to humans.

Still, while scientists were closer to understanding life cycles and transmission of these diseases, by the turn of the 20th century, vector-borne diseases were among the most serious public and animal health problems in the world. Gubler notes that the problem of vector-borne diseases delayed development of major areas. Tens of thousands of men contracted yellow fever and malaria while working on the Panama Canal, the 47.9 mile

(77.1 km) ship canal in Panama that connects the Atlantic Ocean to the Pacific Ocean. In order to attack the problem, scientists and public health officials mounted control and prevention programs aimed at the arthropod vector. The canal was not completed until such diseases were controlled by programs begun in 1905 that hired workers to install mesh screens and fumigate households in the area, as well as eliminating or spraying insecticides in cesspools, standing water, and other breeding grounds for mosquitoes.

Several other areas followed suit, and thus began 50 years of controlling some of the most significant insect-borne diseases. The majority of the programs focused on eliminating the insect breeding sites primarily through the use of DDT (dichlorodiphenyltrichloroethane, a synthetic pesticide) and other residual insecticides to interrupt the transmission cycle.

According to Gubler, by the 1960s, Africa was the only continent still plagued by vector-borne diseases. In North America yellow fever and dengue were eradicated, and both were well-controlled in Central and South America. Malaria was very close to being eliminated in the Americas, the Pacific Islands, and Asia at this time. However, this success did not last long.

By the 1970s, many of these insect-borne diseases began to reemerge and spread into new areas in the ensuing decades. Gubler states that there were a number of interconnected reasons for this decline in control, but two major contributing factors were: "1) the diversion of financial support and subsequent loss of public health infrastructure and 2) reliance on quick-fix solutions such as insecticides and drugs."

⊕ Impacts and Issues

According to the WHO, every year more than 1 billion people are infected with a vector-borne disease. Of those, 1 million people die from these diseases. In a brief written for 2014 World Health Day titled "A Global Brief on Vector-Borne Diseases," the director-general of the WHO, Dr. Margaret Chan, writes in the foreword, "but death counts, though alarming, vastly underestimate the human misery and hardship caused by these diseases, as many people who survive infection are left permanently debilitated, disfigured, maimed, or blind."

For example, in 2014, the WHO estimated that 120 million people were infected with lymphatic filariasis, a parasitic disease caused by microscopic, threadlike worms that live in the lymph system, which maintains the body's fluid balance and fights infections. Of those infected, about 40 million of them had been disfigured and incapacitated by the disease. Chan also notes that other significant consequences include lost productivity, stigma, and social exclusion, particularly for women.

Reported Cases of Human African Trypanosomiasis (*T. b. gambiense*) in 2013

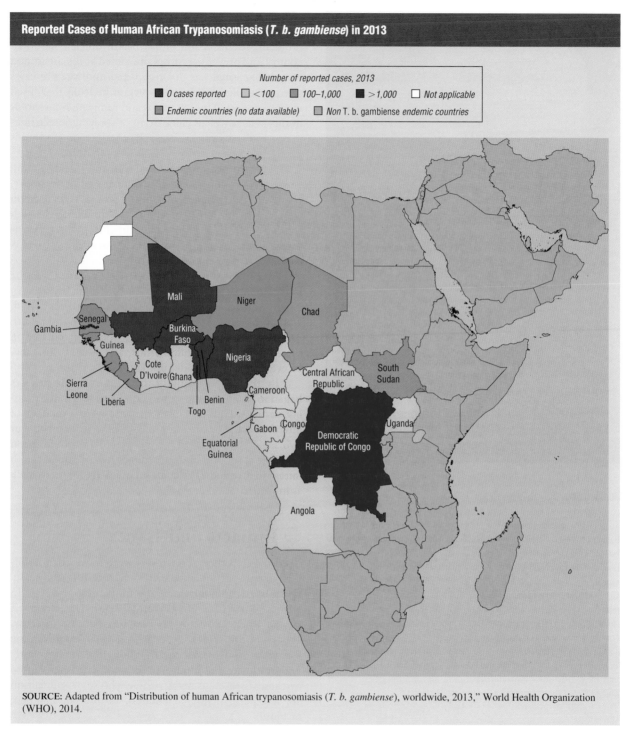

Number of reported cases, 2013

■ 0 cases reported   □ <100   ▨ 100–1,000   ■ >1,000   □ *Not applicable*

▨ *Endemic countries (no data available)*   □ *Non* T. b. gambiense *endemic countries*

SOURCE: Adapted from "Distribution of human African trypanosomiasis (*T. b. gambiense*), worldwide, 2013," World Health Organization (WHO), 2014.

Human African trypanosomiasis is an insect-borne disease carried by tsetse flies that is usually fatal if left untreated. It occurs in 36 countries in sub-Saharan Africa, but the incidence has been decreasing. According to the WHO, in 2009 there were fewer than 10,000 cases reported "for the first time in 50 years." In 2012 the reported number dropped to 7,216 (though the WHO estimates there were 30,000, with many case going unreported).

Vector-borne diseases strike most often in impoverished areas where access to clean water is insufficient, housing is substandard, resources to combat the insects that cause the diseases are limited, and health care infrastructure to provide treatment to those who contract the diseases is absent. This leaves the poorest populations to bear the heaviest burden of these diseases.

What frustrates many public health officials is that many of these diseases were largely eradicated or under control just a few decades ago because of insecticide-based control programs. However, once the diseases were under control and no longer considered a public health threat, resources dried up and the programs abandoned. This enabled several diseases to come back stronger than ever. Now that they have returned, scientists and researchers are starting to see vectors in several countries developing a resistance to the most effective (and affordable) class of insecticides.

Furthermore, historically many of these diseases tended to remain confined to their respective geographic areas. However, this is changing; diseases are showing up in places where they were unknown before. The WHO lists multiple factors in the changes in insect habitat, including "climate change, intensive farming, dams, irrigation, deforestation, population movements, rapid

unplanned urbanization, and phenomenal increases in international travel and trade."

The economic burden of insect-borne diseases is significant for individuals, businesses, and governments. Medical costs and working days lost due to illness are two measurable factors in the calculation of costs. The WHO reports that according to studies from eight countries, 14.8 days and US$514 are lost for each patient who can be treated outside the hospital, and an average of 18.9 days and US$1,491 are lost on each hospitalized patient. When such costs are extrapolated to all vector-borne diseases, including many that are chronic (lingering), the global costs are staggering.

The Diseases

There are dozens of vector-borne diseases, but a handful have a tremendous global impact. The most common have been malaria, leishmaniasis, dengue, and yellow fever.

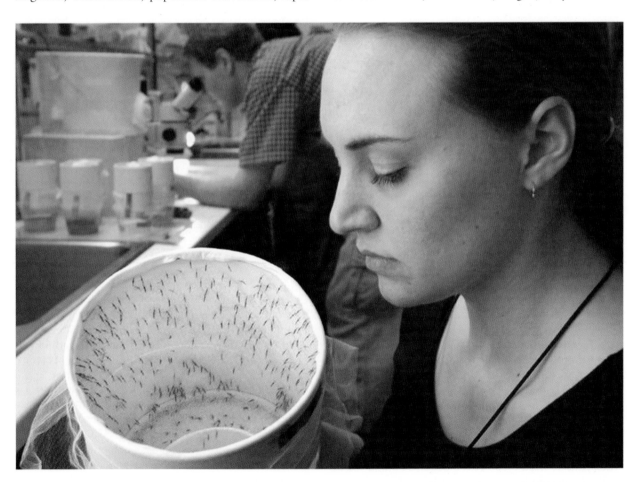

A laboratory technician looks into a sealed cylindrical cardboard container holding a large number of mosquitoes scheduled to undergo testing in a U.S. Centers for Disease Control and Prevention laboratory environment. The container is covered by a thin netting, and the mosquitoes inside alighted on its interior surface, desiring to escape in order to obtain their requisite meal of blood. Although mosquitoes may bite at any time of day, peak biting activity for vectors of some diseases (such as dengue and chikungunya) is during daylight hours. Vectors of other diseases (such as malaria) are most active in twilight periods (dawn and dusk) or in the evening after dark. Avoiding the outdoors or taking preventive actions (such as using repellent) during peak biting hours may reduce risk. Place also matters; ticks and chiggers are often found in grasses and other vegetated areas. Local health officials or guides may be able to point out areas with increased arthropod activity. *James Gathany/U.S. Centers for Disease Control and Prevention.*

GENETICALLY MANIPULATED MOSQUITOES

Research continues into controlling insect populations through the use of pesticides and the proliferation of insect-borne disease through vaccines. However, some other scientists are attempting to manipulate certain insect populations, primarily mosquitoes, genetically to prevent the spread of insect-borne diseases.

There are a few methods for accomplishing this. One of the oldest methods, developed in 1937 and known as the sterile insect technique, uses chemical or physical means to disrupt the natural reproductive process of the insect, rendering it sterile. Early on, this often was done through radiation. Large numbers of these sterilized insects were then released to mate with females in the wild. Although this coupling would produce eggs, the eggs would not hatch. Therefore, over time, the native population of insects would dwindle to the point of extinction as the sterile population grew. Although this method was proven effective, its use was limited because the sterile insects essentially would be carrying carcinogenic materials into the environment.

Another method involves genetically modifying the insect to pass on a lethal gene to its offspring. This has been attempted on male *Aedes aegypti* and *Aedes albopictus*, the mosquitoes responsible for dengue and chikungunya, respectively. To do this, researchers in one study modified the males by inserting protein fragments from coral, cabbage, the herpes virus, and *Escherichia coli* bacteria into the insects. This created a lethal gene that was passed on to the male's offspring when it mated with a native female in the wild. The female would lay eggs, but the offspring would die before reaching maturity.

The British company Oxitec, associated with Oxford University in England, built a facility to develop the genetically modified mosquitoes in Campinas, Brazil. After a series of field trials in 2012 and 2013 during which it released modified male mosquitoes

in several locations, the company claimed to have substantially reduced (in some cases by more than 90 percent) the native population of mosquitoes in the areas tested. The Brazilian government approved the commercial release of the insects in 2014.

Yet another technique being tested focuses on the pathogen itself as opposed to the vector. Female mosquitoes are the only ones that bite, and so they are the ones that spread disease. Dengue, for example, is carried in the mid-gut of the mosquito and then gets pushed up to the salivary glands when the mosquito goes for a blood meal. This is how the pathogen is transmitted to the human host. However, scientists have found a way to modify the mosquito genetically so that the dengue pathogen does not move to the salivary glands. So far studies have shown this method to be effective.

Still another method being used injects naturally occurring bacteria called *Wolbachia* to try to curb the spread of dengue. This bacteria, which is actually present in 60 percent of insects, essentially vaccinates the mosquito against the virus. The idea then is to release the males but also vaccinated females for them to mate with in the hopes that eventually the modified, vaccinated population will overtake and replace the native dengue-ridden bunch.

With the first ever reports to the WHO of dengue in Croatia and France in 2010, and an outbreak on the Madeira Islands of Portugal in 2012, there is cause for concern of outbreaks in Europe. Cases also were reported in Florida (United States) and the Yunnan Province of China in 2013.

Many of these techniques have received criticism from those who are concerned about the unintended consequences of creating a genetically modified species of bug and releasing it in the wild. For them, questions remain about what effects these insects will have on humans and native ecology.

Malaria   Malaria is caused by the *Plasmodium* parasite (any of five different species) and is transmitted by female *Anopheles* mosquitoes. Early symptoms typically include fever, headache, chills, and vomiting. There are a variety of drugs available for treatment of malaria, however, treatment should begin as soon as possible. If not treated within the first 24 hours, the most serious form of the diseases (*P. falciparum* malaria) can worsen the symptoms and lead to death. Children with severe malaria frequently develop symptoms that include anemia, respiratory distress, or cerebral malaria, which is when parasite-filled blood cells block small blood vessels to the brain, causing swelling and brain damage. Even with effective treatment, relapses can occur.

About 3.4 billion people in 97 countries are at risk of acquiring malaria. Most deaths occur among children living in Africa. And, according to the WHO, the risk is greatest in sub-Saharan Africa, an area that accounts for an estimated 90 percent of all malaria deaths. The Democratic Republic of the Congo and Nigeria alone account

for 40 percent of all malaria deaths. There were about 198 million cases of malaria in 2013 and an estimated 584,000 deaths. However, malaria mortality rates among children in Africa were reduced by an estimated 58 percent between 2000 and 2013, according to the WHO.

Leishmaniasis   Annually there are an estimated 1.3 million new cases and 20,000 to 30,000 deaths from leishmaniasis. Infected sand flies are the carriers of the *Leishmania* parasite, which causes leishmaniasis. The disease has three main forms. The most common form is cutaneous leishmaniasis, which causes skin lesions (either under the skin or ulcerative) that can last from weeks to years. In some cases, when the lesions become ulcerative they may become infected with bacteria. The lesions usually heal on their own, but often leave scars. The mucocutaneous form of leishmaniasis affects the mucous membranes, and if left untreated can lead to partial or total destruction of mucous membranes of the nose, mouth, and throat. Visceral leishmaniases, also known as kala-azar, is the most

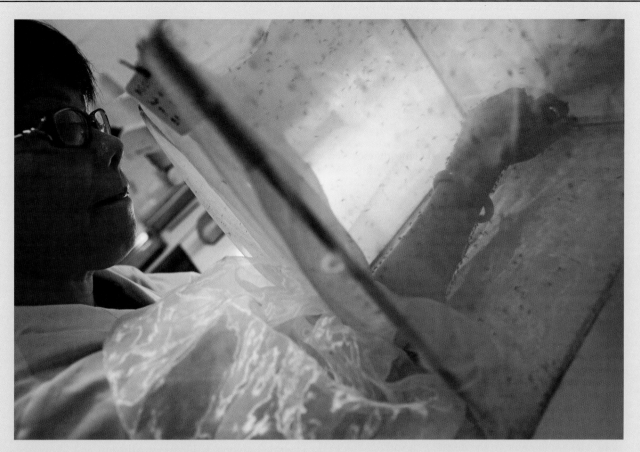

In this photo taken on September 1, 2013, scientist Nguyen Thi Yen blood feeds a cage of mosquitoes in her lab in Hanoi, Vietnam. The mosquitoes are being reared with *Wolbachia* bacteria that works as a natural vaccine to keep them from becoming infected with the virus that causes dengue. About 2.5 billion are at risk globally for dengue, with 70 percent of those living in the WHO Western Pacific Region, according to the WHO. © *Na Son Nguyen/AP Photo.*

serious form of leishmaniasis. Symptoms include fever, weight loss, and swelling of the spleen and liver. This form of the disease is fatal without treatment.

According to the WHO, leishmaniasis generally is associated with people are malnourished or have weak immune systems, displaced populations, people who live in areas with substandard housing or sleep outside or on the ground, and people living in areas in which resources such as indoor spraying with pesticides are not available. In addition to poverty increasing the risk of acquiring the disease, it can also impact the progression of the disease. People who are already impoverished and do not have the economic means to afford food or shelter also may not be able to pay to seek treatment.

Dengue Fever Dengue fever is transmitted by the *Aedes aegypti* and *Aedes albopictus* mosquitoes. Symptoms include high fever; severe headache; nausea and vomiting; swollen glands; rash; and joint, muscle, and bone pain. The latter has led to dengue's nickname,

"break-bone fever." Though only about 2.5 percent of affected people die of dengue itself, dengue infection can progress to dengue hemorrhagic fever (DHF), which is potentially fatal. DHF starts with a high fever then progresses to persistent vomiting, severe abdominal pain, difficulty breathing, circulatory system failure, shock, and death. According to the U.S. Centers for Disease Control and Prevention (CDC), there is no specific medication available to treat dengue fever or DHF, though patients are usually given fluid replacement therapy, preferably under medical supervision in a hospital.

The WHO estimates that an estimated 40 percent of the world's population (2.5 billion people) are at risk of dengue. An estimated 100 million dengue infections occur worldwide every year, with about 500,000 people with DHF requiring hospitalization.

According to the WHO, dengue "is the most rapidly spreading mosquito-borne viral disease in the world." In addition, it tends to erupt in large outbreaks, overwhelming health systems in the areas that are impacted.

The number of cases has increased dramatically since the 1960s—more than 30 times by some estimates. Dengue epidemics also have become prevalent in more countries (traveling from about nine countries in the 1970s to more than 100 as of 2014) and moved from rural into urban areas. The Americas, Southeast Asia, and the Western Pacific Regions are the most seriously affected, with more than 2.3 million cases reported in 2010, according to the WHO.

Yellow Fever Yellow fever is a viral hemorrhagic fever transmitted by mosquitoes in the *Haemagogus* and *Aedes* genera between monkeys and humans. The first phase of the disease is characterized by fever, muscle pain, headache, shivers, loss of appetite, nausea, and vomiting. After three to four days, most of those infected improve and eventually get better. Those that do not, about 15 percent, enter a toxic phase where the fever returns, the person develops jaundice and sometimes bleeding along with bloody vomit, and the kidneys begin to fail. Treatment for yellow fever is limited; the CDC recommends fluids, rest, and medications to help with fever and pain, preferably administered in a hospital setting where a patient can be observed. About 50 percent of patients who enter the toxic phase die within a two-week period.

Though there is a vaccine for yellow fever, about 200,000 cases of illness and 30,000 deaths are reported every year. Yellow fever has become much more common over the past few decades as a result of decreasing populations who are immune to the disease as it spreads due to climate change and other factors. According to the WHO, outbreaks have occurred in seasonal workers and in nomadic and displaced people in several African countries.

⊕ Future Implications

Climate change is expected to have a significant impact on the transmission and proliferation of insect-borne diseases, although how much remains to be seen. What is known is that variations in temperature and rainfall can affect the transmission of vector-borne diseases along with changes in agricultural practices based on those same factors. More study is needed in this area to determine the precise impact of climate change on vector-borne diseases into the future.

The most effective method thus far for controlling insect-borne diseases is targeting the vectors themselves. This is especially effective against diseases that already can be prevented by vaccine or easily treated. In these cases, vector control acts as a complementary measure that can shrink the disease burden faster. For those diseases that do not yet have vaccines, such as dengue and chikungunya, vector control is especially important. Vector-control programs typically use a variety of interventions, including indoor residual spraying and releasing natural insect predators.

However, one of the challenges to vector-control programs is the spread of vectors that have increasing insecticide resistance. In fact, most species of insects are showing some resistance to four out of six classes of insecticides. If new insecticides or alternate and effective options for controlling vector populations are not forthcoming, it could have a devastating effect on the successful efforts previously made in combating malaria and other vector-borne diseases. More research is needed in these areas to find effective alternatives.

In addition to reemerging insect-borne diseases, public health officials also are contending with diseases such as dengue, chikungunya, and West Nile virus emerging in new areas. For example, the primary vector for dengue, the *Aedes aegypti* mosquito, has been found in more than 20 European countries whereas previously it was seen only in Africa, Asia, and the Indian subcontinent. Furthermore, this same mosquito species carried chikungunya to the Caribbean islands, and in July 2014, the first non-travel-related case was reported in the United States, in Florida, according to the CDC.

In addition, some new insect-borne diseases have been discovered. One such disease, the Heartland virus, was discovered in 2012 in the state of Missouri. Scientists assert that the Lone Star tick, naturally occurring primarily in the southeastern and eastern United States, is the vector of this disease. According to the CDC, as of March 2014, eight cases of Heartland virus disease were identified among residents of Missouri and Tennessee. Most patients required hospitalization, and one died.

Scientists still are attempting to learn more about the disease, but so far they report that all of victims were sickened between May and September; had a fever; felt very tired; and complained of headaches, muscle aches, diarrhea, loss of appetite, or feeling sick to their stomach. Additionally, they all had low numbers of cells that fight infection and that help blood clot.

PRIMARY SOURCE

Malaria

SOURCE *Wellcome Library, London. From* The Prevention of Malaria *by Ronald Ross; with contributions by L. O. Howard [and others]. London: John Murray, 1910.*

INTRODUCTION *This primary source from 1910 shows an advertisement for wire gauze mosquito screens to keep out the insects, which carry a variety of insect-borne diseases, including malaria. Such preventive measures are still effectively utilized over 100 years after this advertisement was printed to keep mosquitos and other carriers of insect-borne diseases at bay.*

WIRE GAUZE
MOSQUITO SCREENS

CHRISTIE'S OXYDIZED BRONZE MOSQUITO GAUZE

Strongest and most Durable

Outlasts many renewals of any other quality

BRASS AND GALVANIZED GAUZE
for Windows, Doors, etc.

SAMPLES AND FULL PARTICULARS FROM

GEORGE CHRISTIE, LTD.
LADYWELL WIRE WORKS
GOVAN, GLASGOW

Telegrams and Cables:
"LADYWELL, GLASGOW."

SEE ALSO *Dengue; Malaria*

BIBLIOGRAPHY

Books

Lemon, Stanley M., et al. *Vector-Borne Diseases: Understanding the Environmental, Human Health, and Ecological Connections: Workshop Summary.* Washington, DC: National Academies Press, 2008.

Sree Hari Rao, Vadrevu, and Ravi Durvasula, eds. *Dynamic Models of Infectious Disease,* Vol. 1: *Vector-Borne Diseases.* London: Springer, 2013.

Periodicals

Berg, Henk Van Den, et al. "Global Trends in the Use of Insecticides to Control Vector-Borne Diseases." *Environmental Health Perspectives* 120, no. 4 (April 1, 2012): 577–582.

Bezirtzoglou, C., K. Dekas, and E. Charvalos. "Climate Changes, Environment and Infection: Facts, Scenarios and Growing Awareness from the Public Health Community within Europe." *Anaerobe* 17, no. 6 (December 2011): 347–340. Available online at http://www.ncbi.nlm.nih.gov/pubmed/21664978 (accessed January 30, 2015).

Gubler, Duane J. "Resurgent Vector-Borne Diseases as a Global Health Problem." *Emerging Infectious Diseases* 4, no. 3 (July 1998): 442–450. Available online at http://wwwnc.cdc.gov/eid/article/4/3/98-0326_article (accessed February 5, 2015).

Sutherst, Robert W. "Global Change and Human Vulnerability to Vector-Borne Diseases." *Clinical Microbiology Reviews* 17, no. 1 (January 2004): 136–173. Available online at http://www.ncbi.nlm.nih.gov/pmc/articles/PMC321469/ (accessed January 30, 2015).

Websites

Alexander, Renée. "Engineering Mosquitoes to Spread Health." *Atlantic,* September 13, 2014. http://www.theatlantic.com/health/archive/2014/09/engineering-mosquitoes-to-stop-disease/379247/ (accessed January 30, 2015).

"Division of Vector-Borne Diseases (DVBD)." *U.S. Centers for Disease Control and Prevention (CDC).* http://www.cdc.gov/ncezid/dvbd/ (accessed January 30, 2015).

Ellis, Brett, and Bruce A. Wilcox. "The Ecological Dimensions of Vector-Borne Disease Research and Control." *Cadernos De Saúde Pública* 25, suppl. 1, 2009. http://www.scielo.br/scielo.php?script=sci_arttext&pid=S0102-311X2009001300015 (accessed January 30, 2015).

European Centre for Disease Prevention and Control (ECDC) and WHO Regional Office for Europe. "Lyme Borreliosis in Europe." *European Centre for Disease Prevention and Control (ECDC).* http://ecdc.europa.eu/en/healthtopics/vectors/world-health-day-2014/Documents/factsheet-lyme-borreliosis.pdf (accessed April 29, 2015).

"A Global Brief on Vector-Borne Diseases." *World Health Organization (WHO),* 2014. http://apps.who.int/iris/bitstream/10665/111008/1/WHO_DCO_WHD_2014.1_eng.pdf (accessed January 30, 2015).

"Heartland Virus." *U.S. Centers for Disease Control and Prevention (CDC).* http://www.cdc.gov/ncezid/dvbd/heartland/ (accessed January 30, 2015).

"Leishmaniasis," Fact Sheet No. 375. *World Health Organization (WHO),* Updated February 2015. http://www.who.int/mediacentre/factsheets/fs375/en/ (accessed January 30, 2015).

"Leishmaniasis FAQs." *U.S. Centers for Disease Control and Prevention (CDC).* http://www.cdc.gov/parasites/leishmaniasis/gen_info/faqs.html (accessed January 30, 2015).

"Malaria," Fact Sheet No. 94. *World Health Organization (WHO)*, Updated December 2014. http://www.who.int/mediacentre/factsheets/fs094/en/ (accessed January 30, 2015).

"Oxitec's Genetically Engineered Mosquitoes in Panama Pilot Achieve over 90 Percent Control of the Mosquito Responsible for Outbreaks of Dengue Fever and Chikungunya." *PR Newswire*. http://www.prnewswire.com/news-releases/oxitecs-genetically-engineered-mosquitoes-in-panama-pilot-achieve-over-90-control-of-the-mosquito-responsible-for-outbreaks-of-dengue-fever-and-chikungunya-289887861.html (accessed January 30, 2015.

St. Fleur, Nicholas. "The Genetically-Modified Mosquito Bite." *Atlantic*, January 27, 2015. http://www.theatlantic.com/health/archive/2015/01/Genetically-Modified-Mosquitoes-May-Be-Released-in-Florida-Keys/384859/ (accessed January 30, 2015).

"Vector-Borne Diseases," Fact Sheet No. 387. *World Health Organization (WHO)*, March 2014. http://www.who.int/mediacentre/factsheets/fs387/en/ (accessed January 30, 2015).

Melanie R. Plenda

International Health Regulations, Surveillance, and Enforcement

⊕ Introduction

The International Health Regulations (IHR), adopted as an international treaty by the World Health Organization (WHO) in 2005, represented a shift in international law that addressed a variety of public health risks that were increasingly regarded as global concerns. IHR is a legally binding framework for 194 countries across the world to cooperate in monitoring, preventing, controlling, and responding to threats to their citizens' health.

Throughout history, diseases have known no borders and have spread and killed without prejudice. Now, in a globalized society, where people and goods cross borders routinely and rapidly, diseases can spread across the globe with ease, putting all populations at risk. In response, IHR is designed to strengthen collective defenses and facilitate information exchange, without impeding international travel and commerce.

As infectious diseases continue to emerge and reemerge, surveillance of public health risks is crucial to detecting potential threats and formulating a coordinated response. IHR implements a new and far-reaching surveillance regime that enhances the WHO's authority while placing more obligations on its member states. IHR requires countries to greatly boost their national surveillance and reporting systems, as it also strengthens international surveillance and response capacity. In addition, IHR establishes new provisions to make enforcement easier, while applying humanitarian principles to public health interventions and responses.

IHR is a critical contribution to global public health safety and represents a major departure from previous international health law regimes. The global community now has a legal system for working together to combat threats to public health, making surveillance and cooperation its touchstone. Though IHR has many facets, dimensions, and provisions, they can broadly be divided into two areas: rebuilding and reordering of the international surveillance infrastructure and implementing new actions by states to report and respond to public health

risks. Since the adoption of the new regulations, existing public health programs have been improved while new activities have been successfully established. With its surveillance enhancements, international legal framework, and respect for human rights, IHR characterizes a new era of global cooperation in public health safety.

⊕ Historical Background

The origins of IHR can be traced back to 19th-century efforts to combat diseases. Specifically, the cholera epidemics that ravaged Europe between 1830 and 1847 demonstrated the need for diplomatic and international cooperation to prevent and control outbreaks, according to David Fidler's article, "From International Sanitary Conventions to Global Health Security: The New International Health Regulations" in the *Chinese Journal of International Law*. At the time, merchants and traders encountered a patchwork of national quarantine regulations that impaired commerce and travel. These international efforts manifested themselves in the first International Sanitary Conference in Paris in 1851. At the conference, organized by the French government, standardized international regulations and quarantine procedures for cholera, yellow fever, and plague were proposed.

On the first World Health Day on April 7, 1948, the constitution of the WHO came into force, making the WHO the first specialized agency of the United Nations to which every member subscribed. Prior to the WHO, states had negotiated ad-hoc treaties that were cumbersome and difficult to adapt to different circumstances and new science. Throughout the history of the WHO, member states have had the ability, through the World Health Assembly (WHA), to create and adopt new regulations designed to prevent the spread of disease. According to the WHO's "Frequently Asked Questions about the International Health Regulations (2005)," in 1951, the first of these new regulations, the International Sanitary

Regulations, were adopted by the member states. In 1969, the 22nd WHA revised the International Sanitary Regulations and renamed them the International Health Regulations.

In 1969, IHR was designed to monitor cholera, plague, yellow fever, smallpox, relapsing fever, and typhus. However, member states were required to notify the WHO only if cholera, plague, and yellow fever had been reported. Minor changes were made to IHR in 1973 and 1981, but it would only be in the 1990s that calls for revisions and modification would grow.

According to the WHO, in the early 1990s, the resurgence of infectious diseases, including the reappearance of plague in India and cholera in South America and emergence of new diseases like Ebola virus disease, highlighted deficiencies in the decades-old regulations. In addition, the 1969 regulations were inapplicable in cases of spreading endemic diseases, such as malaria and tuberculosis, and also failed to address new diseases including HIV/AIDS. In 1995, WHA, the main policy-making organ of the WHO, began the process of revising existing regulations because of doubts about their ability to monitor and contain the international spread of disease.

The limitations of the 1969 regulations included a narrow purview, dependence upon official country notification of spreading diseases, and lack of an international mechanism to coordinate efforts to halt the spread of diseases and threats to public health. The increase of trade and travel in recent decades has given rise to increased risks and a multitude of new challenges to public health safety, necessitating revision of the decades-old regulations. In addition, notification proved difficult under the old international health regime; countries lacking confidence in the system were reluctant to disrupt trade and travel with new regulations, according to the WHO.

As a result, the WHO began to approach the issue of public health safety with a broader view of globalized society and the challenges that come with it, according to David P. Fidler and Lawrence Gostin in their article, "The New International Health Regulations: An Historic Development for International Law and Public Health" in the *Journal of Law, Medicine, and Ethics*. In 1998, the WHO proposed using nongovernmental data sources to improve detection; in 2001, the WHA passed a resolution calling on the WHO to support member states in building their capacity to identify and respond to health threats and possible emergencies. In May 2003, a WHA resolution established an intergovernmental work group (IGWG), open to all member states, to study and recommend revisions to the existing international health regulations. The 2003 outbreak of severe acute respiratory syndrome (SARS) caused the revision process to accelerate, as the WHO's response to SARS was seen as a testrun for the ideas being proposed in the revision process. After two sessions of IGWG, WHA voted to adopt IHR on May 23 2005, and the regulations came into force on June 15, 2007.

⊕ Impacts and Issues

Characteristics of the International Health Regulations

The new IHR consists of 66 articles divided into 10 parts with 9 appendexes. Although aspects of the new regulations may resemble older iterations of global public health regimes, IHR offers a comprehensive change to classical international health law. Through a new legal framework, IHR facilitates rapid information gathering and clarifies what constitutes a public health emergency along with the appropriate international response.

According to Article 2, the purpose and scope of IHR is "to prevent, protect against, control, and provide a public health response to the international spread of disease in ways that are commensurate with and restricted to public health risks, and which avoid unnecessary interference with international traffic and trade." Unlike previous regulations, which only applied to a short list of infectious diseases, the new regulations address public health risks regardless of their origin. This catchall strategy embodies a shift in public health, as the risk to human life plays a larger role in calculations than trade and economic considerations.

In addition, the IHR outlines core capacities that each of the countries should have had in place by 2012. The WHO monitors the progress toward each capacity through reports provided by the countries. Some of these capacities, according to the "IHR Core Capacity Monitoring Framework" include:

1. National legislation, policy and financing
2. Coordination and national focal point (NFP) communications
3. Surveillance
4. Response
5. Preparedness
6. Risk communication
7. Human resources
8. Laboratory services

Other core capacities are shown in the graph, along with the percent of countries reporting implementation of each.

Human Rights Principles

In addition to the expansion of its scope, IHR also represents the inclusion and primacy of international human rights. Now, the enforcement of IHR must be done "with full respect for the dignity, human rights, and fundamental freedoms of persons," according to Article 3. As a result, the regulations require states to identify public health risks that justify the imposition of health measures, which should be undertaken in a transparent

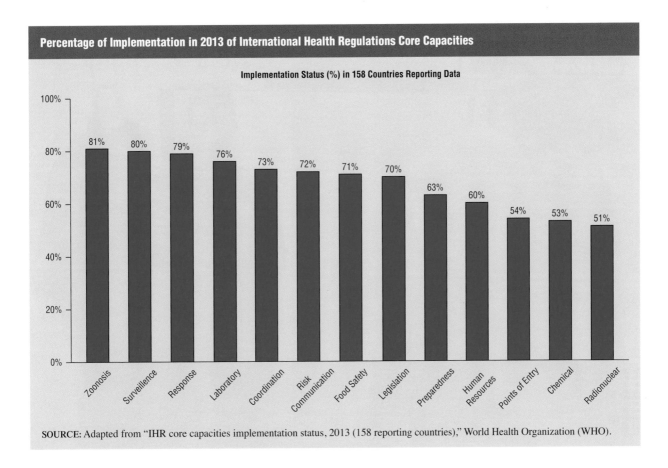

Percentage of Implementation in 2013 of International Health Regulations Core Capacities

Implementation Status (%) in 158 Countries Reporting Data

SOURCE: Adapted from "IHR core capacities implementation status, 2013 (158 reporting countries)," World Health Organization (WHO).

and nondiscriminatory fashion. States must also respect the rights, dignities, and freedom of travelers, taking measures to treat them courteously and to minimize their inconvenience. In addition, states should consider the traveler's gender, sociocultural, ethnic, or religious concerns. They must provide "adequate food and water, appropriate accommodation and clothing, protection for baggage and other possessions, appropriate medical treatment, means of necessary communication … and other appropriate assistance for travellers who are quarantined, isolated or subject to medical examinations or other procedures for public health purposes," according to Article 32. This means that human rights principles should now be applied to any implementation of the IHR laws.

IHR also espouses the principles of informed consent and respect. Under the new regulations, states must get consent from travelers before implementing any health measures, except when quarantine is required, according to Article 23. In the case of compulsory health measures, states must still offer the least invasive medical examinations, while being free to vaccinate and take other actions under their own prerogative.

The right to privacy is also protected in the new regulations. States are required to maintain confidentiality of personal information and records received from other states, international health organizations, and the WHO,

according to Article 45. The WHO is also required to maintain confidential records and, upon request, must allow individuals to access and review any personal identifying information. In addition, states must ensure that any disclosure or use of personal information to address risks to public health will be done with protection of individual privacy in mind.

Main Functions: Notification

IHR requires states to notify the WHO of any events or threats that might constitute a public health emergency, in addition to responding to requests for international cooperation and verification. This allows the WHO to ensure collaboration and cooperation between member states in situations when public health is at risk. Also, in serious circumstances, notification informs states of required actions to be taken in response to a health emergency. States use a decision instrument to determine whether an disease outbreak or event constitutes a public health emergency that warrants international notification.

The new notification provisions reflect a more rigorous approach to addressing the spread of international diseases. The requirements place great emphasis on states' abilities to use surveillance to locate potential public health risks, make determinations about best practices for response, and effectively manage such threats.

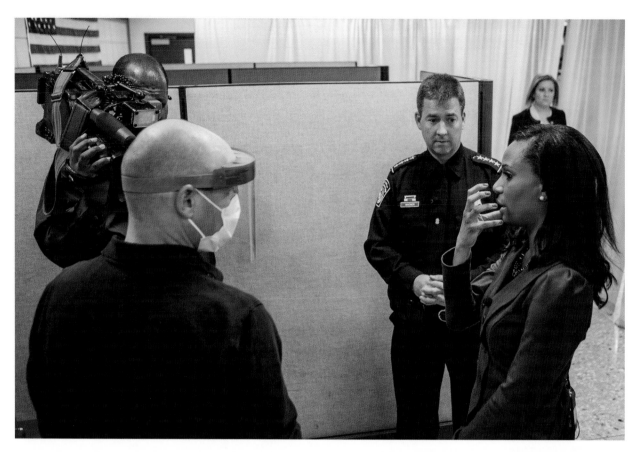

In October 2014, White House communications reporters get a facility tour of Washington, D.C.'s Dulles International Airport from representatives from U.S. Customs and Border Protection (CBP) and Centers for Disease Control and Prevention. They showed them the process a passenger would go through if he or she were flagged as possibly having Ebola, or flying in from a country where Ebola is prevalent. Wearing his protective face mask and face shield, a CBP officer demonstrates how a passenger interview would be conducted. In October, CBP began enhanced passenger processing protocols at Chicago O'Hare International Airport, Dulles International Airport, Hartsfield-Jackson Atlanta International Airport, and Newark International Airport to allow for enhanced screening of more than 94 percent of travelers from Ebola-affected regions to the United States. *Josh Denmark/U.S. Customs and Border Protection/U.S. Centers for Disease Control and Prevention.*

Main Functions: Surveillance

The new IHR Article 5 regarding surveillance requires states "to develop, strengthen, and maintain ... the capacity to detect, assess, notify and report events." Surveillance is central to guiding international action for prevention and response to global public health risks and threats. According to Article 1 of IHR, surveillance is "the systematic ongoing collection, collation, and analysis of data for public health purposes and the timely dissemination of public health information for assessment and public health response as necessary." The new surveillance provisions and obligations far outpace the 1969 regulations, which did not require building a surveillance infrastructure, only requiring states to notify the WHO of a disease outbreak, according to Michael Baker and David Fidler in their article, "Global Public Health Surveillance under New International Health Regulations" in the journal *Emerging Infectious Diseases.*

The new IHR also identifies health-related events that require member states to notify the WHO. States must notify the WHO of all events that might constitute a public health emergency of international concern, regardless of its origin or source, according to Articles 6 and 7. IHR also requires states to inform the WHO of any public health risks identified outside their territories that might cause international disease to spread through exported or imported human cases, vectors that may carry infection or contamination, or contaminated goods, according to Article 9. IHR defines a "public health emergency of international concern" (PHEIC) as a "public health risk to other States through the international spread of disease," which potentially requires a "coordinated international response."

Unlike previous regulations, which encompassed only three communicable diseases, the new IHR defines disease as an "illness or medical condition, irrespective of origin or source, that presents or could present significant harm to humans," according to Article 1. This includes communicable and noncommunicable diseases that are naturally occurring, accidentally caused, or created deliberately (as in the case of bioterrorism). IHR provides guidance for states to comply with its surveillance provisions by means of a decision instrument that helps states identify PHEICs. The decision instrument helps determine the public health impact of a disease event and how likely it is to spread internationally.

IHR also guides countries in making public health assessments by providing a list of diseases, including smallpox, poliomyelitis (polio), human influenza caused by new subtypes, and SARS, for which even a single case is a PHEIC and requires reporting to the WHO. Several other diseases appear on a list for which a single case would require use of the decision instrument to determine the next steps. In addition, IHR also encourages states to communicate with the WHO about any events that might be relevant to public health, even though they do not warrant notification, according to Article 8.

Baker and Fidler argue that the new IHR's expansion of public health events under surveillance and its risk-oriented decision tools enhance effective surveillance of

emerging infectious diseases (diseases that have appeared recently or have been expanding rapidly). In addition to notifying the WHO about events that may constitute a PHEIC within 24 hours of assessment, IHR also requires states to report any "health measure implemented in response to those events," according to Article 6. In addition, according to Article 43, states must inform the WHO within 48 hours if they implement health measures that interfere with international trade and travel, unless recommended by the WHO director-general.

Components of the IHR surveillance regime include requirements for states to develop capabilities to detect, assess, and report diseases from local to national level. Officials must also be able to report notifications via national focal points (NFP), mandated national centers designed to communicate with the WHO and disseminate relevant information throughout the country. This creates a global network for rapidly delivering and communicating real-time public health information about potential communicable disease outbreaks and other threats.

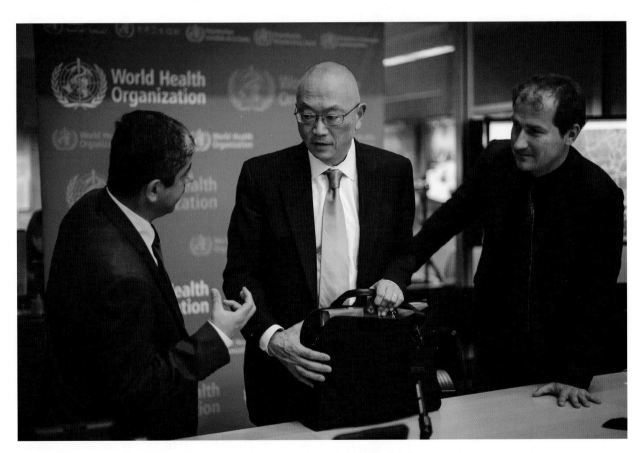

World Health Organization (WHO) assistant director-general for health security Keiji Fukuda (center) speaks with a journalist on May 14, 2014, in Geneva, Switzerland, at the end of a press conference following closed-door emergency talks on the deadly MERS virus. At that time, the Middle East respiratory syndrome coronavirus (MERS-CoV) had killed 152 people in Saudi Arabia and sparked alarm over its spread elsewhere, the United Nations health agency said. Though several IHR emergency meetings regarding the disease were held in the next several months, in February 2015, after the 8th IHR Emergency Committee regarding MERS-CoV, it was again "unanimously concluded that the conditions for a Public Health Emergency of International Concern (PHEIC) have not been met." *© Fabrice Coffrini/AFP/Getty Images.*

H1N1

Few diseases pose a greater threat of becoming a pandemic than influenza. The International Health Regulations (IHR) were designed with influenza in mind. The outbreak of SARS in 2002 helped shape the creation of IHR and its response specifications, and the 2009 outbreak of H1N1, a subtype of influenza A virus, was the first event to activate provisions of IHR. The regulations describe the roles and responsibilities of an individual country and the World Health Organization (WHO) in determining how to manage public health emergencies that may spread internationally. The WHO's response to H1N1 serves as a case study for the implementation of IHR, according to Harvey V. Fineberg in his article, "Pandemic Preparedness and Response—Lessons from the H1N1 Influenza of 2009" in the *New England Journal of Medicine*.

The disease was first detected in February and March 2009 in the United States, Canada, and Mexico, where patients were showing novel flu symptoms. By the end of April, the virus was detected in several countries across the globe, leading the WHO to convene an emergency committee, declare a public health emergency, and call for regulations under its new IHR powers. By June 2009, the disease had spread to more than 70 countries and 26,000 cases were laboratory-confirmed, leading the WHO to declare that H1N1 had become a full-fledged pandemic. According to Fineberg, the WHO offered advice and coordination to national influenza-preparedness plans, which the majority of countries had developed by the first outbreak in North America; such plans assisted with monitoring IHR core capacities. Fineberg also notes that the "WHO Global Influenza Surveillance Network detected, identified, and characterized the virus in a timely manner and monitored the course of the pandemic." In addition, the WHO provided early recommendations for vaccines and offered critical organization and field assistance, distributing more than 3 million antiviral drugs in affected countries.

IHR also provided a framework and legal guidance to deal with the H1N1 outbreak. Mandated surveillance, response, and early-warning systems all proved essential to the public health effort. Crucially, the national focal points (NFPs) provided hubs in member states where countries could communicate easily and plan an international response. The new decision instrument for deciding what warrants a public health emergency was implemented with ease, allowing the WHO to work quickly in confirming the global scope of the problem.

Though IHR aided the identification and response to the H1N1 pandemic, difficulties with its implementation also offer lessons for the future. Few countries responded to the WHO's questionnaire on building their core capacities, and of those that did respond, Fineberg notes that "only 10% claimed to have fully established the capacities called for by IHR."

IHR also failed to specify a program for vaccine sharing and virus sharing, which would allow countries to share pandemic influenza virus samples to facilitate preparedness and international vaccine development. However, this was subsequently addressed in the pandemic-influenza preparedness framework adopted in 2011. IHR's most significant shortcoming remains its inability to offer an enforcement mechanism, such as sanctions, to confirm and build the capacities that IHR requires.

Creating and maintaining such surveillance capabilities requires significant financial resources, which states must allocate on their own. However, the WHO is required to assist states in meeting core surveillance obligations, though the regulations do not allocate funds for this purpose. States are also required to collaborate with each other, providing logistical support and financial means to maintain national and international surveillance capabilities.

Main Functions: Information Verification, Declaration, and Recommendations

In the past, the WHO was required to use information provided by states, which made response difficult when states refused to provide proper notification or did not cooperate. Under the new regulations, states are required to comply with verification requests, and the WHO is allowed to consider information from nongovernmental sources and other state parties. Globalization has greatly decreased the ability of states to restrict and control information about diseases and public health threats, making nongovernmental sources crucial to constructing a cooperative and sharing global surveillance infrastructure.

For the first time, IHR also empowers the WHO to declare a PHEIC, while requiring states to notify the WHO of any disease events that might constitute a PHEIC. Once a PHEIC has been declared, the WHO has the power to issue temporary, nonbinding recommendations for ways to respond. The director-general also has the ability to issue standing recommendations for routine application to specific ongoing public health risks. States are not bound by WHO recommendations, but responses to health risks and emergencies must not be overly invasive and must demonstrate a basis in science and respect for human rights. IHR also contains provisions for obtaining independent technical advice to implement the regulations but does not authorize an enforcement mechanism to confirm compliance. As a result, the lack of enforceable sanctions allows countries to not comply with the IHR without fear of any financial penalties or trade sanctions.

Implementation

Though the regulations were adopted in 2005, they only came into force in 2007. Since then, existing programs have been enhanced, national capacities have been boosted, and new activities have been tested and adopted, according to Maxwell Charles Hardiman and the WHO Department of Global Capacities, Alert, and Response. Their article, "World Health Organization Perspective on Implementation of International Health Regulations" appeared in the journal *Emerging Infectious Diseases*. One example of the world's commitment to successful implementation of IHR is the establishment of NFPs in all but one of the WHA member states. Critical to the regulations, NFPs have provided proactive and diligent engagement and communication between member states, the WHO, and the international community.

In addition to NFPs, IHR rules on monitoring national surveillance and response capacities have been successfully adopted with the use of checklists and an annual technical questionnaire. IHR has also fostered international collaboration at points of entry and cooperation in dealing with pandemic influenza. In addition, the WHO tested three pilot IHR-implementation courses over the course of several years. According to Hardiman and colleagues, the courses created "a global harmonized understanding and application of the IHR framework." The content of the courses was evaluated, showing it "was relevant to participants' work, improved their understanding of IHR, and increased their confidence when dealing with the topic." However, the fourth of such courses, scheduled for March 2013, was canceled due to what the WHO termed "unexpected financial constraints." However, it appears that the direct effects of IHR implementation have increased surveillance capacities, international communication, and coordination.

⊕ Future Implications

By the end of 2014, 63 countries out of 195 WHO member states had declared that core capacity requirements mandated by IHR had been met; the remainder either asked for extensions or had yet to communicate their intentions to the WHO. An IHR Review Committee considered extension requests and advised the director-general on technical matters such as standing recommendations, functioning of the regulations, and possible amendments. Progress is being made slowly in fostering collaboration through the WHO, while building national surveillance and response capabilities.

The IHR Emergency Committee, a group of independent experts that offers advice and helps the director-general determine whether a particular event is a PHEIC, convened three times in 2014 to address the threat of Ebola across the globe. The committee focused on the outbreaks in Guinea, Liberia, and Sierra Leone, where the number of Ebola cases continued into early 2015. By May 2015, the Ebola outbreak was declared over in Liberia, and was waning in the other two countries. As part of its commitment to facilitating travel and

trade while safeguarding public health, the committee urged member states not to adopt travel bans, arguing that such restrictions would cause economic difficulty and increase the uncontrolled migration of people from affected countries, raising the risk of Ebola spreading internationally. The committee and the collaboration between countries with the WHO exemplify the best of what IHR represents: international cooperation and concern for public health.

PRIMARY SOURCE

International Health Regulations (2005), 2nd Edition

SOURCE International Health Regulations (2005), 2nd Edition. *Geneva: World Health Organization (WHO), 2008, 10–12. http://whqlibdoc. who.int/publications/2008/9789241580410_ eng.pdf?ua=1 (accessed January 25, 2015).*

INTRODUCTION *This primary source is excerpted from the second edition of the International Health Regulations put forth by the World Health Organization (WHO), which is responsible for "the management of the global regime for the control of the international spread of disease." All WHO member states are bound by these regulations in their handling of public health risks. The excerpted sections define the purpose and scope and guiding principles of the regulations and give information regarding some of the surveillance and notification measures put in place by the WHO.*

INTERNATIONAL HEALTH REGULATIONS (2005)

PART I—DEFINITIONS, PURPOSE AND SCOPE, PRINCIPLES AND RESPONSIBLE AUTHORITIES

Article 2 Purpose and scope
The purpose and scope of these Regulations are to prevent, protect against, control and provide a public health response to the international spread of disease in ways that are commensurate with and restricted to public health risks, and which avoid unnecessary interference with international traffic and trade.

Article 3 Principles

1. The implementation of these Regulations shall be with full respect for the dignity, human rights and fundamental freedoms of persons.

2. The implementation of these Regulations shall be guided by the Charter of the United Nations and the Constitution of the World Health Organization.

3. The implementation of these Regulations shall be guided by the goal of their universal application for the protection of all people of the world from the international spread of disease.

4. States have, in accordance with the Charter of the United Nations and the principles of international law, the sovereign right to legislate and to implement legislation in pursuance of their health policies. In doing so they should uphold the purpose of these Regulations.

…

PART II—INFORMATION AND PUBLIC HEALTH RESPONSE

Article 5 Surveillance

1. Each State Party shall develop, strengthen and maintain, as soon as possible but no later than five years from the entry into force of these Regulations for that State Party, the capacity to detect, assess, notify and report events in accordance with these Regulations, as specified in Annex 1....

3. WHO shall assist States Parties, upon request, to develop, strengthen and maintain the capacities referred to in paragraph 1 of this Article.

4. WHO shall collect information regarding events through its surveillance activities and assess their potential to cause international disease spread and possible interference with international traffic....

Article 6 Notification

1. Each State Party shall assess events occurring within its territory by using the decision instrument in Annex 2. Each State Party shall notify WHO, by the most efficient means of communication available, by way of the National IHR Focal Point, and within 24 hours of assessment of public health information, of all events which may constitute a public health emergency of international concern within its territory in accordance with the decision instrument, as well as any health measure implemented in response to those events. If the notification received by WHO involves the competency of the International Atomic Energy Agency (IAEA), WHO shall immediately notify the IAEA.

2. Following a notification, a State Party shall continue to communicate to WHO timely, accurate and sufficiently detailed public health information available to it on the notified event, where possible including case definitions, laboratory results, source and type of the risk, number of cases and deaths, conditions affecting the spread of the disease and the health measures employed; and report, when necessary, the difficulties faced and support needed in responding to the potential public health emergency of international concern.

SEE ALSO *Epidemiology: Surveillance for Emerging Infectious Diseases; Pandemic Preparedness; World Health Organization: Organization, Funding, and Enforcement Powers*

BIBLIOGRAPHY

Books

Farmer, Paul, et al. *Reimagining Global Health: An Introduction.* Berkeley: University of California Press, 2013.

Gostin, Lawrence. *Global Health Law.* Cambridge, MA: Harvard University Press, 2014.

Youde, Jeremy. *Global Health Governance.* Malden, MA: Polity Press, 2012.

Periodicals

Baker, Michael, and David Fidler. "Global Public Health Surveillance under New International Health Regulations." *Emerging Infectious Diseases* 12, no. 7 (July 2006): 1058–1065.

Fidler, David. "Emerging Trends." *Chinese Journal of International Law* 4, no. 2 (September 2005): 325–392.

Fidler, David. "From International Sanitary Conventions to Global Health Security: The New International Health Regulations." *Chinese Journal of International Law* 4, no. 2 (September 2005): 325–392.

Fidler, David, and Lawrence Gostin. "The New International Health Regulations: An Historic Development for International Law and Public Health." *Journal of Law, Medicine and Ethics* 34, no. 1 (February 2006): 84–95.

Fineberg, Harvey V. "Pandemic Preparedness and Response—Lessons from the H1N1 Influenza of 2009." *New England Journal of Medicine* 370, no. 14 (April 2014): 1335–1342. Available online at http://www.nejm.org/doi/full/10.1056/NEJMra 1208802 (accessed January 23, 2015).

Hardiman, Maxwell Charles, and World Health Organization Department of Global Capacities, Alert and Response. "World Health Organization Perspective on Implementation of International Health Regulations." *Emerging Infectious Diseases* 18, no. 7 (July 2012): 1041–1046. Available online at http://wwwnc.cdc.gov/eid/article/18/7/12-0395_article (accessed April 23, 2015).

Websites

"Frequently Asked Questions about the International Health Regulations (2005)." *World Health Organization (WHO).* http://www.who.int/ihr/about/FAQ2009.pdf?ua=1 (accessed January 23, 2015).

"IHR Review Committee on Second Extensions for Establishing National Public Health Capacities and on IHR Implementation." *World Health*

Organization (WHO). http://www.who.int/ihr/qa-ihr-rc–11nov.pdf (accessed January 24, 2015).

"International Health Regulations (2005)," 2nd ed. *World Health Organization (WHO)*, 2008. http://whqlibdoc.who.int/publications/2008/9789241580410_eng.pdf?q=international (accessed January 23, 2015).

"International Health Regulations (2005): Toolkit for Implementation in National Legislation: The National IHR Focal Point." *World Health Organization (WHO)*, January 2009. http://http://www.who.int/ihr/NFP_Toolkit.pdf (accessed January 24, 2014).

"Statement on the 3rd Meeting of the IHR Emergency Committee Regarding the 2014 Ebola Outbreak in West Africa." *World Health Organization (WHO)*, October 23, 2014. http://www.who.int/mediacentre/news/statements/2014/ebola-3rd-ihr-meeting/en/ (accessed January 4, 2014).

Yahya Zaffir Chaudhry

Isolation and Quarantine

⊕ Introduction

Isolation and quarantine are methods used to prevent the exposure of the public to people who may have a contagious disease. Isolation separates sick people who have a contagious disease from people who are not sick. Quarantine separates and restricts the movement of people who may have been exposed to a contagious disease to see if they become sick.

Transmission of infectious diseases occurs in numerous ways. Germs are passed from animals to humans, such as those that cause malaria; botulism is contracted via contaminated food or water; human immunodeficiency virus/acquired immune deficiency syndrome (HIV/AIDS) is contracted through infected bodily fluids. Diseases like measles, tuberculosis, influenza (flu), severe acute respiratory syndrome (SARS), and Ebola virus disease are transmitted directly from person to person.

From the Black Death in the 14th century to the SARS epidemic in 2003 to the Ebola epidemic that began in 2014, quarantine has been part of the public health tool kit as a way to reduce contact between the infected and those vulnerable to infection. When treatment is unavailable, these measures work. Diseases for which insolation or quarantine are indicated include cholera, diphtheria, infectious tuberculosis, plague, smallpox, yellow fever, viral hemorrhagic fevers (like Ebola), SARS, and influenza. Quarantine is typically used in conjunction with other traditional strategies, including quick detection and diagnosis and antibiotic or antiviral treatment.

For all its benefits, there have always been critics of quarantine, particularly when the quarantine is involuntary. Primary arguments made by critics are the potential for abuse of power, unfair stigmatization of those infected, marginalization of minority groups, and violation of civil liberties. When instituting these measures, government and public health officials must consider both the interests of the community and the rights of individuals.

⊕ Historical Background

There are recorded examples of isolation and quarantine dating back to biblical times (the book of Leviticus gives instructions on how to quarantine lepers) and Hippocrates (c. 460–c. 377 BCE). However, the concept of isolating people, animals, and goods that had potentially been exposed to a contagious disease began to develop in an organized way during the 14th century.

The word quarantine derives from the Italian word meaning 40, because that is how long ships, crews, and cargo were detained in ports during the plague epidemic of 1347 to 1352. The plague, which is believed to have been brought from the eastern Mediterranean to Sicily via infected fleas on shipboard rats, caused fever, delirium, and large growths in the groin and underarm known as buboes. The plague quickly spread across Italy before hitting ports in Spain and France, heading over the Alps into Austria, and moving into Central Europe.

There was no treatment or cure for the plague, later found to be caused by the bacterium *Yersinia pestis*. To avoid infection and certain death the healthy had to eliminate all contact with the infected. This led to city-states barring strangers, mostly merchants and the marginalized, from entering the city. To enforce the quarantine, armed guards were stationed along transit routes and access points to city with orders to kill anyone who tried to cross the cordon.

Makeshift camps served as a rudimentary way of keeping the sick isolated from the healthy. These eventually evolved into permanent plague hospitals, also known as lazarettos. These hospitals were usually far from communities and further barricaded with either a lake or river. When natural barriers were not available, a moat or ditch was dug around the facility.

Over the next few centuries, isolation and quarantine practices improved slightly, although for years ships would have to provide bills of health, documents stating they came from ports free of contagious diseases. The concept eventually made its way from Venice to England

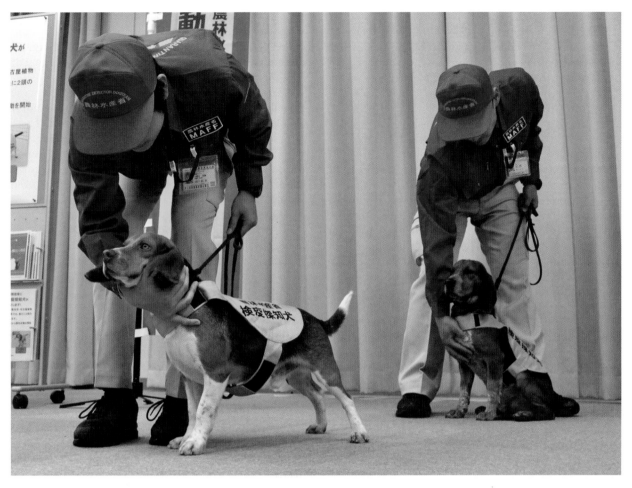

Male beagle dogs Little Man (left) and Hunter are shown to reporters at the Central Japan International Airport, or Centrair, near Nagoya, Aichi Prefecture, central Japan. It is the canines' job to sniff out products that must be quarantined from airplane passengers' luggage. In addition to quarantining people to prevent the spread of human-to-human transmission, most countries regulate the importation of certain foods, plants, and animals to limit spread of diseases or animal and insect vectors for diseases. Quarantine rules for animals are generally strict to prevent the importation of diseases like rabies. © *Kyodo/AP Images.*

and France, and settled in North America when yellow fever first appeared in New York and Boston. Meanwhile in the colonies, health authorities started dabbling in home isolation for people with smallpox. The 18th century brought some of the first legislation to address quarantines, including the Quarantine Act of 1710 in England.

By the 19th century, the new fear was cholera, which spread to Europe in 1830 and to the United States in 1832 with devastating results. Transmission of cholera was aided by globalization, faster modes of transportation like steamships and railroads, and a boost in trade. Fearful authorities quarantined travelers who had been anywhere cholera was present and forced sick people into lazarettos. Those on the fringes of society, particularly beggars and prostitutes, were thought to be natural carriers of cholera and so were kept out of cities.

Quarantine was even used as a means of stopping political opposition. However, the people of the 19th century were not like those in previous centuries. Communities balked at what they viewed as a violation of their personal freedoms. Rebellions and uprisings broke out.

Meanwhile, scientists and health officials were making new discoveries; old rationales and means of quarantine and isolation became obsolete. The 40-day quarantine for those suspected of plague infection was criticized because it exceeded the incubation period of the plague bacillus. Further, it was argued that the use of quarantine was dangerous because the public would believe no further actions would be needed and would not feel inclined to take proper precautions against disease. Travel of persons wishing to pass through towns was impinged by the required fumigation and disinfection of clothes.

While there was scientific progress and movement toward more reasonable methods of containing diseases, countries could not agree about the use of quarantine. Progress stalled as debates continued for decades.

Eventually, the International Sanitary Conferences, a series of 14 meetings from 1851 to 1938, would change that. By 1903, the countries represented at these meetings were able to begin standardizing quarantine regulations against the spread of cholera, plague, and yellow fever. These conferences were also instrumental in establishing the World Health Organization (WHO), which adopted the standards as International Sanitary Regulations in 1951. They would be modified in 1969 and again in 2005 to establish the legal framework within which countries are obligated to mitigate the spread of disease across borders.

The first real test of the regulations was 1918 with the onset of the Spanish flu pandemic. It was a failure, according to Eugenia Tognotti, in her 2013 historical review, "Lessons from the History of Quarantine, from Plague to Influenza A" published in the journal, *Emerging Infectious Diseases*. The world was divided by war, so the international systems put in place earlier were useless. In an attempt to contain the virus, Tognotti explains that medical officers isolated soldiers; health authorities in major cities around the world shut down schools, churches, and theaters, and suspended public gatherings; universities canceled public meetings; and Italian churches stopped holding confessions and funeral ceremonies. The intervention was unsuccessful because measures were difficult to put in practice in war zones and the interventions came too late. She goes on to say that many of the measures adopted by countries, once again, disproportionately affected ethnic and minority groups.

In the decades following the end of the Spanish flu pandemic, isolation and quarantine have, for the most part, been used more judiciously. However, there were times when government officials would once again return to the patterns of the past.

⊕ Impacts and Issues

While steps have been taken to make quarantine, social distancing and isolation less restrictive and more respectful of human rights and civil liberties, fear and social pressure often bring back some of the traditional methods of keeping suspected or actually sick people away from those in good health.

According to the U.S. Centers for Disease Control and Prevention (CDC), modern quarantine is instituted when the individual or group that has been exposed is easily identified and when resources are available to take care of the group that has been isolated. Quarantines are usually just partial containment of many but not all exposed persons. According to the CDC, research shows that in some cases partial quarantine can still effectively slow the rate of the spread of disease, particularly in combination with a vaccine. In fact, quarantines are more likely to involve limited numbers of people, such as those on a plane or cruise shop where a passenger falls ill, or a crowd in a public but contained place where a biological attack with a contagious disease has just occurred, rather than whole cities or neighborhoods.

Health officials, state governments, and even the federal government, according to the CDC, can employ a range of strategies when it comes to quarantine. These include short-term, voluntary home curfew; restrictions on public gatherings and closing of public meeting places, such as theaters; and travel restrictions, including mass transit systems and being able to come and go from the area.

Quarantines do not occur in a vacuum and, as noted by the CDC, should be done in combination with other public health methods, including: "enhanced disease surveillance and symptom monitoring; rapid diagnosis and treatment for those who fall ill; and preventive treatment for quarantined individuals, including vaccination or prophylactic treatment, depending on the disease."

As for those who are sick and need to be isolated, the CDC says that their quarantine, along with that of people with whom they have had contact, should be voluntary to the greatest extent possible. The CDC directive goes on to recommend that mandatory quarantine should only be instituted as a last resort, when voluntary measures cannot reasonably be expected to succeed, and that failure to institute mandatory measures is likely to have a substantial impact on public health.

Once isolated, people must be kept in safe, habitable, and humane conditions of confinement, which includes the provision of basics such as food, water, clothing, medical care and, if feasible, psychosocial support. Health and government officials are also supposed to protect the interests of household members of individuals who are isolated. For example, they are advised to recommend or provide alternative housing for household members if living with the isolated patient presents a significant risk.

Above all, the CDC recommends that procedures for making decisions about affected individuals must be fair. In extraordinary circumstances, exceptions to normal procedural protections may be taken if immediate action is essential to protect the health of others. Even in that situation, legal recourse should be available in all cases for individuals to challenge their isolation or quarantine.

While there are many good reasons to use quarantines, they can also cause a considerable amount of controversy related to civil liberty issues. This was certainly true when some doctors and nurses who volunteered to care for the sick during the Ebola outbreak in Africa were involuntarily quarantined upon returning to the United States. The health-care workers were quarantined despite the fact that they were not showing symptoms of the disease. Many of these health-care workers and other critics of the practice protested that they were quarantined without substantial scientific reason.

Jeffrey Drazen and coauthors explain in their 2014 review, "Ebola and Quarantine" in the *New England Journal of Medicine* that Ebola is transmitted by contact with the bodily fluids of a person showing symptoms of the disease, which include fever, vomiting, diarrhea, and malaise. A person not showing symptoms is not contagious. Therefore, the health-care workers, along with Drazen and coauthors, argued they should not have been quarantined.

Those in favor of the quarantines argued that it is still better to be safe than sorry. After all, it only costs the quarantined person the inconvenience of staying away from the public for 21 days (the incubation period of Ebola).

Drazen and colleagues argue that the only way to stop an epidemic is to control it at the source, which is the job of health-care workers in the field, of whom there is a shortage. The authors assert, "If we add barriers

making it harder for volunteers to return to their community, we are hurting ourselves," because presumably no one will want to volunteer under those circumstances.

Some quarantine critics also point to historical overreach, misuse of power, and use of public fear to further ostracize marginalized people as reasons to use this strategy sparingly. An often-cited example is how the SARS epidemic in 2003 was handled by governments of affected countries.

The rapid transmission and high mortality rate of SARS caused panic among the public and officials. Tognotti observes the approach to containing the disease varied among the countries with the most SARS cases. Those who may have been exposed to the disease were requested by the Canadian public health authorities to self-quarantine, whereas in the People's Republic of China, the public health response was more coordinated. Police serveyed private homes with web cams, blocked off buildings, and set up vehicle checkpoints to contain the spread of SARS. Even further controls were placed on rural areas where workers were isolated.

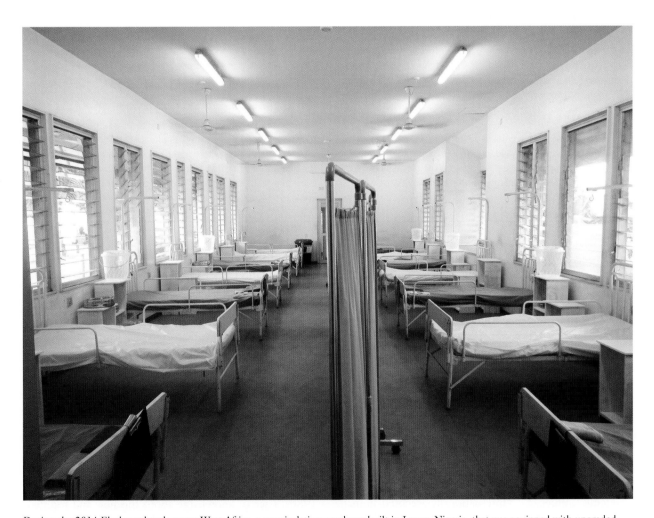

During the 2014 Ebola outbreak across West Africa, a new isolation ward was built in Lagos, Nigeria, that was equipped with upgraded facilities and made ready for Ebola hemorrhagic fever patients. *Bryan Christensen/U.S. Centers for Disease Control.*

QUARANTINE CAUSES VIOLENCE IN LIBERIA

Small-scale quarantines in conjunction with other measures have proven to help contain contagious disease. There is no evidence that such quarantines work on a large scale, yet in August 2014, the president of Liberia ordered security forces to barricade more than 60,000 people into a slum of the capital city of Monrovia in an attempt to contain spread of the Ebola virus.

Cases of Ebola began turning up in West Africa in March 2014 and quickly spread to major cities in Guinea, Sierra Leone, and Liberia. According to the WHO, the disease is caused by the *Filoviridae* virus, naturally occurring in fruit bats and transmitted to humans "through close contact with the blood, secretions, organs, or other bodily fluids of infected animals such as chimpanzees, gorillas, fruit bats, monkeys, forest antelope, and porcupines found ill or dead or in the rainforest." Human-to-human transmission occurs via direct contact with the blood, secretions, or other bodily fluids of the infected, as well as contact with surfaces and materials such as bedding and clothing contaminated with these fluids. The average Ebola case fatality rate is around 50 percent, according to the WHO. Case fatality rates have varied from 25 to 90 percent in past outbreaks. As of January 2015, there were more than 21,724 cases of Ebola in Africa and 8,641 deaths.

In late August 2014, with health-care officials overwhelmed and no space to put the sick or those suspected to be sick, officials decided to turn a local school in the sprawling slum of West Point just outside of Monrovia into a makeshift sick ward. However, they did not warn West Point residents before they started moving sick people in.

According to news reports at the time, West Point was an urban neighborhood of 60,000 to 120,000 people living in close quarters and experiencing crippling poverty. The residents of West Point had only a few years of respite from brutal civil wars when Ebola hit.

As the epidemic made its way through the country in the spring and summer of 2014, Liberia was hard hit. Within the first months of the outbreak, scores of people were getting sick, and many chose to stay in their homes out of fear of stigma as well as a deep mistrust of local government officials and outside agencies. So when health officials brought more sick people into their community, residents were angry. According to news accounts, men, women, and children stormed the school and freed patients inside. Some also resorted to looting the building, running off into the streets with soiled mattresses and supplies, likely contaminated with Ebola.

Police managed to calm the initial rebellion at the school. But just days later, residents woke to armed guards in the streets and boats patrolling the 70 miles (113 kilometers) of West Point's coastline. Liberian president Ellen Johnson Sirleaf, in the middle of the night, had put West Point under quarantine without notifying residents in advance. The people once again acted in violence, attempting to force their way through police barricades. Police fired their weapons to disperse the crowd. Before the fighting ended, several people were shot by security forces, including a 15-year-old boy who was fatally wounded.

In the wake of the quarantine, many public health officials came out against the measure, pointing out that there is little evidence to support the effectiveness of a mass quarantine, particularly in populations that are not showing symptoms of disease. Instead, officials recommended isolation and good health care for those who showed symptoms of being sick. The move, said many experts after the fact, likely fomented greater mistrust of the government, creating a humanitarian crisis since the quarantine cut off West Pointers from food and water supplies, and made the threat of people contracting and spreading Ebola even worse.

In some areas, public health officials were allowed to threaten penalty of death for anyone who violated quarantine. Tognotti asserts, "As had occurred in the past, the strategies adopted in some countries during this public health emergency contributed to the discrimination and stigmatization of persons and communities and raised protests and complaints against limitations and travel restrictions."

⊕ Future Implications

It is generally agreed that quarantine and isolations should be carried out in the least restrictive manner possible. According to the 2007 WHO report "Ethical Considerations in Developing a Public Health Response to Pandemic Influenza," "Internationally-accepted human rights principles provide the framework for evaluating the ethical acceptability of public health measures that limit individual freedom, just as human rights provide the foundation for other pandemic-related policies." Some of these principles include the idea that any limitations on human rights must be lawful, based on a legitimate objective (such as curtailing a contagious disease), necessary in a democratic society, the least restrictive and intrusive means available, and not arbitrary, unreasonable, or discriminatory.

These public health measures cannot place unfair burdens on particular segments of the population. The WHO report notes that, "Policy-makers should pay specific attention to groups that are the most vulnerable to discrimination, stigmatization or isolation, including racial and ethnic minorities, elderly people, prisoners, disabled persons, migrants and the homeless."

This was evident as HIV/AIDS emerged in the early 1980s. Lack of knowledge about this new and frightening disease was used by some as a reason to discriminate against and ostracize homosexuals, hemophiliacs, and Haitians, all of whom were thought to be carriers of the disease. Children who were HIV positive were kept out of schools, and one U.S. official even suggested that those infected should be tattooed to better be identified and avoided.

While the world has learned from some of these past missteps, the WHO in its ethics report asserts, "These measures, by their nature, require vigilant attention to avoid causing prejudice and intolerance. Public trust must be gained through regular, transparent, and comprehensive communications that balance the risks and benefits of public health interventions."

SEE ALSO *Avian (Bird) and Swine Influenzas; Centers for Disease Control and Prevention (CDC); Cholera and Dysentery; Ebola Virus Disease; Epidemiology: Surveillance for Emerging Infectious Diseases; Hemorrhagic Diseases; Influenza; Pandemic Preparedness; SARS, MERS, and the Emergence of Coronaviruses; Smallpox Eradication and Storage of Infectious Agents; Tuberculosis (TB); Viral Diseases; Viral Hepatitis*

BIBLIOGRAPHY

Books

Cliff, Andrew, and Matthew Smallman-Raynor. *Oxford Textbook of Infectious Disease Control: A Geographical Analysis from Medieval Quarantine to Global Eradication.* Oxford: Oxford University Press, 2013.

Selgelid, Michael J., Angela McLean, Nimalan Arinaminpathy, and Julian Savulescu, eds. *Infectious Disease Ethics: Limiting Liberty in Contexts of Contagion.* Dordrecht, Netherlands: Springer, 2011.

Periodicals

Day, T., et al. "When Is Quarantine a Useful Control Strategy for Emerging Infectious Diseases?" *American Journal of Epidemiology* 163, no. 5 (March 1, 2006): 479–485.

Drazen, Jeffrey M., et al. "Ebola and Quarantine." *New England Journal of Medicine* 371, no. 21 (2014): 2029–2030.

Gonsalves, Gregg, and Peter Staley. "Panic, Paranoia, and Public Health—The AIDS Epidemic's Lessons for Ebola." *New England Journal of Medicine* 371, no. 25 (December 18, 2014): 2348–2349.

Tognotti, Eugenia. "Lessons from the History of Quarantine, from Plague to Influenza A." *Emerging Infectious Diseases* 19, no. 2 (2013): 254–259.

Websites

"Ebola Outbreak: Why Liberia's Quarantine in West Point Slum Will Fail." *CBCnews*, August 25, 2014. http://www.cbc.ca/news/world/ebola-outbreak-why-liberia-s-quarantine-in-west-point-slum-will-fail-1.2744292 (accessed January 31, 2015).

"Ebola Situation Reports." *World Health Organization.* http://www.who.int/csr/disease/ebola/situation-reports/en/ (accessed January 30, 2015).

"Ebola Virus Disease," Fact Sheet No. 103. *World Health Organization (WHO)*, Updated September 2014. http://www.who.int/mediacentre/factsheets/fs103/en/ (accessed January 30, 2015).

"History of Quarantine." *U.S. Centers for Disease Control and Prevention.* http://www.cdc.gov/quarantine/HistoryQuarantine.html (accessed January 30, 2015).

Klibanoff, Eleanor. "Awful Moments In Quarantine History: Remember Typhoid Mary?" *NPR*, October 30, 2014. http://www.npr.org/blogs/goatsandsoda/2014/10/30/360120406/awful-moments-in-quarantine-history-remember-typhoid-mary (accessed January 30, 2015).

"Legal Authorities for Isolation and Quarantine." *Centers for Disease Control and Prevention.* http://www.cdc.gov/quarantine/AboutLawsRegulationsQuarantineIsolation.html (accessed January 30, 2015).

Onishi, Norimitsu. "As Ebola Grips Liberia's Capital, a Quarantine Sows Social Chaos." *New York Times*, August 28, 2014. http://www.nytimes.com/2014/08/29/world/africa/in-liberias-capital-an-ebola-outbreak-like-no-other.html?_r=0 (accessed March 4, 2015).

Pope, Sarah, Nisha Sherry, and Elizabeth Webster. "Protecting Civil Liberties during Quarantine and Isolation in Public Health Emergencies." *Law Practice Today*, April 2011. http://www.americanbar.org/publications/law_practice_today_home/law_practice_today_archive/april11/protecting_civil_liberties_during_quarantine_and_isolation_in_public_health_emergencies.html (accessed March 4, 2015).

"Quarantine." *Centers for Disease Control and Prevention.* http://www.cdc.gov/quarantine/ (accessed January 30, 2015).

"State Quarantine and Isolation Statutes." *National Conference of State Legislatures*, October 29, 2014. http://www.ncsl.org/research/health/state-quarantine-and-isolation-statutes.aspx (accessed January 30, 2015).

Melanie R. Plenda

Life Expectancy and Aging Populations

⊕ Introduction

Life expectancy is the average length of time that a person might expect to live. A person's life expectancy is affected by numerous factors, and differs across demographics. For example, in most countries women live longer than men. People in Japan, the country with the longest life expectancy, can expect to live twice as long as people in Sierra Leone, the country with the shortest. Life expectancy has a significant effect on numerous sociopolitical issues. As populations age and as life expectancies increase, issues arise such as population aging and the economic impact on younger populations of caring for the elderly.

As life expectancies change over time, so do the issues surrounding them. Population aging, which occurs when life expectancy increases, also brings with it a number of issues. For example, modern day Japan is facing unprecedented economic pressure from a combination of an aging population and a negative birthrate leading to a shrinking workforce. As the number of people working decreases, so do the resources to take care of the increasing number of elderly people.

The factors that determine both life expectancy and population aging are numerous, and can include disease and health care, and conflict and war. It is rare for a single issue to alter life expectancy by itself, although wars and epidemics have caused drops to both national and international life expectancies for various amounts of time.

The global life expectancy in 2012 was about 70 years. The 10 countries with the longest life expectancies that year were Monaco (89.57 years), Japan (84.46), Singapore (84.38), San Marino (83.18), Andorra (82.65), Switzerland (82.39), Australia (82.07), Italy (82.03), Sweden (81.89), and Liechtenstein (81.68). (See graphic.)

The 10 countries with the lowest life expectancies were Chad (49.44), South Africa (49.56), Guinea-Bissau (49.87), Afghanistan (50.49), Swaziland (50.54), the Central African Republic (51.35), Somalia (51.58), Zambia (51.83), Namibia (51.85), and Gabon (52.06).

⊕ Historical Background

Throughout history, life expectancies have fluctuated with the events and health care of their times. For most of human history, child mortality drastically lowered overall life expectancy statistics. For example, although the life expectancy in Britain during the Middle Ages (500–1500 CE was just 30, people who lived to 21 had a life expectancy of 64.

The United Nations (UN) expects that the worldwide life expectancy will increase to 76 years by 2050, and to 82 years by 2100. In developed countries, the life expectancy is expected to increase to 89 years by the end of the century. In developing countries, disease and conflict are the primary factors causing low life expectancies. According to the UN, reducing the spread of human immunodeficiency virus (HIV) and other diseases is necessary to increase the life expectancy of developing nations. In countries where HIV remains an epidemic, life expectancies remain very low. In southern African countries, for example, the life expectancy from 2005 to 2010 was just 52 years, a drop of 10 years from 1995 to 2000 levels.

1918 Flu Pandemic

No event since the beginning of the 20th century has had so profound an effect on international life expectancy as the 1918 influenza pandemic. Life expectancy in the United States plummeted by more than 10 years. The disease affected young people at a significantly greater rate than is typical of influenza; about half of all deaths from the disease were young adults aged 20 to 40. Its mortality rate was 2.5 percent, staggeringly high compared to the usual influenza mortality rate of .01 percent.

However, life expectancy recovered quickly, and in 1919 actually surpassed the life expectancies of 1917. Even before the flu pandemic, communicable diseases were significantly widespread. Children were particularly susceptible to illness; one of five children in the United States did not live past the age of five. During the pandemic, there

Years of Life Expectancy at Birth, by Country, in 2012

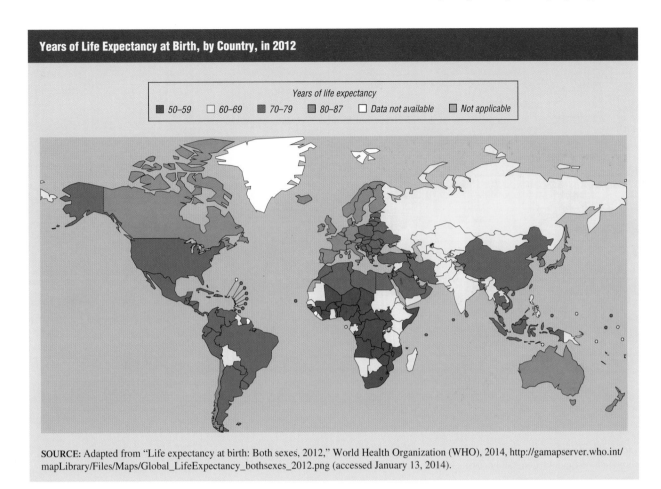

Years of life expectancy

■ 50–59   □ 60–69   ■ 70–79   ■ 80–87   □ Data not available   ■ Not applicable

SOURCE: Adapted from "Life expectancy at birth: Both sexes, 2012," World Health Organization (WHO), 2014, http://gamapserver.who.int/mapLibrary/Files/Maps/Global_LifeExpectancy_bothsexes_2012.png (accessed January 13, 2014).

were widespread educational campaigns to teach Americans how to avoid getting sick. These campaigns increased national awareness that germs caused disease, and that personal hygiene was an effective way to avoid germs. The pandemic also led to more concerted governmental efforts to provide health care. Public health nurses became essential community figures, providing firsthand instruction in hygienic living. By the end of the flu pandemic, many survivors knew better how to avoid getting sick in the future.

Historical Factors for Life Expectancy

Up until the 1920s, infant and child mortality was the single biggest factor affecting life expectancy. In *Demography: Analysis and Synthesis; A Treatise in Population Studies*, Graziella Caselli and colleagues write "from 1740–1749 to 1925, the life expectancy of males gained 29 years, and that of women gained 32 years. In both cases, 23 years can be ascribed to the mortality decline of children younger than 15 years." Gains dropped steeply in the 19th century from previous years as the decline of child mortality slowed.

From the 1920s through the 1940s, the primary factor affecting life expectancy was the decline of adult mortality. According to Caselli and colleagues, the decrease in deaths from infectious diseases and deaths from childbirth

in the 20th century were the primary reasons that life expectancies around the world increased. After World War II (1939–1945), there were more major advances in reducing child mortality. The rise of child vaccinations and antibiotics helped prevent deaths from childhood infectious diseases and once again led to gains in life expectancy.

Since the 1960s, child mortality rates have mostly leveled out. Today, advances in life expectancy have been primarily led by the elderly. From 1968 to 1996, the mortality rate for people older than 60 declined by 60 percent for women and 50 percent for men.

⊕ Impacts and Issues

Although epidemics and conflicts can cause reductions in life expectancy, population aging is not necessarily caused by the absence of these factors. Population aging can also be caused by a reduced birthrate and basic advancements in medical care. And although population aging might sound like an inherently positive thing, it can carry with it a wide range of negative effects on a country's future, particularly its economy, and especially when the primary cause of population aging is a combination of low birthrate and rising numbers of elderly.

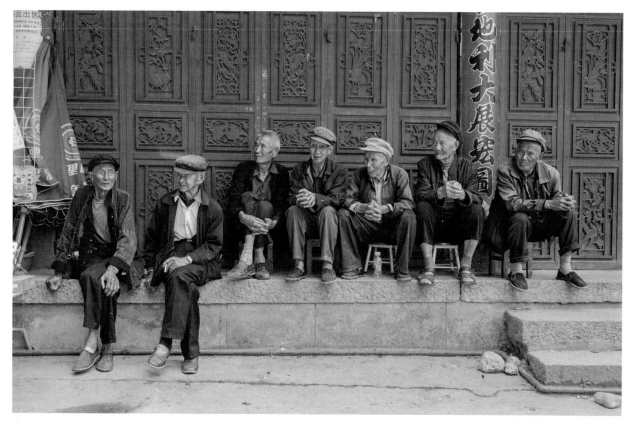

Elderly people sit in front of a social welfare home on July 8, 2013, in Dali, China. In China there is a shortage of elder care, with thousands of applicants on waiting lists. *© Hung Chung Chih/Shutterstock.com.*

According to the U.S. National Institutes of Health, the population over age 65 will soon surpass the number of children under age five for the first time in human history. Around the world, life expectancies are increasing. People older than the age of 85 are one of the world's fastest-growing demographics. As populations age, new issues arise that affect everyone.

Medical issues have always been a significant aspect of aging. With the growth of the elderly as a percentage of the population, these issues take on a greater scope. According to the World Health Organization (WHO), 2 billion people will be aged 60 or older by 2050. Care of the elderly will be a significant international issue in the coming decades.

Noncommunicable diseases, such as heart disease, lung disease, and stroke, are the biggest threat to the elderly. According to a UN report, heart disease and stroke are the primary causes of death for people aged 60 or older in both developed and developing nations. Other major health threats include lung cancer, diabetes, and chronic obstructive pulmonary disease. The UN measures the rate of premature deaths caused by diseases with the statistic "years of life lost." Heart disease alone costs nearly 10,000 years of life lost for every 100,000 adults over the age of 60. Cognitive decline, including dementia and Alzheimer's disease, is also debilitating

and expensive to manage as populations grow older. Alzheimer's disease is the fifth-leading cause of death among people age 65 and older.

Falls are one of the greatest health risks for elderly people. According to the aforementioned report, 28 to 35 percent of people over the age of 65 suffer injuries sustained from falls each year. That number increases to up to 42 percent for people over the age of 70. The health hazards do not end with the fall itself. A person injured from a fall might then suffer from post-fall syndrome, in which a loss of personal autonomy and immobilization from injury can lead to depression. Twenty percent of elderly people who break their hips from falls die within a year of their injuries. The danger of falls is exacerbated by how many older people are isolated. According to the U.S. Department of Health and Human Services, 29 percent of noninstitutionalized older people live by themselves, including 47 percent of women older than 75. According to the UN, in some European countries more than 40 percent of women older than 65 live alone.

As life expectancies increase, so do the costs of staying healthy into old age. Cancer incidences in particular are expected to rise significantly. The National Institute on Aging expects 17 million new cancer cases by 2020, up from 13 million in 2009. That number is expected to reach 27 million by 2030. Developing countries will make up a growing proportion of this population, as life expectancies increase in countries with fewer resources to diagnose and treat cancer effectively.

Other noncommunicable diseases such as heart disease, stroke, and diabetes will have a significant global economic impact. These diseases cost an estimated US$84 billion around the world between 2006 and 2015.

⊕ Future Implications

As populations age, a number of issues arise for their respective nations. Caring for large elderly populations, shrinking workforce numbers, and age-dependency are all issues that countries with significant aging populations face.

The international working-age population is generally considered to be between the ages of 15 and 64. Children from birth to age 14 and persons age 65 and older are considered dependent on the working-age population to have their needs met. High-income nations with low birthrates currently have the highest risk of old-age dependency. In Japan, the old-age dependency ratio, or the number of persons age 65 and older for every working-age person, is 36 percent as of the mid-2010s. That figure is expected to rise to 72 percent by 2050. Other countries that are projected to have substantial old-age dependencies by 2050 include Spain (67 percent), South Korea (66 percent), Italy (62 percent), and Germany (60 percent). The most common worry about aging populations is that an unbalanced proportion of older persons to working persons will force the increasingly smaller working population to save more rather than spend, thus hurting economic growth.

However, projecting the impact of aging populations in different countries can be difficult. Different countries have different cultural views on how best to care for the elderly. In a report on population aging, Harvard University professors David Bloom, David Canning, and Günther Fink write: "The economic impacts of aging are unlikely to be uniform across societies. In the developed world, longer lifespans have been accompanied by a shift in support for older generations from families to the state. In many developing countries, families remain pivotal to elder care and as lifespans becomes longer there may be disruption to family structures, leading to a move towards public transfer systems and savings similar to that experienced in wealthier parts of the world."

Predicting how population aging will affect economies is difficult because each country adapts to aging populaces differently. This is also reflected in how different the concern over population aging is from country to country. A Pew Research Center poll found that 87 percent of people in Japan and 79 percent in South Korea believe that the growing number of older people in their country is a major problem. Perhaps not surprisingly, both Japan and Korea have among the world's

DEMENTIA

More than 25 percent of people older than 85 experience some degree of cognitive decline. No neurological disease is likely to have a widespread impact in the near future than dementia. According to a UN report, dementia alone affects more than 35 million people in the mid-2010s. That number will increase to more than 65 million in 2030 and more 115 million by 2050. There is a new case of dementia diagnosed every four seconds.

The most common form of dementia is Alzheimer's disease. Typically the first symptom of Alzheimer's disease is memory loss, followed by declines in other mental functions, such as decision making.

Vascular dementia (VaD) is widely considered to be the second-most-prevalent form of dementia. Vascular dementia is caused by brain damage stemming from cerebrovascular or cardiovascular issues, such as stroke or endocarditis.

Dementia is one of the costliest cognitive illnesses. In 2010, the worldwide costs of dementia exceeded $600 billion. In addition to drastically lowering the quality of life for those who have it, dementia also leads to shortened lives. The median survival for those with Alzheimer's disease is 7.1 years. For those with VaD, it is 3.9 years.

Many countries have instituted initiatives to address concerns that dementia will become an international problem. These initiatives include providing care packages for people with dementia, training and supporting caregivers, raising public awareness of dementia, and diagnosing dementia early.

Recognizing and treating dementia effectively remains an area of concern for many countries. Mental and neurological health is often given low priority, especially in low- and middle-income countries. According to the World Health Organization (WHO), 40 percent of countries do not have a dedicated mental health policy, and 29 percent of countries do not possess a mental health plan. In poor and middle-income countries, preventing communicable diseases often takes top priority over other health concerns, leaving people in those countries without the resources to diagnose or treat dementia.

In countries that do not have welfare, people with dementia often have no financial recourse. These countries often do not have the budget to spare for focusing on caring for dementia patients and dementia prevention. According to the WHO report, low-cost strategies for dementia care and prevention will be necessary going forward into the coming decades.

highest old-age dependency ratios, at 72 percent and 66 percent, respectively. However, in Spain, where the old-age dependency ratio is 67 percent, 52 percent of people think population aging is a major concern. In Italy, only 41 percent of people are significantly concerned about population aging, despite an old-age dependency ratio of 62 percent. In the United States, just 26 percent of the population is concerned.

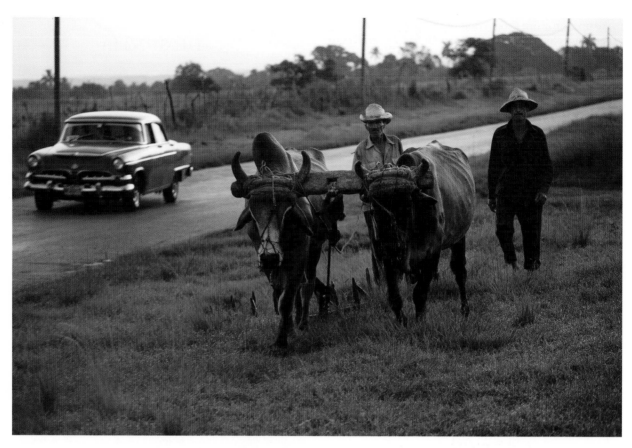

Rogelio Alonso, 74, center, works a plow led by a pair of oxen in Los Palos, Cuba. Cuba grapples with having the oldest citizenry in Latin America, a phenomenon fueled by low birthrates and long life expectancies, plus the migration of young people and women. The government has already postponed the retirement age and is trying to create more homes and programs for the elderly, but still will have to handle the economic consequences and increased need for health care of its increasingly graying population. © *Ramon Espinosa/AP Images.*

SEE ALSO *Nutrition; Vulnerable Populations*

BIBLIOGRAPHY

Books

Caselli, Graziella, Jacques Vallin, and Guillaume Wunsch. *Demography: Analysis and Synthesis.* Amsterdam: Elsevier, 2005.

Lancaster, H. O. *Expectations of Life: A Study in the Demography, Statistics, and History of World Mortality.* New York: Springer-Verlag, 1990.

Magnus, George. *The Age of Aging: How Demographics Are Changing the Global Economy and Our World.* Hoboken, NJ: Wiley, 2009.

Pirages, Dennis, and Ken Cousins, eds. *From Resource Scarcity to Ecological Security: Exploring New Limits to Growth.* Cambridge, MA: MIT Press, 2005.

Robinson, Mary, et al., eds. *Global Health and Global Aging.* San Francisco, CA: Jossey-Bass, 2007.

Periodicals

Bauer, Jürgen, et al. "Evidence-Based Recommendations for Optimal Dietary Protein Intake in Older People: A Position Paper from the PROT-AGE Study Group." *Journal of the American Medical Directors Association* 14, no. 8 (February 4, 2013): 542–559.

Sugiura, Yasuo, et al. "Rapid Increase in Japanese Life Expectancy after World War II." *Biosci Trends* 4, no. 1 (February 2014): 9–16.

Websites

"Ageing and Life Course." *World Health Organization (WHO).* http://www.who.int/ageing/en/ (accessed January 30, 2015).

"Ageing in the Twenty-First Century: A Celebration and A Challenge." *United Nations Populations Fund Division.* http://www.unfpa.org/sites/default/files/pub-pdf/Ageing%20report.pdf (accessed March 22, 2015).

Bloom, David E., David Canning, and Günther Fink. "Implications of Population Aging for Economic Growth." *Harvard School of Public Health,* January 2011. http://www.hsph.harvard.edu/program-on-the-global-demography-of-aging/WorkingPapers/2011/PGDA_WP_64.pdf/ (accessed March 22, 2015).

"Covering Pandemic Flu." *Nieman Foundation for Journalism at Harvard University.* http://www.nieman.harvard.edu/wp-content/uploads/pod-assets/microsites/NiemanGuideToCovering PandemicFlu/AHistoryOfPandemics/TheWorst FluPandemicOnRecord.aspx.html#mother (accessed March 21, 2015).

"The Countries That Will Be Most Impacted by Aging Population." *Pew Research Center.* http://www.pewresearch.org/fact-tank/2014/02/04/the-countries-that-will-be-most-impacted-by-aging-population/ (accessed March 21, 2015).

"Dementia: Life Expectancy." *World Health Organization (WHO).* http://www.who.int/gho/mortality_burden_disease/life_tables/situation_trends/en/ (accessed March 23, 2015).

"Dementia/Alzheimer's Disease." *U.S. Centers for Disease Control and Prevention (CDC).* http://www.cdc.gov/mentalhealth/basics/mental-illness/dementia.htm (accessed January 30, 2015).

"Faststats: Life Expectancy." *U.S. Centers for Disease Control and Prevention.* http://www.cdc.gov/nchs/fastats/life-expectancy.htm (accessed January 30, 2015).

"Global Health Observatory Data Repository: Life Expectancy: Data by Country." *World Health Organization (WHO).* http://apps.who.int/gho/data/node.main.688?lang=en (accessed March 2, 2015).

"The Great Pandemic." *Flu.gov.* http://www.flu.gov/pandemic/history/1918/life_in_1918/ (accessed March 21, 2015).

Kaplan, Karen. "Baby Boomers May Live Longer, but Their Elders Were Healthier." *Los Angeles Times,* February 4, 2013. http://articles.latimes.com/2013/feb/04/news/la-heb-baby-boomers-poor-health-20130204 (accessed March 22, 2015).

"A Profile of Older Americans: 2011." *U.S. Department of Health and Human Services.* http://www.aoa.gov/Aging_Statistics/Profile/2011/docs/2011profile.pdf (accessed March 22, 2015).

"Vascular Dementia (VaD)." *Alzheimer's Association.* https://www.alz.org/cincinnati/documents/vascular.pdf/ (accessed March 22, 2015).

"WHO Global Report on Falls Prevention in Older Age." *World Health Organization (WHO).* http://www.who.int/ageing/publications/Falls_prevention 7March.pdf?ua=1 (accessed March 2, 2015).

"Why Population Aging Matters: A Global Perspective." *U.S. National Institute on Aging.* http://www.nia.nih.gov/sites/default/files/WPAM.pdf/ (accessed March 21, 2015).

"The World Factbook: Country Comparison Life Expectancy At Birth" *U.S. Central Intelligence Agency (CIA).* https://www.cia.gov/library/publications/the-world-factbook/rankorder/2102rank.html/ (accessed March 21, 2015).

World Health Organization and Alzheimer's Disease International. "Dementia: A Public Health Priority." *World Health Organization (WHO),* 2012. http://www.who.int/mental_health/publications/dementia_report_2012/en/ (accessed March 2, 2015).

"World Population Prospects: The 2012 Revision." *United Nations.* http://esa.un.org/unpd/wpp/Documentation/pdf/WPP2012_%20KEY%20 FINDINGS.pdf/ (accessed March 21, 2015).

"World Population Prospects: The 2012 Revision, Key Findings and Advance Tables." *United Nations Department of Economic and Social Affairs/Population Division.* http://esa.un.org/unpd/wpp/Documentation/pdf/WPP2012_%20KEY%20 FINDINGS.pdf (accessed March 27, 2015).

John Michael Bell

Malaria

⊕ Introduction

Malaria is a disease caused by one of several strains of the *Plasmodium* protozoan, a one-celled parasite that is transmitted by the bite of the *Anopheles* mosquito.

Malaria affects hundreds of millions of people worldwide and is endemic in tropical and subtropical regions, including sub-Saharan Africa, South-east Asia, Papua New Guinea, the Pacific States, Haiti, and parts of South America. The World Health Organization (WHO) estimates that in 2013, there were 198 million cases of malaria worldwide, resulting in more than 580,000 deaths. About 77 percent of those who died were children; those under age five are especially vulnerable to the disease. In the developing world, malaria contributes to a high infant mortality rate and a heavy loss of work time.

In response to aggressive global eradication campaigns, as of 2012, the WHO estimated the global malaria rate had fallen by 42 percent for all age groups and 48 percent in children under 5. (See graphic.) By 2014, it was estimated the decrease was continuing on target to 47 percent from 2000 to 2013.

⊕ Historical Background

A connection between swampy areas and fever was made centuries ago, and the word malaria reflects the popular belief that the illness was caused by bad air (Italian, *mal aria*). During the 16th century, people discovered that the disease could be treated using quinine, a compound derived from the bark of the tropical cinchona tree.

Alphonse Laveran, a French Army physician working in North Africa in the 1880s, was the first to observe malarial parasites in human blood. Their mode of transmission was not understood, however, until Ronald Ross (1857–1932), a British medical officer in India, found the organisms within the bodies of *Anopheles* mosquitoes.

Malaria is caused by four species of parasitic protozoa: *Plasmodium vivax*, *P. ovale*, *P. malariae*, and *P. falciparum*. These organisms have complex life cycles involving several different developmental stages in both human and mosquito hosts. Present as infective sporozoites in the salivary glands of the mosquito, they are transferred by the mosquito's bite to the human blood stream, where they travel to the liver. There, each sporozoite divides into thousands of merozoites, which emerge into the blood once again and begin invading the host's red blood cells. This event triggers the onset of disease symptoms, as the merozoites consume proteins necessary for proper red blood cell function, including hemoglobin. The merozoites mature into the trophozoite phase and reproduce by division. As a result, many more merozoites are released into the blood when the host cell finally ruptures. In *P. vivax* and *P. ovale* infection, some sporozoites may delay their development in the liver, lingering in a dormant phase, but emerging later and causing the characteristic recurrence of symptoms.

The cycle of red blood cell invasion and parasite multiplication repeats itself many times during a bout of malaria. If a mosquito bites the affected person, the insect takes up merozoites, which reproduce sexually within its gut. The cycle completes itself as the larval parasites pass through the gut wall and make their way to the mosquito's salivary glands, from whence they may again be transferred to a human host as sporozoites.

The pattern of chills and fever characteristic of malaria is caused by the massive destruction of the red blood cells by the merozoites and the accompanying release of parasitic waste products. The attacks subside as the immune response of the human host slows the further development of the parasites in the blood. People who are repeatedly infected gradually develop a limited immunity. Relapses of malaria long after the original infection can occur from parasites that have remained in the liver, because treatment with drugs kills only the parasites in the blood cells and not in the liver.

Malaria is easily misdiagnosed because it resembles many other diseases. Early symptoms include malaise, fatigue, headache, nausea and vomiting, and muscular

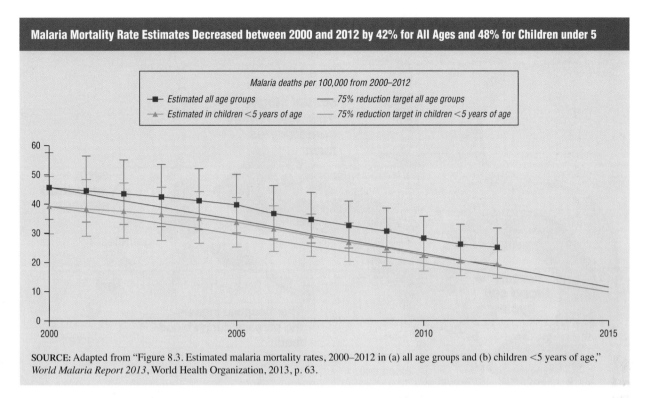

Malaria Mortality Rate Estimates Decreased between 2000 and 2012 by 42% for All Ages and 48% for Children under 5

Malaria deaths per 100,000 from 2000–2012

- ■— *Estimated all age groups*
- —— *75% reduction target all age groups*
- ▲— *Estimated in children <5 years of age*
- —— *75% reduction target in children <5 years of age*

SOURCE: Adapted from "Figure 8.3. Estimated malaria mortality rates, 2000–2012 in (a) all age groups and (b) children <5 years of age," *World Malaria Report 2013*, World Health Organization, 2013, p. 63.

Though malaria mortality rates have dropped since 2000, malaria continues to be a global public health concern. About half the world's population is at risk, especially children under five years old in sub-Saharan Africa.

aches; after several hours, the characteristic high fever and chills occur. The body's principal defenses are fever and filtration of infected red blood cells in the spleen. Neither of these mechanisms, however, is completely effective in ridding the body of the parasite.

Malaria Control

Malaria is controlled either by preventing contact between humans and mosquitoes or by eliminating the mosquito vector.

In 1905, construction on the Panama Canal was interrupted by epidemics of malaria and yellow fever. During the 1950s and 1960s, the WHO launched a worldwide campaign to eradicate malaria using the insecticide DDT (full name, dichlorodiphenyltrichloroethane) to kill *Anopheles*. The disease disappeared in several countries where it had been endemic and was greatly reduced in others, but it began to return as *Anopheles* developed resistance to DDT (which was banned in the United States in 1972 due to its environmental side effects). Other areas—particularly tropical areas where mosquitoes inhabit large spaces, making control by insecticide inefficient—were relatively unaffected by these measures, and research was begun into biological or genetic means of control.

Individuals may protect themselves from mosquito bites by wearing protective clothing, applying mosquito repellents to the skin, or by burning mosquito coils that produce smoke containing insecticidal pyrethrins. Inside houses, mosquito-proof screens and nets keep the vectors out, while insecticides (including the previously banned use of DDT) applied inside the house kill those that enter. The aquatic stages of the mosquito can be destroyed by eliminating temporary breeding pools, by spraying ponds with synthetic insecticides, or by applying a layer of oil to the surface waters. Biological control includes introducing fish (*Gambusia*) that feed on mosquito larvae into small ponds.

⊕ Impacts and Issues

Malaria has been described as the world's greatest public health concern. About half the world's population is at risk, especialy children under five years old in sub-Saharan Africa, though rates dropped in the WHO African Region by 54 percent from 2000 to 2013. Those living in Asia, Latin America, and parts of the Middle East are also at risk. Malaria has essentially been eradicated in most parts of North America, Europe, and Australia, although infected travelers and immigrants can reintroduce the disease if bitten by an infected mosquito. Although eliminated from the United States, an estimated 1,400 travelers to malaria-endemic areas return to the United States each year carrying malarial infections. The cases of malaria are ultimately fatal in, on average,

Life Cycle of the Malaria Parasite

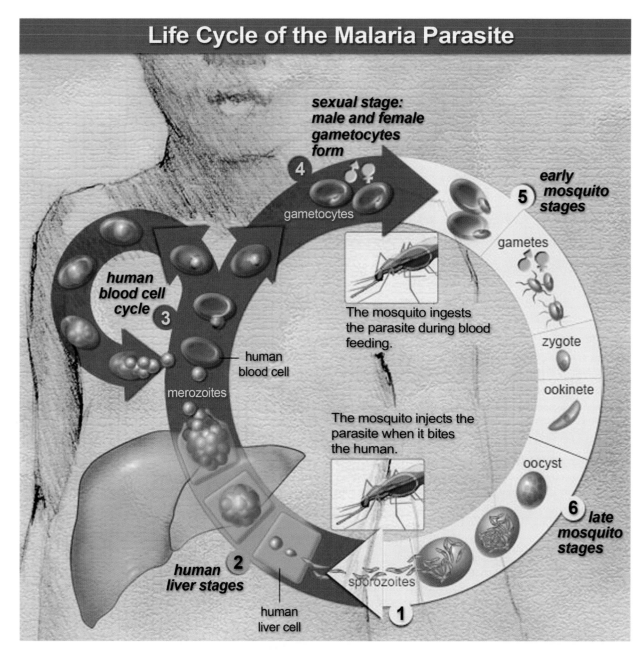

Produced by the National Institute of Allergy and Infectious Diseases (NIAID), this illustration depicts the life cycle of the malaria parasite, differentiating between the parasite's development inside the mosquito vector and development inside the human host, specifically inside the liver hepatocytes, and red blood cells circulating in the blood. In 2010 an estimated 219 million cases of malaria occurred worldwide and 660,000 people died, most (91 percent) in the WHO African Region. *National Institute of Allergy and Infectious Diseases (NIAID)/U.S. Centers for Disease Control and Prevention.*

seven such travelers each year. Malaria presents a major burden for tropical communities and travelers, particularly in areas where the parasite has evolved resistance to the first-line drugs used to treat it.

Malaria can be prevented or cured by a wide variety of drugs (quinine, chloroquine, mefloquine, atovaquone and proguanil, hydroxychloroquine, or pyrimethamine). However, resistant strains of the common species of *Plasmodium* mean that some prophylactic drugs (chloroquine and pyrimethamine) are no longer totally effective.

Organized local campaigns to reduce or temporarily eradicate malaria are usually successful, but the disease is sure to return unless the measures are vigilantly maintained. Some climatologists have argued that the changing global climate of the 21st century could see malaria spread to more temperate parts of the world.

Environmental efforts at preventing the disease have been directed at draining swampy areas and spraying for mosquitoes in areas where they breed. An insecticide spraying campaign undertaken in India was effective for several years, until the mosquitoes evolved resistance to the insecticide used against them and rebounded. The insecticide DDT is used effectively again in targeted areas where mosquitoes carrying resistant malaria are present. In areas where malaria is a constant threat, including many countries in Africa and areas of India, DDT is sprayed inside the dwellings of humans and animals along the walls and roofs in order to reduce the number of insects that carry the malaria parasite. Called indoor residual spraying, the technique is recommended by the WHO as an inexpensive and effective measure to eliminate malaria-carrying mosquitoes where they are most likely to encounter their human hosts, and when used properly, causes no harm to humans or other animals and the surrounding environment.

People in malarial areas are advised to avoid the outdoors during peak mosquito feeding times (dusk and dawn), to use window screens, and to sleep under nets treated with insecticide. However, there are millions of people in malaria-infested regions who are too poor to acquire window screens or netting. In 2007, the WHO encouraged governments where malaria is endemic to make insecticide-treated mosquito nets available rapidly and without cost. After health officials in Kenya distributed over 3 million nets to houses with children in malaria-affected districts, health officials there noted a significant decrease in malaria deaths among children.

The fact that Europe and North America have not been afflicted by malaria since the early 20th century has meant that for decades relatively little research was done on malaria vaccines, new malarial drugs, or specialized insecticides. However, world funding for malaria research has increased dramatically since the mid-1990s and in 2002, researchers announced that they had completely characterized the genomes of the *P. falciparum* parasite and its vector (means of transmission), the *Anopheles gambiae* mosquito. It is hoped that this knowledge will increase understanding of parasite-host and parasite-vector relationships, symptom causation, and drug responses, and will accelerate vaccine development and suggest possibilities for new drugs.

⊕ Future Implications

Studies published in the journal *The Lancet* in 2012 used computer modeling and historical malaria data to show that malaria deaths peaked in 2004 at 1.8 million.

It is uncertain how climate change will affect malaria models. The parasites require a temperature of at least 68 degrees Fahrenheit (20 degrees Celsius) to complete their life cycles. Besides temperature, humidity and rainfall are factors affecting the transmission of malaria.

PLASMODIUM IMMUNITY

In areas where malaria is endemic (normally present), many individuals appear to be immune to the disease. In some populations, including those of India, Latin America, southern Europe, and especially Africa, the gene causing sickle-cell anemia is present.

This gene is directly correlated with malaria immunity: a person possessing one copy of the sickle-cell gene will be malaria-resistant, while a person possessing two copies of the gene will be both malaria-resistant and sickle-cell anemic. Further, even among people who do not have the sickle-cell gene at all, not all infected individuals have symptoms; many individuals will host parasites within their bodies for months and years without showing symptoms. This suggests that a vaccine could be developed, if the mechanism of host immunity could be identified. Thus far, however, the complexity of the immune response and the diversity of the parasite's evasive mechanisms have prevented researchers from clinically assessing immunity. Evidently, each of the protozoan's developmental stages bears different antigens (the molecules that trigger the development of immunity in the host). What is more, these factors are different for each of the four strains of the parasite. This explains why no individual is known to be immune to all four malarial strains.

While global temperatures are predicted to rise, the rise is unequal geographically (i.e., with regard to malaria prone regions). It is likely that more areas of a warming world will become habitats for the *Anopheles* mosquito and its parasites.

As part of the Malaria Vaccine Initiative launched in 1999, candidates for a vaccine against malaria are in various stages of advanced research. The WHO, along with other world health authorities, announced their intention to accelerate the development and licensing of an effective malaria vaccine. Called the Malaria Vaccine Technology Roadmap, this set of strategies calls for vaccines to be developed in stages; the first goal is to introduce a vaccine that will protect against malaria for one year or more and have a 50 percent or greater effectiveness rate. By 2025, the Roadmap calls for a vaccine that can prevent more than 80 percent of malaria cases and is effective for more than four years.

Many people experience side effects from antimalarial medications. Further, chloroquine-resistant strains of falciparum malaria are on the increase worldwide. *P. falciparum* is the most dangerous of the four malaria strains, and can kill a healthy adult within 48 hours. This type is so dangerous because the parasitized red blood cells can become sequestered in the deep vascular beds of the brain—called cerebral malaria for severe malaria infection with this strain.

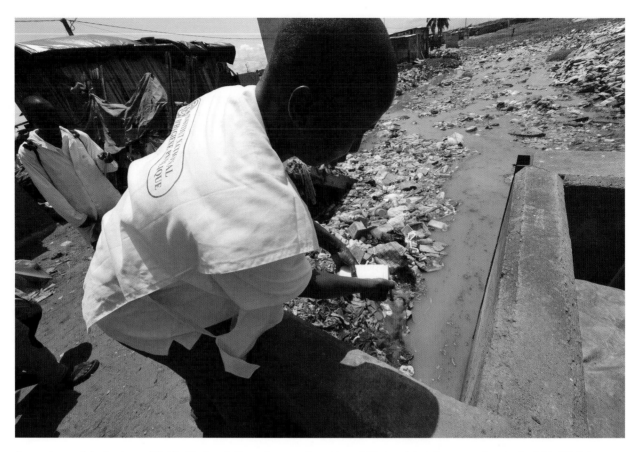

An employee of the Institute of Public Hygiene in Ivory Coast applies an insecticide powder against mosquitos on April 28, 2014, in Koumassi, a popular district in the south of Abidjan, Ivory Coast, during an operation to prevent malaria as part of the World Malaria Day. © *Sia Kambou/AFP/Getty Images.*

Malaria continues to be a global health problem. The disease has reemerged in places where it was assumed the disease had been eradicated. For instance, Sri Lanka and India were virtually free of malaria at the end of the 1970s, but from the 1980s, the number of cases began to increase, reaching levels not seen since before World War II (1939–1945) by the 1990s. Resistance of the parasites to antimalarial drugs, and resistance of *Anopheles* mosquitoes to insecticides are the major factors in the resurgence of the disease. Moreover, increased movements by travelers and migrants on a global scale are likely to add to the risk of reintroducing malaria to countries where it had previously been eradicated.

The results of several studies show a deadly connection between two diseases that are already among the leading causes of disease-related death in Africa. Individuals already infected with human immunodeficiency virus (HIV) show increased levels of the virus in their blood when they also contract malaria. The higher levels of virus make it more likely that they can pass on the HIV infection. In addition, people who are HIV infected show a greater susceptibility to malaria.

The Global Malaria Action Plan, endorsed by the WHO, aims to reduce malaria worldwide and eventually eradicate the disease. The United States is the largest donor to the Global Malaria Action Plan and overall malaria control efforts worldwide. In addition, philanthropic organizations such as the Bill & Melinda Gates Foundation have made conquering malaria among their top priorities.

PRIMARY SOURCE

This Day Relenting God

SOURCE Ross, Ronald. *"This Day Relenting God,"* Memoirs with a Full Account of the Great Malaria Problem and Its Solution. *London: John Murray, 1923, 226.*

INTRODUCTION *This primary source is a poem written by Sir Ronald Ross (1857–1932), a physician in the Indian Medical Service who received Nobel Prize for Physiology or Medicine in 1902 for his work on discovering that malaria*

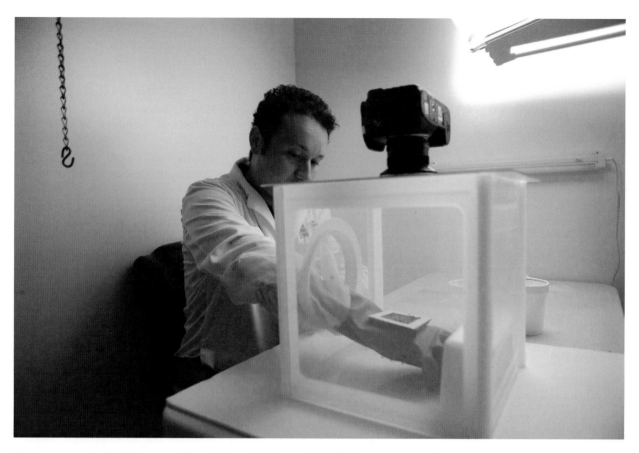

Testing was ongoing in 2014 on a small patch that makes humans "invisible" to mosquitoes, which could prove a powerful weapon against malaria and other mosquito-borne diseases. The Kite patch boasts 48 hours of protection as it disperses nontoxic compounds (safe for even pregnant mothers and children) that block mosquitoes' human-hunting sensors, limiting their ability to detect carbon dioxide and smell skin odors. Cheaper than existing highly toxic repellents, the disposable square patch measures just 1.5 inches (38 millimeters) on each side, and is applied to clothing like a sticker. Initially funded by the Bill & Melinda Gates Foundation, it was created after three years of work at Olfactor Laboratories and research at the University of California, Riverside. It is also being tested in Uganda after it reached its fund-raising target through crowdsourcing, where donations and contributions were asked for online. There are global plans to distribute patches, making it affordable in developing economies and regions impacted most by mosquito-borne diseases. © *Kite/Rex Features/AP Images.*

was transmitted by mosquitoes. In addition to his scientific achievements, Ross was a published novelist, playwright, and poet. He composed the following poem after discovering the malaria parasite inside the mosquito.

This day relenting God
Hath placed within my hand
A wondrous thing; and God
Be praised. At His command,

Seeking His secret deeds
With tears and toiling breath,
I find thy cunning seeds,
O million-murdering Death,

I know this little thing
A myriad man will save.
O Death, where is they sting?
Thy victory, O Grave?

PRIMARY SOURCE

Reliable Quinine

SOURCE *"Reliable Quinine," Advertisement. From* The Prevention of Malaria. *Ronald Ross; with contributions by L. O. Howard [and others]. London: J. Murray, 1910. Wellcome Library, London. http://wellcomeimages.org (accessed January 25, 2015).*

INTRODUCTION *This primary source is a vintage advertisement for quinine, offered in different forms as a treatment for malaria. Quinine, an alkaloid, was the first known antimalarial drug in Western medicine. It is still found on the World Health Organization's Model List of Essential Medicines.*

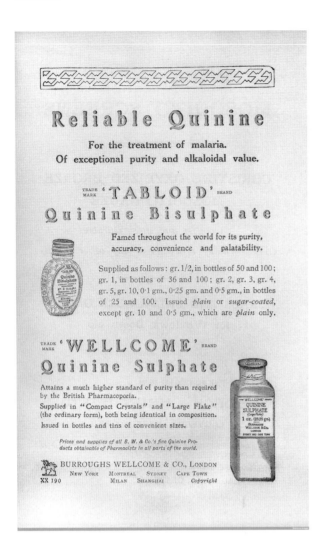

Vector Borne Diseases. Chichester, UK: Wiley-Blackwell, 2011.

Müller, Olaf. *Malaria in Africa: Challenges for Control and Elimination in the 21st Century.* Frankfurt am Main, Germany: Peter Lang, 2011.

Packard, Randall M. *The Making of a Tropical Disease: A Short History of Malaria.* Baltimore: Johns Hopkins University Press, 2011.

Peterson, Anna Margrét, and Gerald E. Calamandrei, eds. *Malaria: Etiology, Pathogenesis, and Treatments.* New York: Nova Science, 2012.

Shah, Sonia. *The Fever: How Malaria Has Ruled Humankind for 500,000 Years.* New York: Sarah Crichton Books/Farrar, Straus and Giroux, 2010.

Sherman, Irwin W. *The Malaria Genome Projects: Promise, Progress, and Prospects.* London: Imperial College Press, 2012.

Shore, William H. *The Imaginations of Unreasonable Men: Inspiration, Vision, and Purpose in the Quest to End Malaria.* New York: PublicAffairs, 2010.

Snowden, Frank M., and Richard Bucala, eds. *The Global Challenge of Malaria Past Lessons and Future Prospects.* Singapore: World Scientific, 2014.

Staines, Henry M., and Sanjeev Krishna, eds. *Treatment and Prevention of Malaria Antimalarial Drug Chemistry, Action and Use.* Basel: Springer, 2012.

Webb, James L. A., Jr. *The Long Struggle against Malaria in Tropical Africa.* New York: Cambridge University Press, 2014.

Periodicals

Fletcher, T. E., and N. J. Beeching. "Malaria." *Journal of the Royal Army Medical Corps* 159, no. 3 (2013): 158–166.

Grayson, M. "Malaria." *Nature* 484, no. 7395 (2012): S13.

Killeen, Gerry F. "Characterizing, Controlling and Eliminating Residual Malaria Transmission." *Malaria Journal* 13 (August 23, 2014): 330

Roach, R. R. "Malaria." *International Public Health Journal* 4, no. 2 (2012): 141–147.

Sinka, Marianne E., et al. "A Global Map of Dominant Malaria Vectors." *Parasites & Vectors* 5 (April 4, 2012): 69.

Smith, Thomas A., Nakul Chitnis, and Erin M. Stuckey. "Estimating Malaria Transmission through Mathematical Models." *Trends in Parasitology* 29, no. 10 (2013): 477–482.

White, Nicholas J., et al. "Malaria." *The Lancet* 383, no. 9918 (2014): 723–735.

Websites

"About Malaria." *Malaria Foundation International.* http://www.malaria.org/index.php?option=com_content&task=section&id=8&Itemid=32 (accessed March 18, 2015).

SEE ALSO *Avian (Bird) and Swine Influenzas; Child Health; Climate Change: Health Impacts; Global Health Initiatives; Insect-Borne Diseases; Pan-American Interoceanic Highway or Transoceanic Highway: Health Impacts; Parasitic Diseases*

BIBLIOGRAPHY

Books

Carter, Eric D. *Enemy in the Blood: Malaria, Environment, and Development in Argentina.* Tuscaloosa: University of Alabama Press, 2012.

Kamat, Vinay R. *Silent Violence: Global Health, Malaria, and Child Survival in Tanzania.* Tucson: University of Arizona Press, 2013.

Lobo, Lancy. *Malaria in the Social Context: A Study in Western India.* London: Routledge, 2010.

Matthews, Graham. *Integrated Vector Management: Controlling Vectors of Malaria and Other Insect*

"Malaria." *U.S. Centers for Disease Control and Prevention (CDC).* http://www.cdc.gov/malaria (accessed March 18, 2015).

"Malaria." Fact Sheet No. 94. *World Health Organization (WHO),* December 2014. http://www.who.int/entity/mediacentre/factsheets/fs094/en/index.html (accessed March 18, 2015).

Malaria No More. http://www.malarianomore.org (accessed March 18, 2015).

"Malaria: Strategy Overview." *Bill & Melinda Gates Foundation.* http://www.gatesfoundation.org/What-We-Do/Global-Health/Malaria (accessed March 18, 2015).

"World Malaria Report 2014." *World Health Organization (WHO),* 2014. http://www.who.int/malaria/publications/world_malaria_report_2014/en/ (accessed March 18, 2015).

K. Lee Lerner

Malnutrition

⊕ Introduction

Malnutrition describes a diet that includes inadequate quantities of protein, vitamins, and other micronutrients needed for human well-being. The symptoms of malnutrition include low energy, reduced physical and mental development, and the susceptibility to disease. Approximately 2 billion to 3 billion people suffer from some form of malnutrition. Malnutrition is most prevalent in poorer developing countries, although it also occurs among poor people living in rich countries. Hunger kills more people than AIDS, tuberculosis, and malaria combined in Africa, Asia, Latin America, the Caribbean, and the Pacific regions.

Hunger and a lack of food are indicators of malnutrition. The United Nations World Food Programme (WFP) states that approximately 800 million people in the world suffer from hunger, lacking consistent and reliable levels of nutritious food to lead a healthy and active life. The World Health Organization (WHO) also considers the growing number of overweight individuals a problem of malnutrition. Approximately 1.5 billion people in the world are obese, including more than 43 million children. Globally, obesity causes more than 2.5 million deaths each year.

Approximately 18 percent of those suffering from hunger are children, with poor nutrition accounting for approximately half of the deaths of children under the age of five. There is also a gender disparity with malnutrition: more than 60 percent of those who are hungry are female. Girls are more likely to die from malnutrition than boys. Pregnant women have particular dietary needs, including the need for higher amounts of protein and iron. Maternal malnutrition is common in developing countries, which increases the risks of poor child development and complications in pregnancy.

Ongoing hunger and resulting chronic malnutrition are common problems for people in poverty. Shorter-term periods of acute hunger and malnutrition may also occur following poor harvests, natural disasters, war, or other calamities. In extreme cases, famines may occur, when more than 30 percent of the population, and 20 percent of households, are faced with acute food shortages.

⊕ Historical Background

Malnutrition was the norm around the world prior to the Industrial Revolution, with life expectancy less than 35 years of age for most countries. Numerous improvements to human health and nutrition occurred with the Industrial Revolution in the 18th and 19th centuries. Although life expectancy had risen, half of the world's population faced malnourishment in all regions of the world at the beginning of the 20th century.

Overcoming malnutrition on a large scale in the Western world became a more possible goal in the 1900s. Better nutrition was the result of improved economic growth and increased agricultural productivity. Also important were the strengthening of government institutions, policies, and social programs that enabled the poor to access nutritious food more easily. In addition, a better understanding of the science of nutrition helped to improve nutrition quality.

A reduction in malnutrition also occurred in developing countries during the 1900s, although at a slower pace than developed countries. Increased food production in developing countries beginning in the 1960s was due in part to the Green Revolution, a worldwide effort that accelerated agriculture production through research, development, and implementation of modern technology including improved management strategies, irrigation technology, and better seeds and fertilizer application. Poverty in developing countries has been a major contributor to slower reductions in malnutrition.

Hunger and Famine

The Great Irish Famine is one of the most familiar instances of widespread hunger in Western history, killing an estimated 1 million people during the period from 1845 to 1849. This famine was caused by potato blight and failed government policies. During the Great Irish Famine, many people died from an inadequate intake of calories and protein, particularly infants and young children. A large number of people emigrated from Ireland to escape the famine.

Many deaths in Ireland resulted from infectious diseases, including dysentery, triggered by poor immunity associated with malnutrition. Others died from poisoning due to the ingestion of poor-quality food. Approximately one-third of the deaths during the Great Irish Famine resulted from cholera, malaria, influenza, and other infectious diseases indirectly attributed to a lack of food. Rates of these infectious diseases increase during famines due to a breakdown in social structures, particularly the ability to maintain sanitary conditions and provide medical care to the sick.

There are numerous examples of famines in human history before and after the Great Irish Famine. Cormac Ó Gráda discusses the numerous famines recorded over the centuries in the text *Famine: A Short History.* Both the Old and New Testaments of the Bible mention hunger and famine. One of the first recorded famines happened in Rome in 441 BCE. Hunger was common throughout the Middle Ages (c. 500–c. 1500), with nearly 100 famines occurring in Britain alone. A famine due to crop failures from 1693 to 1694 killed 1.5 million people in France.

Russia and the Soviet Union also experienced famine in the 20th century, including the starvation of up to 9 million people during 1921–1922 due to drought and civil war. The Soviet famine of the 1930s killed between 4 million and 5 million people in the Ukraine and other regions under Joseph Stalin's (1879–1953) control.

India and its Bengal Province (present-day Bangladesh) experienced a deadly famine in 1943, with estimates of 2 million to 3 million deaths following a year when a pathogen in the rice fields led to poor harvests. This Bengali famine struck working-class people particularly hard because rising food costs made it difficult for them to purchase food. Weakening relations between Britain and India, along with the ongoing World War II (1939–1945), aggravated the impacts of the famine. Author Thomas Keneally discusses the Bengali famine, along with the Great Irish Famine and Ethiopian famine in *Three Famines: Starvation and Politics.*

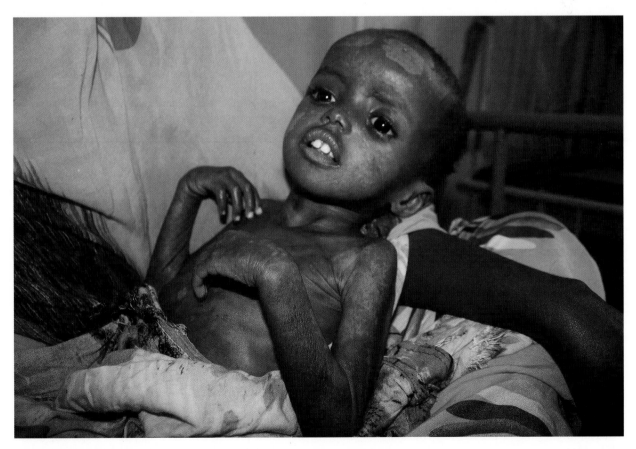

A malnourished girl rests in her mother's arms on a bed at Banadir hospital in Mogadishu, Somalia, in July 2014. The United Nations Food and Agriculture Organization issued a stark warning in June 2014 over food security in war-torn Somalia, launching an urgent appeal for US$18 million to stop hunger spreading. The agency estimated there were 860,000 people in need of humanitarian assistance in Somalia at the time, including 200,000 malnourished children under the age of five. Prices for staples such as maize and sorghum had risen by as much as 60 and 80 percent compared to April 2013.   © *Abdifitah Hashi Nor/AFP/Getty Images.*

GLOBAL FIGHT AGAINST MALNUTRITION

The global community identified reducing hunger and malnutrition as an important development objective in the creation of the Millennium Development Goals (MDGs) in 2000. Under the goal to reduce extreme poverty, a target of the MDGs was to halve the number of people who suffer from hunger between 1990 and 2015. Although hunger persists in certain parts of the world, this goal nearly was reached by 2015.

The number of malnourished individuals declined significantly, from 24 percent in the early 1990s to 14 percent in 2013. However, the rate of decline has slowed since 2005. Areas of eastern and Central Asia, North Africa, and Latin America and the Caribbean saw big improvements in fighting hunger. The rates of improvements have not been as great in southern Asia and sub-Saharan Africa.

Overall, the world has seen strong improvements in childhood nutrition since 1990. The rate of children under five years of age who are underweight decreased from 25 percent to 15 percent by 2013. Although this is an improvement, millions of children continue to suffer from malnutrition. One important indicator of malnutrition, stunting in children, has improved greatly. In 1990, 40 percent of children under the age of five were stunted. This number dropped to less than 25 percent in 2013. (See graphic.) However, there were still 162 million children under five who suffered from stunting due to inadequate nutrition in 2013.

Improving childhood nutrition is important for decreasing rates of infections and other diseases, promoting physical growth, and aiding cognitive development. Improving nutrition in children is seen to improve school attendance and educational achievement. The nutrition children receive while developing as embryos, along with the nutrition quality during the first two years of life, is critical for improving the health of children.

Improving nutrition is not only a matter of increasing the amount of food provided to households, but also requires addressing other public health problems. Poor health conditions and high incidence of diseases including HIV/AIDS, diarrhea, malaria, and tuberculosis exacerbate nutritional problems. Similarly, the prognosis of these diseases is improved with improved nutrition. Many of the deaths of children under the age of five occur when they are weakened by malnutrition and susceptible to infectious disease.

Under guidance of the World Health Organization, the World Health Assembly (WHA) adopted a plan in 2012 to meet six global nutrition targets by 2025. The goals are: (1) Decrease the number of children under five who are stunted by 40 percent. (2) Decrease the rate of anemia in women of reproductive age by 50 percent. (3) Decrease the number of babies born with low birth weight by 30 percent. (4) Have no increase in childhood obesity. (5) Increase the number of babies breast-fed during the first six months of life by 50 percent. (6) Decrease the rates of wasting to less than 5 percent of all children.

These objectives were designed with the recognition that governments will have the primary responsibility to create policies and programs to realize the targets. Also, donor countries, development agencies, and community groups need to be active participants in developing strategies to meet the WHA goals. Achieving these goals is expected to be difficult, yet success could greatly improve the nutritional status of people in developing countries.

China is perhaps the country most familiar with famine, with more than 1,800 documented famines over the last 2,000 years. Estimates range from between 20 million and 43 million people dead from malnutrition and starvation throughout China between 1958 and 1961. Historians blame these deaths in part on the policies of Mao Zedong (1893–1976) that mandated rapid industrialization of rural areas, which collectively were named the Great Leap Forward.

War, drought, and inadequate government policy have caused sub-Saharan Africa to become one of the world's regions where rates of hunger increased during the late 20th and early 21st centuries. The Western world paid close attention to the Ethiopian famine of 1983–1985 due to comprehensive media coverage. That famine killed more than 400,000 people. Approximately 3.8 million died from malnutrition and hunger from 1998 to 2004 during a time of war in the Democratic Republic of the Congo.

Science and Medicine

Medical research understanding the links between nutrition, the immune system, and human development was primitive prior to the 1950s. Since the mid-20th century there has been a growing understanding of the relationship between poor nutrition and disease susceptibility. In 1968, Nevin Scrimshaw (1918–2013), Carl Taylor (1916–2010), and John Gordon (1890–1983) published an important monograph for the WHO titled *Interactions of Nutrition and Infection*. Following this work was the development of the concept of the malnutrition infection cycle, in which inadequate nutritional intake leads to weight loss and poor growth, which in turn leads to an increase in the occurrence of disease. There is then further appetite loss and loss of nutrients, continuing the cycle.

Initial investigations into the link between malnutrition and human immunodeficiency virus/acquired immune deficiency syndrome (HIV/AIDS) occurred in the 1980s. Both malnutrition and HIV suppress the immune system in similar ways. Malnutrition became an important predictor of HIV to AIDS. Typically, undernourished HIV/AIDS patients will have much quicker weight loss than patients with proper nourishment. The WHO recognized the importance of treating issues of malnutrition in patients suffering from HIV/AIDS following a technical review of the literature in 2003 and 2004.

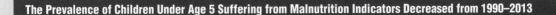

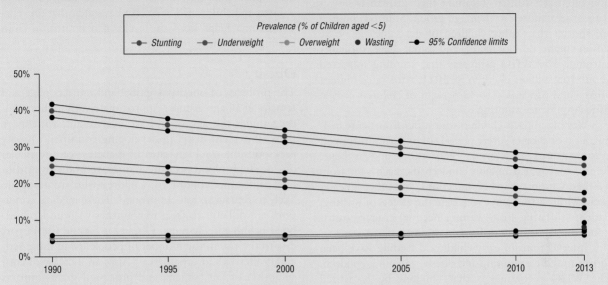

The Prevalence of Children Under Age 5 Suffering from Malnutrition Indicators Decreased from 1990–2013

Prevalence (% of Children aged <5)

● Stunting   ● Underweight   ● Overweight   ● Wasting   ● 95% Confidence limits

SOURCE: Adapted from "Global Child Malnutrition Trends (1990–2013)," *UNICEF-WHO-World Bank Child Malnutrition Dashboard*, United Nations Children's Fund (UNICEF), World Bank, and World Health Organization (WHO), 2014.

Health-care workers use growth charts to track the weight and height of children and adolescents as they age. Body mass index (BMI), a ratio of weight and height also used to track growth and health, is another measure to monitor obesity. The opportunity for nutritional intervention arises if a child is not following a healthy growth pattern based on accepted growth standards. The WHO, the U.S. government, and other national governments adopted standardized height-for-age and weight-for-age growth charts in 1977 based on a large multiyear study of childhood growth. The WHO recommended that the data in these charts serve as a reference for malnutrition.

The growth charts have been used widely throughout the world, but not without some criticism. There has been concern of a lack of racial diversity in the data that are used to construct the chart. Also, the original charts were based on children who were fed strictly with infant formula rather than being breast-fed. The global charts have been revised and refined to address these concerns and make them more useful for health-care workers. New data collected in 1994 and from 1997 to 2003 aimed to include a more global picture of healthy growth rates.

Subsequent charts released by the WHO allow growth of children to be monitored in relation to regional and countrywide standards.

Global Response and Food Aid

The organization of countries with surpluses of food to provide hunger relief to those countries suffering from hunger did not begin to occur regularly until the middle of the 20th century. However, food aid was provided in earlier times, including during the Great Irish Famine when the United Kingdom purchased maize (corn) from the United States as relief for the Irish people. In the mid-2010s, the WFP coordinates and delivers the majority of food aid to hungry communities around the world.

Established by the UN General Assembly and Food and Agricultural Organization (FAO), the WFP began operations in 1963. However, at that time the United States and Canada delivered 90 percent of all food aid outside of the WFP. In 1974, the global community agreed that it would be more effective to reach those in need by coordinating food aid through one organization. Although many organizations provide technical assistance to hunger relief efforts and agriculture development projects, the WFP has assumed coordination of the majority of food aid distribution.

🌐 Impacts and Issues

Children suffering from chronic, longer-term malnutrition often are stunted, meaning their growth is slower than other children in their age group. Stunted children are shorter than other children of the same age, have slower brain development, and often have difficulty learning. The WHO estimates that stunting impacted about 165 million children in 2011, with rates highest in Asia and Africa. Up to 42 percent of children in East Africa experience stunting.

Wasting impacts children who suffer from acute malnutrition or shorter severe periods of undernourishment. Wasting causes the deterioration of muscle and fat tissue. Approximately 1.5 million children die each year from wasting. Chronic diarrhea, infections, and other illnesses occur with wasting and exacerbate the effects of wasting. Patients suffering from wasting need emergency nutritional supplements in order to stay alive.

Interventions in early childhood feeding have been shown to reduce stunting and obesity in young children. The WHO recommends that children be breast-fed exclusively for the first six months of life. Breast-feeding should continue for at least two years, in conjunction with appropriate complementary foods. Approximately 20 percent of deaths of children under the age of five could be eliminated if these nutrition guidelines are followed.

Vitamins and Minerals

The WHO reports that iron, iodine, vitamin A, and zinc are the most common vitamin and mineral deficiencies observed. The most common nutrient deficiency is iron, which often occurs as a result of diets consisting of only grains and legumes without any animal products. Iron deficiency is the primary cause of anemia, a condition in which blood cells do not carry enough oxygen to all of the tissues in the body. Anemia symptoms include fatigue, weakness, and dizziness. Left untreated, it can lead to higher rates of illness, poor cognitive development in children, and lower physical abilities. The prevalence of anemia increases when other diseases are present, including malaria and gastrointestinal infections caused by poor water quality.

Researchers estimate that nearly 2 billion people have deficient iodine levels in their diet, resulting in problems related to the thyroid, including goiters. Iodine is added to table salt in many countries to improve iodine consumption levels. More than one-third of preschool-age children have a deficiency in vitamin A, the primary cause of preventable childhood blindness. Vitamins and minerals are important for improving immunity and fostering proper physical and mental development.

Anemia impacts all genders and age groups, but is a particular problem for adolescent girls and pregnant women. Forty-two percent of pregnant women suffer from anemia. Increasing iron absorption and including additional micronutrients in the diet such as folic acid, vitamin A, and vitamin B12 can help prevent development problems in fetuses, and reduce death rates of women and children. The WHO has stated that preventing anemia helps keep the cycle of malnutrition from passing to the next generation.

Obesity

The problem of obesity is global and impacts male and females in all age groups. Approximately 43 million children under the age of five are overweight, with more than 70 percent living in developing countries. Obesity is responsible for high rates of diabetes, cardiovascular disease, high blood pressure, cancer, reproductive problems, and other conditions. Children who are obese are likely to remain so into adulthood. These medical conditions are difficult to treat in countries with underdeveloped health-care systems. Obesity is on the rise in part due to the rise in the number of people living more sedentary lifestyles in urban areas. Also, an increase in consumption of fats, sugars, and processed grains impacts rates of obesity.

The WHO has implemented a special commission to address issues of obesity, particularly for children. This commission has identified key factors for reducing obesity, particularly the creation of supportive school and community environments that encourage parents and children to make more healthful food choices and increase physical activities. The WHO has suggested policies aimed at improving the availability of affordable and healthful food choices for all consumers. The marketing of unhealthful food options toward children and teenagers may contribute to obesity.

Food Assistance

Providing assistance to fight against malnutrition requires the coordination of many entities including government organizations, community groups, nongovernmental organizations (NGOs), religious groups, other countries, and international humanitarian groups. In some cases, coordination also involves military organizations, and private companies are vital to alleviating hunger and malnutrition. When communities and local governments are unable to provide adequate assistance to those in need, international organizations that specialize in hunger alleviation and issues related to malnutrition often are asked to coordinate relief efforts. The WHO, the United Nations Children's Fund (UNICEF), and Médecins Sans Frontières (MSF, or Doctors Without Borders) are examples of key international organizations providing malnutrition related programs and assistance.

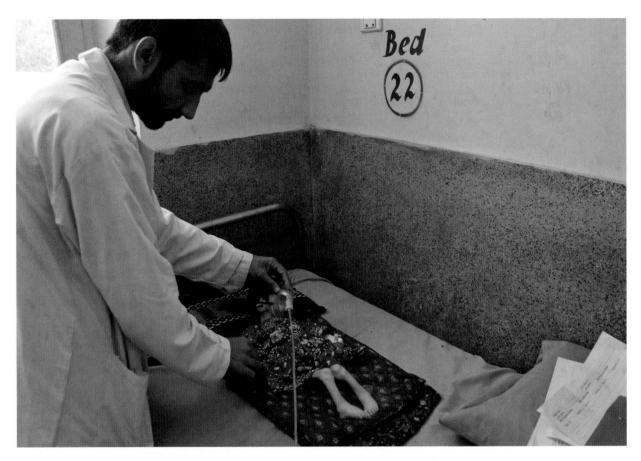

An Afghan child suffering from severe malnutrition receives treatment at a regional hospital in Jalalabad, Afghanistan, in 2014. A study on the situation of nutrition in Afghanistan showed that over 6 percent of children under the age of five suffer from acute malnutrition (low ratio of weight to height), with 40 to 60 percent of children in the same age group suffering from chronic malnutrition.   *© Noorullah Shirzada/AFP/Getty Images.*

Emergency food aid consists of that aid used to meet the acute food needs of individuals struck by natural disasters, epidemics, and war. The WFP describes emergency aid as short-term food aid provided to targeted needy people on a grant basis, meaning the countries receiving it are not required to pay for it. Emergency food aid is distributed to households in the community to minimize instances of malnutrition. Pregnant women, children, individuals suffering from HIV/AIDS, and others experiencing extreme malnutrition receive emergency therapeutic food assistance.

Assistance also is provided to deal with chronic, ongoing issues of malnutrition. The organization Action Against Hunger (Action Contre la Faim, or ACF) discusses the need to provide assistance that addresses social, organizational, and technical concerns of communities that keep them from providing proper nutrition to all members. The ACF provides technical training, mentorship, and other programs that improve local capacity to fight malnutrition. Other organizations assist with building hospitals, providing food to children at schools and improving farming production.

Food Security and Nutrition

Hunger and famine can result from long-term poverty, crop failure, natural disasters, war, and the displacement of people within countries and across international borders. Government policies may further exacerbate situations of hunger. For example, the colonial government of India was criticized for triggering a famine in 1873 because it adopted policies to promote the exportation of commodity food crops. There were accusations that the Ethiopian government could have avoided the famine in 2003 if it had reduced expenditures on military equipment to fight Eritrea. Many issues of hunger do not arise because of a lack of food in a given country or region. Instead, when the ability of people to access food is compromised due to natural disasters, political unrest, or high prices, hunger may become widespread.

Amartya Sen's (1933–) seminal book published in 1981, *Poverty and Famines: An Essay on Entitlement,* is credited with moving the focus toward the ability of people to access food. Sen recognized that people are not deprived of nutritious food because it is not available in the market, but because their access is constrained by other factors. These factors may include lack of income, living far from markets, and weak social networks to assist with coping with a death or other shock faced by a household. Prior to Sen, most policy solutions aimed at avoiding famine and other hunger problems focused on increasing the food supply. Sen's pointed out the limitations of investing in agricultural improvements as the sole way to combat issues of hunger.

⊕ Future Implications

The International Food Policy Research Institute (IFPRI) published the *Global Nutrition Report* in 2014 with nutrition experts from the WHO and other institutions in part to identify global needs to fight malnutrition. The report indicates the nutrition targets set by the World Health Assembly (WHA, which sets global health policies, priorities, and goals for the WHO) are at risk of not being met given the status of policy and intervention. There should be research to understand the ability of some locations to meet nutrition targets while others struggle. The report states that nutrition indicators need to be included more extensively in sustainable development targets because nutrition is important for countries to develop sustainably.

Many countries have pledged funds to address issues of malnutrition. For example, the countries of the European Union announced an investment of 3.5 billion euros to fight malnutrition in developing countries between 2014 and 2020. This pledge is directed to the poorest developing countries. The European Union pledge recognizes the need not only to address issues of hunger but to support programs to improve nutrition, which do not always get the attention needed to be successful.

Malnutrition interventions need to address effectively the variety of malnourishment problems faced by given locations, including stunting, wasting, and obesity. It is necessary for policy makers, development workers, and communities to understand that countries may face one of these problems or combinations of these problems. Intervention programs need to be flexible to address the particular needs of women, children, and other groups particularly vulnerable to the effects of malnutrition. It is necessary to expand efforts to collect and analyze data related to malnutrition, and make these data publicly available, in order to best understand the nutrition needs of a given location. There are data gaps that keep financial resources from being used in the most effective manner.

The worldwide distribution of food aid is tracked by the Food Aid Information System, an international effort coordinated by the WFP to provide data on all food aid donated and received by countries and organizations. This information helps researchers and policy analysts understand whether or not assistance is reaching those who need it the most. For example, the data may indicate whether or not the international community is responding effectively with food aid to lessen human suffering and assist countries in long-term recovery efforts during times of disaster.

Funding for malnutrition problems needs to be focused toward the underlying issues that lead to poor nutrition. For example, investments that increase sanitation and provide access to clean water have been shown to improve nutrition outcomes. Also, investments in agriculture improvements need to be sensitive to the nutrition needs of the population. Improvements in education access, particularly women's enrollment in secondary school, assist with reaching nutrition goals. The WHO has developed a nutrition landscape information system to profile the key indicators of nutrition and related factors, including access to food and health care.

Monitoring of malnutrition programs is needed to track the effectiveness of financial resources. Guatemala is a country in Latin America that has successfully implemented a system to monitor and track nutrition related spending and outcomes. Such monitoring systems are critical, but their implementation requires strong political will, technical knowledge, and coordination of institutions and departments. At times, there are countries that pledge financial resources to fight malnutrition. The IFPRI report suggests the need to hold donor countries accountable for pledges, as well as to better track financial resources and provide targets for the financing of nutrition support programs.

Nutrition experts, motivated institutions, coordinated policies, and strong leadership are critical for achieving nutritional goals. An example of all of these factors working together occurred in the state of Maharashtra in central India, which saw large reductions in child stunting rates in a short time. In 2005, 36.5 of children under age five (39 percent of children under age two) were stunted, but this number fell to 24 percent (23 percent for those under two) in 2012, mainly due to overall economic growth and food security and service delivery through the state-level Nutrition Mission and the national Integrated Child Development Services and the National Rural Health Mission, programs for child nutrition, health, and development. The regional and national programs focused on maternal nutrition and education, expanded postnatal care, and nutrition programs for children under age two, according to UNICEF and the Institute of Development Studies. There is a need to support the training of experts, provide resources to employ a nutrition-related workforce, and to ensure countries implement nutrition-related research programs.

Biofortification of crops may increase the presence of micronutrients such as zinc, iron, vitamin A, and protein in the staple crops grown in various parts of the world. Biofortification can be done through plant breeding or through genetic modification. More research is needed to understand whether biofortification is a cost-effective approach to improving the nutritional quality of food.

PRIMARY SOURCE

The State of Food Insecurity in the World 2014

SOURCE *FAO, IFAD, and WFP. 2014. "Foreword," in The State of Food Insecurity in the World 2014. Strengthening the Enabling Environment for Food Security and Nutrition. Rome: Food and Agriculture Organization of the United Nations, 2014, 4–5. Reproduced with permission. http://www.fao.org/3/a-i4030e.pdf (accessed January 30, 2015).*

INTRODUCTION *This primary source is the foreword from the 2014 version of an annual publication by the Food and Agriculture Organization of the United Nations, the International Fund for Agricultural Development, and the World Food Programme. Its purpose, as outlined in the 2013 publication, is to "raise awareness about global hunger issues, discuss underlying causes of hunger and malnutrition and monitor progress towards hunger reduction targets." The bulletin is aimed at a broad range of readers, including "policy-makers, international organizations, academic institutions and the general public."*

FOREWORD

When the 69th United Nations General Assembly begins its General Debate on 23 September 2014, 464 days will remain to the end of 2015, the target date for achieving the Millennium Development Goals (MDG).

A stock-taking of where we stand on reducing hunger and malnutrition shows that progress in hunger reduction at the global level has continued but that food insecurity is still a challenge to be conquered.

The latest estimates show that, since 1990–92, the prevalence of undernourishment has fallen from 18.7 to 11.3 percent in 2012–14 for the world as a whole, and from 23.4 to 13.5 percent for the developing regions. The global MDG target 1c of reducing *by half* the *proportion* of undernourished people is within reach, if appropriate and immediate efforts are stepped up. Not only is MDG 1c within reach at the global level, but it has already been achieved by many countries. Sixty-three developing countries have already reached the target, 11 of which have maintained the prevalence of undernourishment below 5 percent since 1990–92, while another six are on track to do so by 2015. Twenty-five of the 63 countries have also accomplished the more ambitious 1996 World Food Summit (WFS) goal of halving the *number* of chronically underfed people.

Since 1990–92, the number of hungry people has fallen by over 200 million. This is proof that we can win the war against hunger and should inspire countries to move forward, with the assistance of the international community as needed, by finding individual sets of action that respond to their national needs and specificities. This is the first step to achieving the other MDGs.

Despite this progress, however, the number of hungry people in the world is still unacceptably high: at least 805 million people, or one in nine, worldwide do not have enough to eat. Global trends in hunger reduction mask disparities within and among regions.

While Northern Africa has had a consistently low prevalence of hunger at less than 5 percent, in sub-Saharan Africa, one in four people remain chronically hungry. Reversing this trend is our greatest challenge and requires transforming into concrete progress the growing political will in the region shown by the commitment made at the June 2014 African Union Summit to end hunger by 2025.

The sheer size of Asia makes it a region of extremes: 217 million Asians have overcome hunger since 1990–92; yet, it is still the region where two-thirds of the world's hungry live. Significant reductions in global hunger numbers require even greater progress in the region. While the MDG hunger target has already been achieved in Eastern and South-Eastern Asia, hunger prevalence in Southern Asia has declined, but insufficiently, since 1990–92.

Latin America and the Caribbean is the region that has shown the greatest progress in hunger reduction, with the prevalence of hunger reduced by almost two-thirds since the early 1990s. As a whole, it has already reached the MDG hunger target and is very close to meeting the WFS target. Government-led efforts combining support for production with social protection have been supported by much wider commitment: societies have decided to end hunger; parliaments are taking responsibility, and national efforts have been pushed forward by the strong commitment of the region as a whole that became the first region to commit to the goal of zero hunger by adopting the Hunger-Free Latin America and the Caribbean Initiative 2025 nearly ten years ago–a commitment reaffirmed by the region's leaders at recent Summits of the Community of Latin America and the Caribbean States (CELAC).

A most welcome message emerging from this year's report is that accelerated, substantial and sustainable hunger reduction is possible with the requisite political commitment. This has to be well informed by sound understanding of national challenges, relevant policy options, broad participation and lessons from other experiences. This year's report includes seven case studies that summarize how and to what extent some countries have sought to create an "enabling environment for food security and nutrition". Food insecurity and malnutrition are complex problems that cannot be solved by one sector or stakeholder alone, but need to be tackled in a coordinated way, with the necessary political commitment and integrated leadership. A critical appreciation of lessons learned is essential for hunger reduction.

We, as heads of the Rome-based food and agriculture agencies, will continue working with our member countries to support their efforts to accelerate progress in improving food security and nutrition by strengthening their capacities and capabilities to realize their commitments to make hunger a part of history and not of our future.

SEE ALSO   *Child Health; Global Health Initiatives; Health-Related Education and Information Access; High Blood Pressure; Noncommunicable Diseases (Lifestyle Diseases); Nutrition; Population Issues; Vulnerable Populations; Water Supplies and Access to Clean Water*

BIBLIOGRAPHY

Books

Haddad, Lawrence, Nick Nisbett, Inka Barnett, and Elsa Valli. *Maharashtra's Child Stunting Declines: What Is Driving Them? Findings of a Multidisciplinary Analysis.* Brighton, UK: Institute of Development Studies, 2014. Available online at http://www.cmamforum .org/Pool/Resources/Maharashtra-child-stunting-declines-IDS-2014.pdf (accessed February 13, 2015).

International Food Policy Research Institute (IFPRI). *Global Nutrition Report: Actions and Accountability to Accelerate the World's Progress on Nutrition.* Washington, DC: IFPRI, 2014.

Keneally, Thomas. *Three Famines: Starvation and Politics.* New York: PublicAffairs, 2011.

Ó Gráda, Cormac. *Famine: A Short History.* Princeton, NJ: Princeton University Press, 2009.

Scrimshaw, Nevin, Carl Taylor, and John Everett Gordon. *Interactions of Nutrition and Infection.* Geneva: World Health Organization, 1968.

Sen, Amartya. *Poverty and Famines: An Essay on Entitlement.* Oxford: Oxford University Press, 1981.

UNICEF. *Improving Child Nutrition: The Achievable Imperative for Global Progress.* New York: UNICEF, 2013. Available online at http://www.unicef.org/ publications/files/Nutrition_Report_final_lo_res_8_ April.pdf (accessed February 13, 2015).

Periodicals

Lachat, Carl, et al. "A Decade of Nutrition Research in Africa: Assessment of the Evidence Base and Academic Collaboration." *Public Health Nutrition* (October 2014): 1–8.

Stenberg, Karin, et al. "Advancing Social and Economic Development by Investing in Women's and Children's Health: A New Global Investment Framework." *The Lancet* 383, no. 9925 (April 2014): 1333–1354.

Websites

"Malnutrition." *Médecins Sans Frontières/Doctors Without Borders.* http://www.doctorswithoutborders .org/our-work/medical-issues/malnutrition (accessed January 14, 2015).

"Malnutrition." *Organisation mondiale de la Santé (WHO).* http://www.who.int/maternal_child_ adolescent/topics/child/malnutrition/fr/ (accessed January 14, 2015).

"Nutrition." *United Nations Children's Fund (UNICEF).* http://www.unicef.org/nutrition/ (accessed January 14, 2015).

"Nutrition." *World Food Programme.* http://www.wfp .org/nutrition (accessed January 14, 2015).

"Nutrition Global Targets 2025." *World Health Organization.* http://www.who.int/nutrition/topics/ nutrition_globaltargets2025/en/ (accessed January 7, 2015).

Steven Joseph Archambault

Marine Toxins and Pollution

⊕ Introduction

Marine toxins are produced by algae, bacteria, or pollution from chemicals and compounds in aquatic environments and are harmful to human health in concentrated doses. The toxins are concentrated in marine organisms that consume the toxins without apparent harm, after which the toxins are transmitted to humans who ingest contaminated seafood. When marine toxins are consumed by humans, they can impact human health adversely, causing neurological, gastrointestinal, and cardiovascular syndromes, which can sometimes result in death.

Marine algae, also known as phytoplankton, are single cell organisms that require sunlight and inorganic nutrients to grow. Some marine algae make toxins that then accumulate in organisms such as shellfish and fish through a process known as bioaccumulation, or the buildup of toxins in successive levels in the food chain.

Of the more than 4,000 species of marine algae, only 70 to 80 species are known to produce toxins, according to the United Nations Food and Agriculture Organization. Most of those toxin-producing algae are dinoflagellates, motile organisms that are normal components of the marine ecosystem. Ciguatera poisoning caused by dinoflagellates, for example, is the world's most common marine toxin disease, with about 50,000 cases reported per year.

Under the right environmental conditions, marine algae can experience rapid population booms. Marine biologists know of only around 300 species of marine algae that are involved in algal blooms. Shellfish that filter feed on these algal blooms can accumulate sufficient marine toxin in 24 hours to cause human illness, though not all algal blooms produce toxin. Algal blooms sometimes can be tinted brown or red, hence the name red tide. The frequency and geographic distribution of algal blooms are increasing due to climate change and the globalization of trade and travel. Agricultural runoff and other sources of pollution also have exacerbated algal blooms and thus instances of shellfish poisoning.

Other forms of marine pollution can pose a risk to human health as well. These include residential and industrial runoff and sewage, plastics, heavy metals such as mercury and lead, pesticides, and pharmaceutical compounds, among others. Persistent bioaccumulative toxic substances (PBTs) are amplified as they ascend in the food chain, thus posing a threat to human health.

In addition to toxins caused by algae and pollution, marine bacteria can produce toxins harmful to human health. Bacteria such as *Vibrio vulnificus* produce a toxin that can accumulate in oysters. Puffer fish poisoning has been linked to a bacterial toxin that when consumed can produce sudden death.

⊕ Historical Background

Shellfish Poisoning

Though shellfish poisoning has been recorded in humans as long as medical records have been kept, scientists did not determine the cause of the poisoning until 1927. During a shellfish poisoning outbreak on the coast of California, Dr. Hermann Sommer (1899–1950) and other scientists from the University of California at San Francisco observed and later identified a bloom of marine plankton that coincided with the cases of poisoning. The researchers characterized the marine plankton, the dinoflagellate *Gonyaulax catenella*, and showed that its toxins could be transmitted to and between mussels in the laboratory.

Sommer and his colleagues were able to estimate the dose of toxin needed to cause death in humans. For *Gonyaulax catenella* in mussels, this dose was 20,000 mouse units (MU) of toxin, as measured in mice to which the toxin was administered. Later work in Canada showed that only 5,000 MU of toxin was sufficient for a lethal dose in humans from the dinoflagellate *Gonyaulax tamarensis*. The work of Sommer and colleagues helped establish quarantine measures to minimize the public health risk posed by algal blooms and shellfish.

The geographic distribution of marine algae has been expanding due to globalized trade routes and travel. Along with goods, ships transport invasive marine algae in ballast tanks, which are used to maintain buoyancy. Ships discharge ballast water in ports, thus bringing in marine algae from other parts of the world.

Marine Pollution

For decades the maxim regarding pollution was "the solution to pollution is dilution." Industry and cities legally pumped their waste into the oceans thinking it would be dispersed such that its dilution would render it harmless to the oceans and human health. But in the 1960s and 1970s, pollution became a public and therefore political issue. In 1962 Rachel Carson (1907–1964) published her book *Silent Spring*, which outlined the environmental effects of the pesticide DDT (dichlorodiphenyltrichloroethane). In 1967, the world watched as the S.S. *Torrey Canyon* oil tanker shipwrecked on the shores of Cornwall, England, spilling almost 120,000 tons of crude oil into the Atlantic Ocean.

Increased awareness of human effects on the environment made pollution a public and political issue. In 1972, the United Nations Conference on the Human Environment in Stockholm, Sweden, helped develop guidelines for controlling pollution and maintaining the quality of seawater. "Problems with pollution of the marine environment received considerable attention at the conference," writes Folkert de Jong in *Marine Eutrophication in Perspective: On the Relevance of Ecology for Environmental Policy.*

The Oslo Convention was an international agreement adopted initially by seven countries in February 1972 that called for the control of marine pollution caused by dumping from ships and aircraft. In 1975, the London Dumping Convention was put into effect to control pollution at sea. Since the 1970s, the Environmental Protection Agency of the United States, the International Maritime Organization, and other groups have encouraged the adoption of measures to prevent and control marine pollution. Nevertheless, ballast discharge, oil spills, sewage discharge, and industrial and residential runoff continue to be major sources of marine pollution. Many countries, particularly developing countries, have not passed the regulatory legislation needed to help avoid these sources of marine pollution.

⊕ Impacts and Issues

Marine Toxins and Pathogens

The most common diseases caused by marine toxins are ciguatera poisoning, paralytic shellfish poisoning, neurotoxic shellfish poisoning, and amnesic shellfish poisoning. Other marine toxin diseases include puffer fish poisoning, *Vibrio vulnificus* infection, scombroid fish poisoning, and diarrhetic shellfish poisoning.

With improved molecular techniques, scientists increasingly are finding that viruses in the marine environment also pose a hazard to human health. The viruses they have isolated include adenoviruses, Norwalk viruses, polioviruses, coxsackieviruses, the hepatitis A virus, and other enteric viruses that cause a variety of diseases from respiratory infections to gastroenteritis, hepatitis, and meningitis. Viruses can infect humans exposed in the marine environment and subsequently are transmitted from human to human.

Many of these viruses make their way into coastal marine environments through the discharge of sewage. Even treated sewage contains viral pathogens, because they are small enough to pass through filters designed to remove larger particles such as bacteria and waste. "The discharge of viral pathogens in treated sewage is not regulated," write Dale Griffin and his colleagues in the scientific review "Pathogenic Human Viruses in Coastal Waters" in the journal *Clinical Microbiology Reviews.*

Algal Toxins

Ciguatera Poisoning Ciguatera poisoning is caused by ciguatoxin and can manifest itself as gastrointestinal, neurological, and cardiovascular symptoms. According to Jeremy Sobel and John Painter in "Illnesses Caused by Marine Toxins" in the journal *Clinical Infectious Diseases*, ciguatoxin opens the sodium channels of the nervous system, resulting in spontaneous neurotransmitter release, blockage of synaptic transmission, and depletion of synaptic vesicles. Symptoms start six hours after exposure. Diarrhea, vomiting, and cramping occur in half of patients and precede neurological symptoms that occur in 90 percent of cases. Severe cases of ciguatera poisoning can manifest symptoms for months or years. There is no antidote.

Ciguatoxin is caused by two dinoflagellate species that are consumed by herbivorous reef fish that in turn are consumed by larger carnivorous fish. This is the process by which the toxin is bioaccumulated up the food chain. Human consumption of large tropical reef fish such as barracuda, grouper, sea bass, snapper, and amberjack, among hundreds of other species, has been linked to ciguatera poisoning. Researchers have recorded cases of ciguatoxin poisoning in the tropics worldwide between latitudes 35° north and south of the equator.

Paralytic Shellfish Poisoning Paralytic shellfish poisoning (PSP) is caused by saxitoxin. It is a severe disease that is exclusively neurological and can be fatal. Saxitoxin blocks the sodium channels of the membranes of nerve and muscle cells. Nerve signal transmission eventually is blocked by saxitoxin. Symptoms start to occur 30 minutes after exposure with tingling around the mouth spreading to the face and neck. Usually this numbness is followed by headache, nausea, diarrhea, and vomiting. Death can result within two hours of exposure from paralysis of the respiratory muscles. No antidote exists.

PSP is transmitted by mussels, scallops, cockles, and clams, though it has also been associated with crustaceans, such as oysters and lobsters, and fish including the puffer fish. PSP has been observed in cold water coasts along the East and West Coast of the United States, southern Chile, the North Sea, and Japan. Some seafood and shellfish that have fed on the toxin can clear the toxin before the algal bloom is over whereas others retain the toxin for years.

Neurotoxic Shellfish Poisoning Neurotoxic shellfish poisoning (NSP) is caused by a brevetoxin produced by the dinoflagellate *Gymnodinium breve*, which is known to cause explosive algal blooms. Symptoms of NSP are gastrointestinal and neurological in character and usually resolve within 48 hours of exposure. Diarrhea, difficulty with coordinated movements such as walking, and reversal of temperature sensation are symptoms of NSP. No

deaths have been reported from NSP, and hospitalization is rarely necessary.

The NSP toxin can result in massive fish kills and can even be aerosolized in seawater and cause an inhalational syndrome in humans. The toxin is accumulated in oysters, clams, and mussels. The NSP-causing dinoflagellate typically is found in the Gulf of Mexico, New Zealand, and the Caribbean.

Diarrhetic Shellfish Poisoning Diarrhetic shellfish poisoning (DSP) is caused by three different groups of toxins produced by the dinoflagellates of the genus *Dinophysis* and *Prorocentrum*. Symptoms of DSP are diarrhea, nausea, vomiting, and abdominal pain starting 30 minutes after exposure to mussels, clams, cockles, oysters, and scallops that have fed on the dinoflagellates.

Diarrhetic shellfish poisoning occurs all over the world, with occurrences reported in Japan, China, India, the Philippines, Europe, North and South America, Australia, Indonesia, Australia, and New Zealand. Hospitalization is rare.

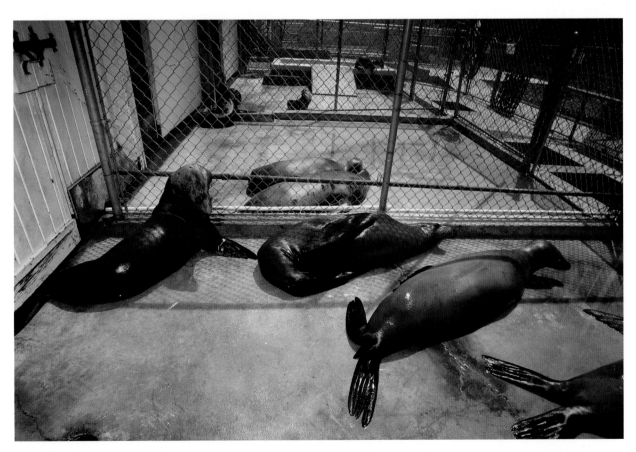

Sea lions, poisoned by toxic domoic acid, the result of an unusually large bloom of microscopic ocean algae, are treated at the Pacific Marine Mammal Center on April 30, 2007, in Laguna Beach, California. The toxin sickened and killed California birds, sea lions, and dolphins from San Francisco to San Diego. About 50 domoic-sickened animals arrived at the facility and nearly all died or had to be euthanized. Little can be done to save them once the toxin causes brain damage. The algae increases, or "blooms," each year as the seasonal ocean water temperature rises. In 2007 the bloom occurred early and was extremely dense. Birds, sea mammals, and humans eat the fish and shellfish that feed on the algae and ingest the toxin as it rises through the food chain. *© David McNew/Getty Images.*

Amnesic Shellfish Poisoning Amnesic shellfish poisoning (ASP) is caused by an amino acid toxin called domoic acid made by the algae *Nitzchia pungens.* Within 24 hours of exposure, gastrointestinal symptoms such as diarrhea, vomiting, and cramps appear. Other symptoms include dizziness, headache, and short-term memory loss. Severe cases result in seizures, focal weakness, and death.

The domoic acid toxin implicated in amnesic shellfish poisoning is accumulated in shellfish such as mussels. The algae that produce the toxin have been isolated worldwide. Scientists first documented the disease in Canada in 1987.

Bacterial Toxins

Other marine pathogens that pose a threat to human health include bacteria that cause cholera, typhoid fever, salmonella, and other food-borne illnesses. Additional pathogens present in the marine ecosystem that cause human illness include *Giardia lamblia* and *Pfisteria* complex organisms.

Scombroid Fish Poisoning Scombroid fish poisoning, also known as histamine fish poisoning, is the most common seafood-related intoxication. The symptoms include rash, diarrhea, flushing, sweating, abdominal pain, and burning or tingling around the mouth. The onset of symptoms can occur as quickly as two minutes after consumption of spoiled fish.

Scombroid fish poisoning is caused by bacterial spoilage of dark-fleshed fish such as tuna, mackerel, and bonito, though it can also be caught from blue fish, sardines, anchovies, amberjack, and mahi-mahi. The spoilage occurs as a result of bacteria growing on fish, which produces a toxin that catalyzes histamines. High histamine levels can exist without a perceptible change in sight or smell of the fish. Producers and consumers can prevent poisoning by rapid refrigeration or freezing of fish after it is caught. For patients with histamine fish poisoning, prompt antihistamine treatment has been shown to be effective.

Puffer Fish Poisoning Puffer fish poisoning results from the consumption of the puffer fish, also known as fugu, globefish, or blowfish. It is caused by tetrodotoxin, which blocks sodium channels and interferes with nerve transmission in skeletal muscle. Symptoms begin 30 minutes after exposure and include lightheadedness, dizziness, vomiting, and ascending paralysis. In cases of severe poisoning, respiratory muscle paralysis leads to death and can occur within six hours of exposure. Mortality rates from puffer fish poisoning have dropped since the early 20th century, mostly due to rapid medical treatment including gastric lavage and administration of activated charcoal.

Researchers once thought tetrodotoxin was produced by the puffer fish, but it now is known to be made by bacteria living within the gonads, liver, and spleen of the puffer fish. In some regions, the puffer fish can contain saxitoxin, the cause of paralytic shellfish poisoning. Puffer fish poisoning is rare outside of Japan, where puffer fish consumption is used in ceremonial meals.

Vibrio Infection *Vibrio vulnificus* can cause illness in humans who consume raw or undercooked seafood laden with the bacteria. Humans also can be exposed if an open wound comes into contact with contaminated seawater. Symptoms include vomiting, diarrhea, and abdominal pain. In severe cases, infection of the bloodstream can cause septic shock, skin lesions, and death. More than 70 percent of infected individuals exhibit bulbous skin lesions. Antibiotics are an effective treatment for *Vibrio vulnificus* infections.

Found in warm coastal waters, *Vibrio vulnificus* is from the same family as the bacteria that causes cholera. The bacterium is naturally present in the marine environment but can accumulate in oysters during summer months. *Vibrio vulnificus* does not alter the taste or smell of oysters. Surveillance and detection of the bacterium is required to ensure public safety.

Marine Pollution

Eutrophication A common consequence of marine pollution is eutrophication, the process by which a body of water receives excessive nutrients, which results in dense plant and algae growth. Algal blooms, some of which can produce fatal levels of marine toxins in seafood, are one consequence of eutrophication. Scientists have linked nitrogen and phosphorous, two chemical elements used heavily in agricultural fertilizers, to algal blooms and fish die-offs. Other pollutants in the marine environment can come from airborne pollution in the form of nitrogen oxides and sulfur oxides expelled from power plants and cars.

"Nitrogen inputs represent the largest pollution problem in the nation's coastal waters and one of the greatest threats to the ecological integrity of these ecosystems," writes Cornell scientist Robert Howarth in a chapter titled "Atmospheric Deposition and Nitrogen Pollution in Coastal Marine Ecosystems" in the book *Acid in the Environment.*

Eutrophication can create algal blooms that not only pose a risk to human health due to their marine toxins but also have ramifications for coastal marine ecosystems. Though eutrophication initially can lead to greater fish production because of an increase in their food supply, namely plankton, deleterious ecological changes can ensue. Algal blooms deplete the water of oxygen when the algae die and are eaten by bacteria, creating conditions such as hypoxia and anoxia. Conditions where low levels of oxygen exist are referred to as hypoxic. Anoxia means no oxygen exists. Anoxic and hypoxic conditions can distress and kill marine organisms such as fish and

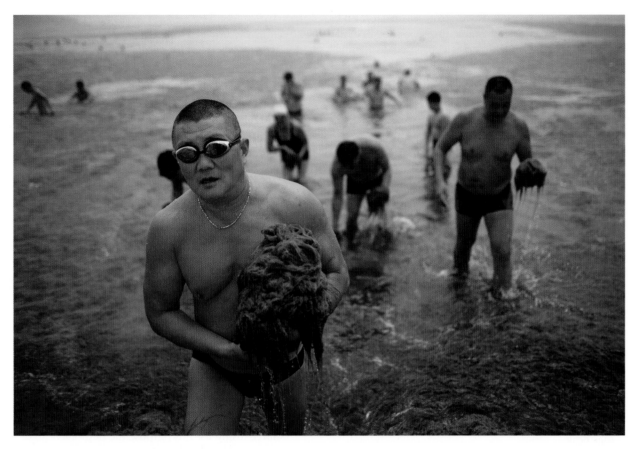

Swimmers clean up the seaweed in seawater covered in a thick layer of green algae in Qingdao, China. A large quantity of nonpoisonous green seaweed, *Enteromorpha prolifera*, arrived on the coast of Qingdao and neighboring cities in Shandong Province. The seaweed grew at a rapid rate due to marine water eutrophication and warm weather. More than 40,000 tons of such seaweed was removed from the city's beaches to lessen the damage caused to tourism and aquatic farming. © *Hong Wu/Getty Images.*

lead to alterations of the ecosystem, including degradation of habitat and community structure and loss of biodiversity.

Sewage The dumping of sewage, both treated and untreated, into the marine environment is a persistent global problem. In addition to treated sewage getting dumped into the marine environment, untreated sewage continues to make its way into marine ecosystems, too. Storm water and combined sewer overflow (CSO) pollution is a major input of pollution into the marine environment. Periodically, heavy storms overwhelm municipal water treatment and sewer systems, forcing them to release runoff and untreated sewage directly into the marine environment, resulting in beach closings, red tides, and public health threats. Gastrointestinal diseases can be a consequence of swimming near sources of urban runoff and storm drains and ingesting polluted water.

Cruise ships consistently dump sewage into the oceans. When this occurs near shore, the sewage can cause algal blooms and introduce other pathogens hazardous to human health. Technicians have installed wastewater treatment technology on some cruise ships.

Heavy Metals, POPs, and PBTs Many toxins remain in an ecosystem for a long time. Like algal and bacterial toxins, inorganic and organic toxins can accumulate in marine organisms or settle in sediment and persist in the environment. Heavy metals are inorganic pollutants that can accumulate in seafood and pose a risk to human health. These metals include mercury, cadmium, zinc, copper, and lead. There has been a significant reduction in the amounts of heavy metals making it into the marine environment thanks to environmental regulation and the efforts of bodies such as the Baltic Marine Environment Protection Commission—Helsinki Commission.

Persistent organic pollutants (POPs) in the marine environment can travel great distances and bioaccumulate in seafood, thus posing a risk to human health. POPs are human-made organic chemicals that include pesticides, industrial chemicals, chemicals in consumer products, and by-products of manufacturing. POPs include DDT, dioxins, and dioxin-like compounds such as polychlorinated biphenyls (PCBs). Human exposure to POPs results in adverse reproductive, developmental, behavioral, neurologic, endocrine, and immunological health effects.

Persistent bioaccumulative toxic substance (PBT) is the name given to a chemical that does not degrade easily in the environment and is consumed and amplified in animals. PBTs typically accumulate in fatty tissues and can bioaccumulate in marine organisms and animals that prey on marine organisms. Therefore, PBTs pose a threat to human health. PBTs include pesticides such as aldrin, chlordane, DDT, dieldrin, endrin, heptachlor, hexachlorobenzene, mirex, and toxaphere. PBTs also include industrial chemicals such as PCBs, dioxins, and furans. Scientists first noted the effects of PBTs during the 1970s when large birds of prey started dying off. The scientists found that PBTs (in that case, DDT) were accumulated low in the food chain and amplified into more toxic amounts the higher the trophic level (level within the food chain). Consuming PBT-containing organisms higher on the food chain is most risky for human health.

⊕ Future Implications

The global demand for seafood has increased the risk of illnesses caused by marine toxins. Medical attention and diagnosis has improved, but most of the marine toxins have no antidotes or specialized treatment. Warming oceans and increased sewage, runoff, and eutrophication will lead to more harmful algal blooms and therefore a higher risk to public health.

Some environmental regulations and safeguards have been put in place to stymie marine pollutants from industrial, agricultural, and residential sources. However, without solidifying these guidelines into law, pollutants will continue to make their way into the marine environment and pose a threat to human health. Public health surveillance and improved case reporting will ward off marine toxin disease outbreaks, but tackling other marine pollution will be much more difficult. Bioaccumulative toxic substances, heavy metals, and sewage will persist in the marine environment for a long time. Controlling their leaching into the environment is one task; cleaning up the decades of pollution currently in the marine environment is another.

PRIMARY SOURCE

United Nations Convention on the Law of the Seas

SOURCE *"Part XII: Protection and Preservation of the Marine Environment," in* United Nations Convention on the Law of the Seas. *New York: United Nations, 1982, 100–101. Copyright © United Nations. http://www.un.org/depts/los/ convention_agreements/texts/unclos/unclos_e .pdf (accessed January 25, 2015).*

INTRODUCTION *This primary source, taken from the United Nations Convention on the Law of the Sea, pertains to environmental protection.*

PART XII

PROTECTION AND PRESERVATION OF THE MARINE ENVIRONMENT

SECTION 1. GENERAL PROVISIONS

Article 192
General obligation

States have the obligation to protect and preserve the marine environment.

Article 193
Sovereign right of States to exploit their natural resources

States have the sovereign right to exploit their natural resources pursuant to their environmental policies and in accordance with their duty to protect and preserve the marine environment.

Article 194
Measures to prevent, reduce and control pollution of the marine environment

1. States shall take, individually or jointly as appropriate, all measures consistent with this Convention that are necessary to prevent, reduce and control pollution of the marine environment from any source, using for this purpose the best practicable means at their disposal and in accordance with their capabilities, and they shall endeavour to harmonize their policies in this connection.

2. States shall take all measures necessary to ensure that activities under their jurisdiction or control are so conducted as not to cause damage by pollution to other States and their environment, and that pollution arising from incidents or activities under their jurisdiction or control does not spread beyond the areas where they exercise sovereign rights in accordance with this Convention.

3. The measures taken pursuant to this Part shall deal with all sources of pollution of the marine environment. These measures shall include, *inter alia*, those designed to minimize to the fullest possible extent:

   a. the release of toxic, harmful or noxious substances, especially those which are persistent, from land-based sources, from or through the atmosphere or by dumping;

   b. pollution from vessels, in particular measures for preventing accidents and dealing with emergencies, ensuring the safety of operations at sea, preventing intentional and unintentional discharges, and regulating the design, construction, equipment, operation and manning of vessels;

c. pollution from installations and devices used in exploration or exploitation of the natural resources of the seabed and subsoil, in particular measures for preventing accidents and dealing with emergencies, ensuring the safety of operations at sea, and regulating the design, construction, equipment, operation and manning of such installations or devices;

d. pollution from other installations and devices operating in the marine environment, in particular measures for preventing accidents and dealing with emergencies, ensuring the safety of operations at sea, and regulating the design, construction, equipment, operation and manning of such installations or devices.

4. In taking measures to prevent, reduce or control pollution of the marine environment, States shall refrain from unjustifiable interference with activities carried out by other States in the exercise of their rights and in pursuance of their duties in conformity with this Convention.

5. The measures taken in accordance with this Part shall include those necessary to protect and preserve rare or fragile ecosystems as well as the habitat of depleted, threatened or endangered species and other forms of marine life.

Article 195
Duty not to transfer damage or hazards or transform one type of pollution into another

In taking measures to prevent, reduce and control pollution of the marine environment, States shall act so as not to transfer, directly or indirectly, damage or hazards from one area to another or transform one type of pollution into another.

Article 196
Use of technologies or introduction of alien or new species

1. States shall take all measures necessary to prevent, reduce and control pollution of the marine environment resulting from the use of technologies under their jurisdiction or control, or the intentional or accidental introduction of species, alien or new, to a particular part of the marine environment, which may cause significant and harmful changes thereto.

2. This article does not affect the application of this Convention regarding the prevention, reduction and control of pollution of the marine environment.

SEE ALSO *Air Pollution: Urban, Industrial, and Transborder; Water Supplies and Access to Clean Water; Waterborne Diseases*

BIBLIOGRAPHY

Books

Basedow, Jürgen, and Ulrich Magnus, eds. *Pollution of the Sea: Prevention and Compensation.* New York: Springer Science & Business Media, 2007.

Howarth, Robert. "Atmospheric Deposition and Nitrogen Pollution in Coastal Marine Ecosystems." In *Acid in the Environment: Lessons Learned and Future Prospects*, edited by Gerald Visgilio and Diana M. Whitelaw. New York: Springer, 2007.

Huss, Hans Henrik, Lahsen Ababouch, and Lone Gram. *Assessment and Management of Seafood Safety and Quality.* Rome: Food and Agriculture Organization of the United Nations, 2004.

Jong, Folkert de. *Marine Eutrophication in Perspective: On the Relevance of Ecology for Environmental Policy.* Berlin: Springer, 2006.

Loganathan, Bommanna, and Paul K. S. Lam, eds. *Global Contamination Trends of Persistent Organic Chemicals.* Boca Raton, FL: CRC Press, 2012.

Visgilio, Gerald R., and Diana M. Whitelaw. *Acid in the Environment: Lessons Learned and Future Prospects.* New York: Springer, 2007.

Periodicals

Andrady, Anthony L. "Microplastics in the Marine Environment." *Marine Pollution Bulletin* 62, no. 8 (August 2011): 1936–1841.

Chen, Tingrui, et al. "Food-Borne Disease Outbreak of Diarrhetic Shellfish Poisoning Due to Toxic Mussel Consumption: The First Recorded Outbreak in China." *PLOS ONE* 8, no. 5 (May 21, 2013). Available online at http://www.plosone.org/article/info%3Adoi%2F10.1371%2Fjournal.pone.0065049 (accessed October 24, 2014).

Griffin, Dale, et al. "Pathogenic Human Viruses in Coastal Waters." *Clinical Microbiology Reviews* 16, no. 1 (January 2003): 129–143.

Rochman, Chelsea, et al. "Ingested Plastic Transfers Hazardous Chemicals to Fish and Induces Hepatic Stress." *Scientific Reports* 3, no. 3263 (November 21, 2013). Available online at http://www.nature.com/srep/2013/131121/srep03263/full/srep03263.html (accessed October 24, 2014).

Sobel, Jeremy, and John Painter. "Illnesses Caused by Marine Toxins." *Clinical Infectious Diseases* 41, no. 9 (November 1, 2005): 1290–1296. Available online at http://cid.oxfordjournals.org/content/41/9/1290.full (accessed April 10, 2015).

Websites

Dell'Amore, Christine. "New Diseases, Toxins Harming Wildlife." *National Geographic News*, April 12, 2013. http://news.nationalgeographic.com/news/2012/04/130412-diseases-health-animals-science-environment-oceans (accessed September 5, 2014).

"HABs and Marine Biotoxins." *National Oceanic and Atmospheric Administration. Northwest Fisheries Science Center.* http://www.nwfsc.noaa.gov/hab/habs_toxins/index.html (accessed September 5, 2014).

"Harmful Algal Blooms and Marine Toxins." *National Oceanic and Atmospheric Administration (NOAA) Northwest Fisheries and Science Center.* http://www.nwfsc.noaa.gov/hab/habs_toxins/index.html (accessed September 5, 2014).

"History of the Negotiations of the Stockholm Convention." *Stockholm Convention: Protecting Human Health and the Environment from Persistent Organic Pollutants.* http://chm.pops.int/TheConvention/Overview/History/Overview/tabid/3549/Default.aspx (accessed October 24, 2014).

"Marine Toxins." *Centers for Disease Control and Prevention (CDC).* http://www.cdc.gov/ncidod/dbmd/diseaseinfo/marinetoxins_g.htm (accessed September 5, 2014).

Aleszu Bajak

Maternal and Infant Health

⊕ Introduction

According to a report by the World Health Organization (WHO), the United Nations Children's Fund (UNICEF), the United Nations Population Fund, the World Bank, and the United Nations Population Division, there were approximately 289,000 maternal deaths—deaths during pregnancy and childbirth—worldwide in 2013. More than half (62 percent) of these deaths occurred in sub-Saharan Africa, and 24 percent occurred in southern Asia. The joint report on child mortality found that 4.6 million deaths occurred worldwide in 2014 during the first year of life (infancy), accounting for the vast majority—nearly three-quarters—of all under-five deaths.

Recognizing these statistics as a tremendous global health issue, two of the eight United Nations (UN) Millennium Development Goals from 2000 focus on maternal and child health: (1) to reduce by three-quarters, between 1990 and 2015, the maternal mortality ratio (MMR) and (2) to reduce by two-thirds, between 1990 and 2015, the under-five mortality rate. Progress on these goals is being made: the global MMR decreased from 380 maternal deaths per 100,000 live births in 1990 to 210 maternal deaths per 100,000 live births in 2013. Similarly, progress has been achieved with regard to the global infant mortality rate, which has decreased from 63 deaths per 1,000 live births in 1990 to 34 deaths per 1,000 live births in 2013. However, the MMR in developing regions was 14 times higher than that in developed regions (230 versus 16 deaths per 100,000 live births, respectively), and the infant mortality rate was seven times higher in less developed regions compared to more developed regions (37 versus 5 deaths per 1,000 live births, respectively), highlighting the existence of enormous maternal and infant health disparities.

The focus of this entry is on maternal and infant health. Maternal health is the health of women during pregnancy, childbirth, and the postpartum period (the six weeks following delivery). Direct causes of maternal mortality, a key indicator of maternal health, include hemorrhage (rapid, uncontrolled loss of blood), infection, high blood pressure, obstructed labor, and unsafe abortion. Underlying these causes are issues of access to skilled care and family planning. According to the Bill & Melinda Gates Foundation's website, satisfying the unmet need for contraception could decrease the number of maternal deaths worldwide by a third. Thus, reproductive health is a key component of maternal health.

Infant health refers to children's health through the first year of life, including the especially vulnerable neonatal period (the 28 days following birth). According to a fact sheet published by the WHO in May 2012, 80 percent of neonatal deaths are the result of just four factors: prematurity and low birth weight, infections, asphyxia (lack of oxygen at birth), and birth trauma. Again, access to skilled care during pregnancy, delivery, and the postpartum period is a key underlying cause of infant mortality.

⊕ Historical Background

In 2008, a leading global health journal, *The Lancet*, published a series of articles focused on maternal and child undernutrition. This series highlighted the importance of improving health in the first 1,000 days of life (pregnancy through two years of age) and concluded that "Nutrition is a desperately neglected aspect of maternal, newborn, and child health. The reasons for this neglect are understandable but not justifiable." The series also reported that 11 percent of the global disease burden was due to maternal and child undernutrition.

Five years later, in 2013, *The Lancet* published a second series on maternal and child nutrition. Emphasis on the importance of health during the first 1,000 days of life continued, maternal and child undernutrition were re-evaluated, and the growing issue of overnutrition—overweight and obesity—was added to the discussion. Indeed, the 2013 series reported that many low- and middle-income countries had come to face what experts

Maternal Mortality Ratio (MMR), by Country, 2013

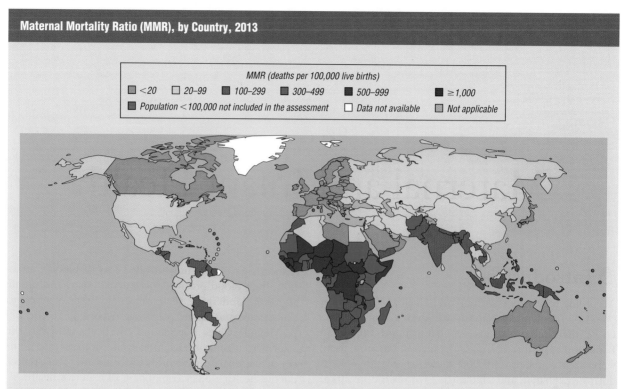

SOURCE: Adapted from "Figure 1. Map with countries by category according to their maternal mortality ratio (MMR, death per 100,000 live births), 2013," in *Trends in Maternal Mortality: 1990 to 2013*, World Health Organization (WHO), United Nations Children's Fund (UNICEF), United Nations Population Fund (UNFPA), The World Bank, and the United Nations Population Division, 2014, p. 23, http://data.unicef.org/corecode/uploads/document6/uploaded_pdfs/corecode/MMR2013_117.pdf (accessed January 13, 2014).

are calling the "dual burden": continued stunting of growth and micronutrient deficiencies and the rising problem of overweight and obesity.

Despite the substantial global burden of maternal and infant malnutrition, and the far-reaching implications of maternal and infant health for future adult health and national economic progress, official development assistance to maternal, newborn, and child health has slowed since the financial crisis of 2007–2009. According to an analysis published in *The Lancet* in 2012 by Justine Hsu and colleagues, in 2010, donor disbursements to this area slightly decreased for the first time since monitoring began: from $6.51 billion in 2009 to $6.48 billion in 2010. However, they also found that targeting of assistance to high-risk countries (i.e., countries with high maternal mortality rates) improved, lending support for the continued tracking of donor aid.

⊕ Impacts and Issues

One of the key components of maternal and infant health is breast-feeding, which is important for the healthy development of infants and the reproductive process for mothers. The WHO and UNICEF's Global Strategy for Infant and Young Child Feeding (2003) recommends

that infants be breast-fed exclusively for the first six months of life, starting within one hour of birth. Thereafter, adequate and safe complementary foods should be introduced while breast-feeding continues up to two years of age. According to a WHO fact sheet updated in February 2014, globally, only 38 percent of infants up to six months old are breast-fed exclusively. The WHO estimates that 800,000 lives of children less than five years of age could be saved every year if all children up to 23 months old were breast-fed optimally.

The primary benefit of early initiation and exclusivity of breast-feeding during the first six months of life is reduced risk of diarrheal infections. According to a meta-analysis by Laura M. Lamberti and colleagues published in the journal *BMC Public Health* in 2011, infants zero to five months old who were not breast-fed were 10.52 times more likely to die of diarrheal infections compared to exclusively breast-fed infants. Furthermore, infants 6 months to 23 months old who were not breast-fed were 2.18 times more likely to die of diarrheal infections compared to infants of that age with some breast-feeding, thus supporting the WHO/UNICEF recommendations. Other infant benefits of breast-feeding are that breast milk is a good source of energy and nutrients; breast-feeding improves performance on intelligence tests; and breast-feeding reduces the risk of being overweight or obese in adulthood.

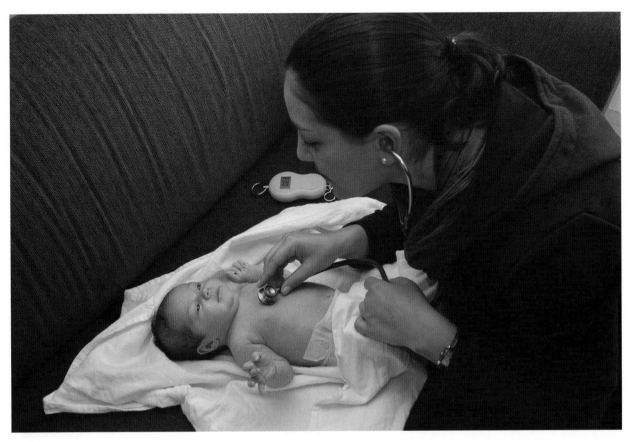

A midwife checks a newborn baby in Auckland, New Zealand. Skilled care during pregnancy, labor, childbirth, and postpartum are necessary for maternal and infant health.   © *ChameleonsEye/Shutterstock.com.*

There are also maternal health benefits from breast-feeding, including reduced risk of ovarian and breast cancer, and family planning. Breast-feeding can induce a lack of menstruation, helping to space pregnancies, though this method of family planning is not fail-proof.

Interventions to improve adherence to breast-feeding recommendations often involve community-based health promotion and education as well as mother support groups. The WHO recommends implementation of the "Ten Steps to Successful Breastfeeding" from the Baby-Friendly Hospital Initiative (1998). These steps include, for example, showing mothers how to breast-feed, breast-feeding on demand, and not giving infants any other food or drinks, including water. In 2014, Valerie L. Flax and colleagues published results of an innovative intervention integrated into a microfinance program in Nigeria in the *Journal of Nutrition*. Women who received the intervention, which included monthly breast-feeding learning sessions and weekly text and voice messages about breast-feeding, were significantly more likely to breast-feed exclusively compared to women who did not receive the intervention.

After six months of age, breast milk alone is not sufficient to meet the energy and nutrient needs of infants, and so complementary foods must be introduced. It is important to note that the WHO still recommends continued, on-demand breast-feeding during this period, especially when the infant is sick. Proper food handling, good hygiene, and access to clean water are also critical during this period. Coinciding with the introduction of complementary foods from 6 months to 24 months is the peak incidence of infections, micronutrient deficiencies, and growth faltering, so this is an especially vulnerable period for infants.

Infant feeding behaviors are receiving increased attention, particularly responsive feeding, which involves directly feeding infants and being patient and encouraging throughout the feeding session. Parental feeding styles may influence infant dietary intake, and subsequent nutrient status and growth. A systematic review of the literature conducted by Margaret E. Bentley and colleagues and published in the *Journal of Nutrition* in 2011 found evidence that positive verbalizations during feeding increase acceptance of food, but that randomized controlled trials are needed to isolate the exact effects of feeding styles, particularly responsive feeding, on infant nutrition.

More traditionally, complementary feeding interventions have focused on introducing fortified complementary

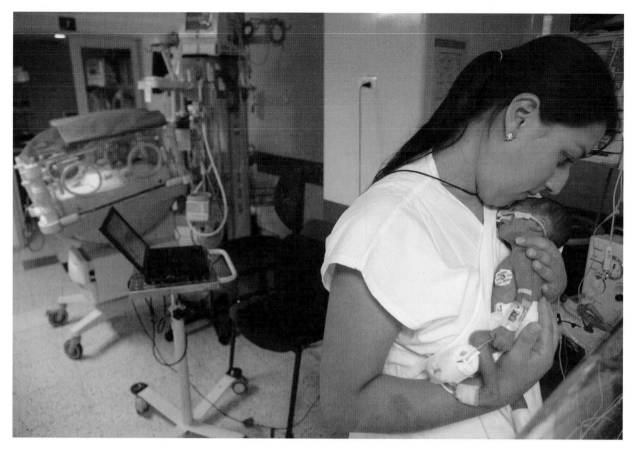

A Colombian mother holds a premature baby after feeding him with milk during the first day of donation of human milk at Medellín's General hospital on August 20, 2014, in Medellin, Antioquia department, Colombia. The region's first Human Milk Bank opened recently, with the aim of reducing the mortality rate in premature infants, preventing disease, ensuring normal growth of newborns and promoting breast-feeding. © *Raul Arboleda/AFP/Getty Images.*

foods or supplements. Food-based approaches are gaining favor because they may be more effective and sustainable, especially when traditional, nutrient-dense foods, including especially animal-source foods, are used. A comprehensive scientific literature review by Kathryn G. Dewey and Seth Adu-Afarwuah conducted in 2008 and published in the journal *Maternal and Child Nutrition* concluded that such interventions need to be context specific. As an example, an intervention published in 2013 in the journal *Maternal and Child Nutrition* by Melissa Bauserman and colleagues found that a complementary food cereal made from dried caterpillars and other local ingredients (corn, palm oil, sugar, and salt) in the Democratic Republic of the Congo was an appropriate source of macro- and micronutrients and was acceptable to mothers and infants.

Micronutrient Deficiencies

Whereas the UN Millennium Development Goals focus on maternal and infant mortality, other outcomes are critical to consider when trying to improve maternal and infant health. Key among these outcomes in low- and middle-income countries is that of micronutrient deficiencies. Nutritional supplements and therapeutic foods have been an important component of improving global maternal and infant health, especially in pregnant women with HIV/AIDS and tuberculosis. Recognizing that food-based approaches may be more effective and sustainable than single-nutrient interventions, and emphasizing that diets containing bioavailable forms of micronutrients should underpin all prevention efforts, this section highlights the four most common micronutrient deficiencies: iron, iodine, vitamin A, and zinc.

Iron According to a 2014 policy brief published by the WHO on anemia, in 2011, 38 percent (32.4 million) of pregnant women aged 15 to 49 years worldwide were anemic, with an estimated half of those cases being due to iron deficiency. (Other causes of anemia include severe malaria, other nutritional deficiencies [folic acid, vitamin B12, vitamin A, and vitamin C], and genetic conditions [sickle-cell disease].) Given that maternal anemia is associated with adverse pregnancy outcomes including, for example, stillbirths, premature birth, and low birth weight, as well as long-term adverse outcomes in off-spring such as poor school performance, this statistic is particularly alarming.

To address this issue, the WHO recommends a multifaceted approach including: iron and folic acid supplementation as part of prenatal care and during the postpartum period (for at least three months); fortification of staples such as wheat and maize flours and rice with iron, folic acid, and other micronutrients; malaria control; deworming; delayed cord clamping (not earlier than one minute after birth); and exclusive breast-feeding up to six months of age.

Iodine Globally, iodine deficiency is the most common cause of preventable mental impairment. This stems from the fact that iodine is needed to produce thyroid hormone, which is essential for proper growth and development. Thus, pregnant women and children are at particularly high risk. According to a 2012 analysis by Maria Andersson and colleagues published in the *Journal of Nutrition*, 29.8 percent (240.9 million) of school-aged children (usually serves as a proxy for the general population) worldwide have insufficient iodine intakes, and 5.2 percent have severely deficient iodine intakes. The vast majority of these children live in Southeast Asia (76 million) and Africa (58 million).

Addressing this global health issue will be difficult for several reasons. Iodization of salt by small-scale, local producers is a goal for reaching populations in remote, rural areas but will not be easy to implement. Furthermore, moving forward, all salt iodization policies will need to consider somewhat conflicting policies to reduce salt consumption in an effort to prevent and control high blood pressure.

Vitamin A Globally, vitamin A deficiency is the most common cause of night blindness in pregnant women and children and is associated with increased mortality. According to the WHO's Global Database on Vitamin A Deficiency (2009), 15.3 percent (19.1 million) of pregnant women and 33.3 percent (190 million) of preschool-aged children worldwide have low serum vitamin A concentrations. As seen with iodine deficiency, the vast majority of vitamin A deficiency cases are in Southeast Asia (6.69 million pregnant women and 91.5 million preschool-aged children) and Africa (4.18 million pregnant women and 56.4 million preschool-aged children).

The promotion of exclusive breast-feeding is one of the best ways to prevent vitamin A deficiency in infants given that breast milk is a good source of vitamin A. High-dose vitamin A supplements also are recommended for deficient children and have been associated with reduced mortality. According to the WHO's 2009 publication, *Global Prevalence of Vitamin A Deficiency in Populations at Risk 1995–2005*, neonatal vitamin A supplementation has been associated with a 21 percent reduction in mortality in the first six months of life.

Routine vitamin supplementation in pregnant women also has been associated with a substantial reduction in mortality: approximately 40 percent. Beyond vitamin supplements, food fortification is recommended as a more long-term, sustainable solution to vitamin A deficiencies. For example, sugar in Central and South America has been vitamin A–fortified since the mid-1990s. Finally, as with all micronutrient deficiencies, increasing dietary diversity should underpin all single-nutrient interventions.

Zinc According to the WHO World Health Report (2013), zinc deficiency may be associated with 800,000 deaths in children under five years of age, particularly deaths attributable to infections (diarrhea, pneumonia, and malaria). In 2004, the WHO and UNICEF issued a statement that all children with diarrheal infections in developing countries should be treated with zinc, and the 2013 World Health Report extended this to include respiratory disease control such as pneumonia.

In regard to zinc supplementation during pregnancy, a review by Sonya Y. Hess and Janet C. King published in the WHO's *Food and Nutrition Bulletin* in 2009 concluded that there may be possible benefits in undernourished (e.g., underweight or zinc-deficient) women, including reducing the risk of preterm birth. The authors of that review also emphasized that the available scientific literature on this topic is limited, particularly for postnatal/infant outcomes, and that more research is needed to inform recommendations on this topic. As of July 2013, a statement by Ian Darnton-Hill on the WHO's website refers to two meta-analyses on zinc supplementation during pregnancy that also found no positive effects on outcomes other than preterm birth. His statement concluded by saying that while there do not appear to be harmful effects of zinc supplementation, the overall public health benefit in pregnancy appears to be limited.

HIV/AIDS

The importance of breast-feeding for both maternal and infant health was discussed above. A key issue related to this is the fact that human immunodeficiency virus (HIV) can pass from mother to child at multiple points, including pregnancy, delivery, and through breast milk. According to the WHO in 2006, without preventive intervention, approximately 35 percent of HIV-infected mothers will pass it on to their child during pregnancy, delivery, or breast-feeding, and 10–20 percent of infants born to HIV-infected mothers will contract the virus over two years of breast-feeding. Furthermore, according to a study published by Hoosen M. Coovadia and colleagues a year later, the risk of mother-to-child transmission of HIV increases with mixed feeding (e.g. breast milk and formula) as compared to exclusive breast-feeding. Thus, breast-feeding and HIV transmission has been an important area of research and debate. Prior to the advent of antiretroviral drugs, global health

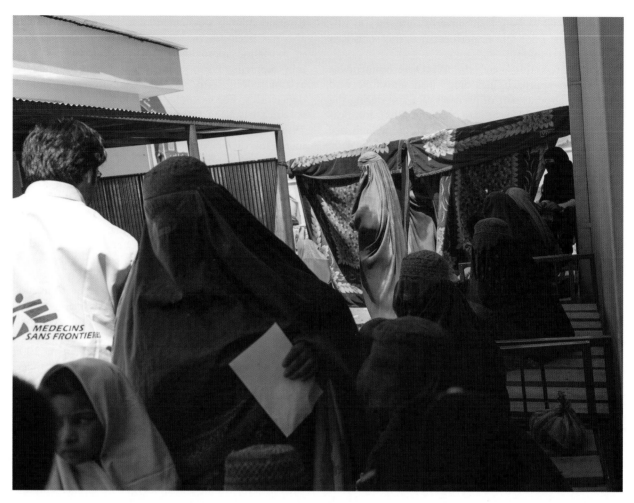

A Médecins Sans Frontières (MSF; Doctors Without Borders) staff person walks through the women's section of a small Afghan government clinic on the eastern outskirts of Kabul, Afghanistan. The local clinic is administered by the Afghan Ministry of Public Health and visited by MSF staff. The clinic offers pre- and post-natal care for women, vaccinations for children, some pharmaceuticals, and minor surgery but offers no operating theater. By some estimates, Afghanistan has the highest infant mortality rate in the world, and tens of thousands of women and children die each year in Afghanistan because of lack of access to medical care and malnutrition.   *© Robert Nickelsberg/Getty Images.*

recommendations had to balance the risk of transmitting HIV to the child with the risks associated with not breast-feeding, including diarrheal infections and undernutrition.

Scientific evidence has shown that giving mothers antiretroviral drugs can reduce significantly the risk of transmission of HIV through breast-feeding. According to the WHO in 2009, the risk of mother-to-child transmission of HIV can be lowered to less than 5 percent among breast-fed infants when antiretroviral drugs are provided. In response to this scientific evidence, the WHO recommended in 2010 that HIV-infected mothers take antiretroviral drugs and exclusively breast-feed until six months of age, continuing up to 12 months of age with the introduction of complementary foods. Furthermore, given the substantial benefits of breast-feeding and substantial risks of not breast-feeding in some parts of the world, the WHO recommends that even when

antiretroviral drugs are not available, HIV-infected mothers should still exclusively breast-feed for six months.

Other Issues Related to Improving Maternal and Infant Health

In addition to the issues surrounding maternal and infant nutrition discussed above—namely, breast-feeding, complementary feeding, and micronutrient deficiencies—several other strategies are available for reducing mortality and improving health. As mentioned, early initiation of breast-feeding, exclusive breast-feeding up to six months of age, and continued breast-feeding up to two years of age are key preventive measures against diarrheal diseases. Rehydration treatment is also an affordable and evidence-based approach to reducing infant mortality from diarrheal diseases.

Immunizations are another key area of intervention for reducing infant mortality and improving infant health. According to the U.S. Agency for International Development's (USAID) June 2014 publication titled "Acting on the Call: Ending Preventable Child and Maternal Death," vaccination prevents an estimated 2.5 million deaths every year. The introduction of new vaccines against rotavirus and pneumococcus in particular contributed to the 72 percent reduction in child risk of dying from diarrhea or pneumonia between 1990 and 2012. Measles, rubella, and polio vaccines, among others, are also important areas needing expansion highlighted in the USAID report. Indoor residual spraying and proper use of insecticide-treated bed nets are key areas of intervention to prevent insect-borne diseases, such as malaria, in this population.

🌐 Future Implications

The 2013 *Partnership for Maternal, Newborn and Child Health Progress Report* highlighted four key areas moving forward: (1) achieving political commitment for maternal and child health in the post-2015 development agenda; (2) improving coverage of interventions for maternal and child health; (3) promoting accountability for commitments to maternal and child health; and (4) strengthening global, regional, and national partnerships. The United Nations secretary-general's Global Strategy for Women's and Children's Health (2010) further aims to prevent unwanted pregnancies and highlights the importance of improving access to family planning in the global maternal and infant health agenda. Clearly, a multifaceted approach involving stakeholders from multiple areas (governments, nongovernmental organizations, scientists and researchers, industry, etc.) will be needed to address this important aspect of global health.

PRIMARY SOURCE

The Millennium Development Goals Report 2014

SOURCE *"Goal 4: Reduce Child Mortality," in* The Millennium Development Goals Report 2014. *New York: United Nations, 2014, 24–27. Copyright © 2014 United Nations. http://www .un.org/millenniumgoals/2014%20MDG%20 report/MDG%202014%20English%20web.pdf (accessed January 31, 2015).*

INTRODUCTION *This primary source is taken from a progress report on the Millennium Development Goals (MDGs) of the United Nations. The MDGs "were a pledge to uphold the principles of human dignity, equality and equity, and free the world from extreme poverty."*

OBSTETRIC FISTULA

Obstetric fistula is a complication of delivery that occurs when a hole forms in the birth canal. According to the WHO Fact Sheet on Obstetric Fistula updated in May 2014, worldwide, between 50,000 and 100,000 women are affected by obstetric fistula annually. Given that this estimate includes only women who seek care, many experts believe that this number is underestimated.

The direct cause of obstetric fistula is obstructed labor, and the direct result is incontinence (continuous leakage of urine). This in turn leads to stigmatization, shame, and often social segregation and poverty. Key underlying causes include lack of skilled birth attendants and emergency obstetric care. A review published in the *Mount Sinai Journal of Medicine* by Tracy Capes and colleagues (2011) found that most cases of obstetric fistula result in stillbirths, most labor durations are two days or longer, and most labors start at home but eventually additional care is sought at hospitals. With regard to the women who experience obstetric fistula, most are young, primiparous (one baby), and of short stature (though it also is reported in older, multiparous [multiple babies] women). Many women report subsequent separation or divorce after presenting at a fistula center.

Key aspects of preventing obstetric fistula include delaying the age of first pregnancy, which is closely related to providing family planning services, and access to obstetric care (distance to care and cost of care remain significant barriers to access). While obstetric fistula is treatable, the WHO Fact Sheet estimates that more than 2 million women live untreated in sub-Saharan Africa and Asia. Rapid management and closure of the hole is essential, yet, according to the aforementioned review by Capes and colleagues, wait times can be substantial. Thus, moving forward on this issue will require training of surgeons, nurses, and social workers devoted to obstetric fistula repairs (masters), provision of infrastructure (specialized clinics, clinics integrated into district hospitals, and/or smaller local units with referrals to larger centers), operating theaters with adequate supplies, and long-term funding, all of which will require government commitment and support.

GOAL 4:

Reduce child mortality

TARGET 4.A
Reduce by two thirds, between 1990 and 2015, the under-five mortality rate

Quick facts

- The child mortality rate has almost halved since 1990; six million fewer children died in 2012 than in 1990.
- During the period from 2005 to 2012, the annual rate of reduction in under-five mortality was more than three times faster than between 1990 and 1995.

- Globally, four out of every five deaths of children under age five continue to occur in sub-Saharan Africa and Southern Asia.

- Immunization against measles helped prevent nearly 14 million deaths between 2000 and 2012.

The global rate of under-five mortality in 2012 was almost half of its 1990 rate, dropping from 90 to 48 deaths per thousand live births. The estimated number of under-five deaths fell from about 12.6 million to 6.6 million over the same period: about 17,000 fewer children died each day in 2012 than in 1990. All regions, with the exception of sub-Saharan Africa and Oceania, have reduced their under-five mortality rate by more than half.

Currently, the world is reducing under-five mortality faster than at any other time during the past two decades. The global annual rate of reduction in under-five mortality has accelerated steadily from 1.2 per cent between 1990 and 1995 to 3.9 per cent between 2005 and 2012. However, regions such as Oceania, sub-Saharan Africa, Caucasus and Central Asia, and Southern Asia still fall short of the 2015 target. It will take until 2028 to reach Goal 4 globally at the current rate. The pace of reduction would need to quadruple in the period from 2013 to 2015 to meet the target of a two-thirds reduction in the under-five mortality rate.

Most of the 6.6 million deaths in children under age five in 2012 were from leading infectious diseases such as pneumonia, diarrhoea and malaria. Moreover, 2.9 million deaths occurred during the first 28 days of life (0–27 days)—the neonatal period. Many under-five deaths occur in children already weakened by undernutrition—a contributing factor in around half of global under-five deaths, mainly in low-income countries where malnutrition and infectious diseases are highly concentrated, predominantly among the poor.

Encouragingly, neonatal mortality is on the decline worldwide. Between 1990 and 2012, the world neonatal mortality rate fell by almost one-third, from 33 to 21 deaths for every thousand live births. However, the pace of decline has fallen behind that of post-neonatal mortality. As a result, the proportion of deaths occurring in the first 28 days of life has increased, from 37 per cent in 1990 to 44 percent in 2012.

Most neonatal deaths are preventable. The best possible way of reducing neonatal mortality is through greater investment in maternal care during the first 24 hours after birth, particularly in labour and delivery care and other high-impact interventions. Far too many births—more than half in some countries—occur outside health facilities, despite the increase in institutional deliveries globally.

Sub-Saharan Africa continues to confront a tremendous challenge. Not only does the region have the highest mortality rate in the world for children under age five—more than 16 times the average for developed regions—but it is also the only region where both the number of live births and the under-five population are expected to rise substantially over the next two decades. In 2012, one child in ten in sub-Saharan Africa did not live until their fifth birthday.

Nevertheless, the region has made remarkable progress since 1990, reducing child mortality rates by 45 per cent. However, its progress continues to lag behind that of every other region except Oceania: nearly half of global under-five deaths in 2012—3.2 million children under age five—occurred in sub-Saharan Africa.

Yet, the signs are that rapid progress is possible. Sub-Saharan Africa, despite its relatively high rate of under-five mortality, was able to step up the rate of decline from 0.8 per cent per year to 4.1 per cent per year—over five times faster during 2005–2012 than during 1990–1995.

Southern Asia has also made strong and steady progress in reducing child deaths, more than halving its under-five mortality rate. Yet, nearly one in every three under-five deaths still takes place there. India had the highest number of under-five deaths in the world in 2012, with 1.4 million children dying before reaching their fifth birthday.

High-income countries had the lowest rates of under-five mortality on average, at six deaths per thousand live births in 2012. Upper-middle-income countries were the most successful in reducing under-five mortality rates between 1990 and 2012, registering a 63 per cent decrease over the period. Countries at all income levels have been getting steadily better at saving children's lives. The annual rate of reduction in the under-five mortality rate has accelerated since 1995 at all levels of national income, except in high-income countries.

Low income need not be an impediment to saving children's lives, despite evidence of a link between a country's income level and its child mortality. There have been notable reductions in the under-five mortality rate since 1990 and particularly since 2000 in some low-income countries such as Bangladesh, Cambodia, Eritrea, Ethiopia, Guinea, Liberia, Madagascar, Malawi, Mozambique, Nepal, Niger, Rwanda, Uganda and the United Republic of Tanzania. Even high- and middle-income countries with low mortality rates can continue to make considerable progress. There were 53 countries in 1990 that had an under-five mortality rate of twenty or fewer deaths per thousand live births, of which 36 countries had—at least—halved their under-five mortality rate, and 11 had reduced it by at least two thirds by 2012.

New analysis has suggested a comprehensive drop in under-five mortality rates among the poorest households in all regions. Disparities in under-five mortality between the richest and the poorest households have declined in most regions of the world, with the exception of sub-Saharan Africa. Hence, it is possible to curb preventable child deaths regardless of the income level of country or household.

Reducing under-five mortality requires political will, applied consistently in support of child and maternal health through concerted action, sound strategies and adequate resources. The success of a significant number of countries in achieving Goal 4 should encourage all global health actors to commit to achieving a fairer and more equitable world for all children.

Measles deaths have declined by more than three-quarters in the past twelve years, from 562,000 deaths in 2000 to 122,000 in 2012, mostly among children under five years of age. Measles deaths in sub-Saharan Africa (56,000) and Southern Asia (53,000) accounted for 89 per cent of the estimated total global measles deaths during 2012. Compared with estimated mortality in the complete absence of a measles vaccination programme, 13.8 million deaths were averted by measles vaccination between 2000 and 2012.

There has been substantial progress in most regions, particularly Oceania which decreased measles deaths by an estimated 89 per cent between 2000 and 2012. Unfortunately, continued measles outbreaks in Europe, sub-Saharan Africa and Southern Asia—due to weak routine immunization systems and delayed implementation of accelerated disease control—have stalled momentum towards regional and global targets in control and elimination.

Measles can be prevented through the application of two doses of a safe, effective and inexpensive vaccine. Reductions in measles-related mortality have been due—in part—both to improvements in routine coverage among children in the appropriate age group who received the first dose of measles containing vaccine (MCV1), and to the success of supplementary immunization activities in vaccinating children outside the reach of existing health services.

Between 2000 and 2009, global coverage with MCV1 increased from 72 per cent to 84 per cent, and then stagnated at 84 per cent between 2009 and 2012. Recommended MCV1 coverage levels—at least 90 per cent at the national level and at least 80 per cent in all districts—were reached in 58 countries with available data in 2012. However, during the same time period, there were 35 countries with less than 80 per cent MCV1 coverage. An estimated 21.2 million infants—many of them from the poorest, most marginalized populations residing in especially hard-to-reach areas—did not receive MCV1 in 2012.

Addressing the decline in political and financial commitment to measles control is the key to making further progress towards the measles objectives established in 2010 by the World Health Assembly....

PRIMARY SOURCE

Message by UN Secretary-General Ban Ki-moon on International Fistula Day

SOURCE Ban Ki-moon. *"Message by UN Secretary-General Ban Ki-moon on International Fistula Day." United Nations Population Fund, Campaign to End Fistula, May 23, 2014. http://www.endfistula.org/public/pid/7441?feedEntryId=31748 (accessed January 25, 2015).*

INTRODUCTION *This primary source is a release from the Campaign to End Fistula, a division of the United Nations Population Fund. It is a message from UN Secretary-General Ban Ki-moon, briefly describing the condition and its consequences, and calling for action to eliminate it.*

Message by UN Secretary-General Ban Ki-moon on International Fistula Day

It is an appalling fact that in our world of modern medical advances, nearly 800 women still die from pregnancy-related complications each day, and for every woman who dies, almost 20 more are injured or disabled with severe or life-shattering, long-term conditions, such as obstetric fistula.

This International Day to End Obstetric Fistula is an opportunity to sound the alarm on this tragedy so that we may galvanize action to end it. Progress is possible. Over the past dozen years, some 47,000 women and girls have received surgical treatment supported by the United Nations Population Fund (UNFPA).

Registering and tracking each woman and girl with fistula can help ensure that more individuals receive treatment, survivors stay healthy and their future babies thrive. The "Every woman, every child" initiative can help advance progress by mobilizing partners to support all those who need help.

Addressing obstetric fistula is more than a matter of health; it is a human rights imperative. This condition is one of the most devastating consequences of neglected childbirth and a stark reflection of inequality at its worst. Although fistula is now virtually unheard of in industrialized countries, it continues to afflict the most impoverished women and adolescent girls in many developing countries. If left untreated, it can contribute to social isolation and depression and lead to chronic medical problems, even the loss of the child.

Fistula is fully preventable when all women and girls have access to high-quality, comprehensive sexual and reproductive health services, especially family planning, maternal health care and emergency obstetric care.

On this International Day, I call on partners to support the UNFPA-led global Campaign to End Fistula. Let us join forces to eliminate this global social injustice.

SEE ALSO *Child Health; Family Planning; HIV/AIDS; Malnutrition; Nutrition; Pregnancy Termination; Vaccines; Water Supplies and Access to Clean Water*

BIBLIOGRAPHY

Books

Ban, Ki-moon. *Global Strategy for Women's and Children's Health.* New York: United Nations, 2010. Available online at http://www.who.int/pmnch/activities/advocacy/fulldocument_globalstrategy/en/ (accessed February 11, 2015).

Partnership for Maternal, Newborn & Child Health. *PMNCH Progress Report 2013.* Geneva: World Health Organization, 2014. Available online at http://www.who.int/pmnch/knowledge/publications/pmnch_2013_report/en/ (accessed February 11, 2015).

World Health Organization. *Antiretroviral Drugs for Treating Pregnant Women and Preventing HIV Infection in Infants: Recommendations for a Public Health Approach.* Geneva: World Health Organization, 2006. Available online at http://www.who.int/hiv/pub/mtct/arv_guidelines_mtct.pdf?ua=1 (accessed February 11, 2015).

World Health Organization. *Evidence for the Ten Steps to Successful Breastfeeding.* Geneva: World Health Organization, 1998. Available online at http://whqlibdoc.who.int/publications/2004/9241591544_eng.pdf?ua=1 (accessed February 11, 2015).

World Health Organization. *Global Nutrition Targets 2025: Anaemia Policy Brief.* Geneva: World Health Organization, 2014. Available online at http://www.who.int/nutrition/publications/globaltargets2025_policybrief_anaemia/en/ (accessed February 11, 2015).

World Health Organization. *Global Prevalence of Vitamin A Deficiency in Populations at Risk 1995–2005: WHO Global Database on Vitamin A Deficiency.* Geneva: World Health Organization, 2009. Available online at http://whqlibdoc.who.int/publications/2009/9789241598019_eng.pdf?ua=1 (accessed February 11, 2015).

World Health Organization. *HIV and Infant Feeding: Guidelines on Principles and Recommendations for Infant Feeding in the Context of HIV and a Summary of Evidence.* Geneva: World Health Organization, 2010. Available online at http://whqlibdoc.who.int/publications/2010/9789241599535_eng.pdf?ua=1 (accessed February 11, 2015).

World Health Organization. *Use of Antiretroviral Drugs for Treating Pregnant Women and Preventing HIV Infection in Infants.* Geneva: World Health Organization, 2009. Available online at http://whqlibdoc.who.int/publications/2010/9789241599818_eng.pdf (accessed February 11, 2015).

World Health Organization. *The World Health Report 2013: Research for Universal Health Coverage.* Geneva: World Health Organization, 2013. Available online at http://www.who.int/whr/2013/report/en/ (accessed February 11, 2015).

World Health Organization and United Nations Children's Fund. *Global Strategy for Infant and Young Child Feeding.* Geneva: World Health Organization, 2003. Available online at http://whqlibdoc.who.int/publications/2003/9241562218.pdf (accessed February 11, 2015).

World Health Organization and United Nations Children's Fund. *Joint Statement: Clinical Management of Acute Diarrhea.* Geneva: World Health Organization, 2004. Available online at http://whqlibdoc.who.int/hq/2004/WHO_FCH_CAH_04.7.pdf (accessed February 11, 2015).

World Health Organization, United Nations Children's Fund, United Nations Population Fund, the World Bank, and the United Nations Population Division. *Trends in Maternal Mortality, 1990 to 2013.* Geneva: World Health Organization, 2014. Available online at http://www.who.int/reproductivehealth/publications/monitoring/maternal-mortality-2013/en/ (accessed February 11, 2015).

World Health Organization, United Nations Children's Fund, the World Bank, and the United Nations Department of Economic and Social Affairs Population Division. *Levels and Trends in Child Mortality 2014.* Geneva: World Health Organization, 2014. Available online at http://www.who.int/maternal_child_adolescent/documents/levels_trends_child_mortality_2014/en/ (accessed February 11, 2015).

Periodicals

Andersson, Maria, Vallikkannu Karumbunathan, and Michael B. Zimmermann. "Global Iodine Status in 2011 and Trends over the Past Decade." *Journal of Nutrition* 142, no. 4 (April 2012): 744–750.

Bauserman, Melissa, et al. "Caterpillar Cereal as a Potential Complementary Feeding Product for Infants and Young Children: Nutritional Content and Acceptability." *Maternal & Child Nutrition,* April 5, 2013.

Bentley, Margaret E., Heather M. Wasser, and Hilary M. Creed-Kanashiro. "Responsive Feeding and Child Undernutrition in Low- and Middle- Income Countries." *Journal of Nutrition* 141, no. 3 (March 2011): 502–507.

Capes, Tracy, Charles Ascher-Walsh, Idrissa Abdoulaye, and Michael Brodman. "Obstetric Fistula in Low and Middle Income Countries." *Mount Sinai Journal of Medicine* 78, no. 3 (May–June 2011): 352–361.

Coovadia, Hoosen M., et al. "Mother-to-Child Transmission of HIV-1 Infection during Exclusive Breastfeeding in the First 6 Months of Life: An Intervention Cohort Study." *The Lancet* 369, no. 9567 (March 31, 2007): 1107–1116.

Dewey, Kathryn G., and Seth Adu-Afarwuah. "Systematic Review of the Efficacy and Effectiveness of Complementary Feeding Interventions in Developing Countries." *Maternal & Child Nutrition* 4, suppl. S1 (April 2008): 24–85.

Flax, Valerie L., et al. "Integrating Group Counseling, Cell Phone Messaging, and Participant-Generated Songs and Dramas into a Microcredit Program Increases Nigerian Women's Adherence to International Breastfeeding Recommendations." *Journal of Nutrition* 144, no. 7 (July 2014): 1120–1124.

Hess, Sonya Y., and Janet C. King. "Effects of Maternal Zinc Supplementation on Pregnancy and Lactation Outcomes." *Food and Nutrition Bulletin* 30, suppl. 1 (March 2009): S60–S78.

Hsu, Justine, et al. "Countdown to 2015: Changes in Official Development Assistance to Maternal, Newborn, and Child Health in 2009–10, and Assessment of Progress since 2003." *The Lancet* 380, no. 9848 (September 29, 2012): 1157–1168.

Lamberti, Laura M., et al. "Breastfeeding and the Risk for Diarrhea Morbidity and Mortality." *BMC Public Health* 11, suppl. 3 (April 2011): S15.

Websites

"Acting on the Call: Ending Preventable Child and Maternal Death." *U.S. Agency for International Development.* http://www.usaid.gov/ActingOn-TheCall (accessed February 11, 2015).

Darnton-Hill, Ian. "Zinc Supplementation during Pregnancy: Biological, Behavioural and Contextual Rationale." *World Health Organization*, July 2013. http://www.who.int/elena/bbc/zinc_pregnancy/en/ (accessed January 29, 2015).

"Infant and Young Child Feeding," Fact Sheet No. 342. *World Health Organization*, Updated February 2014. http://www.who.int/mediacentre/factsheets/fs342/en/ (accessed January 29, 2015).

"Maternal and Child Health." *GlobalHealth.gov*. http://www.globalhealth.gov/global-health-topics/maternal-and-child-health/#birth-defects (accessed January 29, 2015).

"Maternal and Child Nutrition." *The Lancet*, June 6, 2013. http://www.thelancet.com/series/maternal-and-child-nutrition (accessed January 29, 2015).

"Maternal and Child Undernutrition." *The Lancet*, January 16, 2008. http://www.thelancet.com/series/maternal-and-child-undernutrition (accessed January 29, 2015).

"Newborns: Reducing Mortality," Fact Sheet No. 333. *World Health Organization*, May 2012. http://www.who.int/mediacentre/factsheets/fs333/en/ (accessed January 29, 2015).

"10 Facts on Maternal Health." *World Health Organization*, Updated May 2014. http://www.who.int/features/factfiles/maternal_health/en/ (accessed January 29, 2015).

"10 Facts on Obstetric Fistula." *World Health Organization*, Updated May 2014. http://www.who.int/features/factfiles/obstetric_fistula/en/ (accessed January 29, 2015).

"What We Do: Maternal, Newborn & Child Health: Strategy Overview." *Bill & Melinda Gates Foundation.* http://www.gatesfoundation.org/What-We-Do/Global-Development/Maternal-Newborn-and-Child-Health (accessed January 29, 2015).

"WHO PMTCT Guidelines." *AVERT: AVERTing HIV and AIDS* http://www.avert.org/world-health-organisation-who-pmtct-guidelines.htm (accessed January 29, 2015).

Lindsay M. Jaacks

Médecins Sans Frontières

🌐 Introduction

Médecins Sans Frontières (MSF), known in English as Doctors Without Borders, is an international, independent/private, nonprofit humanitarian organization designed to provide assistance in emergency situations caused by war, drought, famine, epidemics, disasters (either natural or humanmade), or lack of available health care. MSF was awarded the Nobel Peace Prize in 1999.

MSF routinely maintains an active presence in areas of need, comprising 67 countries as of 2013. A majority of MSF activities are undertaken in challenging areas where dangers from government and civil instability are common.

In addition to their emergency operations, MSF operates longer-term projects to treat infectious and communicable diseases such as human immunodeficiency virus/acquired immune deficiency syndrome (HIV/AIDS) and tuberculosis. MSF also provides physical and mental health treatment for marginalized groups and street children.

🌐 Historical Background

Since its inception in 1971, when a group of young French physicians founded MSF, the organization has mobilized to help injured victims of earthquakes and hurricanes in Central America, drought in Africa, and war in the Middle East, Africa, and Eastern Europe.

Among the characteristics that distinguish MSF from other charitable organizations are its independence from individual governments and its ability and willingness to make public opinion statements. MSF volunteers and officials frequently grant media interviews and make presentations to raise awareness of populations whose safety and security are at risk and to bring pressure upon governments that might restrict their relief efforts, especially in areas where MSF staff observe violations of a population's basic human rights. By 2015 MSF was

composed of 23 associations with 19 national offices scattered around the world. Roughly 80 percent of its funding comes from public and private donations, while the remaining 20 percent is received from governmental and international humanitarian agencies.

MSF also created 10 specialized satellite organizations to oversee specific areas of operations such as the procurement and delivery of humanitarian relief supplies, epidemiological research, and research on special humanitarian and social issues.

During emergencies, MSF volunteers perform surgery, run nutrition, vaccination, and sanitation programs, and deliver basic health care, often from tented field hospitals. Longer-term goals for an area in crisis might include rehabilitating existing hospitals and training local medical personnel. Basic MSF volunteer field teams usually include a physician, nurse, and logistician.

MSF also has an expert epidemiology section that has been utilized around the world to diagnose, treat, monitor, and contain epidemics. In addition to care and aid to those displaced by violence, MSF epidemiological (medical and statistical) surveys in the field from war-torn areas often provide early warning to the world of major humanitarian catastrophes.

MSF workers often labor under dangerous conditions, and surrounding violence often hampers the efforts of MSF and other relief agencies. Relief supply lines may be cut, with food and medical supplies intended for refugees routinely stolen or confiscated. MSF medical staff have also been abducted and taken captive. When faced with severe and increasing security risks, MSF has been forced to abandon or close medical relief centers.

MSF's primary tasks are the provision of basic and emergency physical and mental health care; the provision of vaccinations and immunizations; and the operation of feeding centers, primarily for children and mothers of infants. MSF also employs infrastructure experts who are able to dig and construct wells or bring in potable (safe to drink) water, in order to establish a means of supplying clean drinking water. When necessary, MSF also assists in creating temporary shelters and can supply necessities such as blankets and plastic sheeting materials.

In addition to their emergency operations, MSF operates longer-term projects to treat infectious and communicable diseases such as HIV/AIDS, tuberculosis, and sleeping sickness, and to provide physical and mental health treatment for marginalized groups and street children. MSF's expert epidemiology section has been utilized around the world to diagnose, treat, monitor, and contain epidemics of cholera, meningitis, and measles, among other diseases.

⊕ Impacts and Issues

Because MSF is an independent international organization, it has no political ties or limitations to prevent it from responding to any situation thought likely to benefit from its assistance. It was not designed to become involved in international governmental affairs. For those involved in the local response of MSF, the effort is a humanitarian one. Traveling staff are primarily volunteers (although their personal expenses are paid and they may receive a small stipend) who are willing to make themselves available with very little notice; they are typically deployed in an area for 6 to 12 months. Assigned locations may be remote and dangerous. MSF hires local staff and provides them with training and materials, and all personnel (MSF core and local staff) work in cooperation with other local and international emergency and relief organizations.

MSF is staffed by physicians, nurses, health-care providers, logisticians, technicians, technical and non-medical personnel, sanitation and water experts, and administrative workers. There is a small core of paid staff, a large number of volunteer workers, and a significant number of local staffers hired at each major site. MSF participates in thousands of medically related missions around the globe each year. By traveling in small teams and enlisting local resources, MSF teams have penetrated war zones and reached refugee groups and epidemic epicenters.

Because of its size, well-trained staff, and ability to hire significant numbers of local people in order to meet personnel needs, MSF is generally able to respond extremely quickly to emergencies. They utilize highly specialized kits and equipment packs that enable them to carry all needed supplies with them when they mobilize, so they are literally able to "hit the ground running," with no delay before they are able to begin emergency operations.

Environmental Emergencies

MSF is active in more than natural disaster areas and war zones. MSF also responds to what it classifies as environmental emergencies. In July 2010, for example, MSF rushed emergency personnel and equipment to Nigeria

MSF RESPONSE TO 2010 EARTHQUAKE IN HAITI

On January 12, 2010, Haiti was rocked by the strongest quake there in more than 200 years, with a 7.0 magnitude. The damage was catastrophic. The official death toll according to the Haitian government was 316,000, but other estimates are closer to 160,000.

An estimated 400,000 people from the Port-au-Prince metropolitan area alone were displaced. Some fled to the mountainous regions of Haiti, while others camped in streets and parks. Most had limited access to water and sanitation. Haiti was already the poorest nation in the Western world by many estimates, with few resources to devote to care of its displaced citizens. After the earthquake, already limited supplies and destruction of infrastructure created drastic shortages of food and medicine.

At the time of the earthquake, MSF had 800 staff already working in the impoverished nation. Prior to the quake, MSF provided emergency care at three primary treatment centers and general health care at a number of other locations. All of the existing MSF facilities were destroyed or rendered unusable by the earthquake, and MSF staff established temporary shelters and moved operations outside. MSF officials confirmed that four employees had died in the Haiti earthquake and that six others remained missing. Within two weeks of the earthquake, MSF health-care providers treated more than 5,000 people in Haiti and performed more than 900 surgeries, often in brutal and primitive conditions.

In October 2010, MSF also responded to a cholera outbreak in Haiti. Cholera is primarily a waterborne and food-borne disease that causes diarrhea and vomiting. Without treatment, cholera can lead to rapid dehydration, which may result in death. MSF mobilized hundreds of staff members to establish more than 50 cholera treatment centers in Haiti. In the first months of the cholera outbreak, MSF treated more than 100,000 patients. The disease became endemic in Haiti.

to treat more than 2,000 lead-poisoning victims. MSF officials reported treating children with lead blood levels more than one dozen times normal levels. The severity of the poisonings required emergency treatment to alleviate life-threatening and brain-damaging seizures.

MSF and World Health Organization (WHO) officials called the poisonings an "unprecedented environmental emergency" caused by unsafe mining and dangerous environmental disposal practices related to the extraction of gold from lead-rich ore. MSF established and supported chelation treatment units in local hospitals. In May 2012, MSF noted that the number of children with lead poisoning in northern Nigeria had risen to 4,000. MSF also reported that 400 children had died of lead poisoning in Nigeria since 2010 because of mining practices.

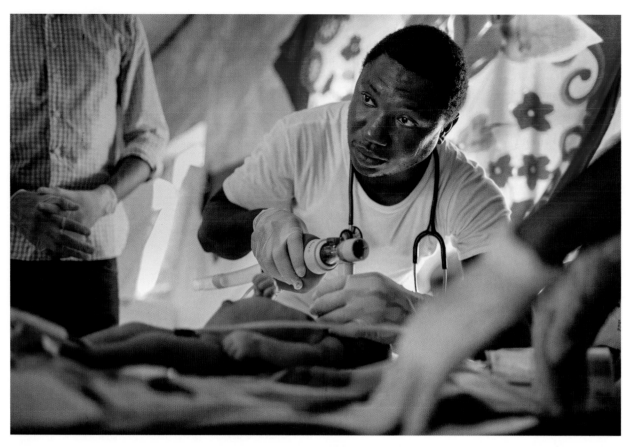

Doctors at Médecins Sans Frontières (MSF; Doctors Without Borders) try to reanimate Marhazu Sa'adu, 9 days old, a child suffering from blood lead level of 49.6 micrograms per deciliter, as well as tetanus and septicemia, inside the MSF clinic in Anka, Zamfara State, Nigeria. Marhazu passed away within the day. The MSF facility handles serious cases of lead poisoning referred to them by local clinics in the surrounding villages. It is mainly caused by ingestion and breathing of lead particles related to unsafe mining and ore processing, according to MSF. An estimated 400 children died of lead poisoning in the area in 2010. © *Alex Masi/Corbis.*

MSF Range of Operations

Along with the International Red Cross and Red Crescent, MSF is one of the few organizations that can respond to simultaneous and widely separated global crises. While still deeply engaged in recovery efforts in Haiti, in late July 2010, MSF responded to massive flooding in Pakistan. Heavy monsoon rains produced flooding that covered over one-fifth of Pakistan at its peak. The floods persisted throughout August and September, displacing over 20 million people and eroding Pakistan's most productive farmland. By December 2010, MSF provided medical care to more than 80,000 Pakistanis, distributed 528,344 gallons (2 million liters) of water, and provided 65,000 relief kits.

MSF workers in the Philippines shifted their mission to provide critical post-disaster care in the wake of Super Typhoon Haiyan (called Yolanda in the Philippines) on November 8, 2013. Medical teams entered the hardest-hit areas as soon as they could arrange transport for doctors and supplies and within days were operating field hospitals in Panay, Guiuan, Ormoc, Tacloban, and Burauen. Doctors had difficulty maintaining adequate

stores of medicines, antibiotics, sterilization equipment, and basic hospital supplies. Teams reported high numbers of patients seeking treatment for infected wounds and noted a steady increase in diarrheal illnesses caused by contaminated water.

MSF workers were among the first international health workers to respond to the 2014 Ebola outbreak in West Africa. MSF warned that local health systems, especially in Liberia, were unequipped to handle a large outbreak of the virus.

Drug Delivery

MSF is a major contributor and coordinating body for the delivery of drugs to and within developing countries. In cooperation with the International Network for the Rational Use of Drugs (INRUD), MSF aims to improve the global availability of drugs for the treatment of infectious diseases like malaria and tuberculosis (TB). MSF works with partner organizations to find ways of lowering the price of essential medicines and bringing certain cheap and effective drugs back into production. MSF continues to lobby for increased research funding

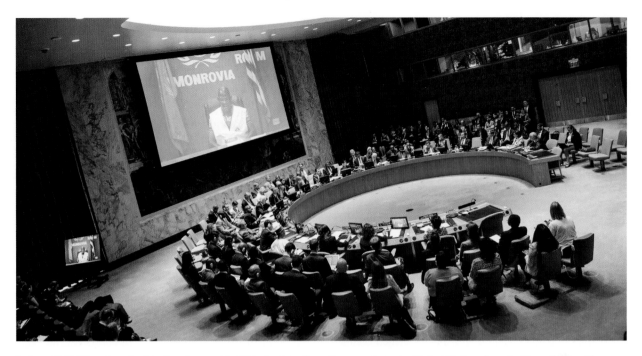

Jackson K. P. Niamah, a physician's assistant with Médecins Sans Frontières, speaks to the United Nations Security Council via a videoconference call from Monrovia, Liberia, during a meeting on the Ebola outbreak in West Africa on September 18, 2014, in New York City. © *Andrew Burton/Getty Images.*

to study malaria, TB, sleeping sickness, leishmaniasis, and other diseases.

Most of the effort in improving drug delivery in developing countries has been focused on the major infectious diseases. Regarding malaria, for instance, MSF has been persuading governments to consider funding the artemisinin-based combination therapy favored by the WHO. This will help address the growing problem of chloroquine resistance. Chloroquine is a drug that is commonly used as a treatment for malaria. Although chloroquine is relatively inexpensive, it is not effective in the areas where the malaria parasites are resistant, therefore, there is a need for alternative drugs to be made available.

It is now well established that antiretroviral (ARV) therapy for HIV/AIDS is effective treatment, enabling people to live with the condition rather than almost inevitably dying from it, as they would without the treatment. Therefore, improving access to ARV to persons with HIV in developing countries has become a top priority for MSF.

A program begun by MSF in 2003 showed that giving ARV therapy in even the poorest countries of the world was feasible; people adhered to the complex treatment regiments and benefited from them, just as HIV/AIDS patients in the West did. Therefore, the United Nations World Summit in 2005 made a pledge to achieve universal access to ARV therapy by 2010. However, this goal was not achieved. WHO studies continue to show a widespread lack of access to ARV drugs in developing countries.

Influence

One of the unique aspects of MSF, in contrast to nearly all other relief and aid organizations, is its commitment to combining humanitarian medical care with outspoken opinion on the causes of worldwide suffering. It is equally vocal on perceived impediments to the provision of effective medical care. For example, MSF has spoken publicly against pharmaceutical companies that refuse to manufacture pediatric dosages of AIDS-related drugs or to provide affordable and appropriate medications to African countries hardest hit by the AIDS pandemic.

MSF has sought (and received) audiences with the United Nations, various international and governmental organizations, and the worldwide media, in an effort to communicate both the needs of their various patient groups and to educate the world on violations of international humanitarian doctrines that they have witnessed or that they argue have been perpetrated across the globe. Researchers, academics, and scientists associated with MSF publish scholarly articles, create media campaigns, engage in public education programs, and offer presentations and exhibits at local and international conferences.

In response to the civil war in Syria, MSF called international attention to the use of force by government troops against medical facilities and doctors in Syria. Although the Syrian government did not authorize MSF to operate in its country, the organization sent doctors into Syria to assist local medical personnel. However, some rebel groups pushed MSF workers out of critical areas. MSF also worked with Syrian doctors and aid groups to smuggle medicine and other supplies from neighboring Jordan. MSF also provides medical assistance to refugee camps across the Syrian border in several neighboring countries.

⊕ Future Implications

International aid workers, including those working for MSF, have traditionally been afforded special protections under international law or custom. Since the mid-1990s, however, international aid workers have increasingly become targets of military, police, paramilitary, or other armed groups. Since the mid-1990s, international aid workers have been the victims of a generally increasing number of targeted attacks globally. The exact number and nature of attacks on international health workers is difficult to quantify. Many nongovernmental organizations (NGOs) do not release detailed information about attacks on medical facilities or health workers. Heightened areas of danger traditionally include armed conflict zones and area of widespread civil unrest.

In 2011, the International Committee of the Red Cross (ICRC) released "Health Care in Danger: Making the Case," a comprehensive report on the extent of attacks on international health workers. The ICRC analyzed media reports, NGO reports, and other sources from armed conflict zones. The report revealed that with regard to violent incident attacks on those delivering medical services, state-sponsored armed forces, local police, paramilitary forces, criminal gangs, and recognized terrorist organizations were collectively responsible for the majority of attacks. The report concluded that one reason for the upsurge in violence against health-care workers generally is the perception among some governments and armed groups that aid workers are affiliated ideologically with Western political agendas, Accordingly, the attacks are not random acts of violence but rather deliberately targeted acts against international aid workers.

SEE ALSO *Conflict, Violence, and Terrorism: Health Impacts; Ebola Virus Disease; Food Security and Hunger; Health as a Human Right and Health-Care Access; Health-Care Worker Safety and Shortages; NGOs and Health Care: Deliverance or Dependence; Social Theory and Global Health; Vulnerable Populations*

BIBLIOGRAPHY

Books

Abu-Sada, Caroline, ed. *Dilemmas, Challenges, and Ethics of Humanitarian Action: Reflections on Médecins Sans Frontières' Perception Project.* Montreal: McGill-Queen's University. Press, 2012.

Biehl, João, and Adriana Petryna, eds. *When People Come First: Critical Studies in Global Health.* Princeton, NJ: Princeton University Press, 2013.

Crisp, Nigel. *Turning the World Upside Down: The Search for Global Health in the Twenty-First Century.* London: Royal Society of Medicine Press, 2010.

De Maio, Fernando. *Global Health Inequities: A Sociological Perspective.* Houndsmill, UK: Palgrave Macmillan, 2014.

Fox, Renée C. *Doctors Without Borders: Humanitarian Quests, Impossible Dreams.* Baltimore: Johns Hopkins University Press, 2014.

Hubbard, Nyla Jo Jones. *Doctors Without Borders in Ethiopia: Among the Afar.* New York: Algora, 2011.

Médecins Sans Frontières/Doctors Without Borders. *World in Crisis: Populations in Danger at the End of the 20th Century.* Hoboken, NJ: Taylor and Francis, 1996.

Ratcliffe, John. *Biting through: Five Years in Afghanistan.* Brunswick, Australia: Scribe, 2014.

Redfield, Peter. *Life in Crisis: The Ethical Journey of Doctors Without Borders.* Berkeley: University of California Press, 2013.

Periodicals

Cerón, Alejandro. "Review of *Life in Crisis: The Ethical Journey of Doctors Without Borders.*" *Global Public Health* 8, no. 10 (2013): 1180–1181.

Chen, K. "Review of *Doctors Without Borders.*" *Science* 346, no. 6215 (2014): 1304.

Duggan, L. "Treating Cholera Patients in Africa with 'Doctors Without Borders.'" *World of Irish Nursing and Midwifery* 20, no. 2 (2012): 52–53.

Ko, J., and B. Kung. "A Doctor Without Borders: Dr. Fan Ning—His Medical Adventures and Inspiring Thoughts." *Hong Kong Medical Journal* 18, no. 6 (2012): 552–553.

"Médecins Sans Frontières: Doctors Without Borders." *Australian Journal of Medical Science* 35, no. 4 (2014): 142.

Rasool, Sabahat, and Omar Salim Akhtar. "Doctors Without Borders." *International Journal of User-Driven Healthcare* 3, no. 4 (2013): 92–95.

Zacher, Meghan, Hollie Nyseth Brehm, and Joachim J. Savelsberg. "NGOs, IOs, and the ICC: Diagnosing and Framing Darfur." *Sociological Forum* 29, no. 1 (March 2014): 29–51.

Websites

Cooper, Anderson. "Doctors Without Borders Help Typhoon Survivors." *CNN: Anderson Cooper 360,* November 15, 2013. http://ac360.blogs.cnn.com/2013/11/15/doctors-without-borders-help-typhoon-survivors/?iref=allsearch (accessed March 1, 2015).

"Doctor on the Front Line." *BBC World Service*, February 12, 2015. http://www.bbc.co.uk/programmes/p02jcqmw (accessed March 1, 2015).

"Doctors Without Borders." *PBS Religion & Ethics Newsweekly*, October 3, 2014. http://www.pbs.org/wnet/religionandethics/2014/10/03/october-3-2014-doctors-without-borders/24264/ (accessed March 1, 2015).

Drehle, David von, and Aryn Baker. "Person of the Year 2014: The Ebola Fighters." *Time*, December 10, 2014. http://time.com/time-person-of-the-year-ebola-fighters/ (accessed March 1, 2015).

Médecins Sans Frontières/Doctors Without Borders. http://www.doctorswithoutborders.org (accessed March 1, 2015).

K. Lee Lerner

Mental Health Treatment Access

⊕ Introduction

Access to timely, effective, evidence-based, mental health care is a global issue and a human right, and it disproportionately affects the most vulnerable populations. Mental illness affects people from all cultures and countries and occurs among persons of all ages and socioeconomic status. However, persons in the poorest areas and those with the least education are least likely to be able to obtain needed mental health care.

According to the World Health Organization (WHO) roughly 14 percent of the global disease burden is attributable to mental illness. Of those affected, 7 to 80 percent, many of whom live in poor countries, do not have any access to quality mental health treatment. Ensuring access to, and availability of, mental health care is a fundamental mental health policy issue, however as the graph based on the WHO data shows, just 60 percent of countries have dedicated mental health policies.

The relationship between physical and mental health and illness is a complex and dynamic one—the two are interrelated, inseparable, and continuously interact with one another. Mental health issues are often associated with, and can improve or worsen, physical illnesses. There is a significant relationship between projected life span with chronic and life-threatening illnesses and mental health, such as human immunodeficiency virus/acquired immune deficiency syndrome (HIV/AIDS), tuberculosis, many forms of cancer, autoimmune disorders (illness that occurs when the body tissues are attacked by its own immune system), diabetes, and heart disease.

To lead full and productive lives, it is important to have physical and mental health. Persons with untreated, or inadequately treated, mental health disorders may have great difficulty attending school, obtaining and keeping gainful employment, securing stable housing, and becoming functioning members of society.

⊕ Historical Background

Since the dawn of civilization, people have experienced mental illness, and there have been efforts to treat or cure it. Mental illness was thought by the ancient Greeks, Romans, and Egyptians to be caused by demonic possession or by other types of religious or spiritual maladies, such as being cursed, angering the gods, dark magic, or sorcery. As a result, early treatment involved efforts to rid the body of the demons or other negative spirits. When mental illness was thought to have been caused by demons or other spiritual maladies, it was treated by priests and other clergy through the use of exorcism, prayer, incantations, and other types of rituals.

Sometimes, treatment for mental illness utilized an approach referred to as trepanation, which involved boring one or two small holes into the skull in order to relieve pressure on the brain or release the negative energy or spirits. The earliest evidence of the practice was found in skulls dating from the Neolithic period. There is some archaeological evidence that Stone Age cave dwellers may have used trepanation to treat mental illness, and the medical practice of trepanation continued up to the present century. Ancient cultures considered it an effective way to relieve pressure on the brain or release the demons that possessed it. Later the purpose of trepanation was described as offering the closed skull of the adult an expansion window to restore the blood flow that was diminished when, during the course of normal development, the skull sealed in infancy.

The early Greek physician Hippocrates (c. 460–c. 377 BCE), who lived during the 5th century BCE, believed that mental illness had physiological underpinnings. He advocated the use of rest, moving to a different locale, change of job, or other life or environmental shifts as a means of cure.

The first documented self-contained facility for housing and treating the mentally ill was located in Valencia, Spain, and was created in 1407 CE. Between the 1400s and the 1700s, the mentally ill were typically

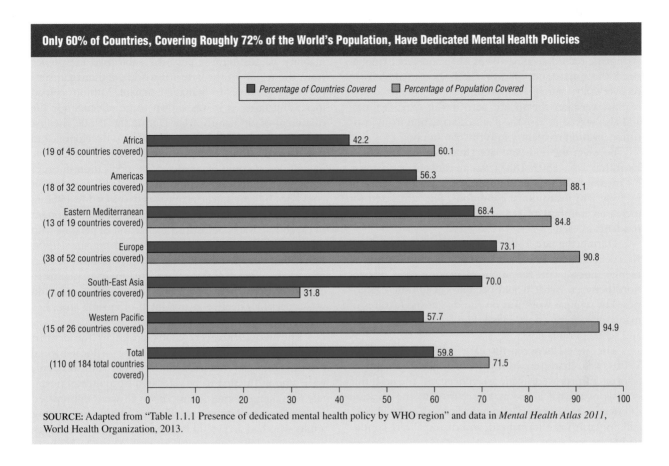

Only 60% of Countries, Covering Roughly 72% of the World's Population, Have Dedicated Mental Health Policies

■ *Percentage of Countries Covered*　　■ *Percentage of Population Covered*

Africa (19 of 45 countries covered): 42.2 / 60.1
Americas (18 of 32 countries covered): 56.3 / 88.1
Eastern Mediterranean (13 of 19 countries covered): 68.4 / 84.8
Europe (38 of 52 countries covered): 73.1 / 90.8
South-East Asia (7 of 10 countries covered): 70.0 / 31.8
Western Pacific (15 of 26 countries covered): 57.7 / 94.9
Total (110 of 184 total countries covered): 59.8 / 71.5

SOURCE: Adapted from "Table 1.1.1 Presence of dedicated mental health policy by WHO region" and data in *Mental Health Atlas 2011*, World Health Organization, 2013.

housed in asylums, where they were often isolated from the rest of society. Sometimes beaten, starved, shackled and chained, treatment that would now be considered inhumane was the norm. Because the etiology (causes) and mental illness itself were poorly understood, there were few efforts made to treat affected people.

During the latter part of the 18th century, growing acceptance of scientific and biological explanations of mental illness inspired more enlightened, humane understanding and treatment of sufferers. A new approach to the treatment of persons with mental illness known as "moral management" emerged in Europe. Those who championed this approach posited that the mentally ill were affected by their surroundings and that a soothing environment was helpful in treatment. In Italy, Vincenzo Chiarugi (1759–1820) was appointed by the Grand Duke Leopold I (1747–1792) to design the new hospital of St. Bonifacio, which would become one of the first facilities devoted to the humane care of people with mental illness. With Chiarugi serving as its director, St. Bonifacio opened in 1788.

Around the same time, William Tuke (1732–1822) a merchant living in England, was horrified by the abusive treatment of patients in asylums. Tuke opened the York Retreat in 1796. The retreat was a country house in which patients were treated with kindness and understanding in a supportive environment, without any form of physical restraint. Comfortable beds, pictures, and curtains replaced shackles, chains, and barren cement cells. Tuke believed that recovery would be more likely in sheltered, homelike surroundings. Patients worked in the house and garden as part of their treatment. Like modern-day therapeutic communities, the retreat combined work with exercise, walks, conversations, reading, games, arts, and crafts. The retreat pioneered another novel therapeutic approach—patients' privileges increased incrementally in response to their progress. This approach was the forerunner of using positive reinforcement to promote behavior modification.

In France, the psychiatrist Philippe Pinel (1745–1826) advocated for changes in what he viewed as cruel mental health treatment. He believed that those housed in asylums should have clean and pleasant living conditions conducive to increasing health, that residents should be able to be outside in good weather, and that they should not be restrained or shackled in any way.

In addition to promoting understanding and compassionate treatment of persons with mental illness, Pinel contributed to the advancement of mental health treatment by classifying types of mental illness based on categories of symptoms. He described four classes of mental illness: melancholia (feelings of severe depression), mania (excessive nervous excitement with or without delirium), dementia (disturbance in thought processes), and idiocy (defective intellectual functions). Pinel also introduced the practice of documenting individual case histories and systematic record keeping. Both Tuke and Pinel emphasized the importance of work and vocational skills in recovery. Structured work programs and organized recreation were key therapeutic activities in their facilities, and also served to ease the planned transition from institutionalization to reentry into the community.

Between the mid- and late 1800s, American activist Dorothea Dix (1802–1887) was an outspoken advocate for mental health system reform, particularly in terms of housing and institutional conditions. She advocated for increased numbers of state-run facilities with far fewer residents in each.

During the late 1800s in Germany, physician Emil Kraepelin (1856–1926) undertook a scientific study of mental illness, with the intent of making clear distinctions between (what would become) diagnostic categories. His seminal work was on the diagnostic features of manic-depressive (now called bipolar disorder) illness and schizophrenia.

The period between the early 1800s and the early 1900s was characterized by mental health treatment reform. Efforts were made to understand the scientific genesis of mental illness as a precursor to the creation of effective treatment. The significantly mentally ill were still primarily institutionalized, and custodial care continued to be prevalent.

Throughout the 19th century biological and psychological explanations of mental illness were put forth by psychiatrists, philosophers, and scientists in Europe and the United States. German psychiatry made the first attempts to combine elements of each in an effort to develop a more integrated philosophy that considered both body and mind as involved in mental illness.

In the early 1900s, the Austrian neurologist Sigmund Freud's (1856–1939) psychoanalytic theories gained widespread popularity, and his treatment methods were widely used. By the 1930s, an increasing variety of treatment protocols had been initiated, with differing degrees of success: drugs were used to treat psychosis; there was a common belief that seizures and severe mental illnesses such as schizophrenia could not coexist, so a number of treatments designed to induce seizures were developed. The precursors to electroconvulsive therapy were evolving by the end of the 1930s; in addition, high fevers created by bacterial injections (malaria-causing bacteria were briefly popular) and insulin-induced comas lasting for several days were sometimes utilized as treatment for mental illness.

During this time, a type of brain surgery called frontal lobotomy, which involved the removal or ablation of brain tissue, was popularized. Lobotomies were used to treat schizophrenia, persistent depression, obsessive disorders, and disabling anxiety.

In 1949, the Australian psychiatrist John F. J. Cade (1912–1980) pioneered the use of lithium to treat the symptoms of psychosis (mental illness characterized by drastic changes in personality, impaired functioning, and inability to distinguish personal subjective experience from the reality of the external world), rather than simply using sedatives to manage behavior. Lithium gained increasing favor as it was shown to be effective for the treatment of bipolar disorder. During the 1950s, the first generation of antipsychotic drugs was developed and popularized, along with an understanding that chronic mental illness could be treated with medication in order to achieve significant symptom reduction, but that it could not be cured. Thorazine was developed in 1952 in France and was found to be beneficial for the treatment of psychosis. Rates of institutionalization of persons with mental illness reached a global peak during the 1950s. Behavioral therapy (also known as behavior modification or cognitive behavioral therapy), treatment that aims to change self-destructive behaviors, came into vogue, and was especially effective at treatment of anxiety and phobias (extreme or irrational fears).

The mid-1960s were characterized by the deinstitutionalization movement and the rise of local mental health clinics and smaller facilities. Older adult residents were among the first to be relocated from mental hospitals to nursing homes, many of which were unprepared to treat persons with mental illnesses. Others were young adults who had grown up in mental institutions and with few coping skills were unable to manage in the community. These young adults often suffered from substance abuse and mental illness and some were homeless or became fixtures in hospital emergency departments, shelters, and correctional facilities.

Despite the problems associated with deinstitutionalization, most observers believe that it was a sound policy choice, and research has demonstrated that with a comprehensive range of community support services including day treatment and residential settings for persons in crisis, job training, employment opportunities, and housing, persons with serious and persistent mental illness can live in the community. For those unable to live in the community, care should be provided in the least restrictive settings.

⊕ Impacts and Issues

Mental illness creates significant disease and disability as well as economic and social burdens worldwide. According to the WHO, the disorders causing the highest rates of disability among adults and older youth are substance use disorders, schizophrenia and psychotic disorders, bipolar disorders, severe anxiety disorders, and clinical depression. The latter is both the most prevalent and the most costly in terms of lost productivity, particularly among females. The WHO estimates that, by 2030, depression will be the most frequently diagnosed and most prevalent form of mental illness, particularly in adult females.

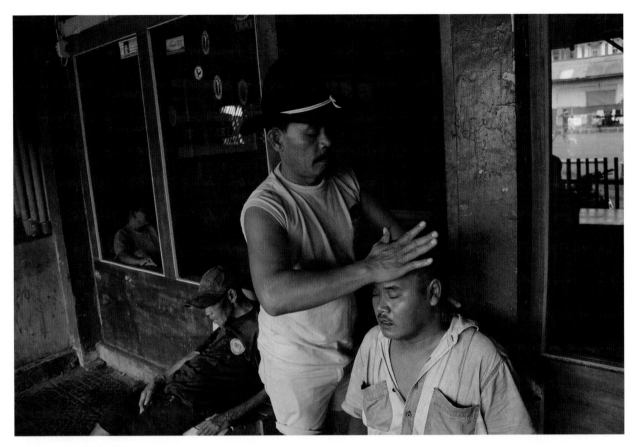

Arbert, a shaman, gives a mental health patient a massage at a clinic in Tasikmalaya, Indonesia. The Mentari Hati Foundation set up the mental health rehabilitation center in a former bus terminal. They largely take in patients with mental health issues who have no support network. A shortage of trained health workers, lack of treatment options, and widespread misconceptions about mental illness in Indonesia have led to reports of abusive treatment, with families often abandoning mentally ill relatives. The Mentari Hati Foundation uses traditional methods such as performing massage on a regular basis for each patient, giving them mineral water, and giving them affection. They claim 178 patients have been cured since the rehabilitation center was founded in 2008. They cared for 170 patients in May 2014.   © *Nurcholis Anhari Lubis/Getty Images.*

Throughout the world, but particularly in developing, low- and middle-income countries, there is very limited access to mental health services. Such services as are available may be impossible to access for reasons of transportation or financial hardship. In many countries, the inequitable distribution of resources between mental and physical health contributes to the burden of disease. Historically, mental health research, prevention and treatment have been underfunded, with fewer resources devoted to these activities than to comparable actions to maintain physical health.

The primary barriers to access include poverty, scarcity of mental health providers, lack of culturally sensitive treatment, and stigma related to mental illness and treatment. In developing countries, there also are commonly shortages of necessary medications for the treatment of mental disorders. According to WHO data, nearly one-fifth of reporting countries lack a minimum of one efficacious antipsychotic drug, one antiseizure medication, or one routinely prescribed antidepressant medication.

Another global issue limiting access to mental health treatment is a dearth of policies and procedures governing the provision of mental health care. More than half of African countries, along with more than one-third of all countries, lack adequate mental health plans, policies, or procedures. The graphic reveals that globally, 40 percent of countries do not have mental health policies in place. Among those countries with published plans, nearly half have not revised their policies since 1990 and therefore do not reflect contemporary trends and developments in mental health care. Nearly 25 percent of the countries in the WHO do not offer any legal protections to persons living with mental illness.

The WHO reports that the treatment gap, which refers to the percentage of the population in need of but not receiving services, ranges from roughly 40 percent to more than 70 percent in developed countries. In developing countries, the gap is reportedly as high as 90 percent. In addition to a significant lack of adequately educated or properly trained mental health professionals,

THE WHO MENTAL HEALTH GAP ACTION PROGRAMME

Because mental illness is ubiquitous—it affects all genders, ages, socioeconomic strata, cultures, and national boundaries—and access to quality mental health services is a growing global concern, world health leaders have developed a plan and program to address access to, and availability of, mental health services worldwide. The WHO Mental Health Gap Action Programme (mhGAP), outlined in 2008, was designed to scale up mental health services and programming after identifying key diagnostic needs and global disease burdens. The mhGAP also identified the most efficient and effective treatments to address the disorders with the greatest disease burdens.

The WHO reports that roughly 14 percent of the overall global disease burden is attributable to mental health issues, and nearly three-fourths of those affected are unable to access necessary and appropriate services. The mhGAP aims to make services available to those in need, with the goal of ensuring access to appropriate treatment to millions of patients worldwide. This involves provision of case management (coordination of all medical, mental health care, and support services to improve continuity of care and efficiency), medications, and life skills for persons with mental illness, as well as those with neurological and substance abuse disorders. The program targets diagnosis and treatment of depression and mood disorders, schizophrenia, and epilepsy and seizure disorders.

The program uses best practice methods in conjunction with epidemiological data (information about the causes and occurrence of disease), to create and then deliver a comprehensive package of services and interventions tailored to cultural and regional needs. Previous WHO analyses identified a series of priority conditions associated with the highest rates of disability, mortality (deaths), and morbidity (illness), as well as those with the most significant social and economic burdens. They also looked at conditions that were most likely to be the focus of human rights violations. The priority list includes psychotic disorders and schizophrenia, depressive disorders, epilepsy, dementia, disorders related to alcohol or illicit drug abuse suicide, and mental health issues affecting children and youth. The mhGAP describes treatment, long-term management, and prevention for these disorders customized to meet the needs of each culture and region. The mhGAP programming targets countries with the greatest disease burden and greatest resource gaps.

The overarching goals of mhGAP are to establish productive partnerships; reinforce commitments with existing partners; and accelerate efforts and increase investments to reduce of the burden of mental health disorders. The mhGAP intends to scale up services by training local health-care workers to provide comprehensive service coverage at the household, community, and health-care facility levels. Scaling up is a social, political, and institutional process that engages a range of stakeholders— governments, health professionals, civil society, communities, and families, with support from the international community.

The mhGAP works to create programming to prevent mental illness, effectively treat existing mental illness, and improve access to timely, effective, and culturally appropriate services. It employs varied strategies to achieve its aims including promotion of widespread professional and public health education about mental illness, recovery, and resiliency, along with programs designed to eliminate barriers to care and to disseminate information about efficient and effective treatment. In order to assess its efficiency and to monitor long-term outcomes, the mhGAP program has an assessment component that will measure objective and subjective improvement in wellness, program development, and implementation.

paraprofessionals, and community service workers, there are economic issues; people who may have access to services may not be able to afford them. In addition, there is often a lack of administrative infrastructure to enforce mental health laws, policies, procedures, and legal protections for persons living with mental illness.

Access to mental health services is frequently hampered for economic reasons; it is generally significantly more expensive to obtain than physical health care, particularly because it often involves an extended period of services or a range of treatment types. Behavioral health medications are often costly and must be taken for extended periods, sometimes throughout the life span. In countries with private or national insurance, there may not be mental health benefits, or they may be inadequate for the cost or duration of services.

The WHO indicates that at least one-fourth of all countries do not provide disability benefits for incapacitating mental illness. Lack of adequate budgetary allocations for the development and provision of mental health services is common, creating significant barriers to care. The WHO observes that about 33 percent of the global population resides in countries that allocate 99 percent of their total health care budget to physical health services and less than 1 percent to mental health services. Nearly one-third of all countries reporting do not even have line items in their budgets related to mental health.

Even in developed countries with stable economies, mental health services are frequently either inadequate for population size, located primarily in population centers rather than in rural or sparsely populated regions, or are underutilized for reasons of cost or stigma. In more-affluent countries, personal, regional, or cultural biases continue to prevent people from seeking services. Mental illnesses are often mistakenly thought to be voluntary,

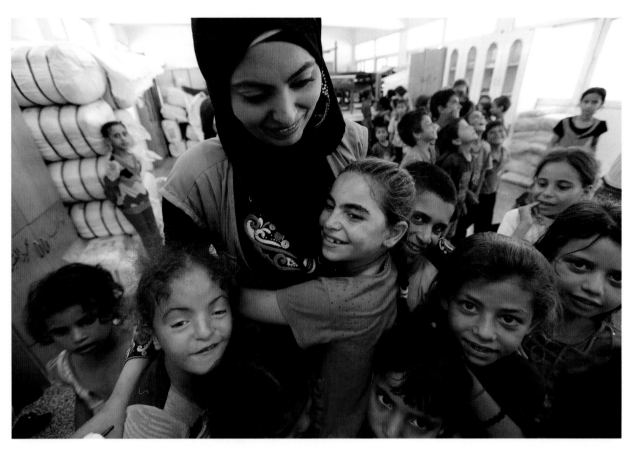

Palestinian children affected by the war gather around a United Nations volunteer during a group class as part of the United Nations community mental health programs in the Gaza Strip at a school converted to a refuge in Jabalia, in the north of the Gaza Strip. "To prevent children from processing and thinking about all these issues we try to distract them, to help them live some joy, to have a little fun inside the shelter," said psychiatrist Dr. Iyad Zaqout, who manages the program. © *Mohammed Abed/AFP/Getty Images.*

reflecting the notion that people with mental health disorders can simply "snap out" of them or that mental illness is a choice or reflects moral weakness or lack of initiative. Stigma associated with a diagnosis of mental illness or seeking mental health treatment remains an issue, even in well-educated, affluent cultures with adequate legal protections and equitable access to services.

In many areas, independent of the level of development, political climate or economic stability, there is often a lack of understanding of the causes, progression, treatments, and outcomes of mental illness. If people do not understand how to recognize mental illness, or do not know how or where to seek treatment, then it is unlikely that they will obtain appropriate treatment. Research reveals that even when people do seek mental health care, fewer than half recognize the need for ongoing treatment.

Compounding these barriers to access is the fact that unlike most physical medical care, which often requires a brief series of interactions and perhaps some follow-up to manage symptoms or cure disease, mental health care often necessitates a substantial investment of time and resources over a protracted period. It also requires access

to and availability of additional social services and supports, such as housing and vocational training.

⊕ Future Implications

In developed countries, there has been a steady increase in the range and efficacy of mental health treatments available—from various forms of therapy to an ever expanding array of pharmaceutical drugs and ancillary services such as clinical homes, life and social skills, and job training, and progressively safer and more beneficial forms of surgery and deep brain stimulation. However, for many people throughout the world, the fundamental issue remains one of access to effective forms of mental health treatment.

In the first decade of the 21st century, various international programs and initiatives catalyzed improvements in global access to mental health care. Global mental health organizations and programs aim to improve overall access to necessary and appropriate services, to reduce inequalities in provision of quality services, and to ensure positive outcomes (how patients fare as a result of treatment) between, within, and across communities, regions and nations. The global mental health community—providers, individuals, institutions and organizations—asserts that human rights must be supported and protected and stigma reduced in order for people to feel safe when seeking mental health services. For example, the Movement for Global Health, an international network launched in 2007, seeks to create a common language and understanding for professionals and the general public to advocate for improving global mental health through scientific research and human rights.

There is currently a global shortage of high-level mental health practitioners, particularly pediatric psychiatrists and psychiatric nurses, and the shortage is especially critical in impoverished and middle-income countries, with a reported 0.05 psychiatrists and 0.16 psychiatric nurses per 100,000 individuals. The WHO reports that the staffing issues are most critical for children and adolescents, with an average of one pediatric psychiatrist for every 1 million to 4 million people. Only about half (52 percent) of low-income countries offer access to community-based mental health centers, compared with nearly 97 percent of upper-income countries. Because services are often concentrated in urban population centers, it may be difficult or impossible for persons living in remote or rural areas to obtain care.

There is much evidence to suggest that shifting service provision from the very limited number of mental health professionals to locally trained paraprofessionals and community workers is socially beneficial and economically sound. Community providers intimately understand the prevailing culture and mores and may be better able to understand the needs and issues of their peers.

The 2010 Grand Challenges in Global Mental Health Initiative, led by the U.S. National Institute of Mental Health (NIMH) and the Global Alliance for Chronic Disease, has worked with Wellcome Trust, the McLaughlin-Rotman Centre for Global Health, and the London School of Hygiene and Tropical Medicine to focus global attention on neuropsychiatric disorders. It not only will distinguish research priorities and mental health interventions with the greatest impact but also will promote interventions that can be scaled up to address the urgent need for mental health care worldwide.

SEE ALSO *Body Image and Eating Disorders; Conflict, Violence, and Terrorism: Health Impacts; Gender and Health; Global Health Initiatives; Post-Traumatic Stress Syndrome; Social Theory and Global Health; Stigma; Universal Health Coverage; Vulnerable Populations*

BIBLIOGRAPHY

Books

Dudley, Michael, Derrick Silove, and Fran Gale, eds. *Mental Health and Human Rights: Vision, Praxis, and Courage.* Oxford, UK: Oxford University Press, 2012.

Eaton, William W., et al., eds. *Public Mental Health.* New York: Oxford University Press, 2012.

Knifton, Lee, and Neil Quinn, eds. *Public Mental Health Global Perspectives.* Maidenhead, UK: McGraw-Hill Education, 2013.

Mills, China. *Decolonizing Global Mental Health: The Psychiatrization of the Majority World.* New York: Routledge, Taylor and Francis Group, 2014.

Nock, Matthew, Guilherme Borges, and Yutaka Ono, eds. *Suicide: Global Perspectives from the WHO World Mental Health Surveys.* Cambridge, UK: Cambridge University Press, 2012.

Okpaku, Samuel O., ed. *Essentials of Global Mental Health.* Cambridge, UK: Cambridge University Press, 2014.

Patel, Vikram, I. H. Minas, Alex Cohen, and Martin Prince, eds. *Global Mental Health: Principles and Practice.* New York: Oxford University Press, 2014.

Thornicroft, Graham, et al. *Global Mental Health: Putting Community Care into Practice.* Chichester, UK: Wiley, 2011.

Thornicroft, Graham, and Vikram Patel, eds. *Global Mental Health Trials.* Oxford: Oxford University Press, 2014.

Thornicroft, Graham, Mirella Ruggeri, and David P. Goldberg, eds. *Improving Mental Health Care: The Global Challenge.* Chichester, UK: Wiley-Blackwell, 2013.

World Health Organization. *mhGAP Mental Health Gap Action Programme: Scaling Up Care for Mental, Neurological, and Substance Use Disorders.* Geneva: WHO Press, 2008.

World Health Organization. *Investing in Mental Health: Evidence for Action.* Geneva: WHO Press, 2013. Available online at http://www.who.int/mental_health/publications/financing/investing_in_mh_2013/en/ (accessed March 17, 2015).

Periodicals

Andrade, L. H., et al. "Barriers to Mental Health Treatment: Results from the WHO World Mental Health Surveys." *Psychological Medicine* 44, no. 6 (April 2014): 1303–1317.

Naik, S. and S. Skeen. "The Movement for Global Mental Health." *British Journal of Psychiatry* 198, no. 2 (February 2011): 88–90.

Hahm, H. C. "Intersection of Race-Ethnicity and Gender in Depression Care: Screening, Access, and Minimally Adequate Treatment." *Psychiatric Services* 66, no. 3 (March 2015): 258–264.

Hensel, J. M., and A. J. Flint. "Addressing the Access Problem for Patients with Serious Mental Illness Who Require Tertiary Medical Care." *Journal of Healthcare for the Poor and Underserved* 26, no. 1 (2015): 35–48.

Kaufman, K. R., and E. S. Hwang. "Culture, Impaired Access to Mental Health Care, and Bipolar Disorder: Case Analysis." *Harvard Review of Psychiatry* 27, no. 1 (2015): 69–73.

Patel, Vikram. "Global Mental Health: From Science to Action." *Harvard Review of Psychiatry* 20, no. 1 (January–February 2012): 6–12.

Wahl, O. F. "Stigma as a Barrier to Recovery from Mental Illness." *Trends in Cognitive Science* 16, no. 1 (2012): 9–10.

Websites

Grand Challenges in Global Mental Health. https://grandchallengesgmh.nimh.nih.gov/ (accessed March 19, 2015).

"Mental Health." *Partners in Health.* http://www.pih.org/priority-programs/mental-health/about (accessed March 1, 2015).

"Mental Health." *World Health Organization (WHO).* http://www.who.int/mental_health/en/ (accessed March 1, 2015).

"Mental Health Gap Action Program (mhGAP)." *World Health Organization (WHO).* http://www.who.int/mental_health/mhgap/en/ (accessed March 1, 2015).

Movement for Global Mental Health. http://www.globalmentalhealth.org (accessed March 1, 2015).

"What Is Mental Health?" *MentalHealth.gov.* http://www.mentalhealth.gov/basics/what-is-mental-health/index.html (accessed March 1, 2015).

Pamela V. Michaels

Methicillin-Resistant
Staphylococcus Aureus (MRSA)

⊕ Introduction

Methicillin-resistant *Staphylococcus aureus* (MRSA or MRSa) is a particular type (bacterial strain) of *S. aureus* that is resistant to the antibiotic methicillin, a synthetic penicillin antibiotic. The bacterium is important because of its antibiotic resistance and because it can cause a number of severe infections. In addition to methicillin, MRSA is also resistant to all of the penicillin class of antibiotics. This wide range of resistance makes the bacterium difficult to treat because commonly used antibiotics will not kill it.

Infection perils include necrotizing fasciitis, more popularly known as "flesh-eating disease." MRSA is also known as oxacillin-resistant *S. aureus* (oxacillin is another antibiotic) and multiple-resistant *S. aureus*.

Until the late 1990s, MRSA infections were almost exclusively found in hospitals (termed hospital-acquired, or HA-MRSA). The use of antibiotics in hospitals provided a powerful selection pressure by creating an environment where only the most resilient bacteria could survive. The prevalence of MRSA outside of hospitals is increasing, and this form of infection from MRSA bacteria has been designated as community-associated- or community-acquired-MRSA (CA-MRSA).

⊕ Historical Background

MRSA infections are actually an old problem, evident almost as long as the use of methicillin itself. Methicillin was first introduced in 1959 to treat strains of *S. aureus* showing resistance to penicillin. By chemically altering the structure of penicillin, scientists were able to produce methicillin, and the penicillin-resistant *S. aureus* were killed by the newly synthesized antibiotic. However, this beneficial effect did not last long. By 1961, MRSA appeared in the United Kingdom (UK) and soon reports of MRSA came from other countries in Europe, Asia, and North America. By 2010, MRSA accounted for about half of all hospital-acquired infections.

Methicillin resistance is caused by the presence of a gene (a section of genetic material responsible for the production of a protein or other compound) that codes for a protein that binds to the antibiotic and prevents the antibiotic from entering the bacteria. The *S. aureus* that is susceptible to methicillin does not have this gene. It is the transfer of this gene from one bacterium to another that has spread resistance through populations of *Staphylococcus* around the globe.

Although MRSA initially was named and characterized by resistance to methicillin, over the years it has also proved resistant to other antibiotics, including cephalosporins, macrolides, and quinolones.

The spread of MRSA has been aided by the fact that *S. aureus* is a common species of bacteria, present in soil and on human bodies. Because *S. aureus* has a worldwide distribution, epidemiologists and infectious disease researchers argue that it is not surprising that MRSA has a similar distribution.

Underuse of an antibiotic, such as when a person does not complete the entire course of a prescribed antibiotic medication, is frequently followed by successive generations of bacteria that show resistance to the antibiotic. This is because those bacteria that have slight genetic differences that confer resistance are able to reproduce in greater numbers than those without the unique set of genes. As a highly simplified example, if an antibiotic were effective against 99 percent of all the bacteria it encountered, the remaining 1 percent would survive to pass on to successive generations whatever unique set of genes created their resistance to the antibiotic and allowed survival. Overuse of antibiotics, such as when antibiotic medications are routinely given to livestock or when they are taken to treat colds, influenza, or other viral illnesses for which antibiotics are not effective, can also contribute to the development of antibiotic resistance.

Antibiotic resistance also arises with overuse of antibiotic drugs. Antibiotics kill off targeted bacterial strains but may leave resistant strains to reproduce.

Future generations of bacteria, often a growing percentage of the bacterial population, then exhibit antibiotic resistance.

Tens of millions, by some estimates nearly 100 million, people carry MRSA on their bodies. In the United States, about a third of people are colonized with *S. aureus* (mostly on the surface of the skin and/or nasal passages). Colonization refers to bacteria (or other pathogens) that establish a presence on a tissue. In these environments, the bacterium is normally harmless. If MRSA enters a wound, however, or if a person's immune system is not functioning efficiently, illness can result.

Although fewer than 1 percent of otherwise healthy individuals colonized with MRSA will ultimately develop MRSA-related disease, studies indicate that a hospitalized patient who acquires MRSA is about five times more likely to die than a patient in the same hospital who does not carry the bacterium. MRSA is capable of causing necrotizing fasciitis, an extremely invasive disease that progresses rapidly. In extreme cases, amputation of the infected limb is the only way to save the patient's life. MRSA can also carry genes that code for the production

COMBATING MRSA

The U.S. Centers for Disease Control and Prevention (CDC) states that "MRSA is transmitted most frequently by direct skin-to-skin contact." The CDC also states that contact precautions, including hand washing, are critical in preventing MRSA infection.

The CDC recommends that in addition to cleaning hands carefully and often with soap and water and/or using a hand sanitizer with an alcohol base, other good hygiene practices should be used. These include (1) covering broken skin or and exposed wounds (cuts and abrasions) with a clean, dry sanitary bandage; (2) avoiding communal use of towels or razors; (3) using clothing and towels as barriers between open skin and shared exercise equipment; (4) disinfecting shared exercise equipment before and after use.

The CDC has estimated that adherence to hand washing guidelines could prevent 30,000 deaths per year caused by nosocomial (hospital acquired) infections, including MRSA infections in the hospital.

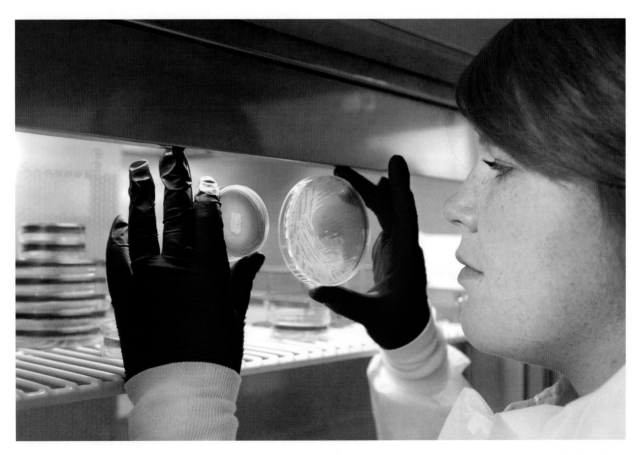

U.S. Centers for Disease Control and Prevention microbiologist Valerie Albrecht holds up two petri dish culture plates inoculated with methicillin-resistant *Staphylococcus aureus* (MRSA) bacteria. MRSA is a bacterium that is resistant to many antibiotics. In the community, most MRSA infections are skin infections. In medical facilities, MRSA causes life-threatening bloodstream infections, pneumonia, and surgical site infections. *James Gathany/U.S. Centers for Disease Control and Prevention.*

of potent toxins. If these toxins enter the bloodstream, the resulting effects can be devastating to the body.

Having another infection can increase the likelihood of developing a MRSA infection. For example, individuals with cystic fibrosis often have recurring lung infections that require treatment with a number of different antibiotics. This situation increases the risk of compromise by MRSA and other resistant bacteria.

The U.S. Centers for Disease Control and Prevention (CDC) has found that direct skin-to-skin contact is the most common way for MRSA to be transmitted, but MRSA can also remain viable on hard surfaces long enough to be transmitted to another person.

Although some antibiotics such as vancomycin currently remain effective against MRSA (especially if treatment begins soon after infection) the search continues for new antibiotics effective against MRSA. New forms of MRSA have emerged that are resistant to vancomycin, called vancomycin intermediate *S. aureus* (VISA) and vancomycin resistant *S. aureus* (VRSA).

A few antibiotics have shown effectiveness against acute bacterial skin and skin structure infections, including linezolid and daptomycin. Several new long-acting treatments—tedizolid, dalbavancin, and oritavancin—were approved by the U.S. Food and Drug Administration in 2014.

⊕ Impacts and Issues

Globally, nonresistant *S. aureus* and MRSA have similar prevalence. The incidence (the number of new cases in the population in a given period) of infection due to MRSA continues to increase in many countries, especially in southern and eastern Europe and southern and eastern Asia. But not all the news is negative. Hand washing and other contact prevention precautions have stabilized HA-MRSA case levels in the United States. Prevention efforts in northern Europe have been so effective that the prevalence of MRSA among patients with skin and soft tissue infections is well under 10 percent.

MRSA countermeasures started prior to 2005 quickly yielded tangible results. A study of hospital-acquired infections in nine metropolitan U.S. areas during a four-year period from 2005 to 2008 found that MRSA was responsible for an average of 28 percent fewer infections in each geographical area than before the study commenced. Recent studies and reports continue to support a decline in such infections. In addition, the U.S. Veterans Administration reported that a "bundle" of actions taken by staff at Veterans Affairs hospitals across the country reduced hospital-acquired MRSA infections by 45 to 62 percent. Actions included nasal-swab testing for MRSA colonization upon admission to the hospital, isolating or cohorting those that test positive, and using such contact precautions as frequent hand washing and wearing gowns and gloves when caring for infected persons.

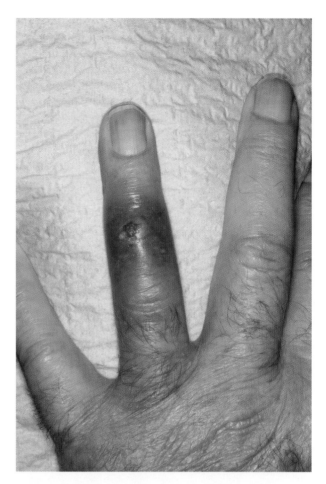

A MRSA infection on the ring finger of a 79 year old male with a history of diabetes. © *Scott Camazine / Alamy.*

A third study released in April 2011 showed that testing everyone upon admission to the hospital for MRSA infection did not help curb hospital-acquired infections, at least in the intensive care unit. These contradicting studies sparked an ongoing debate among infection control experts, who continue to work toward reducing the burden of MRSA infections in hospitals. A 2012 study by researchers at the University of Edinburgh revealed that MRSA infections spread from large city hospitals to smaller hospitals, typically when patients are transferred. The researchers called for increased screening and treatment of infected patients before transfer to other hospitals.

Despite some success, CA-MRSA remains a great concern for public health officials. The organism tends to aggressively invade tissues and often produces a more severe infection than that produced by hospital-acquired MRSA, for reasons that are not yet clear. Whereas in-hospital MRSA infections declined in the United States from 2003 to 2008, a study released in 2012 found that the number of patients checking into U.S. hospitals with active MRSA infections had more than doubled during the same period. In another 2012 report by the CDC on the incidence of invasive MRSA by epidemiological

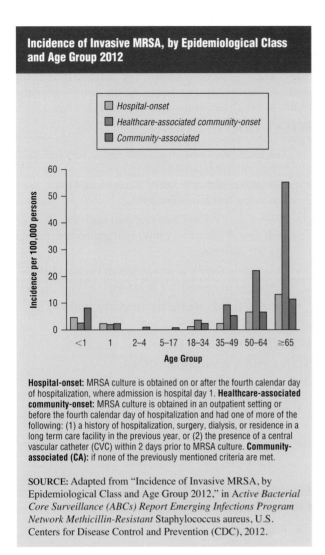

Incidence of Invasive MRSA, by Epidemiological Class and Age Group 2012

- ☐ Hospital-onset
- ☐ Healthcare-associated community-onset
- ☐ Community-associated

Hospital-onset: MRSA culture is obtained on or after the fourth calendar day of hospitalization, where admission is hospital day 1. **Healthcare-associated community-onset:** MRSA culture is obtained in an outpatient setting or before the fourth calendar day of hospitalization and had one of more of the following: (1) a history of hospitalization, surgery, dialysis, or residence in a long term care facility in the previous year, or (2) the presence of a central vascular catheter (CVC) within 2 days prior to MRSA culture. **Community-associated (CA):** if none of the previously mentioned criteria are met.

SOURCE: Adapted from "Incidence of Invasive MRSA, by Epidemiological Class and Age Group 2012," in A*ctive Bacterial Core Surveillance (ABCs) Report Emerging Infections Program Network Methicillin-Resistant* Staphylococcus aureus, U.S. Centers for Disease Control and Prevention (CDC), 2012.

class and age group (see graphic), an increase in MRSA cases with age is well documented. As people age, older populations become more vulnerable to MRSA and, of course, exposure to hospital and health-care facilities dramatically increases with age. The CDC study showed that the incidence of all epidemiological source MRSA infections (hospital-onset, health-care-associated community-onset, and community onset) showed increases with age.

Vectors of infection are also on the increase. Researchers discovered that MRSA can grow and divide inside another microscopic organism called *Acanthamoeba*. *Acanthamoeba* can become airborne and drift for a considerable distance on air currents. This may mean that MRSA is acquiring the ability to spread great distances. Spread of CA-MRSA via sexual contact is possible.

Bedbugs have also been shown to be vectors of MRSA, mechanically transmitting the bacteria from one location to another or acting as a direct vector of infection to a susceptible hosts. In 2011, bedbugs were removed from three infested patients who were admitted

to a hospital in Vancouver, British Columbia. Analysis of the removed bedbugs showed that MRSA was present on the surface of their bodies. Additionally, *Staphylococcus* has been previously identified in the saliva of bedbugs. Both findings lend evidence to the possibility that bedbugs could at least passively transmit MRSA or another *Staphylococcus* bacteria during a blood meal. The findings suggest that increasing bedbug populations, especially in urban areas, might serve as hidden reservoirs of MRSA.

Two additional and unusual sources of CA-MRSA appeared the first decade of the 2000s. In what some scientists termed the "flip-flop" effect, humans who acquired MRSA were found to infect their pets with the organism, and the pets in turn later re-infected their owners. In another study, scientists at the University of Washington found that some public beaches could be a reservoir for MRSA infection. Marine water and beach sand taken from one sampling of Puget Sound, Washington, beaches in 2009 revealed MRSA in 7 of 13 samples. The human contributions to the contamination are unknown because MRSA can also exist as an environmental contaminant, even in salty marine settings.

MRSA often is detected in gyms and sports facilities. In October 2013, physicians diagnosed three players from the Tampa Bay Buccaneers of the U.S. National Football League with MRSA infections. Researchers found MRSA in team training facilities, which were sterilized following detection of the bacteria-resistant infection.

⊕ Future Implications

Research for antibiotics effective against MRSA is in a race against time. Variants of MRSA are appearing that are resistant even to vancomycin and other antibiotics and so the development of new antibiotics must at least keep pace with the evolution of resistance by MRSA.

In 2008, the CDC launched the National MRSA Education Initiative, aimed at helping the public to recognize and prevent MRSA skin infections. Educational materials were made available to students and teachers just as the school year began. The campaign also included continuing education for health-care professionals and MRSA treatment guidelines. Similar programs have been implemented in the United Kingdom and other countries with high rates of MRSA infections.

Similar educational campaigns are carried on globally. Activists and health-care professionals in the United States, Canada, and the United Kingdom coordinate and sponsor World MRSA Day annually in October in order to raise awareness and knowledge about MRSA.

Research continues on other biotechnology options to combat the spread of MRSA. One option is called phage therapy. Phage is short for bacteriophage, which is a virus that specifically infects and forms new phage particles inside of a bacterium. The phage-bacterium association is specific—a certain type of phage infects a certain type of bacterium. In doing so, the phage ultimately destroys the bacterial cell. Scientists are experimenting with a phage that targets MRSA. If this technique proves successful, it would be a powerful treatment because resistance to phages is very rare.

PRIMARY SOURCE

Methicillin-resistant *Staphylococcus aureus* (MRSA)

SOURCE *"Methicillin-Resistant* Staphylococcus aureus *(MRSA)," in* Antibiotic Resistance Threats in the United States, 2013. *Centers for Disease Control and Prevention (CDC). U.S. Department of Health and Human Services, 2013, 77–79. http://www.cdc.gov/drugresistance/ threat-report-2013/pdf/ar-threats-2013-508 .pdf#page=20 (accessed January 25, 2015).*

INTRODUCTION *This primary source is a section from a 2013 publication of the U.S. Centers for Disease Control and Prevention on antibiotic resistance in the United States. MRSA, the topic of this excerpt, is classified in the report as a serious threat.*

METHICILLIN-RESISTANT STAPHYLOCOCCUS AUREUS (MRSA)

Methicillin-resistant *Staphylococcus aureus* (MRSA) causes a range of illnesses, from skin and wound infections to pneumonia and bloodstream infections that can cause sepsis and death. Staph bacteria, including MRSA, are one of the most common causes of healthcare-associated infections.

RESISTANCE OF CONCERN

Resistance to methicillin and related antibiotics (e.g., nafcillin, oxacillin) and resistance to cephalosporins are of concern.

PUBLIC HEALTH THREAT

CDC estimates 80,461 invasive MRSA infections and 11,285 related deaths occurred in 2011. An unknown but much higher number of less severe infections occurred in both the community and in healthcare settings.

FIGHTING THE SPREAD OF RESISTANCE

Although still a common and severe threat to patients, invasive MRSA infections in healthcare settings appear to be declining. Between 2005 and 2011 overall rates of invasive MRSA dropped 31%; the largest declines (54 percent) were observed among infections occurring during hospitalization. Success began with preventing central-line associated bloodstream infections with MRSA, where rates fell nearly 50 percent from 1997 to 2007.

During the past decade, rates of MRSA infections have increased rapidly among the general population (people who have not recently received care in a healthcare setting). There is some evidence that these increases are slowing, but they are not following the same downward trends as healthcare-associated MRSA.

WHAT CDC IS DOING

- Tracking illness and identifying risk factors for drug-resistant infections using two systems, the National Healthcare Safety Network and the Emerging Infections Program.

- Providing states and facilities with outbreak support such as staff expertise, prevention guidelines, tools, and lab assistance.

- Developing tests and prevention recommendations to control drug-resistant infections.

- Helping healthcare facilities improve antibiotic prescribing practices.

WHAT YOU CAN DO
States and Communities Can:

- Know resistance trends in your region.

- Coordinate local and regional infection tracking and control efforts.

- Require facilities to alert each other when transferring patients with any infection.

Healthcare CEOs, Medical Officers, and Other Healthcare Facility Leaders Can:

- Require and strictly enforce CDC guidance for infection detection, prevention, tracking, and reporting.

- Make sure your lab can accurately identify infections and alert clinical and infection prevention staff when these bacteria are present.

- Know infection and resistance trends in your facility and in the facilities around you.

- When transferring a patient, require staff to notify the other facility about all infections.

- Join or start regional infection prevention efforts.

- Promote wise antibiotic use.

Healthcare Providers Can:

- Know when and types of drug-resistant infections are present in your facility and patients.

- Request immediate alerts when the lab identifies drug-resistant infections in your patients.

- Alert the other facility when you transfer a patient with a drug-resistant infection.

- Protect patients from drug-resistant infections.

- Follow relevant guidelines and precautions at every patient encounter.
- Prescribe antibiotics wisely.
- Remove temporary medical devices such as catheters and ventilators as soon as no longer needed.

Patients and Their Loved Ones Can:

- Ask everyone, including doctors, nurses, other medical staff, and visitors, to wash their hands before touching the patient.
- Take antibiotics only and exactly as prescribed.

SEE ALSO *Antibiotic/Antimicrobial Resistance; Epidemiology: Surveillance for Emerging Infectious Diseases; Sanitation and Hygiene*

BIBLIOGRAPHY

Books

Ji, Yinduo, ed. *Methicillin-Resistant* Staphylococcus Aureus *(MRSA) Protocols,* 2nd ed. New York: Springer, 2014.

McKenna, Maryn. *Superbug: The Fatal Menace of MRSA.* New York: Free Press, 2010.

Weigelt, John A., ed. *MRSA,* 2nd ed. New York: Informa Healthcare, 2009.

Periodicals

Chatterjee, Som S., and Michael Otto. "Improved Understanding of Factors Driving Methicillin-Resistant *Staphylococcus Aureus* Epidemic Waves." *Clinical Epidemiology* 5 (July 2013): 205–217. Available online at http://www.ncbi.nlm.nih.gov/pmc/articles/PMC3707418/ (accessed April 1, 2015)

Falagas, Matthew E., Drosos E. Karageorgopoulos, John Leptidis, and Ioanna P. Korbila. "MRSA in Africa: Filling the Global Map of Antimicrobial Resistance." *PLOS ONE* 8, no. 7 (July 29, 2013): e68024, 1–12.

Liu, Catherine, et al. "Clinical Practice Guidelines by the Infectious Diseases Society of America for the Treatment of Methicillin-Resistant *Staphylococcus Aureus* Infections in Adults and Children." *Clinical Infectious Diseases* 52, no. 3 (February 1, 2011): 285–295.

Tang, Sarah S., Anucha Apisarnthanarak, and Li Yang Hsu. "Mechanisms of β-lactam Antimicrobial Resistance and Epidemiology of Major Community- and Healthcare-Associated Multidrug-Resistant Bacteria." *Advanced Drug Delivery Reviews* 78, suppl. 1 (November 30, 2014): 3–13.

Websites

"Methicillin-Resistant *Staphylococcus aureus* (MRSA) Infections." *U.S. Centers for Disease Control and Prevention (CDC).* http://www.cdc.gov/mrsa/ (accessed April 1, 2015).

"MRSA." *U.S. National Institutes of Health (NIH).* http://www.nlm.nih.gov/medlineplus/ency/article/007261.htm (accessed April 1, 2015).

"MRSA Infection." *Mayo Clinic.* http://www.mayoclinic.org/diseases-conditions/mrsa/basics/definition/con-20024479 (accessed April 1, 2015).

"WHO's First Global Report on Antibiotic Resistance Reveals Serious, Worldwide Threat to Public Health." *World Health Organization (WHO).* http://www.who.int/mediacentre/news/releases/2014/amr-report/en/ (accessed April 1, 2015).

K. Lee Lerner

Mobile Health Technologies

⊕ Introduction

Mobile health technology, usually abbreviated as mHealth, is a system of public health sustained by the use of mobile electronic devices such as cellular phones, smartphones, tablet computers, and unique devices created for the tracking and monitoring of health-related data. Applications (apps) for mHealth take many different forms. They have the ability to track a diabetic's glucose level, monitor sleep patterns, check which symptoms indicate specific diseases, and rate patient satisfaction with physicians. Apps for mHealth have become a growing and essential means of accessing health care in developing countries, spurred by the increase in available wireless connectivity in both developing countries and industrialized nations. The increase in available wireless networks, and the shortage of adequate, affordable health care around the world has created the perfect environment for mHealth apps to grow exponentially.

As a relatively new mode of supplying and accessing health-care systems, mHealth has only recently been made possible by a series of advances in technology. Telephone and Internet access had already changed the face of health care, but it was not until the proliferation of smartphones that health care could be delivered into the hands of people all over the world. A smartphone is a mobile phone with additional features similar to those of a traditional computer operating system. Smartphones have apps such as GPS navigation, digital cameras, and Internet access that were not available on traditional cellular phones, but whose data are carried over similar networks. The growth of the mHealth field has been driven by the challenges faced by traditional health-care systems, which both industrialized and developing nations have been unable to overcome. Growing populations, burdensome costs, and the rapid spread of disease in rural areas with an insufficient health-care workforce slow the health-care process. According to the World Health Organization's (WHO) second annual survey on eHealth, there are over 5 billion wireless subscribers, 70 percent of whom live in low- and middle-income countries where the wireless grid covers far more area than the electrical grid.

Despite the availability of apps for mHealth in developing countries, higher-income countries show more mHealth activity, consistent with advanced educational systems and structures. In higher-income countries, more people have expendable income to spend on mobile phones and smartphones, and they are more likely to be educated about their personal health. However, even regions that are industrialized and accustomed to accessing data via mobile phones have considerable hurdles to overcome before mHealth will be able to reach its full potential.

Some of the biggest challenges countries have experienced in integrating various mHealth come from existing health-care systems being unable or unwilling to adapt to rapid changes in the field. Health systems all over the world are chronically underfunded and understaffed. Because of this, funding mHealth initiatives sometimes requires taking the funds from some other, usually vital, area of the existing health-care system. The lack of sufficiently educated employees, funding shortages, diverse disease presentation, and data security requirements make choosing the best methods of treatment difficult. There are a great many priorities with which mHealth must compete, and that competition for resources will likely the be the greatest barrier to mHealth expansion in industrialized regions.

⊕ Historical Background

mHealth is a young field, currently creating its history and determining the ways in which it will incorporate itself into existing and different health-care structures around the world. It faces challenges to expansion, but is almost wholly driven by consumer demand across the globe for cheaper, more efficient access in both

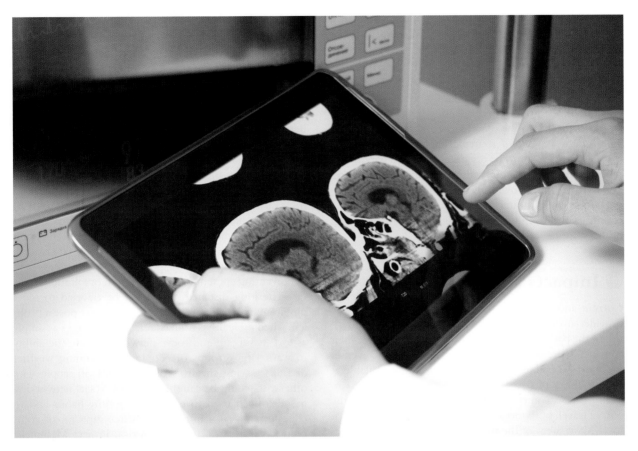

A doctor examines a brain scan on a digital tablet, a sight increasingly seen in hospitals and elsewhere, after the first medical imaging software was approved by the U.S. Food and Drug Administration in 2011. © *sfam_photo/Shutterstock.com.*

industrialized and developing regions. mHealth is sometimes considered a derivative of eHealth, which is a term for health care supported by the Internet, communication devices, and electronics. Even eHealth, which has a longer history than mHealth, has only been a part of the medical repertoire since the 1990s. mHealth's advances would not have been possible were it not for the familiarity health-care practitioners and patients already had with eHealth systems. mHealth apps rely on eHealth data storage that already exists and electronic statistical programs to assess those data. mHealth is a subset of health care that refers only to its relation to mobile electronic devices.

One of the first mHealth initiatives was the emergency/health call center. An emergency call center is a number that a person can call to speak with someone who is able to render help and send additional medical assistance. In the United States this number is 911, and in most European countries it is 112. The use of an emergency number has been in operation since 1937, when the number 999 was employed in London. Even today, however, there are countries, and entire regions, that do not have access to traditional call centers because of the lack of infrastructure, secure roads, or emergency services.

In a survey performed by the WHO, 112 of the 194 member nations reported having at least one existing mHealth initiative within their country, call centers being the most common. Three-quarters of those with at least one initiative reported having four or more types. This indicates that once mHealth is adopted into a country, other initiatives are quickly adopted as well by the population. Although the consumers of mHealth applications are most active in the European region, the region with the greatest number of different initiatives was the Southeast Asia region. The fewest initiatives in reporting countries came from the African region.

In 2009, smartphones were only just beginning to contribute significantly to the telecommunications market, but within five years they became the dominant operating systems. Companies that were once the leading revenue generators in the field were overwhelmed and disappeared from the market completely within those five years. Apps development has grown at an extraordinary rate, making it easier for users to access and track their own health. Soon, with some exceptions for still-developing countries, almost the entire population of the world will be able to supplement their current medical systems with mHealth apps. The growing sophistication of the networks, faster connectivity, and cheaper, more powerful handheld devices create the possibility of a greater level of individualization and patient-centered health.

mHealth apps developed first in higher-income countries, which is consistent with electronic health-care models, and with a population that already uses telephones as a primary form of communication. Source countries seem to be developing these technologies without the benefit of strategic implementation plans. mHealth apps seem to be organically filling a gap in current health-care systems without strong policy-maker involvement, but growth cannot continue without support forever. Without strong leadership in developing countries, mHealth is already struggling with conflicting health priorities and unsure legal footing.

⊕ Impacts and Issues

Current and traditional health-care structures place the provider at the center of a huge array of patients. Oftentimes, the patient must be physically present to have their ailments addressed by a health-care practitioner; even in the most accessible locations, many are only available at specific times of day. In developing countries, access to health care is sometimes a great distance away, and the cost of travel, both monetary and physical, can be prohibitive. Many areas of the world without access to electricity or clean running water already have access to mobile communications. mHealth has the ability to reach out to people who would otherwise have no access to a health-care provider. Having the health-care provider present in the same room as the patient is not always necessary with the growing use of telemedicine.

Developing countries face medical challenges that have been improved in more industrialized nations. Greater economic development is linked to increased life expectancy, a lower rate of malnutrition, better sanitation, and a greater successful birthrate. In countries without a flourishing economy, chronic diseases are becoming more prevalent and communicable diseases have greater impact. The WHO noted in a press release from 2013 that many countries are critically lacking in health-care providers, with a global shortage of 7.2 million health-care providers. This figure is expected to grow to 12.9 million by 2035. The WHO states that 83 countries were below the recommended 23 skilled health professionals per 10,000 people, mainly in Asia and sub-Saharan Africa.

mHealth has the potential to help lower acute communicable disease rates and to assist ongoing treatment of chronic diseases in areas with low clinician density. The leading preventable causes of noncommunicable diseases are tobacco use, poor diet, and sedentary lifestyle. A person who is sedentary has little to no regular physical activity. Poor nutrition can be caused by being unable to afford to obtain healthful, fresh food or by lack of information about what foods are most healthful. It may

result in diseases such as scurvy and can contribute to tooth decay. These three factors contribute to the majority of ailments in the world, such as heart disease, diabetes, malnutrition, lung disease, and cancer. The chronic nature of these diseases requires frequent interventions that can be facilitated by the availability of mHealth apps.

Communicable diseases such as human immunodeficiency virus/acquired immune deficiency syndrome (HIV/AIDS), Ebola, measles, and mumps are spread from person to person and are considerably harder to control without the necessary medical staff and sanitation that are more readily available in developed countries. mHealth cannot stop the spread of disease but can contribute to education about how disease is spread. In areas of the world where knowledge about the way disease is passed from one person to another is rare, educational outreach is the greatest weapon health-care workers have in preventing epidemics that can sicken or kill thousands.

The long distances that must be traveled to see a physician in developing countries no longer pose a problem when mHealth is utilized effectively. Things as simple as text messaging and social networking have the ability to warn large groups of people of impending weather disasters, saving the lives of thousands of people who otherwise would be caught off guard. Social networking has also been used to encourage healthy habits and to educate people on nutrition or the symptoms of communicable diseases. In South Africa, Project Masiluleke sends upward of 1 million text messages daily to promote testing and treatment for HIV/AIDS, with call center numbers attached for additional information. Large-scale educational outreach like this has the potential to prevent or slow the outbreak of epidemics.

In addition to reaching out to possible patients for awareness and treatment purposes, patients can also easily seek out information that was previously inaccessible. Patients are able to learn about conditions with which they may have been diagnosed and check whether symptoms they are experiencing are indicative of serious health concerns. This access to medical information can have its downfalls, especially in regions where the person is able to see a physician. Some people may use the Internet as a way to avoid seeing a physician despite access to one, or may ignore a doctor's advice because of conflicting information found online. Additionally, patients can misinterpret the information they find because of a lack of medical knowledge. Online information about health must come from a trusted source and be verified by a doctor if the patient has access to one.

One of the major challenges posed by traditional health care is the lack of appropriately trained physicians and health-care workers, especially in developing countries. mHealth technologies have the ability to convey web-based learning to people around the globe, without the constraint of needing to be physically present. Decentralized training can help reduce financial barriers for people trying to continue their education, and make community in the future. To be successful, traditional health-care units must adapt to the impact these new health outlets will make on their practices and have a clear understanding of the mHealth market. Currently there is strong resistance from the traditional health-care systems in developed countries, but consumers will ultimately control the products.

There are major areas in which mHealth will likely have great impact. The first is the likelihood for improved treatment outcomes. One of the biggest challenges faced by doctors for successful treatment is the patient's compliance with instructions. Patient compliance is when a doctor suggests changes in a patient's behavior or consumption for relief of a symptom or an ailment, which is then either followed, partially followed, or ignored. Patient compliance is likely to improve if an mHealth app continuously reminds the patient of when to take prescriptions or gives instructions on physical therapy exercises that might otherwise be forgotten. The improvement of preventive medicine and education on medical topics for the general public is also likely to improve drastically with easy access to information. The more educated people are about their own health needs and severity of chronic illnesses the more likely they will be able to address and treat those illnesses appropriately.

mHealth apps have incredible potential to reduce or at least decelerate increasing costs of health care throughout the world. Initially this can be accomplished by diverting people from emergency rooms when hospital care may be unnecessary, or through mHealth apps that schedule appointments or transfer data to the doctor without patient input. The more people take advantage of preventive health measures afforded by mHealth apps, and the greater compliance with medical instructions, the less likely those same patients will end up admitted, or readmitted, for costly hospitalization.

A major critique of health care in industrialized nations is a doctor's lack of "bedside manner." Bedside manner is a doctor or nurse's relationship with or approach to patients in their care. Lack of bedside manner can contribute to a patient avoiding appointments, or even affect compliance with the doctor's instructions. mHealth has the ability to connect doctors, nurses, and patients in a familiar and accessible way. Sometimes patients are embarrassed to answer questions from a doctor honestly. For example, many patients know that they should get regular physical exercise and may exaggerate that amount when a doctor inquires. mHealth apps will be able to more accurately track patient habits and internal functioning (such as glucose level) in a way that is not subjective. Accurate analysis and data collection improves diagnostic accuracy and quality of care.

Improved data collection is another broad way that mHealth has begun, and will continue, to advance medical practice. With so many people logging data manually

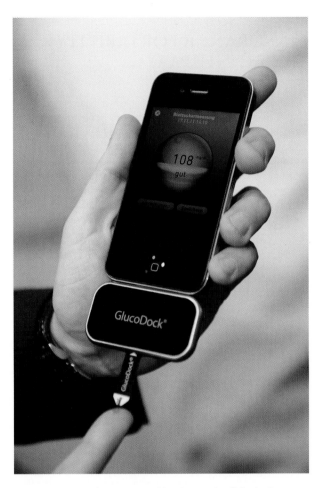

An iPhone device for measuring blood sugar for diabetics is shown. © *Patrik Stollarz/AFP/Getty Images*

it possible for people in rural areas to become more adept at self-treatment. Doctors who are looking for increased knowledge and advanced data can use mHealth's vast catalog of research and advice.

As of 2015 there is no mHealth registration of data. Traditional clinical trials maintain a registration database, and globally interested organizations such as the WHO contribute by fostering research and comparing outcomes. Creation of this sort of registration for mHealth apps would greatly impact their value by educating app developers and improving economic impact forecasts. The more successful mHealth is proven to be through data, the more likely it is that such programs will continue to receive funding, be successful, and advance health objectives globally.

⊕ Future Implications

Based on rate of growth within the first five years of smartphone introduction, it seems clear that mHealth apps will play a much larger role within the medical

DATA SECURITY AND HEALTH INSURANCE PORTABILITY AND ACCOUNTABILITY ACT (HIPAA)

Even though mobile health technology (mHealth) applications (apps) have evolved from eHealth, it is increasingly necessary for policy makers and the creators of these apps to be aware of the risk of privacy breaches, and implement policy accordingly. An enormous amount of highly sensitive and private personal information is contained in mHealth apps. Privacy laws differ from country to country. A company is not required to follow the laws of the country in which users are located but rather the laws of the country in which it is incorporated.

The Health Insurance Portability and Accountability Act (HIPAA) privacy regulations, enacted in the United States in 1996, provide protections for individually identifiable health information and give patients an array of rights with respect to that information if it is disclosed by an entity covered by HIPAA rules. The information protected by HIPAA is any information relating to the type of care, or payment for care, being received by an individual; the law is sometimes interpreted broadly to include the person's entire medical record. However, disclosure rules are balanced so that disclosure of health information needed for patient care and other important purposes is permitted. If an mHealth app is created by a company incorporated in the United States, it is bound to the HIPAA regulations.

Any person who feels his or her information has been inappropriately disclosed by a corporation based in the United States can file a complaint with the Department of Health and Human Services' Office of Civil Rights. The complaint will then be investigated, and both criminal and civil penalties can be imposed, including imprisonment for wrongdoers. However, criminal penalties are only pursued for those individuals or organizations that knowingly disclose individually identifiable health information. Entities that disclose information accidentally or negligently are prosecuted civilly, but can be fined up to US$1.5 million for multiple separate violations. Because mobile apps store patient data and are able to transmit those data over various networks, they raise unique security threats, and there is no standardized system of encryption. Encryption is the process of encoding a message so that it can be read only by the person sending the information and the person receiving it. The same problem existed when the government and private sector began utilizing electronic data, and the Advanced Encryption Standard was created as a result. The same techniques could be used to develop an encryption standard for mHealth apps.

Additionally, it is unclear as to whether only some or all of the information that makes up mHealth apps is subject to HIPAA and other privacy standards. Developers of these apps are not necessarily focused on what may or may not be subject to regulations. For example, a website or app may require patients to enter personal health information such as the symptoms they are experiencing, but if the entity that created the site is not covered by HIPAA, that information is not protected. Or customers may assume their medical data are safe because they reside in a country such as the United States, with strong medical privacy protections, but not realize the app they use is not similarly incorporated.

Without sufficient security measures, mHealth apps risk exposing the data they collect, and the data stored in these apps are not always protected by HIPAA privacy regulations. As the field grows, it must adapt to meet these regulations and protect private information of its users.

or through device sensors, the pool of information for research is limitless. In statistics, the largest data sample collected in answer to a question is the most reliable way to achieve the smallest margin of error (the likelihood that outcome of statistical analysis may have been affected by random chance). The data input by mHealth apps could provide enormous data samples and increase the accuracy of scientific measure.

SEE ALSO *Health as a Human Right and Health-Care Access; Health-Related Education and Information Access*

BIBLIOGRAPHY

Books

Donner, Jonathan, and Patricia Mechael, eds. *mHealth in Practice: Mobile Technology for Health Promotion in the Developing World*. London: Bloomsbury Academic 2013.

Godara, Balwant, and Konstantina S. Nikita, eds. *Wireless Mobile Communication and Healthcare: Third International Conference, MobiHealth*. Berlin: Springer, 2012.

Istepanian, Robert, Swamy Laxminarayan, and Constantinos S. Pattichis, eds. *M-Health: Emerging Mobile Health Systems*. Berlin: Springer, 2005.

WHO Global Observatory for eHealth. *mHealth: New Horizons for Health through Mobile Technologies: Second Global Survey on eHealth (Global Observatory for eHealth)*. Geneva: World Health Organization, 2011.

Periodicals

Estrin, D. "Small Data, Where n = me." *Communications of the ACM* 57, no. 4 (April 2014): 32–34.

Kahn, James G., Joshua S. Yang, and James S. Kahn. "'Mobile' Health Needs and Opportunities in Developing Countries." *Health Affairs* 29, no.2 (2010): 254–261. Available online at http://www.k4health.org/sites/default/files/Kahn,%20Yang,%20Kahn%20Mobile%20Health%20Needs%20 and%20Opportunities%20in%20Developing%20 Countries.pdf (accessed March 5, 2015).

Kumar, S., W. Nilsen, M. Pavel, and M. Srivastava. "Mobile Health: Revolutionizing Healthcare through Transdisciplinary Research." *IEEE Computer Magazine* 46, no. 1 (January 2013): 28–35.

Saranummi, N., et al. "Moving the Science of Behavioral Change in the 21st Century." *IEEE Pulse Magazine* 4, no. 5 (September 2013): 22–34.

Websites

"Density of Physicians (Total Number per 1000 Population, Latest Available Year)." *World Health Organization: Global Health Observatory(GHO).* http:// www.who.int/gho/health_workforce/physicians_ density/en (accessed March 5, 2015).

"mHealth App Developer Economics 2014." *Research-2Guidance.*http://mhealtheconomics.com/mhealth-developer-economics-report/ (accessed March 5, 2015).

"mHealth—Mobile Health Technologies." *National Institutes of Health: Office of Behavioral and Social Sciences Research.* http://obssr.od.nih.gov/ scientific_areas/methodology/mhealth/ (accessed March 5, 2015).

Sullivan, Tom. "Top 10 mHealth News Stories of 2014." *mHealthNews,* December 19, 2014. http://www .mhealthnews.com/news/top-10-mhealth-news-stories-2014 (accessed March 5, 2015).

Margaret Loraine Scott